Prognosis in
Advanced Cancer

Prognosis in Advanced Cancer

Edited by

Paul Glare

Head of Palliative Care,
Sydney Cancer Centre,
Royal Prince Alfred Hospital;

Clinical Associate Professor,
Central Clinical School (Medicine),
Faculty of Medicine,
University of Sydney,
Australia

Nicholas A. Christakis

Professor, Department of Health Care Policy,
Harvard Medical School;

Department of Medicine,
Mount Auburn Hospital,
Boston, USA

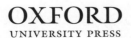

OXFORD
UNIVERSITY PRESS

OXFORD

UNIVERSITY PRESS

Great Clarendon Street, Oxford OX2 6DP

Oxford University Press is a department of the University of Oxford.
It furthers the University's objective of excellence in research, scholarship,
and education by publishing worldwide in

Oxford New York

Auckland Cape Town Dar es Salaam Hong Kong Karachi
Kuala Lumpur Madrid Melbourne Mexico City Nairobi
New Delhi Shanghai Taipei Toronto

With offices in

Argentina Austria Brazil Chile Czech Republic France Greece
Guatemala Hungary Italy Japan Poland Portugal Singapore
South Korea Switzerland Thailand Turkey Ukraine Vietnam

Oxford is a registered trade mark of Oxford University Press
in the UK and in certain other countries

Published in the United States
by Oxford University Press Inc., New York

British Library Cataloguing in Publication Data

Data available

Library of Congress Cataloging in Publication Data

Data available

Typeset by Cepha Imaging Private Ltd., Bangalore, India
Printed in Great Britain
on acid-free paper by
Ashford Colour Press Ltd., Gosport, Hampshire

ISBN 978–0–19–853022–0

10 9 8 7 6 5 4 3 2 1

Whilst every effort has been made to ensure that the contents of this book are as complete, accurate
and up-to-date as possible at the date of writing. Oxford University Press is not able to give any guarantee
or assurance that such is the case. Readers are urged to take appropriately qualified medical advice in all
cases. The information in this book is intended to be useful to the general reader, but should not be used as a
means of self-diagnosis or for the prescription of medication.

Contents

Part 3 **Prognosis in palliative care**

Contributors

Lara Alloway, Consultant in Palliative Medicine, North Hampshire Palliative Care Service, Basingstoke, UK

Laura Biganzoli, Head, Clinical Research Unit, Sandro Pitigliani Medical Oncology Unit, Hospital of Prato, Istituto Toscano Tumori, Italy

Murray F. Brennan, Attending Surgeon, Department of Surgery, Memorial Sloan Kettering Cancer Center, New York, USA

Andrew Broadbent, Director of Palliative Care, Hope Healthcare North, Greenwich, Sydney, Australia

Bert Broeckaert, Professor and Coordinator, Interdisciplinary Centre for the Study of Religion & Worldview, K. U. Leuven, Belgium

Eduardo Bruera, Professor and Chair, Department of Palliative Care and Rehabilitation Medicine, The University of Texas, MD Anderson Cancer Center, Houston, USA

Cinzia Brunelli, Statistician, Unit of Rehabilitation and Palliative Care, Istituto Nazionale Tumori, Milan, Italy

Markus W. Büchler, Head of the Department of Surgery, University Hospital, Heidelberg, Germany

Phyllis Butow, Professor, NHMRC Priniciple Research Fellow and Director Medical Psychology Research Unit, University of Sydney, Australia

Angela Byrne, Fellow in Cross-sectional Imaging, Beaumont Hospital, Dublin, Ireland

Jonathan Carter, Professor Gynaecological Oncology, The University of Sydney; Head, Sydney Gynaecological Oncology Group, Sydney Cancer Centre; Head, Gynaecology Services, Royal Prince Alfred Hospital; Area Director, Gynaecological Oncology, Sydney South West Area Health Service, Sydney, Australia

Eric L. Chang, Associate Professor, Department of Radiation Oncology, The University of Texas, M. D. Anderson Cancer Center, Houston, USA

Edward Chow, Associate Professor, Department of Radiation Oncology, Toronto Sunnybrook Regional Cancer Centre, University of Toronto, Canada

Nicholas A. Christakis, Professor, Department of Health Care Policy, Harvard Medical School; Department of Medicine, Mount Auburn Hospital, Boston, USA

Katherine Clark, Senior Staff Specialist, Department of Palliative Care, Sydney Cancer Centre, Royal Prince Alfred Hospital, Sydney, Australia

David Currow, Director, Southern Adelaide Palliative Services; Chair, Department of Palliative and Supportive Services, Flinders University, Adelaide, Australia

Prajnam Das, Assitant Professor, Department of Radiation Oncology, The University of Texas, MD Anderson Cancer Center, Houston, USA

Mellar P. Davis, The Harry H. Horvitz Center for Palliative Medicine, Taussig Cancer Center, Cleveland Clinic, Cleveland, USA

Jonathan E. Dowell, Chief, Hematology/Oncology, Dallas Veterans Affairs Medical Center; Associate Professor of Internal Medicine, University of Texas-Southwestern, Dallas, USA

Charles Dumontet, Services d'Hématologie, Hopital Edouard Herriot, Centre Hospitalier Lyon Sud, Hospices Civils de Lyon, Université Claude Bernard Lyon, France

Fabio Efficace, Head, Health Outcome Research Unit, Gruppo Italiano Malattie EMatologiche dell'Adulto (GIMEMA), GIMEMA Data Center, University of Rome 'La Sapienza', Department of Cellular Biotechnology and Hematology, Rome, Italy

John Ellershaw, Professor of Palliative Medicine, University of Liverpool, UK, Director, Marie Curie Palliative Care Institute, Liverpool, UK

Miriam Friedlander, Instructor, Department of Psychiatry and Behavioral Sciences, Memorial Sloan-Kettering Cancer Center, New York, USA

Tony Geoghegan, Lecturer in Radiology, The Department of Academic Radiology, Beaumont Hospital, Dublin, Ireland

Timothy Gilligan, Urologic Oncology Program, Cleveland Clinic Taussig Cancer Center, Cleveland, USA

Phyllis A. Gimotty, Professor of Biostatistics, Department of Biostatistics and Epidemiology, University of Pennsylvania, Philadelphia, USA

Paul Glare, Head of Palliative Care, Sydney Cancer Centre, Royal Prince Alfred Hospital; Clinical Associate Professor, Central Clinical School (Medicine), Faculty of Medicine, University of Sydney, Australia

Rebecca Hagerty, Ph.D. Research Co-ordinator, Medical Psychology Research Unit, University of Sydney, Australia

Anne Hamilton, Senior Staff Specialist, Department of Medical Oncology, Sydney Cancer Centre, Royal Prince Alfred Hospital, Sydney, Australia

Irene Higginson, Professor of Palliative Care and Policy, Department of Palliative Care, Policy and Rehabilitation, King's College London, UK

George Hruby, Clinical Senior Lecturer, Department of Radiation Oncology, Sydney Cancer Centre, University of Sydney, Australia

Ceri Hughes, Consultant Maxillofacial / Head and Neck Surgeon, Department of Maxillofacial / Head and Neck Surgery, United Bristol Healthcare Trust, Bristol, UK

Vicki Jackson, MPH Instructor in Medicine, Harvard Medical School; Associate Director of the Palliative Care Service, Massachusetts General Hospital, Boston, USA

Nora Janjan, Professor of Radiation Oncology and Symptom Management, The University of Texas, MD Anderson Cancer Center, Houston, USA

Aminah Jatoi, Professor, Department of Oncology, Mayo Clinic, Rochester, USA

Vaughan Keeley, Consultant in Palliative Medicine, Derby Hospitals NHS Foundation Trust, Nightingale Macmillan Unit, Derby, UK

David Kissane, Chairman, Department of Psychiatry and Behavioral Sciences, Memorial Sloan-Kettering Cancer Center, New York, USA

Moritz Koch, Attending, Department of Surgery, University Hospital, Heidelberg, Germany

Sunil Krishnan, Assistant Professor, Department of Radiation Oncology, The University of Texas, MD Anderson Cancer Center, Houston, USA

Elizabeth B. Lamont, Assistant Physician, Massachusetts General Hospital Cancer Center; Assistant Professor, Departments of Health Care Policy and Medicine, Harvard Medical School, Boston, USA

Michael J. Lee, Professor of Radiology, Department of Radiology, Beaumont Hospital and the Royal College of Surgeons in Ireland, Dublin, Ireland

Edward Lin, Associate Professor, Fred Hutchison Cancer Center, Department of Hematology Oncology, University of Washington, Seattle, USA

William J. Mackillop, Professor and Chair, Department of Community Health and Epidemiology, Queen's Universtity, Kingston, Canada

Anita Mahajan, Associate Professor, Department of Radiation Oncology, The University of Texas, MD Anderson Cancer Center, Houston, USA

Marco Maltoni, Palliative Care Unit, Oncology Department, GB. Morgagni-L. Pierantoni Hospital, Forlì, Italy

Sebastiano Mercadante, Professor of Palliative Medicine, University of Palermo; Director of Anesthesia and Intensive Care and, Pain Relief and Palliative Care, La Maddalena Cancer Center, Palermo, Italy

Ian McCutcheon, Professor, Department of Neurosurgery, University of Texas, MD Anderson Cancer Center, Houston, USA

Maria Montoya, Department of Palliative Care and Rehabilitation Medicine, The University of Texas, MD Anderson Cancer Center, Houston, USA

Katherine T. Morris, Surgical Oncologist and Medical Director of Cancer Research and Hepatobiliary Programs, Legacy Health System, NW Surgical Oncology PC, Portland, USA

Lida Nabati, Instructor in Medicine, Harvard Medical School; Attending Physician, Pain and Palliative Care Service, Dana-Farber Cancer Institute, Boston, USA

Kelvin K. Ng, Associate Consultant, Department of Surgery, Queen Mary Hospital, Hong Kong, China

Phuong L. Nguyen, Associate Professor, Department of Laboratory Medicine and Pathology, Mayo Clinic, Rochester, USA

Hiroko Ohgaki, Head, Pathology Group, International Agency for Research on Cancer, Lyon, France

Martin Pecherstorfer, Specialist in Haematology and Oncology Department of Medicine, Center for Hematology and Oncology, Wilhelminenspital der Stadt Wien, Vienna, Austria

Jay F. Piccirillo, Director, Clinical Outcomes Research Office, Department of Otolaryngology, Head and Neck Surgery, Washington University School of Medicine, St Louis, USA

Ronnie T. Poon, Professor of Surgery, Department of Surgery, The University of Hong Kong, Queen Mary Hospital, Hong Kong, China

Christine Sanderson, Senior Registrar, Southern Adelaide Palliative Services, Australia

Luigi Schips, Associate Professor of Urology Chief, Department of Urology, Ospedale 'S.Pio da Pietrelcina'-Vasto, Italy

James Stevenson, Clinical Fellow, Marie Curie Palliative Care Institute, Liverpool, UK

Martin Stockler, Associate Professor and Co-Director of Cancer Trials, NHMRC Clinical Trials Centre, University of Sydney; Consultant Medical Oncologist, Sydney Cancer Centre – RPA and Concord Hospitals, Sydney, Australia

C. Martin Tammemagi, Associate Professor, (Epidemiology) Department of Community Health Sciences, Brock University, St Catharines, Canada

Martin Tattersall, Professor of Cancer Medicine, University of Sydney, Australia

Catherine Thieblemont, Services d'Hématologie, Hopital Edouard Herriot, Centre Hospitalier Lyon Sud, Hospices Civils de Lyon, Université Claude Bernard Lyon, France

Steven J. Thomas, Consultant Head and Neck Surgeon and Head of Division of Maxillofacial Surgery, University of Bristol and United Bristol Health Care Trust, UK

Anna Vlahiotis, Clinical Outcomes Research Office, Department of Otolaryngology, Head and Neck Surgery, Washington University School of Medicine, St Louis, USA

Jürgen Weitz, Head of Section of Surgical Oncology, Department of Surgery, University Hospital, Heidelberg, Germany

Tugba Yavuzsen, Research Fellow, The Harry H. Horvitz Center for Palliative Medicine, Department of Hematology, Medical Oncology, The Cleveland Clinic Foundation, Cleveland, USA

Albert Yee, Assistant Professor, Department of Surgery, University of Toronto, Division of Orthopaedic Surgery, Sunnybrook Health Sciences Centre; Consultant, Surgical Oncology, Centre for the Study on Bone Metastases, Toronto Sunnybrook Regional Cancer Centre, Canada

Richard Zigeuner, MD, Associate Professor of Urology, Vice Chairman, Department of Urology, Medical University Graz, Austria

Niklas Zojer, Consultant, Department of Medicine, Center for Oncology and Hematology, Wilhelminenspital, Vienna, Austria

Part 1

The science of prognostication

Overview
Advancing the clinical science of prognostication

Paul Glare and Nicholas A. Christakis

Introduction

'Doctor, how long do I have?' is a question dreaded by most physicians. It is also what most physicians think about when they hear the words 'prognosis' and 'prognostication'. While it is true that most patients want this type of information and that this question often gets asked during consultations, there is much more to prognostication than the communication skill required to answer this most difficult of questions. Physicians are prognosticating all of the time at both a conscious and subconscious level. Indeed, arguably, every time a physician chooses one course of therapy over another, it is at least implicitly, if not explicitly, because the one offers a better future than the other. Examples of some typical day-to-day prognostic questions formulated by physicians are shown in Table 1.1. In patients with far advanced cancer, prognostication most commonly involves a prediction of remaining time of survival, but there are many other dimensions to prognosis. The aim of this book is to help physicians and other clinicians to improve their skills at prognostication near the end of life in patient with cancer, a group comprising roughly a third of deaths in most industrialized countries (see Table 1.2 for distribution of cancer deaths).[1]

Traditionally, prognostication was regarded as one of the three cardinal clinical skills, along with diagnosis and therapeutics.[1] In fact, prognostication can be traced at least as far back as Hippocrates, who wrote the *Book of prognostics*.[2] In it he said:

> It appears to me a *most excellent thing for physicians to cultivate Prognosis*; for by foreseeing and fore-telling, in the presence of the sick, the present, the past and the future and explaining the omissions which patients have been guilty of, *he will be the more readily believed to be acquainted with the circumstances of the sick*; so that *men will have the confidence to entrust themselves to such a physician*.

Table 1.1 Some typical day-to-day prognostic encounters,

'I'll operate if you think he'll be alive in 3 months'
'There's a 20% chance of the kidney stones recurring'
'He'll never walk again'
'No, not every one with cancer develops pain'
'The nausea should wear off in 3 days'
'His care will cost more because it was an embolic rather than an ischaemic stroke'

[1] In contemporary medicine, one may add Prevention, Patient Education and Health economics to this list.

Table 1.2 Total deaths in the USA in 2000, all ages, due to malignancy

Malignant neoplasms of lip, oral cavity, and pharynx	5,927
Malignant neoplasm of oesophagus	9,596
Malignant neoplasm of stomach	11,480
Malignant neoplasms of colon, rectum, and anus	48,583
Malignant neoplasms of liver and intrahepatic bile ducts	9,732
Malignant neoplasm of pancreas	24,313
Malignant neoplasm of larynx	3,209
Malignant neoplasms of trachea, bronchus, and lung	131,750
Malignant melanoma of skin	5,941
Malignant neoplasm of breast	38,102
Malignant neoplasm of cervix uteri	3,753
Malignant neoplasms of corpus uteri and uterus part unspecified	5,318
Malignant neoplasm of ovary	11,292
Malignant neoplasm of prostate	30,672
Malignant neoplasms of kidney and renal pelvis	9,521
Malignant neoplasm of bladder	9,563
Malignant neoplasms of meninges, brain, and other parts of the central nervous system	10,039
Hodgkin's disease	1,021
Non-Hodgkin's lymphoma	17,924
Leukaemia	16,600
Multiple myeloma and immunoproliferative neoplasms	9,099
All other and unspecified malignant neoplasms	51,182
Total malignant neoplasms	464,688

In fact, until at least the middle of the nineteenth century, prognosticating was a central task of physicians, for there were few effective treatments available for them to use.

As things changed gradually over the past 150 years, there has been a progressive diminution of prognosis, and information on prognosis largely disappeared from medical textbooks during the last century. Virtually nothing is taught about prognostication in medical schools now. We believe, however, that with the ageing of the population and with the growing prevalence of patients living with chronic diseases, there will be a refocusing on the 'care of the incurables'. When a person has a serious, progressive, and incurable condition, then that person wants much more than acute and preventive services. At this point, the patient seeks longevity, comfort, maintenance of function, protecting family from burdens and bankruptcy, control over decisions, dignity, and so on. The fact that the person will live with a serious chronic condition as it worsens through to death creates the need for a very different care system for this phase of life. Most of the objectives that patients near the end of their lives have could be met more sensitively and more fully if doctors were able to formulate a more reliable prognosis. For a patient to plan how to live their remaining few months in a way most in keeping with their wishes, they must first of all be able to rely on their physician to provide accurate prognostic information.

The hope of living well, even with serious and progressive illness, gives affected people many concerns and needs in common, despite having a variety of medical conditions. Improving care for the end of life might best target those with eventually fatal chronic illness. Restoration of a high level of skill in prognostication will be an inevitable part of improving that care. We hope this book goes some way towards contributing to the renaissance of prognostication.

The clinical science of prognostication

Definition and scope

In its broad sense, prognosis is an epidemiological term defined as the relative probabilities of the various outcomes of the natural history of a disease. Consequently, prognoses can be made about any outcome of an illness. In their book *Prognosis in Contemporary Medicine*,[3] Fries and Ehrlich coined the term 'the 5Ds of prognostication' that address each of the outcomes of the natural history of most illnesses, namely:

1. Disease progression/recurrence
2. Death
3. Disability/discomfort
4. Drug toxicity
5. Dollars (costs of health care).

   We believe a sixth 'D' could be added to the list, namely 'Derivatives' which capture the fact that illnesses can have externalities for the people connected to the sick person. For example, the risk of death in a husband increases by 22 per cent if his elderly wife is hospitalized with a serious illness,[4] and it is important to be able to predict such consequences: and the timely use of palliative care ma have benefits for the patient's spouse, and prolong the spouse's life.[5] All six of these 'Ds' are relevant to patients with far advanced cancer and many will be addressed in this book, although most of the emphasis will be on predicting death.

Reasons for prognosticating in advanced cancer

There are many reasons why we want to be accurate in prognosticating about patients with advanced cancer and other eventually fatal illnesses. As previously mentioned, most patients and their families request this information. In a recent US survey, approximately 80 per cent of patients wanted to know their median survival and 5-year survival rate.[6] Interestingly, substantially less (65 per cent) wanted to know their 1-year survival rate. It is noteworthy, in relation to the 5Ds, that the survey found there was more interest in disease progression/recurrence (Response rate of tumour to chemotherapy, 95 per cent) and drug toxicity (side-effects of chemotherapy, 99 per cent) than death. Other reasons for wanting prognostic information include determining eligibility for services (e.g., hospice benefit in the US), the design and analysis of clinical trials, and the development of health care plans by policy-makers. While all of these are important, we would argue that the most important reason for clinicians to improve their skills in prognostication is that it a technical prerequisite for rational clinical decision-making about therapeutics and other aspects of clinical care (see Table 1.3).

Ways of formulating a prognosis: subjective vs actuarial judgement.

There are two components to prognostication: formulation of the prognosis, or 'foreseeing', and communication of the formulated prognosis, or 'foretelling'.

Table 1.3 Considerations in clinical decision-making in patients with eventually fatal illnesses at an advanced stage

Diagnosis, including extent of disease
Treatment options
Risks and burdens vs benefits of treatments
EBM of effectiveness
Patient's preferences
Relative probabilities of the various outcomes of the disease: prognosis.
– with and without treatment
– short term and long term
– in context of comorbidities and rehabilitation potential

There are a number of ways of formulating a prognosis (Table 1.3). We can refuse or, even worse, just guess; neither is recommended. We could get an 'expert opinion' from a specialist in the field or a textbook. Neither may be available, although this book aims to provide a repository of such information. We could use evidence-based medicine (EBM) and conduct an electronic search to find a systematic review or well designed primary trial – this is certainly feasible, although the evidence base of prognostic studies is (sadly) not as well developed as that of intervention studies. Moreover, there are further limitations to this approach. First, we would have to appraise the study for its validity and applicability to the patient in our care. Second, we would be using population data (e.g. median survivals), but the exponential nature of survival curve in advanced cancer indicates that 20 per cent of individuals will survive < 1/4 or > 3× the median.[7]

Hence, the best alternative is to try to formulate an individualized prognosis for the patient. There are two ways of approaching this: either to rely on our clinical experience and make a subjective judgement, formulating the prognosis in our head, or else use actuarial judgement, using established prognostic factors, determined by multiple regression of survival analysis data, especially if they have been combined in a prognostic model or index.[8]

While actuarial judgement is generally preferred to clinical subjective judgement in most areas of healthcare, clinical prediction of survival (CPS) is consistently retained as an independent survival predictor in multivariate analysis of survival in terminal cancer when it is included as a factor, and there are certain advantages to making subjective prognostic judgements for physicians working at the bedside in the care of the terminally ill (e.g., requisite prognostic factors such as lab tests may not be available, or the prognostic index may not provide information in the format required). Our previous systematic review indicates that physicians can discriminate (between patients who are dying or not) but that these discriminations are not well calibrated.[9] When it comes to making temporal subjective judgements of survival duration in seriously ill patients near the end of life, physicians generally err in the overly optimistic direction, often by a factor of 3–5.[10] Furthermore, there are other factors, such as the experience and specialty of the physician and the nature of the physician–patient relationship, that affect subjective prognostic judgements in this context. Hence, CPS is not a panacea either, at present.

The role of clinical judgement in advanced cancer has been recently reviewed by the EAPC working group on prognostication, who concluded that CPS is generally valid and useful, but that because of the factors that influence its formulation it is best used in conjunction with actuarial judgement.[11] The systematic review also showed that CPS accounted for 51 per cent of the variance in observed survival, while the usual prognostic factors used in actuarial judgement in terminal cancer (performance status, symptoms, abnormal labs) accounted for only 37 per cent of the variance. When the two were combined, this figure increased to 54 per cent. This indicates that clinicians at the bedside use other factors yet to be determined (perhaps comorbidities and psychosocial factors) to estimate survival. Conversely, there are many other factors operating that physicians do not currently take account of.

Cancer prognosis: early vs advanced disease

While the twentieth century saw the ellipsis of prognosis from the medical literature, especially in the case of treatable illnesses such as pneumonia,[12] modern oncology textbooks do contain a lot of prognostic information. In fact, there are now textbooks on prognostic factors in cancer, such as the UICC textbook.[13]

Therefore, it is very important to distinguish between the role of prognostication in *early stage* cancer – including newly diagnosed advanced cancer – and prognosis in *far advanced* disease, which is the aim of this book. In early stage cancer, prognostic information addresses the Fries and Ehrlich's first 'D': disease progression/response to treatment. In this case, tumour-related factors are paramount – not only type, stage and grade, but also cytognetic and molecular markers.

On the other hand in patients with far advanced cancer, these tumour-related factors become much less relevant as patients enter the final common pathway, typified in the cancer 'death trajectory' of anorexia, weight loss, breathlessness, failing performance status, lymphopenia and systemic inflammation.[14, 15] Comorbidities and psychosocial factors may also play a role. Mackillop has developed a conceptual model that captures the difference between these two aspects of oncological prognostication (see Chapter 2).

Prognostication: a dynamic process

An important difference between prognostication and the other two core clinical skills of diagnosis and therapeutics is that it is dynamic while the other two are relatively static. In 2007, once the diagnosis of a particular type of cancer is made (complete with radiology, PET scanning, biopsy and immunocytochemistry), it rarely changes and the treatment protocol is set. The prognosis on the other hand is always conditional and needs to be regularly reviewed, consequent to the response to treatment and other developments. Consider the example of the patient diagnosed with renal cancer metastatic to lung. At this stage his prognosis is grim, with median survival of 6–12 months, extended to 2–3 years if he is otherwise fit and well. He undergoes a cytoreductive nephrectomy and is one of the lucky handful of patients to obtain a spontaneous remission of the metastases. At this stage, his prognosis is revised to uncertain. He is followed up every six months and remains disease free five years later, at which time he may be spoken of as cured. He is now a cancer survivor and his prognosis has been revised again to good.

Overcoming barriers to prognostication

While the clinical science of prognostication is becoming increasingly well established, there remains a reluctance on the part of physicians to prognosticate and there are a number of reasons for this. First, there is the ascedency and centrality of therapy in medical practice, which diverts physicians interest in, and attention to, prognosis. Second, physicians are not, at present, adequately trained in prognostication, and journals and textbooks tend to neglect the topic. Third, there is the objective difficulty of prongostication, and the fact that it is often prone to error (more so than the clinical tasks of diagnosis and therapy): since these errors can be consequential for patients and physicians alike, this quite naturally restrains the practice of prongostication. Fourth, it seems as if prognosis may depend on social factors which physicians typically view as outside their purview, and avoid. Fifth, physicians believe in the self-fulfilling prophecy, and this quite understandably makes them less willing to formulate, let alone communicate, unfavourable prognoses. Finally, prognosis is more emotional than diagnosis and therapy, and more linked to death: both these linkages militate towards its avoidance, in the minds of physicians. The professional norms of prognosis have been described by Christakis (see Table 1.5).[16] These need to be overcome if prognostication is to advance. Education of medical students and house officers in the science of prognostication is the main hope of achieving this.

Future directions in prognostication

Improving the accuracy of CPS

Until validated prognostic indices are available that use simple, readily available prognostic factors to provide precise prognostic information for a range of relevant time points in the trajectory of the cancer illness, subjective judgement will remain important and it is apparent that the CPS contains useful prognostic information. There has been little research into what information physicians take into account when formulating a prognosis, but because it explains approximately half of the variance in actual survival, what they currently assess may not be the most relevant factors.[17] It is possible that the greater accuracy of the survival estimates made by experienced physicians compared to inexperienced ones is that they have learnt to take PS and symptoms into account when prognosticating, although this remains to be proven. Other factors like response to treatment, disease-free intervals, the impact of comorbidities and the attitude of the patient may also be factored in. If this process can be better understood, it could be taught to less experienced physicians.

Novel prognostic markers

Patient-rated measures of PS and psychosocial parameters and serum cytokine levels are candidate prognostic factors with the potential to improve the accuracy of existing prognostic models. Patient-rated measures of subjective sensations like well-being and symptoms have advantages over physician-rated ones and have been incorporated in some tools. The cancer cachexia syndrome is the direct cause of death in approximately one third of patients and contributes to morbidity in up to 80 per cent. Recent preclinical work and some clinical studies indicate that pro-inflammatory cytokines play a role in its genesis.[18] Pro-inflammatory cytokines such as IL-6 may prove to be useful prognostic markers.[19] These two diverse areas (patient-rated psychosocial

Table 1.4 How to formulate a prognosis

◆ Refuse, guess

◆ Get an 'expert opinion'

– specialist

– textbook

◆ Use population data

◆ EBM

– not as well developed as intervention studies

◆ Clinical experience: subjective judgement

◆ Formulate a prognosis: actuarial judgement

---

parameters and cytokines) may be connected as recent research has shown that mood and social support influences levels correlate with levels of the angiogenic cytokine VEGF in women with ovarian cancer.[20] As well as improving prognostication, establishing a link between biobehavioural factors, cytokines, and tumour progression raises the possibility for novel therapies, including combined anti-cytokine agents/psychosocial interventions that may control tumour spread and prolong survival. Identification of these novel biobehavioural pathways may give new insights into the resolution of controversies surrounding the association between psychosocial correlates and cancer survival.

Better prognostic tools

More research is needed to validate the existing tools and demonstrate their usefulness in clinical practice. The type of prognostic information provided by current indices limits their utility. New developments in biostatistics and information technology are resulting in new web-based tools based on algorithms and nomograms derived from large patient databases are currently being constructed (see Chapter 7). This field is being led by groups at the Memorial Sloan Kettering Cancer Center (MSKCC) and Washington University at St Louis (WUSTL). The MSKCC group have web-based nomograms for breast, pancreas, lung, prostate and renal cancers and sarcomas, although many of the predictions are for treatment decisions in early stage disease. The WUSTL group's *Prognostigram* uses SEER data to generate individualized survival curves based on age, gender, race, primary site, extent of disease and comorbidities, but the data have not been widely validated.

Methodological issues and evidence-based medicine

Progress in the field of prognostication will be held up until certain methodological issues that ensure the validity of the work being reported are addressed. These relate to the sample, measurement, and data analysis. With regard to the sample, the results of studies to date indicate that there is a difference in the factors affecting the prognosis of patients with advanced cancer compared to those with terminal cancer. In advanced cancer patients (better performance status, still undergoing therapy, survival 6–12 months), tumour-related factors retain some importance whereas in hospice populations (poor performance status, no further treatment, survival 1–2 months) they do not. It is essential that the characteristics of the sample are clearly described in the Methods section of studies so that the results can be applied to the appropriate clinical populations. Many of the studies in terminal cancer are based on referral to hospice programmes. Clear definitions of appropriate inception cohorts (e.g failing first line palliative chemotherapy) need to be agreed on.

With respect to measurement, studies involving subjective prognostic judgements need to clearly state that the judgement was made before the term of survival observation commenced. Completeness of follow-up needs to be at least 95 per cent. The means of confirming death needs to be clearly stated (e.g., death certificates, cancer registry data, clinical databases).

With regard to evidence-based medicine, prognostic scores can be considered a form of clinical prediction rule. The *JAMA Users Guides* provide the hierarchy for such evidence, with studies to demonstrate that use of the prognostic score changes clinical practice representing Level I evidence. To date no such studies have been undertaken. Most studies provide data on regression analyses of prognostic information nd represent Level III under this hierarchy.

Communication and ethical issues

The current status of foretelling, or communication of the formulated prognosis, is covered in Chapter 4. Physicians tend to paint an even rosier picture to patients than the overly optimistic prognosis they have already formulated. This can have dire consequences for the patient and family if it leads to them seeking treatments that are more suited to patients whose real prognosis is much better than theirs. Patients become twice removed from the reality of their condition – first because of unconscious errors in the prognoses that doctors formulate, and second because of further, additive, conscious errors in the prognoses that doctors communicate. Research needs to be ongoing to understand the optimal way of communicating prognostic information accurately to patients, ensuring that patients have understood it and what they will do with the information provided.

A series of unanswered ethical questions go hand in hand with the rest of the prognosis research agenda. Some of these might include:

- How do the principles of autonomy, beneficence, non-maleficence and justice relate to prognostication?

- How would the virtuous physician foresee and foretell?

- Should prognostication be an explicit part of decision-making?

- What are the medico–legal implications of prognostication?

Prognosis in eventually fatal illness other than cancer

In this era of chronic, progressive, incurable and eventually fatal illness, it has been estimated that approximately two-thirds of all deaths are now predicatble. As the focus of this book is terminal cancer, only one third of these predicatble deaths are specifically covered here. Many of the concepts and principles discussed in the first section of this book are relevant to prognostication in terminal illness, whatever the underlying diagnosis.

Depsite this, formulating a prognosis in patients with other eventually fatal illnesses, such as end-stage congestive heart failure, chronic obstructive pulmonary disease (COPD) and Alzheimer's disease, is more difficult than in cancer patients. This is because the natural history of these illnesses is different to that of terminal cancer. In the case of death from organ failure, the final years of life are characterized by a gradual deterioration punctuated by precipitous declines in health due to acute exacerbations that take the patient close to death but then respond to treatment. As a result, the risk of dying can fluctuate wildly, soaring during acute exacerbations and receding if the process is stabilized.

The general indicators of the terminal phase in these conditions are impaired performance status and impaired nutritional status. Specific predictors have been identified for individual diseases. They are shown in Table 1.4. Similar criteria are also available for HIV/AIDS, chronic liver disease, renal failure, stoke, coma and motor neuron disease. There are currently very few prognostic scores for actuarial judgement of survival in terminal non-cancer illnesses, and more work in this area is needed.

Table 1.5 Factors associated with shortened survival in non-cancer illnesses

Congestive heart failure:
Age greater than 64 years
Chest pain/breathless at rest
Left ventricular ejection fraction < 20%
Dilated cardiomyopathy
Uncontrolled arrhythmias

Table 1.5 (continued) Factors associated with shortened survival in non-cancer illnesses

Systolic hypotension

Chest X-ray signs of left heart failure are all associated with poor short-term survival

Already optimally treated with diuretics and vasodilators

Chronic obstructive pulmonary disese:

Advanced age

Dyspnoeic at rest

Forced expiratory volume at one second (FEV_1) of < 30%

Pulmonary hypertension with cor pulmonale/right heart failure

Alzheimer's disease

Unable to walk unaided and/or hold a meaningful conversation

Onset of medical complications (e.g. aspiration pneumonia, UTI, decubitus ulcers)

References

1. Anderson RN, Miniño AM, Hoyert DL, Rosenberg HM. Comparability of cause of death between ICD–9 and ICD–10. *National Vital Statistics Reports* 2001; 49(2).

2. Hippocrates A. *Book of prognostics* Digireads.com; 2004.

3. Fries JF, Ehrlich GE (eds) *Prognosis. Contemporary outcomes of disease.* Bowie, MD: The Charles Press Publishers, 1981.

4. Christakis NA, Allison PD. Mortality after the hospitalization of a spouse. *N Engl J Med.* 2006; 354(7):719–30.

5. Christakis NA, Iwashyna TJ. The health impact of health care on families: a matched cohort study of hospice use by decedents and mortality outcomes in surviving, widowed spouses. *Soc Sci Med* 2003; 57(3):465–75.

6. Steinhauser K, Christakis NA, Clipp E, McNeilly M, McIntyre L, Tulsky J. Factors considered important at the end of life by patients, family, physicians, and other care providers. *JAMA* 2000; 284(19):2476–82.

7. Stockler MR, Tattersall MH, Boyer MJ, Clarke SJ, Beale PJ, Simes RJ. Disarming the guarded prognosis: predicting survival in newly referred patients with incurable cancer. *Br J Cancer* 2006; 94(2):208–12.

8. Dawes RM, Faust D, Meehl PE. Clinical versus actuarial judgement. *Science* 1989; 243:1668–74.

9. Glare P, Virik K, Jones M *et al.* A systematic review of physicians' survival predictions in terminally ill cancer patients. *BMJ* 2003; 327(7408):195.

10. Christakis NA, Lamont EB. Extent and determinants of error in doctors' prognoses in terminally ill patients: prospective cohort study. *BMJ* 2000; 320:469–73.

11. Maltoni M, Caraceni A, Brunelli C *et al.* Prognostic factors in advanced cancer patients: evidence-based clinical recommendations – a study by the Steering Committee of the European Association for Palliative Care. *J Clin Oncol* 2005; 23(25):6240–8.

12. Christakis NA. The ellipsis of prognosis in modern medical thought. *Soc Sci Med* 1997; 44(3):301–15.

13. Gospodarowicz M, O'Sullivan B, Sobin L. (eds) *Prognostic factors in cancer,* 3rd edn. Hoboken, NJ: Wiley-Liss, 2006.

14. Lunney JR, Lynn J, Foley DJ, Lipson S, Guralnik JM. Patterns of functional decline at the end of life. *JAMA* 2003; 289(18):2387–92.

15. Wachtel T, Allen-Masterson S, Reuben D, Goldberg R, Mor V. The end stage cancer patient: terminal common pathway. *Hospice J* 1988; 4(4):43–78.

16. Christakis N. *Death foretold: prophecy and prognosis in medical care* Chicago, IL: Chicago University Press, 1999.

17. Tannenberger S, Malavasi I, Mariano P, Pannuti F, Strocchi E. Planning palliative or terminal care: the dliemma of doctors' prognoses in terminally ill cancer patients. *Annals of Oncology* 2002; 13:1319–1323.

18. Lee BN, Dantzer R, Langley KE. *et al.* A cytokine-based neuroimmunologic mechanism of cancer-related symptoms. *Neuroimmunomodulation* 2004; 11(5):279–92.

19. Elahi MM, McMillian DC, McArdle CS, Angerson WJ, Sattar N. Score based on hypoalbuminemia and elevated C-reactive protein predicts survival in patients with advanced gastrointestinal cancer. *Nutrition and Cancer* 2004; 48(2):171–3.

20. Lutgendorf SK, Johnsen EL, Cooper B. *et al.* Vascular endothelial growth factor and social support in patients with ovarian carcinoma. *Cancer* 2004; 95(4):808–15.

2

Differences in prognostication between early and advanced cancer

William J. Mackillop

Introduction

Prognosis plays an important role in the management of patients with early, potentially curable cancer, and there is an extensive literature devoted to prognostic factors in that context.[1] Prognosis is perhaps even more important in the management of patients with advanced and incurable cancer, but here it has received much less attention. This is unfortunate because, despite many advances in cancer treatment over the last century, 50 per cent of all cancer patients diagnosed today will die of their disease, and the quality of their end-of life care is often highly dependant on the accuracy of prognostic judgements. Although the art and science of prognosis are fundamentally the same in any situation, the basis of prognostic judgements, the scope of those judgements, and the ways in which they are useful to patients and their caregivers, all vary with the clinical context. The purpose of this paper is to discuss the particular characteristics of prognosis in advanced cancer. The historical evolution of prognosis will first be reviewed to provide a framework for that discussion.

The evolution of the science of prognosis

Prognosis in antiquity

Sick people have always had an interest in their prospects for recovery and *mantic prognosis*, the foretelling of the outcome of an illness based on omens and magic, has been practiced since the earliest recorded history.[2–4] *Semiotic prognosis*, the foretelling of the outcome of an illness based on clinical findings, also has a very long history. It can be traced as far back as the Sumerian civilization of 2,000 BC,[2] and reached a high level of sophistication in Greece in the era of Hippocrates, about 400 BC.[5] The Hippocratic school of medicine recognized complexes of symptoms and signs that predicted a good or bad outcome.[5] Hippocratic knowledge resembled modern medical knowledge in that it was acquired by clinical observation and applied by pattern recognition.[5] Hippocratic prognostication, however, differed significantly from modern prognostication in that the prognosis was based directly on the clinical findings, rather than on the diagnosis of a particular disease.[1, 5] (See Figure 2.1.) Although many of the symptom complexes described by Hippocrates are readily recognizable today as corresponding to specific diseases, Edelstein points out that 'there is, in ancient medicine, no theory of disease per se'.[5]

Prognosis in early scientific medicine

After Hippocrates, there were surprisingly few real advances in the science of medicine for almost 2000 years. Therapeutics flourished, but remedies were almost always directed by theories that had no empirical basis, and often did more harm than good.[2, 3] The transition to modern,

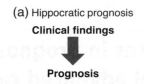

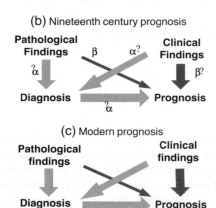

Figure 2.1 The evolution of the science of prognosis. The three diagrams illustrate how the science of prognosis has evolved over the history of medicine.

empirically based medicine began about 300 years ago when it was first clearly recognized that the right way to treat a patient could not be *deduced* from scientific theory, but instead had to be *induced* from clinical observations.[6,7] Induction is the general process of inference that allows us to predict what will happen in a specific set of circumstances in the future, based on observations made in similar circumstances in the past.[6] To apply inductive reasoning in medicine, it was essential to have a means of classifying clinical problems into groups of 'similar' cases. In the seventeenth century, Sydenham provided the first 'nosology', or classification of human diseases into diagnostic groups, based on the symptoms reported by the patient and the signs elicited by the clinicians.[2,3,7] In the eighteenth century, post-mortem studies began to reveal the pathological changes that were responsible for specific clinical syndromes, and this led to a more objective clinico-pathological classification of diseases.[3,7] From then on, the diagnosis served as a link to past experience that provided a rational basis both for prognosis and choice of therapy.

Figure 2.1b shows that two distinct pathways were now available to provide information about the prognosis in the individual patient.[8–11] The first or 'alpha' pathway starts with the assignment of a diagnosis based on clinical and pathological findings.[11] The general prognosis associated with this diagnosis is then induced from past experience in patients with the same diagnosis; this is sometimes referred to as the *ontologic prognosis*.[11] This prognosis is then attributed to the individual case. The second or 'beta' pathway provides additional prognostic information based on the particular characteristics of the case; this is used to modify the ontologic prognosis to provide an *individual prognosis*.[11] Factors that are predictive of outcome, but which are not subsumed into the diagnosis itself, were formerly referred to as 'prognostics'.[12] Today they are usually known as 'prognostic factors'.

The information relevant to the prognosis in the individual case flows from two different sources.[11,12] Much of the information that flows through the (β) pathway, and all the information that flows through the (α) pathway is derived from observations of the course of the illness in similar patients in the past. This may be referred to as the *external frame of reference*.[11]

Observations of the previous course of the illness in the particular patient, including its rate of progression and its response to therapy, may supply additional information that flows through the (β) pathway. This may be referred to as the *internal frame of reference*.[11]

Prognosis in modern medicine

The discovery of effective treatments for many common diseases in the twentieth century was responsible for a major shift in the emphasis in clinical scholarship from the study of the natural history of diseases to the science of therapeutics. Christakis discovered this phenomenon and labeled it the 'ellipsis of prognosis', based on the declining coverage allocated of this topic in the context of pneumonia in successive editions of a standard textbook of medicine.[13] While this trend may not have been uniform across the whole of medical practice, it is certainly true that the prognosis in many contexts is now greatly modified by treatment and scholarly interest in the natural history of diseases seems generally to have declined. Figure 2.1(c) illustrates the factors that contribute to the prognosis in contemporary medicine.

Prognosis in cancer medicine

Notwithstanding the general decline in interest in prognosis, the increasing success of cancer treatment over the last century seems paradoxically to have stimulated an increasing interest in prognostic factors in the field of oncology. Better treatments have been discovered, but none have proved to be universally effective. A particular treatment may greatly improve outcomes in some subgroups of cancer patients, but offer no benefit in others, and prognostic factors have become important as a basis for case selection for treatment. It is conventional to classify prognostic factors in cancer medicine as tumour-related, patient-related, treatment-related and environmental, depending on the source of the information.[1] However, it is also useful to classify prognostic factors based on the way in which they relate to the prognosis. Cancer is a unidirectional, time-dependent process that causes morbidity and mortality by disruption of normal cellular function and organ function through the processes of invasion, metastasis and the secretion of toxic products. At any point in time, the prognosis depends on how far the disease has already progressed and on its rate of progression. Prognostic factors can be broadly grouped into those that reflect the

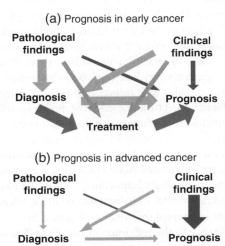

Figure 2.2 Prognosis in cancer medicine. The two diagrams illustrate differences in the information available to establish the prognosis in early and advanced cancer.

current extent of the cancer, and those that reflect its rate of progression. The former we will refer to as *state-related* and the latter as *trait-related prognostic factors*. Tumour volume, for example, is state-related factor while tumour doubling time is a trait-related factor. These two types of prognostic factor are complementary and both types of information are required to provide the best estimate of the prognosis. The effects of different types of treatment on prognosis may also be incorporated into this model. Surgery, for example, is a *state-modifying* therapy while a hormonal agent that retards tumour cell proliferation is a *trait-modifying* therapy.

The basis of prognosis in advanced cancer

The basis of prognosis in advanced cancer differs from that in early disease in three important ways. First, as the disease progresses, the primary diagnosis declines in importance as a determinant of prognosis. The diagnosis, stated in terms of anatomic site and tissue of origin, is strongly predictive of outcome in patients with relatively early cancers, because it determines both the risk of local invasion and/or metastasis and the options for curative treatment. The (α) pathway therefore plays a central role in prognostication in the context of early and potentially curable cancer (see Figure 2.2a). However, in patients with advanced disease, in whom the options for active treatment have been exhausted and extensive local invasion and/or metastasis have already occurred, the (α) pathway provides much less prognostic information (see Figure 2.2b). In support of this, a recent population-based study of patients who were dying of cancer in Ontario described the rate of increase in morbidity towards the end of life using hospitalization as a surrogate for poor health status. It clearly showed that, over the last the six months of life, the patient's health deteriorates almost as rapidly in prostate cancer as it does in cancer of the lung, despite the profoundly different early natural histories of these diseases and their very different prognoses at the time of diagnosis.[14]

Second, disease-related prognostic factors are in general less important in advanced cancer than in early disease. The random cellular mutations and metastatic events that characterize cancer progression make every advanced case unique, and it is therefore inherently difficult to design a classification system that creates prognostically uniform groups of cases. Furthermore, current classification systems were designed primarily to create subgroups of cases that are homogeneous with respect to probability of cure, and not to create subgroups of incurable cases that are homogeneous with respect to life expectancy. The TNM classification, for example, has been carefully designed to reflect even small differences in the extent of the tumour in relatively early cases, where these have been shown to be associated with differences in long-term survival.[15] In contrast, much less effort has been made to refine the classification of the extent of disease in advanced cancer. The TNM Stage 4 groups are generally very heterogeneous with respect to the volume and anatomic distribution of the disease, and also with respect to survival.[15] It remains to be seen if more prognostic information can be extracted from the extent of disease by refining classification systems for advanced cancer. Treatment-related factors also decline in importance as the disease progresses. Prognostic factors that reflect radiosensitivity and chemosensitivity may be powerful determinants of prognosis in early cancer, but are clearly irrelevant in patients who have already failed active treatment. In contrast, patient-related factors including symptoms and measures of functional status appear to become increasingly important.[16] Thus, the basis of prognosis in advanced cancer resembles the Hippocratic model, with diagnosis and therapy being almost irrelevant and clinical signs and symptoms providing most information (Figure 2.2b).

Third, the internal frame of reference to the previous course of the illness in the individual patient becomes increasingly useful as the disease progresses. The rate of progression of the tumour is rarely well documented at the time of diagnosis and initially the prognosis has to be based entirely on the external frame of reference. In contrast, in patients with advanced and recurrent cancers, there may be extensive information available about previous rate of progression, which may provide very useful prognostic information. For example, the PSA doubling time is very closely linked to the risk of early death in patients who have failed local treatment for prostate cancer.[17] The recent vast improvements in imaging make it possible to describe the pace of tumour growth much more precisely than ever before and in future, information about the trajectory of the disease provided by serial observations in the individual case may prove to be very important in determining the prognosis in patients with advanced cancers.[18]

Thus, as the disease progresses:

◆ the importance of the alpha pathway decreases, while that of the beta pathway increases,

◆ the importance of disease-related and treatment-related prognostic factors decreases, while that of patient-related factors increases, and

◆ the importance of the external frame of reference decreases, while that of the internal frame of reference increases.

The scope of prognostic judgements in advanced cancer

The prognosis is multidimensional. Prognosis may concern any aspect of future health or functional status that is of concern to the patient.[19–21] The idea that prognosis relates only to the issue of survival is a modern misconception.[19–21] The following classical description of the types of questions that should be addressed in formulating the prognosis appeared a standard textbook of medicine almost 150 years ago.[21]

1. *Will the disease end in death or recovery or will it continue indefinitely?*

2. *If it proves fatal will death come quickly or slowly and how will the patient die?*

3. *If the patient recovers, will some morbid condition remain either in the form of general ill health or some local problem?*

4. *How long will the illness last?*

5. *What events are likely to take place in its course, such as changes in symptoms, critical phenomena, the occurrence of complications?*

6. *Does having had the illness make the patient more or less susceptible to other illnesses?*

This list of issues remains entirely relevant to contemporary medical practice and surveys have shown that each of these aspects of the prognosis remains relevant to a large number of cancer patients and their caregivers today.[22–25] The relative importance of these different types of prognostic information varies depending on the clinical situation and on the values of the individual patient.

The prognosis is a dynamic quantity that changes over time. Initial prognostic judgements require to be reviewed periodically and revised, if necessary, to take account of progression or response to treatment. Patients should be made aware of this so that they are not taken by surprise when the prognosis is revised and do not assume that the change is indicative of a previous mistake.

Patients should also be aware that, at any point in time, there may be more than one prognosis depending on choice of treatment. Decisions about active treatment for cancer are always based on the comparison of at least two *conditional prognoses*, the prognosis without treatment, and the prognosis with treatment. This, of course, is not true in the final stages of the illness when active treatments are ineffective and the prognosis is dominated entirely by the natural history of the disease.

The value of prognosis in advanced cancer

Medical decision-making

Prognosis is important to the two major strategic decisions that should guide the overall care of a patient with advanced cancer: what are to be our therapeutic goals and what types of intervention should we used to achieve them?

The first question that must be addressed in the care of the patient with advanced cancer is whether the overall goals of care are curative or strictly palliative. Treating a patient with curative intent does not preclude providing appropriate symptomatic and supportive care, but it does often involve paying a definite price in quality of life in the short term, in return for possible gains in survival in the long term. The question, therefore, is not only whether there is any chance of cure or long-term survival, but also whether that chance is worth taking in the face of the expected side-effects of treatment. The answer hinges not only on the probability of cure but also on the probability and expected severity of the toxicity of treatment. The decisions that individual patients make in these fairly common 'close call' situations depend on the patients' individual values and may be highly sensitive to the probabilities of adverse outcomes.[26, 27] Optimizing this type of decision therefore requires accurate information about multiple aspects of the prognosis.

Once the overarching decision has been made that the overall goals of treatment are palliative, there remain other important strategic decisions about whether to use active anti-cancer treatments or to focus entirely on symptomatic and supportive care. The decision to forego or cease one type of active treatment does not necessarily apply to other types of active treatment that may differ in their efficacy, toxicity and convenience. This type of decision must often, therefore, be made repeatedly in the course of the illness. There is a danger that this type of decision will not receive conscious consideration and that patients with advanced and incurable cancer will instead be exposed to an endless series of active interventions. Explicit reconsideration of the prognosis prior to each new active intervention is the only way to guard against this.

Prognostic information is also important to decisions about how best to meet patients' needs for palliative and supportive care. For example, decisions about whether patients should be admitted to a hospice programme are often explicitly predicated on judgements about their life expectancy.

Personal decision-making

Quite apart from its use as a guide to their medical care, patients and their families often need prognostic information for personal reasons. Patients may need to know their prognosis in order to make decisions about their finances, their employment and their housing. Patients also need to know their prognosis in order to make the best use of what remains of their lives, for example to take a trip that they have previously deferred, to reconcile old differences with family members, or to make spiritual preparations for the end of their lives. Relatives may also need prognostic information in order to prepare for a caregiving role, or for future life without the support of the patient. Finally, and perhaps most importantly, many patients want to know their prognosis not to assist them in making any kind of decision, but just for the sake of knowing.[25] Perhaps, in some cases, knowledge of the prognosis allays fear of the unknown, but some observers believe that it simply meets a psychological need to know what the future holds.

The health policy perspective

On a societal level, skill in prognosis is useful as a means of optimizing the use of limited resources. Accurate prognosis is a precondition for good medical decisions; good decisions lead to efficient care, whereas bad decisions waste resources. The use of active cancer treatment when the patient will not live long enough to benefit from it is an expensive error because it consumes resources that could be better used elsewhere. Not providing active treatment for patients who would benefit from it may also have adverse financial as well as medical consequences. The decision not to treat a potentially curable patient, because of an incorrect assessment of the prognosis, is not only a potentially lethal error, it is also an expensive one, because the cost of dying of cancer may greatly exceed the cost of effective treatment. Likewise, the decision not to offer active, palliative treatment for a patient with advanced cancer, based on the incorrect prognostic judgement that they will not live long enough to benefit from it, may be an expensive mistake, because active cancer treatment in the ambulatory care setting may cost less than providing symptomatic and supportive care in hospital.[28]

Prognostic information may also be useful in making decisions about the allocation of resources. Some publicly funded health care systems have now begun to make decisions about which types of care they are willing to provide and for whom, based on economic appraisal of the benefits they achieve in the relationship to their cost. This type of decision-making may be unfair unless the individual characteristics of the case can be factored into the equation. The principle of justice demands not only that like situations be treated alike, but also that situations that are not alike should not be treated as if they were the same.[29] Making decisions about the allocation of resources at the level of the diagnostic group may seem sensible enough, but it may prove to be inequitable when those groups are very heterogeneous, as is the case in advanced cancer. Homogeneous prognostic groups would provide a fairer basis for allocation of resources in this type of situation.

The research perspective

Accurate prognosis also serves societal needs by enhancing the quality of clinical research. An understanding of prognostic factors is important in the design and analysis of clinical trials. In all cancer trials, prognostic factors are used as eligibility criteria to ensure a relatively uniform study population from which it may be possible to draw generalizable conclusions. Stratification based on prognostic factors may also be used to balance the case mix in each arm of a randomized trial, in order to make it easier to detect differences in the effectiveness of the interventions. An understanding of prognostic factors is also important in cancer research because, in some instances, prognostic factors may have a causal relationship to the outcome of the disease, in which case, the prognostic factor itself becomes a potential target for therapy.

Communicating the prognosis in advanced cancer

The question of whether patients should be told their prognosis has received extensive discussion over many generations, but the weight of ethical, legal and professional opinion today is in favour of truth-telling and full disclosure.[29, 30, 31] Modern medical ethics emphasizes the patient's right to self-determination, and doctors therefore have an obligation to provide patients with prognostic information to promote their autonomy and enable them participate effectively in decisions about their care. In practice, however, it has been shown that even diligent attempts to inform patients about their prognosis are not necessarily successful.

It has been shown that many patients hold erroneous views about their prognosis even if their doctors believe they have succeeded in informing them of the facts.[32, 33] This is true across the whole spectrum of cancer but is most common in patients with incurable disease. Occasional patients with early cancers underestimate their chance of being cured, but many patients with advanced cancer greatly overestimate their chances of long-term survival, and some continue to believe that they will be cured even if they have explicitly been told that they are incurable.[32, 33] Some patients accept the general truth of the prognosis as it applies to others in their situation, but regard themselves as exceptions to the rule..[32, 33] This appears to be a common type of coping strategy, and should be respected as such. However, doctors should recognize that this phenomenon may put the patient at risk of accepting aggressive treatments that have very unfavourable risk:benefit ratios. The model of shared decision-making permits and requires doctors to steer such patients gently away from treatments that will do them more harm than good. It is recommended that doctors not only provide patients with prognostic information but also ask them what they believe about their prognosis after that information has been provided.[33]

There is continuing debate about how best to present patients with prognostic information. Some observers recommend answering patients' questions about the prognosis in qualitative terms using words such as 'excellent', 'good' and 'fair', while others recommend the use of numerical values.[34, 35] Proponents of the use of qualitative terms argue that they are readily understood, and that percentages convey a false sense of precision. Proponents of the quantitative approach argue that qualitative terms are too subjective and also lack the necessary precision.[34, 35] In fact, it has been shown that most patients are able to understand percentages or proportions, and can use them in reaching their decisions.[26, 27, 35] Graphical representations of probabilistic information have been shown to facilitate communication and some formats have been shown to be more useful than others. Decision aids based on these findings have been shown to communicate prognostic information more effectively than routine practice.[25, 26]

Practicing prognosis in advanced cancer

Although a good deal is known about how we should, in theory, formulate the prognosis, almost nothing is known about how doctors actually go about this in their day-to-day practice. In the case of a patient with relatively early cancer, doctors have ready access to tabular information about the 5-year survival rates observed in patients with the same type and stage of cancer, and there is often additional quantitative information available about the way in which the average outcome is modified by additional prognostic factors. The literature is replete with this type of information and we are taught to use it in our training. I use this external frame of reference in my own practice and I assume that others do likewise, although I am not aware of any survey that has addressed this question directly. Whatever our collective approach may be, there is evidence that it works reasonably well in this context. It has been shown that oncologists' estimates of long-term survival in routine practice are, in fact, remarkably accurate.[36]

There seems little doubt that, in assigning a prognosis to patients with advanced cancer, doctors are also guided by their experience with similar patients in the past. Here however, there is no external frame of reference to a set of easy to use tables that describe the outcomes observed in well-defined subgroups of very similar patients. There is a growing body of information about prognostic factors in advanced cancer and, in theory, there is additional information available from the internal frame of reference to the previous course of the illness in the individual patient. However, until recently, doctors had little guidance as to how to integrate all this information. Not surprisingly, therefore, doctors' estimates of life expectancy in advanced cancer in the past have been shown to be fairly inaccurate, although they do partly discriminate between patients with better and worse outcomes.[36–43] Several studies have also shown systematic overestimation of life expectancy in this context, although a recent review and meta-analysis of eight previous studies showed that this was not a universal phenomenon.[44]

Recognizing the critical importance of prognosis in the management of advanced cancer and the inadequacy of current practice, a number of investigators have recently started to develop and evaluate prognostic scoring systems with promising results. For example, the Palliative Prognostic (PaP) scoring system,[46] which combines objective information about the patient with the doctor's subjective estimates of expectancy, has been shown to be able to divide patients with advanced cancer into isoprognostic groups.[47]

Conclusions

Medical decisions in patients with advanced cancer rely heavily on prognostic judgements. Patients with advanced cancer may also rely on their doctors' prognostic judgement in making important personal decisions. There is abundant evidence that prognostic judgement in this context is suboptimal. Prognosis in advanced cancer is inherently difficult because of the huge diversity of clinical presentations that fall under this broad heading. Despite its importance and the unique challenge that it represents, prognosis in advanced cancer has received less attention in the past than it deserves. There is now promising work ongoing but the field remains under-researched. There is scope for huge improvement in prognosis through the discovery of new prognostic factors and the development of improved methods for integrating the available information. Improved prognosis would enhance both the quality and the efficiency of patient care, and the field demands much more attention from both clinicians and scientists.

References

1. Gospodarowicz M, Henson E, Hutter VP, O'Sullivan B, Sobin LH, Wittekind C. *Prognostic factors in cancer*, 2nd edn. Wiley-Liss, New York, 2001.

2. Magner LN. *A history of medicine*. New York: Marcel Dekker Inc., 1992.

3. McManus JFA. *The fundamentals of medicine: a brief history of medicine*. Springfield IL: Charles C. Thomas, 1963.

4. Sigerist HE. *History of medicine*. New York: Oxford University Press, 1951–1961.

5. Temkin O and Temkin CL. (eds) *Ancient medicine: selected papers of Ludwig Edelstein*. Johns Hopkins University Press, Baltimore and London, 1967.

6. Howson C and Urbach P. *Scientific reasoning*. LaSalle, IL: Open Court Publishing Company, 1989.

7. Shryock RH. *The development of modern medicine: An interpretation of the social and scientific factors involved*. Madison: University of Wisconsin Press, 1979.

8. Buchanan S. *The doctrine of signatures: a defense of theory in medicine*, 2nd edn. Ed. Peter P. Mayock Jr, Foreword by Edmund D. Pellegrino. Urbana and Chicago, IL: University of Illinois Press, 1991.

9. Gibson AG. *The physician's art: an attempt to expand John Locke's Fragment De Arte Medica*. Oxford: Clarendon Press, 1933.

10. Wiesemann C. The significance of prognosis for a theory of medical practice. *Theoretical Med and Bioethics* 1998; 19:53–261.

11. Mackillop WJ. The importance of prognosis in cancer medicine. measuring the accuracy of prognostic judgements. In M Gospodarowicz, E Henson, VP Hutter, B O'Sullivan, LH Sobin, C Wittekind (eds) *Prognostic factors in cancer*, pp 127–145, UICC 2nd edn. New York: Wiley-Liss, 2001.

12. Ash E. Prognosis. In J Forbes, A Tweedie and J Conolly (eds) *The cyclopaedia of practical medicine*, pp. 699–706, Vol. III. Philadelphia, PA: Blanchard and Lea, 1859.

13. Christakis NA. The ellipsis of prognosis in modern medical thought. *Social Science and Medicine* 1997; 44:301–15.

14. Huang J, Boyd C, Tyldesley S, Zhang-Salomons J, Groome PA, Mackillop WJ. Time spent in hospital in the last six months of life in patients who died of cancer in Ontario. *Clin Oncol* 2002; 20:1584–1592.

15. Sobin LH and Wittekind C. *TNM classification of malignant tumours*, 6th edn. New York: Wiley-Liss, 2002.

16. Reuben DB, Mor V. Clinical symptoms and length of survival in patients with terminal cancer. *Arch Intern Med* 1988; 148:1586–91.

17. Kwan W, Pickles T, Duncan G, Liu M, Agranovich A, Berthelet E, Keyes M, Kim-Sing C, Morris WJ, Paltiel C. PSA failure and the risk of death in prostate cancer patients treated with radiotherapy. *International Journal of Radiation Oncology, Biology, Physics* 2004; 60:1040–6.

18. Mackillop WJ. The growth kinetics of human tumours. *Clin Phys Physiol Meas* 1990; 11:123.

19. Flint A. *A treatise of the principles and practice of medicine*, 5th edn, Henry, C., Lea's Son & Co., Philadelphia: PA, 1881.

20. Hartshorne H. *A system of medicine*. J. Russell Reynolds (ed.) Vol. 1. Philadelphia, PA: Henry C. Lea's Son & Co., 1880.

21. Roberts FT. *A handbook of the theory and practice of medicine*, London: H.K. Lewis, 1885.

22. Chammas S. *An empirical approach to informed consent in ovarian cancer*. MSc Thesis, Department of Community Health and Epidemiology, Queen's University, 1991.

23. Feldman-Stewart D, Chammas S, Hayter C, Pater J, Mackillop WJ. An empirical approach to informed consent in ovarian cancer. *J Clin Epidemiol* 1996; 49:1259–69.

24. Feldman-Stewart D, Brundage MD, Hayter C, Groome P, Nickel JC, Downes H, Mackillop WJ. What prostate cancer patients should know: variations in professionals' opinions. *Radiother and Oncol* 1998; 49:111–23.

25. Feldman-Stewart D, Brundage MD, Hayter C, Groome P, Nickel JC, Downes H, Mackillop WJ. What questions do patients with curable prostate cancer want answered? *Medical Decision Making* 2000; 20:7–19.

26. Brundage MD, Davidson J, Mackillop WJ. Trading treatment toxicity for survival in locally advanced non-small cell lung cancer. *J Clin Oncol* 1997; 15:330–40.

27. Brundage MD, Davidson J, Mackillop WJ, Feldman-Stewart D, Groome P. Using a treatment trade-off method to elicit preferences for the treatment of locally advanced non-small cell lung cancer. *Med Decis Making* 1998; 18:256–7.

28. Huang J, Zhou S, Groome P, Tyldesley S, Zhang-Solomans J, Mackillop WJ. Factors affecting the use of palliative radiotherapy in Ontario. *Journal of Clinical Oncology* 2001; 19:137–44.

29. Veatch RA. *Theory of medical ethics*. New York: Basic Books Inc, 1981.

30. Applebaum PS, Lidz CW, Meisel A. *Informed consent. Legal theory and clinical practice*. New York: Oxford University Press, 1987.

31. Sneiderman B, Irvine JC, Osborne PH. *Canadian medical law*. Ontario: The Carswell Company Limited, 1989.

32. Mackillop WJ, Stewart W, Ginsburg D, Stewart SS. Cancer patients' perceptions of their disease and its treatment. *Br J Ca* 1988; 58:355–8.

33. Quirt CF, Mackillop WJ, Ginsburg AD. Do doctors know when their patients don't? A survey of doctor-patient communication in lung cancer. *Lung Cancer* 1997; 18:1–20.

34. Feldman-Stewart D, Brundage MD. Challenges for designing and implementing decision aids. *Patient Education & Counseling* 2004; 54:265–73.

35. Feldman-Stewart D, Kocovski N, McConnell BA, Brundage MD, Mackillop WJ. Perception of quantitative information for treatment decisions. *Medical Decision Making* 2000; 20:228–38.

36. Mackillop WJ, Quirt CF. Measuring the accuracy of prognostic judgements in oncology. *Journal of Clinical Epidemiology* 1997; 50:21–9.

37. Parkes CM. Accuracy of predictions of survival in later stages of cancer. *BMJ* 1972; ii: 29–31.

38. Evans C, McCarthy M. Prognostic uncertainty in terminal care: can the Karnofsky index help? *Lancet* 1985; i: 1204–6.

39. Heyse-Moore L, Johnson-Bell VE. Can doctors accurately predict the life expectancy of patient with terminal cancer? *Palliat Med* 1987; 1:165–6.

40. Maltoni M, Nanni O, Derni S, Innocenti MP, Fabbri L, Riva N. *et al*. Clinical prediction of survival is more accurate than the KPS in estimating life span of terminally ill cancer patients. *Eur J Cancer* 1994; 30A:764–6.

41. Oxenham D, Cornbleet MA. Accuracy of prediction of survival by different professional groups in a hospice. *Palliat Med* 1998; 12:117–82.

42. Maltoni M, Pirovano M, Scarpi E, Marinari M, Indelli M, Arnolodi E. *et al.* Prediction of survival of patients terminally ill with cancer. *Cancer* 1995; 75:2613–22.

43. Maltoni M, Nanni O, Pirovano M, Scarpi E, Indelli M, Martini C. *et al.* Successful validation of the palliative prognostic score in terminally ill cancer patients. *J Pain Symptom Management* 1999; 17:240–7.

44. Christakis N, Lamont E. Extent and determinants of error in doctors' prognoses. *BMJ* 200; 320:469–73.

45. Glare P, Virik K, Jones M, Hudson M, Eychmuller S, Simes J, Christakis N. A systematic review of physicians' survival predictions in terminally ill cancer patients. *BMJ* 2003; 327:195–8.

46. Pirovano M, Nanni O, Maltoni M, Marinari M, Indelli M, Zaninetta G. *et al.* A new palliative prognostic score: a first step for the staging of terminally ill cancer patients. *J Pain Symptom* 1999; 17:231–9.

47. Glare PA. Eychmueller S. McMahon P. Diagnostic accuracy of the palliative prognostic score in hospitalized patients with advanced cancer. *Journal of Clinical Oncology* 2004; 22:4823–8.

3

Foreseeing
Formulating an accurate prognosis

Elizabeth B. Lamont

Introduction

Physicians are routinely asked to make estimates of patient survival often through the question, 'doc, how long do I have to live?'[1] In responding to such a question, physicians engage in at least two often separate tasks, (1) they must *formulate a prognosis*, or make a mental calculation of the patient's expected survival, and (2) they must *communicate the prognosis* to the inquiring individual. These survival estimates, or *prognoses*, that physicians formulate and then communicate are important to both physicians and patients in all phases of a patient's life because they guide both medical and non-medical decisions. At the end of life, these prognoses can become critically important, as they may signal a change from primarily curative or life-prolonging care to primarily supportive or palliative care, a change that clearly impacts clinical and personal decisions. The irony is that despite its importance, prognostication in advanced cancer is largely inaccurate, both in terms of formulated and communicated prognoses (see Chapter 4). Numerous studies have revealed substantial optimistic bias in the prognoses physicians formulate for their termi- nally ill cancer patients and perhaps further optimistic bias in prognoses they communicate to patients. However, studies have also shown that even if physicians' formulated prognoses are not well calibrated they can discriminate, and thus carry important prognostic information. Future work seeks to incorporate physicians' prognosis with objective measures of patient survival to yield useful algorithms for predicting survival. Because timely awareness of poor prognoses is a precondition for timely initiation of palliative care, accurate prognoses by physicians may attenu- ate the current discrepancy between the idealized home-based, symptom-guided care and the actual institutional-based, invasive care at the end of life.

Importance of prospective identification of the end of life

There is wide agreement among patients, their families, and doctors that the end of life is an impor- tant period to recognize prospectively because, among other things, the type of medical care that one receives during this period should be different from the medical care received at other points in life. Specifically, they are in agreement that the medical care should be supportive in nature, focused on the control of symptoms like pain, rather than invasive in nature, aimed at extending life.[2,3] Consistent with this approach, they agree that the favoured place of death is the home, rather than the hospital.[4,5] Most physicians report that such home-based, symptom-guided care should be ini- tiated at least three months prior to patient death for optimal palliative care.[1]

Despite this broad agreement that home-based, symptom-guided care is the preferred form of medical care at the end of life, epidemiologic and health services research reveals that the current patterns of medical care for the dying in America are far from this ideal.[6–9] For example, study of Medicare claims data (an excellent population-level source of medical treatment and survival data for elderly Americans) show that about half of all Medicare beneficiaries die in acute care hospitals rather than in their homes. Further, fewer than 20 per cent receive hospice care,[7, 8, 10] the most common route to home-based, symptom-guided therapy, prior to death. Finally, among those few who do receive this idealized form of medical care at the end of life, most receive it for a period far shorter than the idealized three months, with most receiving it for less than a month prior to death.[11] The same work reports that fewer than 15 per cent of Medicare beneficiaries enrolled in hospice programmes survive longer than allotted six months.

Inaccuracy of the formulated prognosis

Part of the disparity between idealized and actual care at the end of life may result from the practical problem healthcare providers have of prospectively recognizing the onset of the end of life period. To do this, physicians must accurately formulate prognoses, or determine in their own mind how long they think the patient will live. Within the palliative care literature, there are several studies specifically designed to determine the quality of physicians' formulated prognoses in patients with advanced illness. These studies report quality in the form of physicians' prognostic accuracy in predicting survival of patients following admission to hospice programmes.[12–17] Investigators in these studies have measured physicians' prognostic accuracy by comparing patients' observed survival to their predicted survival (these predictions are not necessarily ones communicated to patients; rather, they are ones physicians formulate for themselves). Results of the studies, summarized in Table 3.1, show that, in aggregate, physicians' overall survival estimates tended to be incorrect by a factor of approximately three, always in the optimistic direction. A representative study documents that physicians over-estimate patient survival by a factor of five and patients, on average, live only 24 days in a hospice (realizing only 13 per cent of the maximal, six month Medicare benefit and only 25 per cent of physicians' idealized three month hospice length of stay).[17]

Studies of physicians' abilities to predict terminally ill patients' survival are not limited to patients in palliative care settings but have also been evaluated in ambulatory patients undergoing anti-cancer therapy. Investigators measured oncologists' prognostic accuracy in the care of their ambulatory cancer patients by asking them to first predict patients' likelihood of cure and then to

Table 3.1 Studies comparing physicians' estimated survival to patients' actual survival

Lead author	Ref	Year	Number of doctors	Number of patients	Median estimated survival (weeks)	Median actual survival	Estimated survival/actual survival
Parkes	12	1972	NR	168	4.5[a]	2.5[a]	1.8
Evans	13	1985	3	42	NR	NR	3.2[c]
Heyse-Moore	14	1987	NR	50	8	2	4
Forster	15	1988	3	108	7[b]	3.5	2
Maltoni	16	1994	4	100	6	5	1.2
Christakis	17	2000	343	468	NR	3.4	5.3[c]

NR, not reported.

[a] Values estimated from graph in paper.

[b] Seven weeks calculated through statement in paper that survival was overestimated by 3.4 weeks on average.

[c] Ratio of mean estimated survival/mean survival.

estimate the duration of survival for those whose likelihood of cure was zero.[18] At the 5-year point, patients who were alive and disease-free were termed 'cured'; the dates of death of the incurable patients also were determined. The researchers reported that oncologists were highly accurate in predicting cure. That is, for subgroups of patients (i.e., not individual patients) the ratio of the observed cure rate at 5 years to the predicted cure rate was quite high, at 0.92. However, the same oncologists had difficulty predicting the length of survival of individual incurable patients. They predicted survival 'correctly' for only one-third of patients, with the errors divided almost equally between optimistic and pessimistic.

Improving the accuracy of formulated prognoses

Prognostication at the end of life is an under-studied aspect of clinical medicine, and this fact may explain part of the difficulty physicians have in predicting their patients' survival.[19] The predictive algorithms that are so common and useful in more narrow organ system-based aspects of clinical medicine (e.g., Goldman criteria, TNM cancer staging system, Glasgow Coma Score) have few parallels in the broad clinical area of end of life care. In fact, the current Medicare and National Hospice Organization guidelines for hospice eligibility for patients with certain highly prevalent non-cancer diagnoses (i.e., dementia, advanced lung, heart and liver disease) have been shown to be inadequate for discerning which patients with these conditions have less than 6 months to live.[20–22] At present, no such formal guidelines exist for the terminal illness of cancer.

However, within palliative oncology research, there is a growing literature focused on identifying predictors of survival of advanced cancer patients that might aid physicians in their prognostic estimates for similar patients. Multiple prospective and retrospective cohort studies have consistently identified three broad classes of survival predictors: patients' performance status, patients' clinical signs and symptoms, and physicians' clinical predictions. Research that can integrate these, and other, prognostically relevant domains through survival models to yield easy metrics for clinicians may help to attenuate the problem of prognostic inaccuracy.

Performance status

With regard to the first broad class of predictors, performance status is a global measure of a patient's functional capacity and has consistently been found to predict survival in cancer patients.[23] Given this survival importance, performance status is frequently used as a selection criteria for patients entering clinical trials and also as an adjustment factor in the subsequent analyses of treatment effect. Several different measures have been developed to quantify performance status, and among them, the Karnofsky performance status (KPS) is the most often used. The KPS ranges from values of 100, signifying fully normal functional status with no complaints, nor evidence of disease, to 0, signifying death. Table 3.2 contains a representation of the complete spectrum of values for the KPS scale.

Multiple studies[13, 16, 24–33] have reported associations between cancer patients' survival and their performance status. The direction of the association is positive; that is, as a patient's performance status declines, so too does their survival. The magnitude of the association is described differently in different studies depending on the statistical methods employed, but several studies report that among patients enrolled in palliative care programmes, a KPS of less than 50 per cent suggests a life expectancy of less than 8 weeks.[13, 16, 25, 32, 34, 35]

Signs and symptoms

With regard to the second broad class of survival predictors, patients' clinical signs and symptoms have also been shown to be associated with survival in the setting of advanced cancer.

Table 3.2 Karnofsky performance status scale

Value	Level of functional capacity
100	Normal, no complaints, no evidence of disease
90	Able to carry on normal activity, minor signs or symptoms of disease
80	Normal activity with effort, some signs or symptoms of disease
70	Cares for self, unable to carry on normal activity or to do active work
60	Requires occasional assistance, but is able to care for most needs
50	Requires considerable assistance and frequent medical care
40	Disabled, requires special care and assistance
30	Severely disabled, hospitalization is indicated although death is not imminent
20	Hospitalization is necessary, very sick, active supportive treatment necessary
10	Moribund, fatal processes progressing rapidly
0	Dead

Several investigative groups have examined the prognostic importance of patients symptoms,[25, 35–39] and Vigano and colleagues have described this importance in their systematic review of prognostic factors in advanced cancer.[40] In examining 136 different variables from 22 studies, they found that, after performance status, specific signs and symptoms were the next best predictors of patient survival. The presence of dyspnoea, dysphagia, weight loss, xerostomia, anorexia, and cognitive impairment had the most compelling evidence for independent association with patient survival in these studies.

Several groups of investigators have evaluated associations between biological markers (i.e., laboratory values) and survival in advanced cancer patients.[24, 41, 42] For example, in their retrospective analysis of 339 phase I chemotherapy patients with advanced cancer at the University of Chicago, Janisch and colleagues found that among routine pretreatment laboratories, only platelet count elevation and serum albumin depression were associated with shorter survivals in a multivariate model that included KPS. Among a sample of 207 consecutive advanced non-small cell lung patients, Meurs and colleagues found that in addition to performance status and symptoms, lymphocyte count, albumin, sodium, and alkaline phosphatase were all predictive of survival. Similarly, Maltoni and colleagues examined 13 haematological and urinary parameters at baseline and every 28 days in a group of 530 patients in Italian palliative care centres. In a multivariate model that included performance status, the investigators describe high total white blood cell count, low lymphocyte percentage and low pseudocholinesterase as associated with diminished survival. From these studies one can conclude that there appears to be negative associations between survival and bone marrow parameters (e.g., platelets, white blood cells) as well as positive associations between survival and synthetic parameters (e.g., serum proteins) in this patient population.

Clinical predictions

With respect to the third broad class of predictors of survival in terminal cancer, physicians' clinical predictions about patient survival are important. As noted previously, numerous studies suggest that physicians' predictions regarding patients' survival in palliative care programmes are frequently inaccurate and systematically optimistic. However, the overly optimistic estimates are well-correlated with actual survival.[16, 17, 43] That is, while physicians are not well calibrated with respect to survival (that is, they are systematically optimistic), they nevertheless have discriminatory abilities.[44]They are able to order patients in terms of how sick they are, or how long they have to live. This fact suggests that physicians' clinical predictions may be a useful, but not exclusive, source of information regarding patient survival. Thus, integration of clinical predictions with other known prognostic factors may be beneficial in predicting patient survival. For example, Muers and colleagues found that the addition of physician clinical prediction to their previously mentioned prognostic model (that contained performance status, symptoms, and laboratory values) improved the model's predictive power.[41] This suggests that physicians are able to measure and quantify factors relevant to survival that are unmeasured by the previously mentioned factors. Similarly, Knaus and colleagues in their study of SUPPORT patients found that multivariate regression models that included physicians' prognostic estimates were more accurate than the models without the physician input.[45] Hence while it is true that statistical models can be more accurate than human intuition alone,[41, 45, 46] it is also true that physicians provide valuable prognostic information that, thus far, has not been captured in the objective models. Such integrated models hold the greatest promise for improving physicians' predictive accuracy in advanced cancer patients. Maltoni and colleagues explicitly combined this information with other known predictors of patient survival in their predictive tool.[47]

Integrated tools

Investigators have also sought to model patient survival by combining and interacting these previously identified clinical predictors.[32, 39] The most recent generation of studies describe integrated models that combine these and other prognostic variables into a single prognostic score. For example, Morita and colleagues developed a regression model predicting survival from performance status and certain clinical signs and symptoms.[38] Coefficients from the regression were then transformed into partial scores and summing the values of each partial score led to a final score termed the Palliative Prognostic Index (PPI). After developing the PPI in a sample of 150 patients, the investigators then tested the approach on a second sample of 95 patients, finding that the PPI predicted 3-week survival with sensitivity of 83 per cent and a specificity of 85 per cent, and 6-week survival with sensitivity of 79 per cent and a specificity of 77 per cent. Several other groups have developed similar scoring systems that rely on integration of all or some of the previously described classes of prognostic indicators of patients with advanced cancer and under palliative care.[47–49] Such scoring systems need to be sensitive to a variety of methodologic concerns.[50–52] The most recent generation of studies in this area seek to determine if these scoring systems are useful in the clinical care of cancer patients and if they are applicable to patients who are not yet enrolled in palliative care programmes or who are dissimilar from such patients.[53, 54] With regard to the clinical utility of the scoring systems, treating physicians will need to determine if the tools' test characteristics (e.g., sensitivity and specificity) fall above certain minimum thresholds for use in clinical decisions.

Other sources of prognostic information

Other sources of information regarding survival in advanced cancer are studies that include cancer patients who do not undergo anti-cancer therapy. Both natural history studies and randomized therapy trials that include a 'best supportive care' arm describe patients who do not undergo anti-cancer therapy. Typically, natural history studies are single institution case series of untreated patients with mortality follow-up. Such reports have been published for a variety of advanced solid tumours.[55–57] Survival information can also be found by examining the survival of patients on the best supportive care arms of randomized clinical trials.[58–61]

Conclusion

Prognostication in advanced cancer is a difficult task that may become easier as physicians become more comfortable with the process and as researchers begin to develop better clinical prediction tools. Such efforts may help to temper the pervasive and systematic optimism in the prognoses physicians formulate regarding their patients who are near the end of life. Ultimately, such improvement would expect to manifest through increasing rates of referral to palliative care programmes and increased survival times after referral to the same programmes. More broadly, however, such improvement may provide patients with a better understanding of their expected survival and thereby allow them to make informed medical and social choices regarding their treatment path at the end of life, whether curative or palliative.[62]

Acknowledgement

This chapter was supported in part by a grant from the National Institutes of Health (EBL, grant #K07 CA93892 to Elizabeth Lamont, MD, MS).

References

1. Christakis NA, Iwashyna TJ. Attitude and self-reported practice regarding prognostication in a national sample of internists. 1998; 158(21):2389–95.
2. Steinhauser KE, Christakis NA, Clipp EC, McNeilly M, McIntyre L, Tulsky JA. Factors considered important at the end of life by patients, families, physicians, and other care providers. *JAMA* 2000; 284(19):2476–82.
3. Steinhauser KE, Clipp EC, McNeilly M, Christakis NA, McIntyre LM, Tulsky JA. In search of a good death: observations of patients, families, and providers. *Annals of Internal Medicine* 2000; 132(10): 825-832.
4. Fried TR, van Doorn C, O'Leary JR, Tinetti ME, Drickamer MA. Older persons' preferences for site of terminal care. *Annals of Internal Medicine* 1999; 131(2):109–12.
5. Gott M, Seymour J, Bellamy G, Clark D, Ahmedzai S. Older people's views about home as a place of care at the end of life. *Palliative Medicine* 2004; 18(5):460–7.
6. SUPPORT Principle Investigators. A controlled trial to improve care for seriously ill hospitalized patients. *JAMA* 1995; 274:1591–98.
7. Emanuel EJ, Ash A, Yu W, Gazelle G, Levinsky NG, Saynina O, McClellan M, Moskowitz M. Managed care, hospice use, site of death, and medical expenditures in the last year of life. *Arch Intern Med* 2002; 162(15):1722–8.
8. McCarthy EP, Burns RB, Ngo-Metzger Q, Davis RB, Phillips RS. Hospice use among Medicare managed care and fee-for-service patients dying with cancer. *JAMA* 2003; 289(17):2238–45.
9. Barnato AE, McClellan MB, Kagay CR, Garber AM. Trends in inpatient treatment intensity among Medicare beneficiaries at the end of life. *Health Services Research* 2004; 39(2):363–75.
10. Iwashyna TJ,. Zhang JX, Christakis NA. Disease-specific patterns of hospice and related healthcare use in an incident cohort of seriously ill elderly patients. *J Palliat Med* 2002; 5(4):531–8.
11. Christakis NA, Escarce JJ. Survival of Medicare patients after enrollment in hospice programs. 1996; 335 (3):172–8.
12. Parkes EM. Accuracy of predictions of survival in later stages of cancer. *BMJ* 1972; 2:29–31.
13. Evans C, McCarthy M. Prognostic uncertainity in terminal care; can the Karnofsky index help? *Lancet* 1985; 1204–6.
14. Heyse-Moore LH, Johnson-Bell VE. Can doctors accurately predict the life expectancy of patients with terminal cancer? *Pall Med* 1987; 1:165–6.
15. Forster LE, Lynn J. Predicting life span for applicants to inpatient hospice. *Arch Intern Med* 1988; 148:2540–3.

16. Maltoni M, Nanni O, Derni S, Innocenti MP, Fabbri L, Riva N, Maltoni R, Amadori D. Clinical prediction of survival is more accurate than the Karnofsky performance status in estimating life span of terminally ill cancer patients. *Eur J Cancer* 1994; 6:764–6.

17. Christakis NA, Lamont EB. Extent and determinants of error in doctors' prognoses in terminally ill patients; prospective cohort study. *BMJ* 2000; 320:469–73.

18. Mackillop WJ, Quirt CF. Measuring the accuracy of prognostic judgements in oncology. *J Clin Epidemiol* 1997; 50:21–9.

19. Christakis NA. The ellipsis of prognosis in modern medical thought. *Social Science in Medicine* 1997; 44(3):301–15.

20. Schonwetter RS, Han B, Small BJ, Martin B, Tope K, Haley WE. Predictors of six-month survival among patients with dementia; an evaluation of hospice Medicare guidelines. *Am J Hosp Palliat Care* 2003; 20(2):105–13.

21. Schonwetter RS, Soendker S, Perron V, Martin B, Robinson BE, Thal A. Review of Medicare's prosposed hospice eligibility criteria for select noncancer patients. *Am J Hosp Palliat Care* 1998; 15(3):155–8.

22. Fox E, Landrum-McNiff K, Zhong Z, Dawson NV, Wu AW, Lynn J. Evaluation of prognostic criteria for determining hospice eligibility in patients with advanced lung, heart, or liver disease. *JAMA* 1999; 282(17):1638–45.

23. Zubrod GC, Schneiderman M, Frei E, Brindley C, Gold GL, Shnider B *et al.* Appraisal of methods for the study of chemotherapy in man; comparative therapeutic trial of nitrogen and mustard and triethylene thiophosphoramide. *J Chron Disease* 1960; 11:7–33.

24. Janisch L, Mick R, Schilsky RL, Vogelzang NJ, O'Brien S, Kut M, Ratain MJ. Prognostic factors for survival in patients treated in phase I clinical trials. *Cancer* 1994; 74:1965–73.

25. Maltoni M, Pirovano M, Scarpi E. *et al.* Prediction of survival or patients terminally ill with cancer. *Cancer* 1995; 75:2613–22.

26. Loprinzi CL, Laurie JA, Wieand S. *et al.* Prospective evaluation of prognostic variables from patient-completed questionnaires. *J Clin Oncol* 1994; 12:601–7.

27. Rosenthal MA, Gebski VJ, Kefford RF. *et al.* Prediction of life-expectancy in hospice patients;identification of novel prognostic factors. *Palliative Medicine* 1993; 7:199–204.

28. Coates A, Porzsolt F, Osoba D. Quality of life in oncology practice;prognostic value of EORTC QLQ-C30 scores in patients with advanced malignancy. *Eur J Cancer* 1997; 33:1025–30.

29. Allard P, Dionne A, Potvin D. Factors associated with length of survival among 1081 terminally ill cancer patients. *J Pall Care* 1995; 11:20–4.

30. Yates JW, Chalmer B, McKegney P. Evaluation of patients with advanced cancer using the Karnofsky performance status. *Cancer* 1980; 45:2220–4.

31. Mor V, Laliberte L, Morris JN. *et al.* The Karnofsky performance status scale. *Cancer* 1984; 53:2002–7.

32. Reuben DB, Mor V, Hiris J. Clinical symptoms and length of survival in patients with terminal cancer. *Arch Intern Med* 1988; 148:1586–91.

33. Christakis NA. Timing of referral of terminally ill patients to an outpatient hospice. *J Gen Intern Med* 1994; 9:314–20.

34. Morita T, Tsundoa J, Inoue S. *et al.* Validity of the palliative performance scale from a survival perspective. *J Pain Symptom Manage* 1999; 18:2–3.

35. Llobera J, Esteva M, Rifa J. *et al.* Terminal cancer;duration and prediction of survival time. *Eur J Cancer* 2000; 36:2036–43.

36. Pirovano M, Maltoni M, Nanni O. *et al.* A new palliative prognostic score;a first step for the staging of terminally ill cancer patients. *J Pain Symptom Manag* 1999; 17:231–9.

37. Hardy JR, Turner R, Saunders M. *et al.* Prediction of survival in a hospital-based continuing care unit. *Eur J Cancer* 1994; 30A:284–8.

38. Morita T, Tsundoa J, Inoue S. *et al.* The Palliative Prognostic Index;a scoring system for survival prediction of terminally ill cancer patients. *Supportive Care Cancer* 1999; 7:128–33.

39. Bruera E, Miller MJ, Kuehn N, MacEachern T, Hanson J. Estimate of survival of patients admitted to a palliative care unit;a prospective study. *J Pain Symptom Manage* 1992; 7:82–6.

40. Vigano A, Dorgan M, Buckingham J. *et al.* Survival prediction in terminal cancer patients; a systematic review of the medical literature. *Palliative Med* 2000; 14:363–74.

41. Muers MF, Shevlin P, Brown J. *et al.* Prognosis in lung cancer; physicians' opinions compared with outcome and a predictive model. *Thorax* 1996; 51:894–902.

42. Maltoni M, Pirovano M, Nanni O. *et al.* Biological indices predictive of survival in 519 Italian terminally ill cancer patients. *J Pain Symptom Manage* 1997; 13:1–9.

43. Vigano A, Dorgan M, Bruera E. *et al.* The relative accuracy of the clinical estimation of the duration of life for patients with end of life cancer. *Cancer* 1999; 86:170–6.

44. Justice AC, Covinsky KE, Berlin JA. Assessing the generalizability of prognostic information. *Ann Intern Med* 1999; 16:515–24.

45. Knaus WA, Harrell FE, Lynn J. *et al.* The SUPPORT prognostic model. Objective estimates of survival for seriously ill hospitalized adults. *Ann Intern Med* 1995; 122:191–203.

46. Lee KL, Pryor DB, Harrell FE. *et al.* Predicting outcome in coronary disease. Statistical models versus expert clinicians. *Am J Med* 1986; 80:553–60.

47. Maltoni M, Nanni O, Pirovano M. *et al.* Successful validation of the Palliative Prognostic Score in terminally ill cancer patients. *J Pain Symptom Manage* 1999; 17:240–7.

48. Shimozuma K, Sonoo H, Ichihara K. *et al.* The prognostic value of quality-of-life scores;preliminary results of an analysis of patients with breast cancer. *Surg Today* 2000; 30:255–61.

49. Tamburini M, Brunelli C, Rosso S. *et al.* Prognostic value of quality of life scores in terminal cancer patients. *J Pain Symptom Manage* 1996; 11:32–41.

50. Walter SD, Feinstein AR, Wells CK. A comparison of multivariable mathematical methods for predicting survival – II. Statistical selection of prognostic variables. *J Clin Epidemiol* 1990; 43:349–59.

51. Feinstein AR, Wells CK, Walter SD. A comparison of multivariable mathematical methods for predicting survival – I. Introduction, rationale, and general strategy. *J Clin Epidemiol* 1990; 43:339–47.

52. Wells CK, Feinstein AR, Walter SD. A comparison of multivariable mathematical methods for predicting survival – III. Accuracy of predictions in generating and challenge sets. *J Clin Epidemiol* 1990; 43:361–72.

53. Glare P, Virik K. Independent prospective validation of the PaP score in terminally ill patients referred to a hospital-based palliative medicine consultation service. *Journal of Pain and Symptom Management* 2001; 22:891–8.

54. Glare PA, Eychmueller S, McMahon P. Diagnostic accuracy of the Palliative Prognostic Score in hospitalized patients with advanced cancer. *Journal of Clinical Oncology* 2004; 22(23):4823–8.

55. Attali P, Prod'homme S, Pelletier G. *et al.* Prognostic factors in patients with hepatocellular carcinoma. *Cancer* 1987; 59:2108–11.

56. Johnstone PA, Norton MS, Riffenburgh RH. Survival of patients with untreated breast cancer. *J Surg Oncol* 2000; 73:273–7.

57. Kowalski LP, Carvalho AL. Natural history of untreated head and neck cancer. *Eur J Cancer* 2000; 36:1032–7.

58. Scheithauer W, Rosen H, Krnek GV. *et al.* Randomised comparison of combination chemotherapy plus supportive care with supportive care alone in patients with metastatic colorectal cancer. *BMJ* 1993; 306:752–5.

59. Glimelius B, Ekstrom K, Hoffman K. *et al.* Randomized comparison between chemotherapy plus best supportive care with best supportive care in advanced gastric cancer. *Annals Oncology* 1997; 163–8.

60. Thongprasert S, Sanguanmitra P, Juthapan W. *et al.* Relationship between quality of life and clinical outcomes in advanced non-small cell lung cancer;best supportive care (BSC) versus best supportive care plus chemotherapy. *Lung Cancer* 1999; 24:17–24.

61. CLIP Group. Tamoxifen in treatment of hepatocellular carcinoma;a randomised controlled trial. *Lancet* 1998; 352:17–20.

62. Weeks JC, Cook EF, O'Day SJ. *et al.* Relationship between cancer patients' predictions of prognosis and their treatment preferences. *JAMA* 1998; 279:1709–14.

4

Foretelling
Communicating the prognosis

Phyllis Butow, Rebecca Hagerty, Martin Tattersall, and Martin Stockler

Introduction

Estimating how long people have to live is hard. Talking to them about it is harder. The purpose of this chapter is to help clinicians better communicate their prognoses to those affected. Knowing 'how long you've got' is important. Appreciating the uncertainty of any forecast is equally important. An individual's life expectancy is dramatically shortened by advanced cancer. Knowing this can help them make the most of what remains. It reduces their risk of having unnecessary and potentially harmful treatments under false pretences and gives them a chance (and an imperative) to get their affairs in order, make peace, and attend to their significant others.

A number of studies have reported that variations in the communication of risk can influence decision-making about medical treatments. For example, people are more likely to choose riskier treatment options if information is worded positively (chances of surviving) rather than negatively (chances of dying).[1] Similarly, treatments offering long-term benefits were more likely to be chosen when a longer discussion had taken place, suggesting that additional explanation can assist understanding.[2] These findings suggest that discussions about prognosis take on a special importance in the context of treatment decision-making. In this context, clear, balanced presentation of facts is imperative, with sufficient time and explanation to assist patients to understand and adjust to the facts being presented.

This chapter is written for clinicians caring for people with advanced cancer. By clinicians, we mean doctors, nurses, counsellors and other professionals looking after people with advanced cancer. We have written it for an interested, experienced audience and sought to keep it clear, practical, and focused on talking with patients and their carers.

Our aim is to provide ideas, frameworks and words for talking about prognosis. The chapter is organised under the following headings:

- Views on prognostication (what the literature tells us)
- The nature of prognosis and prognostication
- Suggestions for discussing prognosis
- Determining what and how people want to know
- How to present prognosis
- Dealing with denial and despair
- Checking, summarizing and recording what has been said

Views on prognostication

Over the past 100 years, there has been an ongoing debate concerning whether information about diagnosis and prognosis harms or benefits patients. However, there has undoubtedly been a shift towards greater provision of medical/health information to cancer patients over the past 20 years in the western world. This is for many reasons, including more and better treatments and better prognoses, less stigmatization of cancer, the development of the medical consumer movement and increasing medico–legal concerns.

What is the legal view?

The legal view pertaining to information provision is that the patient has a basic human right of self-determination which is protected by the written constitutions of Germany and the United States and by the common law of England.[3] This right has, however, been interpreted in various ways in different countries. Perhaps the most paternalistic interpretation is in English law where informational requirements are based on the judgement of the individual *reasonable doctor*.[3] Discretion is allowed in weighing up the potential for causing harm by providing additional information, against the benefit of allowing the patient a totally autonomous choice. In Canada and several states of the United States, the standard of disclosure focuses on the informational needs of the *reasonable patient*, in the particular patient's position. This approach has been criticized because it may fail to protect those whose fears, apprehensions, religious beliefs or superstitions (and therefore information needs) lie outside the mainstream of society. German law goes further still in declaring that

> a doctor will be liable if he fails to supply such information regarding the proposed course of treatment, including the risks attendant thereupon, as he knew or ought to have known the *particular patient* would have required to reach his decision.[3]

The ramifications of these laws are still being tested in court.

In addition to the law, many Health Councils have published guidelines which while not legally binding, may be consulted in disciplinary or civil proceedings. These attempt to take a more flexible, educational approach to influencing information provision. However, in attempting flexibility, the guidelines are often anything but clear. For example, the relevant document produced by the National Health and Medical Research Council (NHMRC) of Australia, states that information provided to patients should cover such aspects as known severe risks of treatment, even when occurrence is rare, the degree of uncertainty of any diagnosis or therapeutic outcome and any significant long-term physical, emotional mental, social, sexual or other outcome which may be associated with a proposed intervention. However, the information should be 'appropriate to the patient's circumstances, personality, expectations, fears, beliefs, values and cultural background' and may be influenced by 'current accepted medical practice'.[4] This leaves considerable latitude on the part of the doctor.

What do patients want?

A clear majority of cancer patients report a preference for detailed information about their disease and prognosis[5–7] and that this information be given in a direct and honest manner.[8–10] Patients rate this information as both important to them and necessary.[11–23]

Most patients want information about:

◆ the chances of cure
◆ the extent of disease spread

◆ life expectancy (e.g. the chances of living one year or five years)

◆ best and worst case scenarios

◆ the possible effects of cancer on their life

◆ possible side-effects of treatment.[17, 21, 24, 25]

However, many patients would like the specialist to *check with them first* if they want prognostic information at all, and also have views on the format for receiving this information.[25, 26] For example, Kaplowitz *et al.* asked 352 patients whether they would like to be given a 'qualitative prognosis' (i.e. patient will/will not die from the disease/probably live a long time) or a 'quantitative prognosis' (i.e. an estimate of their expected survival). They found that 80 per cent wanted a qualitative prognosis but *only one half wanted a quantitative estimate.*[13] Another qualitative study found that patients preferred written prognostic information to be presented using *positively framed language* for example, survival probabilities as opposed to chances of mortality.[20]

A majority of metastatic patients surveyed in Australia recently, preferred words (47 per cent) or percentages (42 per cent) to graphical presentations (21 per cent) which they described as 'too cold, clinical and confronting'. The graphical presentations were also reported as the most difficult to understand.[27]

Patients' views also change. In a study exploring changes in information and involvement preferences over time, 80 patients were followed over a 3–6 months period.[11] Patients whose follow-up visit encompassed a significant deterioration to their condition were significantly more likely to shift towards wanting less information ($p < 0.05$). Thus information preferences need to be renegotiated as disease progresses.

There is limited evidence available regarding preferences of patients with *palliative* stage disease. From the three studies identified, which were conducted in the USA, it was found that most patients wanted to discuss their prognosis truthfully with their doctor, including the impact of the illness on their daily lives.[9, 10] The most recent study conducted in 2003 found that the majority of palliative care patients (55 per cent) and their caregivers (75 per cent) who were interviewed retrospectively, would like to have discussed life expectancy with their clinician.[28]

Which patients want what?

Several studies have identified predictors of prognostic information preferences. In early stage cancer, younger, female and rural patients, those with a better prognosis and those who were less anxious were more likely to want full disclosure of a terminal prognosis.[12] Anxious patients were more likely to prefer the physician to tell a loved one the prognosis,[12] and to avoid thinking about death.[26] Patients who were being treated more radically were more likely to want to know information about treatment side-effects and the chances of cure,[16] perhaps to assist them in making an informed choice about an arduous treatment.

In the advanced cancer setting, patients with higher depression scores were more likely to want to discuss prognosis including the worst news (shortest time to live without treatment),[27] while anxious patients were more likely to want to know the longest time to live without treatment. Patients whose prognosis was better were more likely to want to discuss prognosis upfront, at the first consultation. Patients without children were also more willing to discuss death and dying earlier than those with children, perhaps because they could face these issues more easily without the worry of leaving children behind.[27]

Patients of Anglo-Saxon background were more likely to prefer words when being given survival statistics while those without good English found numbers easier to understand. The more educated patients liked the graphical presentations, probably because they found them easier to process and understand.

Patient understanding of prognostic information

In most studies of patient understanding, wide discrepancies between doctor prognostication and patient understanding have been noted. The literature suggests that cancer patients frequently mis-understand much of what they are told,[24, 25] incorrectly state the extent of their disease and the goal of treatment,[29] and overestimate their prognosis.[24, 30–34]

One early study was conducted in Scotland and found that only one of the 74 patients surveyed was aware of their prognosis.[35] The more recent studies also found that many patients incorrectly state the extent of their disease and the goal of treatment, and overestimate their expected survival.[24, 30, 32, 36] Even when discussions of prognosis reportedly occurred, patients tend to overestimate their expected survival.[37] Such misunderstanding may lead patients to make decisions contrary to their best interests, for example choosing futile life-extending therapy at the expense of quality of life.[38]

In the palliative care setting, an early study found that many incurable cancer patients (73 per cent) were not aware of their disease status and many (40 per cent) had not been given this information.[39] This study compared results with an earlier 1969 study and found that there had been an increase in awareness and disclosure between 1969 and 1987. A more recent study found that most patients (74 per cent) acknowledged their terminal diagnosis and had a realistic understanding of their expected survival. There was a substantial minority (19/200), however, who denied their terminal status and shortened life expectancy.[30]

What are the views of doctors regarding prognostic discussions?

Doctor views on this issue have been influenced by the struggle between different ethical principles within medicine; that of beneficence (acting for the good of others) and paternalism (which requires the doctor to take responsibility for acting in their patients' presumed best interests), versus that of patient autonomy (which recognizes the need to respect the patient's integrity and right to self-determination). Reluctance to provide information to patients is often based on the paternalistic model, which assumes that sickness makes the patient vulnerable, and therefore places the responsibility for deciding what constitutes benefit or harm firmly upon the doctor. Providing information which portrays a gloomy prognosis or offering choice in treatments may cause psychological distress in some patients, albeit temporary; therefore it is advisable to 'first, do no harm' and withhold information. Many doctors from this philosophical stance argue vehemently that the modern practice of full disclosure can be cruel and insensitive, be contrary to patients' wishes or best interests[40, 41] and disrupt the physical and psychological benefits arising from denial and hope.[35, 42]

Those arguing from the principle of patient autonomy take a different stance. This group, now in the majority within the Western world, have argued that patients have a right to control what is done to their body, to be provided with full information about their situation and to make decisions about their care. These ideas have been embodied in the principles of informed consent and shared decision-making. The mechanism of informed consent has been proposed as the way to ensure an ethical dialogue about treatment options between doctor and patient. Informed consent requires that the physician not only communicates the risks and benefits of all treatment options (including prognosis with and without treatment) to the patient but also assures that the patient understands the information and reaches their own conclusion regarding the preferred option.[43] Within this model, information about prognosis is seen as essential to informed decision-making, and therefore an integral part of any medical discussion.

In practice, most doctors argue for a combination of these extremes, suggesting that the *way* in which information is given is as important as the content, and that honest disclosure is only effective when given compassionately and sensitively. We explored health professionals' views in more depth concerning disclosure of prognosis, specifically in the context of metastatic disease.[8] We audio-taped, transcribed and coded interviews with 13 experienced health professionals involved in cancer care, including doctors, nurses, psychologists, psychiatrists and social workers. Seven main themes were identified:

1. Communication within a caring, trusting, long-term relationship
2. Open and repeated negotiations for patient preferences for information
3. Clear, straightforward presentation of prognosis where desired
4. Strategies to ensure patient understanding
5. Encouragement of hope and a sense of control
6. Consistency of communication within the multidisciplinary team
7. Communication with and care of other members of the family, whose needs may differ from those of the patient.

How do doctors and patients discuss prognosis?

In the advanced cancer setting, most studies report that prognosis is infrequently discussed[34, 44–46] and one study found that if a prognostic discussion had occurred, it most commonly had taken place between the doctor and someone other than the patient.[46] Where prognostic discussions had occurred it was found that there was lack of clarity in the information,[44] estimates of expected survival were often not given[46] and that both doctors and patients tended to avoid acknowledging or discussing prognosis by focusing on the treatment plan. Although the most recent study reported that patients were well informed of the aim of their treatment and the incurable status of their disease, fewer were informed of their expected survival.[31]

In early studies conducted in the palliative care setting, it was reported that many physicians mostly did not discuss the diagnosis or prognosis with their terminally ill patients[47, 48] and, if the issue of prognosis was raised, it was usually initiated by the patient and was not directly addressed by the physician.[47] More recent studies have also found that physicians often do not discuss prognosis with the patient or their carer;[49, 50] they present fewer facts and less detail concerning prognostic information as compared with other types of information;[51] and may not provide their best estimate of survival even when asked by patients.[52] A lack of communication to terminally ill patients of impending death has also been reported.[37] One study, however, found that the physicians who did provide a prognosis reportedly did so in a direct manner.[50]

Clearly, prognosis is a difficult area for both patients and doctors to broach, and becomes more difficult, the worse the news to be delivered. Some writers have suggested that health professionals and patients fall into a 'conspiracy of silence' where both are too frightened to raise the issue of prognosis. Doctors face particular difficulties when discussing life expectancy with patients with a poor prognosis. Such information raises immediate issues for the patient, and the information required includes much shorter time frames than the long range forecasting required in early stage disease.

Maintaining hope

Provision of hope is a common theme in the literature.[53, 54] The need for optimism and hope to be sustained in the process of honestly delivering bad news and information about a limited life expectancy is an ideal expressed by both doctors and patients.[8, 14, 26, 55] There is, however, a delicate balance between fostering realistic hope and unethically creating unrealistic expectations of longevity.[8, 10] Furthermore, hope is a broad concept which can hold different meanings for each individual, suggesting that efforts to convey hope may need to be tailored to the individual.[8, 10, 56, 57]

Disclosure of prognosis and family members

Family members often have an intense desire for prognostic information, particularly as the patient becomes sicker and more care is needed, a time when patients may have less need for prognostic information and focus more on daily living.[14, 21, 23, 25, 26, 58, 59]

It is not always easy to meet the needs of family members whilst also respecting those of the patient.[8, 17] Recent Western studies have revealed a general belief in prioritizing the preferences of the patient over those of family members both in terms of what the patient is told and disclosure to family members.[8, 17, 25, 26, 60] The evidence for patient preferences for prognostic information provision to family members is mixed. One study found that patients favoured openness with family members but rejected unconditional disclosure of information without their consent and their family influencing what information they would be given.[26, 60]

One major difficulty is when relatives wished to keep the prognosis a secret from the patient. Butow *et al.* found that health professionals tried to build up a trusting relationship with the family, and to convince them that such a course would not be helpful.[8] However, oncologists in one study reported a greater willingness to withhold prognostic information than diagnostic information from the patient, if the family desired it.[20, 61]

Cultural issues

An important issue in information-giving is that cultural expectations differ, and in some communities it is not considered appropriate for the doctor to disclose prognosis to the patient or involve them in decision-making. Several studies exploring the Greek culture have been conducted in recent years[35, 62] and other cultures examined include that of Israel,[29] Sweden,[63] Norway,[10, 64] Germany,[65] South Africa,[66] Italy,[67] Singapore,[68] Turkey,[69] Spain,[70] Tanzania[71]and Chinese migrants of Australia[72] and one cross-cultural study of Canadian, South American and European physicians.[73]

The evidence suggests that patients of Anglo-Saxon background prefer disclosure[14, 16, 21, 26] whereas those of other cultural background vary[62, 66, 74] with a tendency to favour non-disclosure.[62, 72]

Many health professionals of different cultures, particularly Asian cultures, are in favour of non-disclosure.[68, 71, 75] Patients are also reportedly unaware of their diagnosis and/ or prognosis, which may indicate that it is common for patients not to be given this information.[64, 65, 74]

Members of some cultures may prefer that the family have a high level of involvement in the consultations, and in some cases that the family be informed first of the diagnosis and prognosis and that the patient be either told gradually or not at all.[62, 75]An Australian study found that in many cultures such as the Chinese, the Filipinos and the Greeks, it is proper to discuss the diagnosis and treatment of cancer with the eldest son rather than with the patient.[76] The family should be told, but not the patient, and they then decide what the patient should be told. The family would then prepare and emotionally support the patient before telling them. Conversely Dutch, Poles and Muslims interviewed for this qualitative study believed the patient should be told, whereas Macedonians and Croatians did not want to be told at all.

However, it is important to note that even within ethnic groups, which are perceived by outsiders as being strongly unified in their attitudes, there may be variations in their expectations. The need for doctors to avoid possible cultural stereotypes when discussing diagnosis and prognosis in cancer has also been noted.[76]

Nature of prognosis and prognostication

Biologic processes are inherently unpredictable. Biologic forecasts (prognoses) must be couched in terms of probabilities. Life expectancy is the end product of many such processes. For a given individual, we cannot know where next a tumour will cause problems or whether it will respond to anti-cancer treatment, and if so, for how long. Individuals vary widely even if the clinical picture is precisely defined. A group of 70-year-old men with bone-dominant metastatic prostate cancer, no visceral metastases, and no comorbidities who are treated with androgen deprivation may have a median survival of 3 years, but the group will include some men who will live for only a few months, and others who will live for many years.

Prognoses are probabilistic. Even if we have a good idea of the *average* effect of a disease, prognostic factor, or treatment, this average is made up of variable and idiosyncratic individual responses. We must be satisfied with statements like 'the probability of being alive in 6 months is X, and this can be increased to Y with the addition of treatment C'. The accuracy and precision of our probability estimates are also uncertain because of the effects of chance – random error – and bias – systematic error.

Probabilities can be estimated, but not known in any absolute sense. This is true for both common definitions of probability. The more traditional frequentist definition of probability is that it is the rate of occurrence in the whole (and therefore infinite) population. The more fashionable Bayesian definition of probability is that it represents the strength of belief in a particular proposition. Either way, probabilities are unknowable parameters that can only be estimated from finite samples (less than everybody). The accuracy of any estimate depends on the both the size of the sample, and on how closely the sample resembles the population of interest.

Random error is the effect of chance fluctuations. It is the imprecision that occurs when measurements of a parameter from a random sample of individuals are used to estimate the value of the parameter among all such individuals. The precision of an estimate depends on the size and homogeneity of the sample. The bigger and more homogeneous the sample, the smaller the effect of chance fluctuations and the more precise the estimate.

Confidence intervals can be used to quantify and express random error. Even substantial samples produce estimates with wide ranges of plausible values. For example, an estimated probability of 50 per cent based on a sample of 100 individuals has a 95 per cent confidence interval of 40–60 per cent. The play of chance is important, but relatively innocent because we can always reduce its effect by taking a bigger sample.

Biases are systematic differences that influence our estimate of interest. In the case of prognostication, we want to apply estimates from a research study population to individuals in a clinical target population. Bias will result from any aspect of the study population that differs from the target population *and* affects life expectancy.

Some biases are obvious and can be taken into account. For example, patients meeting strict eligibility criteria for a clinical trial are usually quite different from people in a routine clinical target population, many of whom do not meet the eligibility criteria. Life expectancy in the study population is likely to be longer than in the target population. A clinician who appreciates this bias can adjust an estimate based on the study population before applying it to an individual from a systematically different target population.

Many biases are obscure and can not be taken into account. For example, many patients at 'centres of excellence' are there because they have unusual characteristics. They may have an unusual variant of their disease, may want access to a new treatment, or be unusually wealthy. They are probably quite different from people seen in routine clinical practice, many of whom don't have these characteristics, but the sizes and even directions of these effects on life expectancy are much harder to estimate and account for.

What should we do about the imperfections of our forecasts of life expectancy? The rest of this book is about improving their accuracy by reducing systematic errors that bias our estimates. A key point of this chapter is that substantial uncertainty will remain around even the most accurate estimate. Our forecasts should make this uncertainty explicit by emphasizing pragmatic, plausible ranges rather than falsely precise point estimates.

Survival distributions are usually broad and skewed toward longer survival times. This is because survival times vary substantially, even in homogeneous populations; but the minimum survival time can be no shorter than 0, whereas the maximum survival time can be many years. The shortest survival time in a group is usually much closer to the median than the longest survival time. The same constraints should apply to estimates for an individual. Someone with a predicted survival of 6 months can die no sooner than immediately, but may live for several years. These features have important implications for thinking and talking about life expectancy.

The best simple summary of a survival distribution is its median and interquartile range. Survival curves give more information (see Chapter 00, page 00), but confuse most people (including many doctors!).

The median is the best single number description of a survival distribution. It is has a more obvious meaning, is easier to estimate, and is less susceptible to outliers than the mean (average). The median is the middle value in a group ranked from smallest to biggest. It is the 'typical' value for that sample. Because the median is the middle value, it is unaffected by the size of atypical values at either end of the distribution: it will be the same regardless of how large or small are the maximum and minimum. The mean is substantially affected by atypical values. The median (and mean) tell us where a distribution is centred, but not how widely its individuals are spread around that centre.

Ranges and standard deviations tell us about the spread of a distribution. Standard deviations are unsuitable for survival distributions because of their skewing and asymmetry. The most commonly used ranges are the absolute and interquartile.

Absolute ranges are popular, simple, and remarkably uninformative. They define a distribution's limits (100 per cent of observations are within these values), but the minimum and maximum are often so because they are outliers (atypical examples). Absolute ranges are also unstable – they vary much more from sample to sample than estimates closer to the middle of a distribution, like the median and mean. Repeated samples from the same population often give very different estimates of the absolute range. Narrower ranges including smaller proportions of the distribution are both more stable (less susceptible to outliers) and more informative (tell us more about the distribution).

Interquartile ranges are more informative and less complicated than they seem. The interquartile range extends from the 25th percentile to the 75th percentile of a distribution. This means that 50 per cent of observations are within the range, 25 per cent are higher (than the 75th percentile) and 25 per cent are lower (than the 25th percentile). The interquartile range is also unaffected by outliers so it is also more stable than the absolute range – it varies less from sample to sample.

Suggestions for discussing prognosis

Determining what and how people want to know

Since people vary in whether they want to know their prognosis, and how they want to hear it, you will need to negotiate prognostic discussion. Box 4.1 depicts a short negotiation between a doctor and patient on this topic.

Box 4.1 A discussion between doctor and patient about prognosis

Doctor: Most patients in your situation do very well, but in a small proportion the cancer will come back. Having chemotherapy reduces the chances of the cancer coming back by about one third. Unfortunately we don't know upfront who will do well and who won't. Therefore we have to give chemotherapy to everyone to achieve that reduction in risk. So we would recommend chemotherapy to someone like you. Now, are you the sort of person who likes numbers? Some people like to know what their risk is in numbers, other people don't like that degree of preciseness.

Patient: Well, will it make a difference to the treatment I get?

Doctor: It won't change my recommendation, but this is a trade-off between reducing risk and putting up with the side-effects of chemotherapy for a few months. You may feel differently to me about that trade-off.

Patient: Look, I trust you, and I don't really want to have a number in my head. I'll go with the chemotherapy.

Doctor: OK, but often people change their mind about this sort of thing. Please feel free to ask me questions about this, or anything else about your cancer and the treatment, at anytime.

Patients will often raise prognosis themselves, not necessarily in a straightforward manner. For example, they may comment that they are thinking of selling their house to look for something bigger, and then pause and look at you expectantly. This may be a request for information about whether they will have time to enjoy their new house, or should conserve energy and stay where they are. You may need to explore what the question really is. The method identified so far to facilitate prognostic communication is providing patients with a question prompt list (see Box 4.2). Question prompt lists endorse question asking if and when patients wish, and contain lists of questions patients may want to ask, in categories. They have been shown to increase question asking in oncology and palliative care settings, particularly about prognosis.[77]

Box 4.2 A question prompt list for patients seeing a medical or radiation oncologist for the first time

Most people who see a medical or radiation oncologist for the first time have questions and concerns. Often these get forgotten in the heat of the moment, only to be remembered later. To help you make the most of the consultation with your oncologist we have compiled a list of questions to enable you to get the information you want about your illness, and possible treatments.

These questions have been developed after discussion with many people. Your oncologist is keen to answer any questions you may have, either now or at future consultations. You and your family may choose to use this list at any time. We suggest you tick those that you want to ask, and write down any that you may have thought of which are not listed. In many cases, the oncologist will have answered the questions without you even asking, and in that instance this card can serve as a checklist.

Negotiation of how and when to ask questions

- Do you have time today to discuss my questions?
- Can I ask you to explain any words that I am not familiar with?

Diagnosis

- What kind of cancer do I have?
- Where is the cancer at the moment? Has it spread to other parts of the body?
- How common is my cancer?

Investigations

- Are there any further tests that I need to have? What will they tell us? Will they confirm my diagnosis?
- What will I experience when having the test/s?

Prognosis

- How bad is this cancer and what is it going to mean for me?
- What is the aim of the treatment? To cure the cancer or to control it and manage symptoms?
- How likely is it that the cancer will spread to other parts of the body without any more treatment?
- How likely is it that the cancer will spread to other parts of the body if I do have more treatment?
- What is the expected survival with my type of cancer?
- Is the treatment going to improve my chance of survival; is it worth going through?
- What symptoms will the cancer cause?
- Will my sexual drive diminish due to treatment or the illness?
- How likely is it that the treatment will improve symptoms?

Box 4.2 A question prompt list for patients seeing a medical or radiation oncologist for the first time *(continued)*

Optimal care

- Do you specialize in treating my type of cancer?
- How well established is the treatment you are recommending?
- Are there guidelines on how to treat my cancer?

The multidisciplinary team

- Do you work in a multidisciplinary team and what does this mean?
- Can you explain any advantages of a team approach?
- Is there any other member of your team that I should meet now?
- How do you all communicate with each other and me?
- Who will be in charge of my care?
- What do I do if I get conflicting information?

Options

- What are my options?
- What are the pros and cons of each treatment option?
- Is it necessary to have any treatment?
- What can I expect if I decide not to have treatment?
- How much time do I have to think about this? Do you need my decision today?
- What is your opinion about the best treatment for me?

Treatment information

- What exactly will be done during the treatment and how will it affect me?
- What is the treatment schedule e.g. how many treatments will I have, how often and for how long will I have treatment?
- Are there any advantages/disadvantages of the private versus public health system?

Clinical trials

- Are there any clinical trials that might be relevant for me?
- Will I be treated any differently if I enrol in a trial?

Second opinion

- Is there another specialist who treats this type of cancer that you recommend for a second opinion?

Preparing for treatment

- Is there anything that I can do before or after my treatment that might make it more effective?
- What side-effects should I expect and when are these likely to happen?

Box 4.2 A question prompt list for patients seeing a medical or radiation oncologist for the first time *(continued)*

- Who do I contact if I experience any problems?
- What are the dos and don'ts while having treatment?
- Are there long-term side-effects from the treatment?
- Should I change my diet, work, exercise, etc.?
- Will I require any additional treatment after this; if so what might that be?
- What is my long-term follow-up plan?

Costs

- What costs will I incur throughout my treatment? E.g. medication, chemotherapy etc.
- Am I eligible for any benefits if I cannot work?

Support information

- What information is available about my cancer and its treatment? e.g. books, videos, websites etc.
- In relation to complementary therapies is there anything that you believe may be helpful or that is known to be bad for me?
- Can you give me any advice on how to cope with this?
- Is there someone I can talk to who has been through this treatment?
- Are there services/support groups to help myself and my family deal with this illness?

How can prognosis be best communicated?

The stereotypical question about life expectancy – 'How long have I got?' – begs a simple, single-number answer. Unfortunately, the stereotypical, simple, single-number answer – '6 months' – is misleading and unsympathetic. A single number suggests greater precision than is warranted, and is often interpreted as a hard limit: 'They said I only had 3 months, but that was 6 months ago and I'm still going strong.' Honest disclosure requires words that convey the inherent uncertainty of prognostic forecasts.

Typical, best and worst case scenarios are what many people want and what most research delivers. The problems are: finding data that best matches a particular patient; modifying it to account for any important differences (between the study population and the patient of interest) and then summarizing and conveying it clearly to the patient. We suggest the following approach.

The median of a group of similar people is the best starting point, the more similar the better. The rest of this book is about finding the best groups. Because predictions of life expectancy are imprecise and probabilistic, having found the group and its median (e.g. 6 months), it is probably better to think and talk about ranges around the median (e.g. 3–9 months) than about its point estimate. It is natural to think of ranges that are symmetrical around an estimate, as in the example above. However, because survival distributions are skewed towards longer times, ranges around an estimate should be also be skewed towards longer times with a wider interval above the estimate than below it. So, 3–12 months would be a better range around an estimate of 6 months than 3–9 months. But what range should we use and how should we estimate it?

The interquartile range has several desirable properties discussed above, including its simple interpretation – that half the values lie within this range – but using interquartile ranges from actual studies assumes that we know them by heart, or have them at hand. This is rarely the case, but needn't be a problem if we can guesstimate it.

The interquartile range can be estimated as about half to double the median if we assume an exponential distribution (see Table 4.1). The assumption that survival follows an exponential distribution is the basis of sample size calculations for most trials using survival as an end point. It is also assumed in many cost-effectiveness studies. Few survival distributions are exactly exponential, but it is a reasonable approximation for most groups with advanced cancer, especially given the imprecision of all the other parameters we are working with.

Thinking of the median survival as a half-life helps us remember that the interquartile range is about half to double the median. In an exponential distribution, the median is the time taken for a group to be halved. This means that 50 per cent remain after one half-life, 25 per cent remain after two half-lives, 12.5 per cent remain after three half-lives, and so on. Working backwards, it turns out that 71 per cent of a group remain after 0.5 half-lives. Half to double the median therefore includes the middle 46 per cent in an exponential distribution, but given the imprecision of what we're working with, this is close enough to half!

Best and worst case scenarios can also be estimated using this approach. The absolute worst case scenario is rarely helpful – getting hit by a bus as you leave. The absolute best case scenario is often misleading because it is so atypical. Any choice is arbitrary. We suggest using the 10th and 90th percentiles because they are easy to estimate, describe and understand. Assuming an exponential distribution, the 10th percentile is about one-sixth of the median, and the 90th percentile is about three to four times the median.

Instead of giving a single estimate of the median survival, we suggest giving a range that includes a substantial proportion of similar patients, for example the middle 50 per cent of patients (the interquartile range). The interquartile range is estimated by taking half to double the predicted median. The worst and best case scenarios are estimated as being one-sixth of the estimated median (worst 10 per cent) and three to four times the estimated median (best 10 per cent).

The recommended answer to the question 'How long have I got?' might be something like:

> This is a hard question. The typical person with your kind and stage of cancer lives about 12 months. This means that half the people live longer than 12 months and half live shorter than 12 months. If we had 100 people exactly like you, then we'd expect that the 10 who did worst might only live a few (2) months, but the 10 who did best might still be around in a few (3–4) years, and that most (about half) would live somewhere between 6 months and 2 years.

Table 4.1 Numbers of months and proportions surviving after given multiples of the median survival (half-life) in an exponential distribution

Number of half-lives	Number of months			Proportion who lived this long or longer (%)	Proportion who died this soon or sooner (%)	Proportion dying between this multiple and the medium (%)
1/6	1	2	4	89	11	39
1/2	3	6	12	71	29	21
1 (medium)	6	12	24	50	50	0
2	12	24	48	25	75	25
3.3	20	40	79	10	90	40

Formats for presenting prognosis

Prognosis can be presented in a variety of formats, including, words, numbers and graphs. Figure 4.1 shows a variety of formats for presenting risk. Research suggests that most people find numbers and 100-person diagrams the easiest to understand, although some people find 100-person diagrams confronting. Pie charts and survival graphs are harder to take in, and some people find them too clinical and cold when discussing their own life. The bar graphs generated by adjuvant-online for breast cancer (www.adjuvant_online.com) appear to be well understood by patients.

Research also suggests that the way you discuss prognosis is just as important as what you say about it. It is important to stop often and check that people have understood what you said, invite questions, explore whether the information was as they expected, what this means to them in the context of their lives (for example its impact on holiday, home and work plans) and how they are coping with the news. If they are upset, your support and reassurance that you will be working with them to maximize their chances and quality of life, will be very important. It may assist them if you write things down for them to take home.[14, 78]

Maintaining hope

Most doctors and patients emphasize the importance of maintaining hope when discussing prognosis.

Factors found to influence patient hope are physician willingness to:

- Talk about psychosocial issues.
- Answer questions and provide information honestly and openly.
- Offer the most up-to-date treatment and demonstrate expertise.
- Provide emotional support.
- Discuss outliers.
- Focus on positive and achievable goals
- Couch the patient's prognosis in terms of reaching goals or 'landmarks', or overcoming 'hurdles'.[54]
- Normalize preparations for death, as something that everyone needs to do. Death can come to anyone at short notice, so that discussing death does not make it an inevitable event.[27, 54, 78–81]

Factors reported as potentially decreasing hope include:

- Perceived poor communication.
- A pessimistic attitude.
- An impersonal context for the disclosure.[11, 54, 81]

Dealing with denial and despair

The use of denial may be an adaptive approach to responding to a cancer diagnosis or a poor prognosis. Watson describes denial as usually employed when one feels overwhelmed by events or emotions and a strategy which can be effective in dealing with anxiety and depression.[82] It is only when denial interferes with recommended treatment schedules that it is labelled maladaptive and becomes a concern for medical professionals. Maguire has suggested the following approach to patient denial. Accept the patient's world view, but probe gently for inconsistency ('I understand that you are feeling very optimistic about achieving a cure.[83] But it sounds like you do sometimes wonder if things won't work out. Do you want to talk about that?'). If you are concerned about potential danger arising from denial, tell the patient. ('Of course it is your decision what treatment you have, but I strongly recommend that you have chemotherapy. I believe that this offers you a real chance of cure, which you might lose if you don't have it.')

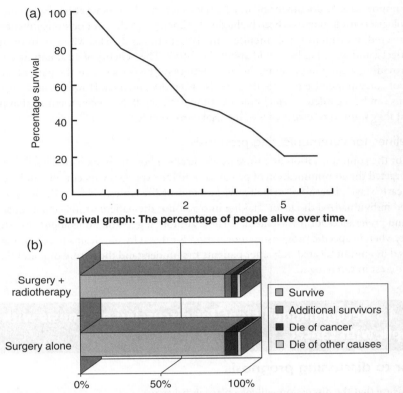

(a) Survival graph: The percentage of people alive over time.

(b) Bar graph: useful for communicating relative prognosis with and without therapy

Figure 4.1 Ways to present prognosis.

Summarizing, recording and communicating to others

The management of persons with advanced cancer is increasingly a multidisciplinary matter, and inevitably there is the potential for inconsistent information being presented by different members of the team, with resulting confusion or misunderstanding. The patient's general practitioner is rarely fully informed of what prognostic information has been given, although they may be involved in the patient's management outside the hospital, and be responsible for coordinating care at home. There has been little research directed at communication within and between multidisciplinary team members caring for patients with far advanced cancer and incurable cancer. Team members' predictions of life expectancy may vary widely. Different means of documenting the outcome of consultations have not been researched though copies of correspondence commonly are sent to different team members, but not usually to the patient. Within the hospital record, there is conventionally notation of patient attendance at multidisciplinary meetings, and sometimes detail is given of management recommended. However, if prognosis is mentioned, it is rare for what has been said to be detailed in the patient record. When palliative care has been consulted in hospital inpatients, the specialist usually completes a consultation sheet making specific recommendations, but prognosis is rarely covered in detail, nor is it always stated what the patient has been told.

There is a need for consistency of information provided by the hospital team and the patient's general practitioner. Inconsistent information is seen as confusing for the patient, destructive of patient–doctor trust and detrimental to patient coping.

The importance of documenting in letters to referring doctors what has been said to patients in oncologist consultations has been highlighted.[84] Topics include mention of treatments considered and rejected, treatment recommended, likely benefits and risks, what to do in the event of side-effects, and what has been said about the future. The benefits of audiotaping consultations and providing a copy to patients, dictating letters in the presence of the patient, and sending copies of correspondence to patients have also been documented. However, none of these interventions can be regarded as usual practice, though the NHS has recommended that patients are asked if they want to receive copies of medical correspondence.

Guidelines for communicating prognosis

Much of the communication literature has focused on how to break bad news.[85–87] Few studies have targeted the communication of prognosis and life expectancy specifically, and these focus on either early stage disease[14, 26] or palliative and end-of-life issues.[9, 10, 29, 88] Reviews have recommended individualized disclosure, taking into account the patient's intellectual capacity, coping style, and preferences for involvement.[17] These authors suggest that oncologists use stepwise disclosure, wherein specific prognostic information is offered by physicians to patients and actually provided or communicated only after patients first understand the nature of it and then indicate their interest in receiving it.

Box 4.3 Recommended steps for discussing prognosis with people with cancer

Prior to discussing prognosis:

- Ensure that the discussion will take place in privacy.
- Ensure as much as possible that there will be no interruptions (e.g. switch off mobile phones and pagers; inform staff).
- Check if the patient would like to have a friend or relative present.
- Check if the patient would like another medical person present (if applicable).

Negotiating

- Ask first if the person wants to be given information about prognosis (e.g. "I can tell you what happens to most people in your situation. Would you like me to do that?") and explore what he or she currently understands and expects.
- Explore and negotiate with the patient the *type* (e.g. staging details; the chances of being cured; short and long-term side-effects of treatment; survival estimates) and *format* (e.g. words, numbers, graphs) of prognostic information desired and adhere to these preferences,

Aspects of prognosis to discuss

- Adhere to the person's stated preference for information about prognosis. If/when desired, the following can be provided:
  - staging details and their implications for prognosis
  - chances of being cured or that cancer will never return

Box 4.3 Recommended steps for discussing prognosis with people with cancer *(continued)*

– likely benefits and risks of treatment

– chances of the cancer shortening the individual's life compared to other life events, e.g. heart disease

– average and longest survival times, emphasizing a range rather than a single time point

How to discuss prognosis

◆ Adopt an honest and straightforward yet sensitive approach.

◆ Encourage a collaborative relationship with the patient (e.g. provide an opportunity to ask questions).

◆ Use the most up-to-date information, and if desired, explain its source. Explain how this may be revised by additional information. Suggest a time frame for when additional prognostic information is likely to be available.

◆ Preface any statement of prognostic estimates with the limitations of prognostic formulations. Explain that you can't predict how the person as an individual will respond to the illness and its treatment

◆ If giving a time frame, emphasize a range and not specific endpoints.

◆ Use mixed framing, i.e. give the chances of cure first, then the chances of relapse.

◆ Present information in a variety of ways (e.g. words, graphs, statistics).

◆ Present absolute risks with and without treatment.

◆ Broaden discussion of the prognosis to include the effect of the cancer on the individual's lifestyle.

◆ Emphasize hope-giving aspects of the information, e.g. extraordinary survivors.

◆ Repeat negotiation of information preferences and needs over time.

◆ When explaining relative risk reduction, provide several examples of the calculations.

◆ Only use statistical terminology, e.g. median, hazard risk ratio, if a person is familiar with these concepts.

Concluding the discussion

◆ Summarize main points of the consultation and reassess the person's understanding.

◆ Emphasize hope-giving aspects of the information, such as extraordinary survivors.

◆ Check the patient's emotional reaction to the information and offer support or referral if needed.

◆ Indicate your availability for contact to address any questions or concerns and arrange a further appointment to review situation with a stated time period.

Adapted frpm Lobb *et al.* Talking prognosis with women who have early breast cancer, National Breast Cancer Centre

The Australian National Breast Cancer Centre has produced a set of evidence-based psychosocial guidelines for clinicians on communicating prognosis, which has been endorsed by the Australian NHMRC. However, these too were developed for the scenario of early stage disease. Recommended steps for discussing prognosis, based on these guidelines, are shown in Box 4.3.

References

1. O'Connor AM. Effects of framing and level of probability on patients' preferences for cancer chemotherapy. *Journal of Clinical Epidemiology* 1989; 42:119–26.

2. Mazur DJ, Jickam DH. The effect of physicians' explanations on patients' treatment preferences. *Medical Decision Making* 1994; 14:255–8.

3. Giesen D. Legal accountability for the provision of medical care: a comparative view. *Journal of the Royal Society of Medicine* 1993; 86:648–652.

4. NHMRC. *General guidelines for medical practitioners on providing information to patients.* Canberra: National Health and Medical Research Council, Commonwealth of Australia, Australian Government Publishing Service; 1993.

5. Cassileth BR, Zupkis RV, Sutton-Smith K, March V. Information and participation preferences among cancer patients. *Annals of Internal Medicine* 1980; 92:832–6.

6. Ravdin PM, Siminoff LA, Harvey JA. Survey of breast cancer patients concerning their knowledge and expectations of adjuvant therapy. *Journal of Clinical Oncology* 1998; 16:515–21.

7. Butow P, Tattersall MHN. Talking prognosis with cancer patients. *Australian Doctor* 2002; (17 May):1–8.

8. Butow PN, Dowsett S, Hagerty RG, Tattersall MH. Communicating prognosis to patients with metastatic disease: what do they really want to know? *Supportive Care in Cancer* 2002; 10(2):161–8.

9. Greisinger AJ, Lorimor RJ, Aday LA, Winn RJ, Baile WF. Terminally ill cancer patients: their most important concerns. *Cancer Practice* 1997; 5(3):147–54.

10. Kutner JS, Steiner JF, Corbett KK, Jahnigen DW, Barton PL. Information needs in terminal illness. *Social Science and Medicine* 1999; 48(10):1341–52.

11. Butow PN, McLean M, Dunn S. *et al.* The dynamics of change: Cancer patients' preferences for information, involvement and support. *Annals of Oncology* 1997; 8(9):857–63.

12. Marwit SJ, Datson SL. Disclosure preferences about terminal illness: an examination of decision-related factors. *Death Studies* 2002; 26(1):1–20.

13. Kaplowitz SA, Osuch JR, Safron D, Campo S. Physician communication with seriously ill cancer patients: results of a survey of physicians. In B de Vries B (ed.) *End of life issues: interdisciplinary and multidimensional perspectives*, pp. 205–27. New York: Springer Publishing Company, 1999.

14. Lobb EA, Kenny DT, Butow PN, Tattersall MHN. Women's preferences for discussion of prognosis in early breast cancer. *Health Expectations* 2001; 4:48–57.

15. Schofield PE, Beeney LJ, Thompson JF, Butow PN, Tattersall MH, Dunn SM. Hearing the bad news of a cancer diagnosis: the Australian melanoma patient's perspective. *Annals of Oncology* 2001; 12(3):365–71.

16. Meredith C, Symonds P, Webster L, Lamont D, Pyper E, Gillis CR. *et al.* Information needs of cancer patients in west Scotland: cross sectional survey of patients' views. *BMJ* 1996; 313(7059):724–6.

17. Butow PN, Kazemi J, Beeney LJ, Griffin AM, Tattersall MHN, Dunn SM. When the diagnosis is cancer: Patient communication experiences and preferences. *Cancer* 1996; 77(12):2630–7.

18. Derdiarian AK. Informational needs of recently diagnosed cancer patients. *Nursing Research* 1986; 35(5):276–81.

19. Reynolds PM, Sanson- Fisher RW, Poole AD, Harker J, Byrne MJ. Cancer and communication: information-giving in an oncology clinic. *BMJ* 1981; 282:1449–51.

20. Davey HM, Butow PN, Armstrong BK. Patient preferences for written prognostic information. *British Journal of Cancer* 2003; 89:1450–6.

21. Degner LF, Kristjanson LJ, Bowman D, Sloan JA, Carriere KC, O'Neil J. *et al.* Information needs and decisional preferences in women with breast cancer. *Journal of the American Medical Association* 1997; 277(18):1485–92.

22. Lind SE, DelVecchio Good MJ, Seidel S, Csordas T, Good BJ. Telling the diagnosis of cancer. *Journal of Clinical Oncology* 1989; 7(5):583–9.

23. Merriman L, Perez DJ, McGee R, Campbell AV. Receiving a diagnosis of cancer: the perceptions of patients. *New Zealand Medical Journal* 1997; 110(1049):297–8.

24. Eidinger RN, Schapira DV. Cancer patients' insight into their treatment, prognosis and unconventional therapies. *Cancer* 1984; 53:2736–40.

25. Lobb EA, Butow PN, Kenny DT, Tattersall MH. Communicating prognosis in early breast cancer: do women understand the language used? *Medical Journal of Australia* 1999; 171(6):290–4.

26. Kaplowitz SA, Campo S, Chui WT. Cancer patients' desire for communication of prognosis information. *Health Communication* 2002; 14(2):221–41.

27. Hagerty RG, Butow PN, Ellis PA, Lobb EA, Pendlebury S, Leighl N. *et al.* Cancer patient preferences for communication of prognosis in the metastatic setting. *J Clin Oncol* 2004; 22(9):1721–30.

28. Fried TR, Bradley EH, O'Leary J. Prognosis communication in serious illness: perceptions of older patients, caregivers, and clinicians. *Journal of the American Geriatrics Society* 2003; 51(10):1398–403.

29. Sapir R, Catane R, Kaufman B, Isacson R, Segal A, Wein S. *et al.* Cancer patient expectations of and communication with oncologists and oncology nurses: the experience of an integrated oncology and palliative care service. *Supportive Care in Cancer* 2000; 8(6):458–63.

30. Gattellari M, Butow PN, Tattersall MH, Dunn SM, MacLeod CA. Misunderstanding in cancer patients: why shoot the messenger? *Annals of Oncology* 1999; 10(1):39–46.

31. Gattellari M, Voigt KJ, Butow PN, Tattersall MH. When the treatment goal is not cure: are cancer patients equipped to make informed decisions? *Journal of Clinical Oncology* 2002; 20(2):503–13.

32. Mackillop WJ, Stewart, WE, Ginsburg AD. *et al.* Cancer patients' perceptions of their disease and its treatment. *British Journal of Cancer* 1988; 50:355–9.

33. Siminoff LA, Fetting JH. Factors affecting treatment decisions for a life-threatening illness: The case of medical treatment of breast cancer. *Social Science & Medicine* 1991; 32(7):813–18.

34. Chan A, Woodruff R. Communicating with patients with advanced cancer. *Journal of Palliative Care* 1997; 13(3):29–33.

35. McIntosh J. Patients' awareness and desire for information about diagnosed but undisclosed malignant disease. *Lancet* 1976; (August 7):300–3.

36. Siminoff LA, Fetting JH, Abeloff MD. Doctor–patient communication about breast cancer adjuvant therapy. *Journal of Clinical Oncology* 1989; 7(9):1192.

37. Seale C. Communication and awareness about death: a study of a random sample of dying people. *Social Science & Medicine* 1991; 32(8):943–52.

38. Weeks JC, Cook EF, O'Day SJ, Peterson LM, Wenger N, Reding D. *et al.* Relationship between cancer patients' predictions of prognosis and their treatment preferences. *Journal of the American Medical Association* 1998; 279:1709–14.

39. Chochinov HM, Tataryn DJ, Wilson KG, Enns M, Lander S. Prognostic awareness and the terminally ill. *Psychosomatics* 2000; 41(6):500–4.

40. Editorial. Your baby is in a trial. *Lancet* 1995; 345:805–6.

41. Tobias JS, Souhami RL. Fully informed consent can be needlessly cruel. *BMJ* 1993; 307:1199–201.

42. Druss RG, Douglas CJ. Adaptive responses to illness and disability: Health denial. *General Hospital Psychiatry* 1988; 10:163–8.

43. Levine RY. *Ethics and regulation of clinical research*, 2nd edn. Baltimore, MD: Verland and Schwarzenburg, 1986.

44. The AM, Hak T, Koeter G, van der Wal G. Collusion in doctor–patient communication about imminent death: an ethnographic study. *Western Journal of Medicine* 2001; 174(4):247–53.

45. Kim MK, Alvi A. Breaking the bad news of cancer: the patient's perspective. *Laryngoscope* 1999; 109 (7 Pt 1):1064–7.

46. Bradley EH, Hallemeier AG, Fried TR, Johnson-Hurzeler R, Cherlin EJ, Kasl SV. *et al*. Documentation of discussions about prognosis with terminally ill patients. *American Journal of Medicine* 2001; 111(3):218–23.

47. Gilmore AJ. The care and management of the patient in general practice. *The Practitioner* 1974; 213:833–42.

48. Noyes R, Travis TA. The care of terminally ill patients. Archives of Internal Medicine 1973; 132:607–611.

49. McGrath P. End-of life care for hematological malignancies: the 'technological imperative' and palliative care. *Journal of Palliative Care* 2002; 18(1):39–47.

50. Prigerson HG. Socialisation to dying: social determinants of death acknowledgement and treatment among terminally ill geriatric patients. *Journal of Health and Human Behaviour* 1992; 33:378–95.

51. Miyaji NT. The power of compassion: truth-telling among American doctors in the care of dying patients. *Social Science and Medicine* 1993; 36(3):249–64.

52. Lamont EB, Christakis NA. Prognostic disclosure to patients with cancer near the end of life. *Annals of Internal Medicine* 2001; 134(12):1096–105.

53. Girgis A, Sanson-Fisher RW, Schofield MJ. Is there consensus between breast cancer patients and providers on guidelines for breaking bad news? *Behavioral Medicine* 1999; 25(2):69–77.

54. Koopmeiners L, Post-White J, Gutknecht S, Ceronsky C, Nickelsom K, Drew D. *et al*. How healthcare professionals contribute to hope in patients with cancer. *Oncology Nursing Forum* 1997; 24(9):1507–13.

55. Christakis NA. *Death foretold: prophecy and prognosis in medical care*. Chicago, IL: University of Chicago Press, 1999.

56. Fallowfield L, Lipkin M, Hall A. Teaching senior oncologists communication skills: results from phase I of a comprehensive longitudinal program in the United Kingdom. *Journal of Clinical Oncology* 1998; 16(5):1961–8.

57. Jevne RN. *It all begins with hope:patients, caregivers and the bereaved speak out*. California: LuraMedia, 1991.

58. Kirk P, Kirk I, Kristjanson LJ. What do patients receiving palliative care for cancer and their families want to be told? A Canadian and Australian qualitative study. *BMJ* 2004; 328(7452):1343.

59. Jenkins V, Fallowfield L, Saul J. Information needs of patients with cancer: results from a large study in UK cancer centres. *British Journal of Cancer* 2001; 84(1):48–51.

60. Benson J, Britten N. Respecting the autonomy of cancer patients when talking with their families: qualitative analysis of semistructured interviews with patients. *BMJ* 1996; 313(7059):729–31.

61. Anderlik MR, Pentz RD, Hess KR. Revisiting the truth-telling debate: a study of disclosure practices at a major cancer center. *Journal of Clinical Ethics* 2000; 11(3):251–9.

62. Goldstein D, Thewes B, Butow PN. Communicating in a multicultural society II: Greek community attitudes towards cancer in Australia. *Internal Medicine Journal* 2002; 32:289–96.

63. Salander P. Bad news from the patient's perspective: an analysis of the written narratives of newly diagnosed cancer patients. *Social Science & Medicine* 2002; 55(5):721–32.

64. Loge JH, Kaasa S, Hytten K. Disclosing the cancer diagnosis: the patients' experiences. *European Journal of Cancer* 1997; 33(6):878–82.

65. Petrasch S, Bauer M, Reinacher-Schick A, Sandmann M, Kissler M, Kuchler T. *et al*. Assessment of satisfaction with the communication process during consultation of cancer patients with potentially curable disease, cancer patients on palliative care, and HIV-positive patients. *Wiener Medizinische Wochenschrift* 1998; 148(21):491–9.

66. McLoughlin HA, Oosthuizen BL. The information needs of cancer patients in the Pretoria and Witwatersrand area. *Curationis* 1996; 19(2):31–5.

67. Pronzato P, Bertelli G, Losardo P, Landucci M. What do advanced cancer patients know of their disease? A report form Italy. *Supportive Care in Cancer* 1994; 2:242–4.

68. Tan TK, Teo FC, Wong K, Lim HL. Cancer: to tell or not to tell? *Singapore Medical Journal* 1993; 34(3):202–3.

69. Derman U, Serbest P. Cancer patients' awareness of disease and satisfaction with services: the influence of their general education level. *Journal of Cancer Education* 1993; 8(2):141–4.

70. Barroso P, Osuna E, Luna A. Doctors' death experience and attitudes towards death, euthanasia and informing terminal patients. *Medicine & Law* 1992; 11(7–8):527–33.

71. Harris JJ, Shao J, Sugarman J. Disclosure of cancer diagnosis and prognosis in Northern Tanzania. *Social Science & Medicine*. 2003; 56(5):905–13.

72. Huang X, Butow P, Meiser B, Goldstein D. Attitudes and information needs of Chinese migrant cancer patients and their relatives. *Australian and New Zealand Journal of Medicine* 1999; 29(2):207–13.

73. Bruera E, Neumann CM, Mazzocato C, Stiefel F, Sala R. Attitudes and beliefs of palliative care physicians regarding communication with terminally ill cancer patients. *Palliative Medicine* 2000; 14(4):287–98.

74. Iconomou G, Viha A, Koutras A, Vagenakis AG, Kalofonos HP. Information needs and awareness of diagnosis in patients with cancer receiving chemotherapy: a report from Greece. *Palliative Medicine* 2002; 16(4):315–21.

75. Georgaki S, Kalaidopoulou O, Liarmakopoulos I, Mystakidou K. Nurses' attitudes toward truthful communication with patients with cancer. A Greek study. *Cancer Nursing* 2002; 25(6):436–41.

76. Norman C. Breaking bad news. *Australian Family Physician* 1996; 25(10):1583–7.

77. Brown RF, Butow PN, Dunn SM, Tattersall MH. Promoting patient participation and shortening cancer consultations: a randomised trial. *British Journal of Cancer* 2001; 85(9):1273–9.

78. Parker PA, Baile WF, de Moor C, Lenzi R, Kudelka AP, Cohen L. Breaking bad news about cancer: patients' preferences for communication. *Journal of Clinical Oncology* 2001; 19(7):2049–56.

79. Ptacek JT, Ptacek JJ. Patients' perceptions of receiving bad news about cancer. *Journal of Clinical Oncology* 2001; 19(21):4160–4.

80. Peteet JR, Abrams HE, Ross DM, Stearns NM. Presenting a diagnosis of cancer: patients' views. *Journal of Family Practice* 1991; 32(6):577–81.

81. Sardell AN, Trierweiler SJ. Disclosing the cancer diagnosis. Procedures that influence patient hopefulness. *Cancer* 1993; 72(11):3355–65.

82. Watson M, Greer S, Blake S, Shrapnell K. Reaction to a diagnosis of breast cancer. Relationship between denial, delay and rates of psychological morbidity. *Cancer* 1984; 53(9):2008–12.

83. Maguire P, Faulkner A. Communicate with cancer patients: 2. Handling uncertainty, collusion, and denial. *BMJ* 1988; 297(6654):972–4.

84. Tattersall MHN, Butow PN, Brown RF, Thompson JF. Improving doctors' letters. *Medical Journal of Australia* 2002; 177(9):516–21.

85. Baile WF, Kudelka AP, Beale EA, Glober GA, Myers EG, Greisinger AJ. *et al*. Communication skills training in oncology. Description and preliminary outcomes of workshops on breaking bad news and managing patient reactions to illness. *Cancer* 1999; 86(5):887–97.

86. Girgis A, Sanson-Fisher RW. Breaking bad news: consensus guidelines for medical practitioners. *Journal of Clinical Oncology* 1995; 13(9):2449–56.

87. Girgis A, Sanson-Fisher RW. Breaking bad news. 1: Current best advice for clinicians. *Behavioral Medicine* 1998; 24(2):53–9.

88. Wenrich MD, Curtis JR, Shannon SE, Carline JD, Ambrozy DM, Ramsey PG. Communicating with dying patients within the spectrum of medical care from terminal diagnosis to death. *Archives of Internal Medicine* 2001; 161(6):868–74.

5

Statistical concepts and issues related to prognostic models

Phyllis A. Gimotty

Prognostic studies have traditionally been used to identify significant prognostic factors that are important for risk prediction to aid in clinical management. These studies have identified relevant prognostic factors for stratification in designs of clinical trials and for development of cancer classification schemes and staging systems. Prognostic factors are patient and tumour characteristics that have been shown to be related to clinical events such as response to treatment, development of metastasis, and survival. Prognostic models are statistical models that are used to characterize and evaluate the relationship between potential prognostic factors and clinical events of interest. Clinically relevant prognostic factors will identify patient risk groups for which prognosis differs. In the first part of this chapter multivariable statistical modelling approaches for use in prognostic modelling are described including logistic regression for binary clinical events, proportional hazards regression and accelerated failure time models for survival outcomes, and tree-based classification for both binary and survival outcomes. The second part of this chapter reviews statistical issues in the assessment of new prognostic factors, prognostic models and their subsequent validation. This chapter concludes with the identification of important questions to ask when considering using a prognostic model.

Alternative prognostic models

Logistic regression for binary events

A logistic regression model[1] is used when the clinical outcome of interest is binary, such as the occurrence of the clinical event or not. A linear logistic regression model that describes the relationship between the probability that the event will occur, $P(X_1, X_2, X_3)$, and a set of three potential prognostic factors (X_1, X_2, and X_3) is given by:

$$P(X_1, X_2, X_3) = \exp[PI] / (1 + \exp[PI]) \qquad [1]$$

where the prognostic index, PI, is equal to a linear function of the prognostic factors,

$$PI = b_0 + b_1X_1 + b_2X_2 + b_3X_3$$

where b_0, b_1, b_2, and b_3 are estimated from the sample data and $\exp(.)$ is the exponential function. Predicted probabilities for each patient are computed using these estimated coefficients and the values of the prognostic factors the patient. A patient's estimated probability is sometimes referred to as 'individualized', however, this estimated probability represent the likelihood of the event in a population of patients who have the same values for the prognostic factors. Confidence intervals can be computed for the predicted probabilities using the standard errors of the estimated coefficients. Logistic regression models are appropriate when all study participants are observed to either have the clinical event or not, with no censored observations (patients for whom the occurrence, or not, of the clinical event cannot be ascertained).

This logistic regression equation can be written in terms the logarithm of the odds of the event (log odds) where the odds is defined to be the ratio of the probability that the event occurs to the probability that it does not occur:

$$\log [P(X_1, X_2, X_3) / (1 - P(X_1, X_2, X_3))] = b_0 + b_1 X_1 + b_2 X_2 + b_3 X_3 \qquad [2]$$

where log (.) is the natural logarithm. Odds ratios for each prognostic factor are obtained by exponentiating each of the coefficients in this model. For a binary prognostic factor (X_1), the odds ratio is equal to $\exp(b_1)$. This odds ratio is the ratio of the odds of the event for those in one group $(X_1 = 1)$ compared to the odds of the event for those in the reference group $(X_1 = 0)$. For a continuous prognostic factor (X_1), this odds ratio is also equal to $\exp(b_1)$. However, in this context it is the ratio of the odds of the clinical for those with $X_1 = x$ compared to the odds of the event for those with $X_1 = x-1$. Odds ratios from a multivariate logistic regression model are referred to as adjusted odds ratios in contrast to unadjusted odds ratios that are computed using only the clinical event and a single prognostic factor. The adjusted odds ratio for a prognostic factor is an estimate of the association between it and the clinical event controlling for all other prognostic factors in the model. Prognostic factors that are statistically significant in a multivariate linear logistic regression model are considered to be independent prognostic factors for the study population.

Alternative logistic regression models can be defined when the relationship between the log odds of the event and one or more prognostic factor is not linear by changing the functional form involving the prognostic factors (e.g. log-odds of treatment response is a non-linear function of dose). In larger samples models can be specified to examine effect modification for specific subgroups. When the association between the event and a prognostic factor differs in subgroups defined by a second prognostic factor (e.g. subgroups of breast cancer patients with positive versus negative oestrogen receptor status), interaction terms for the two prognostic factors are added to the linear model to capture these differences. All of these models can be used to compute predicted probabilities, however, the coefficients in these more complicated models generally no longer have a simple interpretation.

Regression modelling of time to event data

Survival analysis[2] is used when the event of interest is observed over time and, particularly, when there are censored observations. The first objective in a survival analysis is to estimate the survival curve. The observed times to each patient's event, or the censored times if the patient is no longer available to the study, are used to estimate the cumulative proportion of events that have occurred as a function of time. The survival curve is used to estimate survival rates as the probability of survival beyond time t. Three survival curves with different 10 year survival rates are presented in Figure 5.1(a). From top to bottom the ten-year survival rates for groups 1, 2, and 3 are 60 per cent, 30 per cent and 15 per cent. In the survival analysis literature, the term 'survival time' is used generically to refer to any time-to-event. The predicted probabilities of interest are event rates at specific landmark times that are computed from the estimated survival curve.

The hazard function is another function that plays an important role in survival analysis. The hazard can be thought of as the probability of the clinical outcome in the next instant given that the clinical outcome has not yet occurred, and the hazard function characterizes these probabilities over time. For example, when one considers death over a person's lifetime, the hazard function decreases through early childhood, remains constant until 40 years of age or so, and then starts increasing in later life. In contrast, the survival curve characterizing the probability of living beyond a specific time decreases as age increases, and the survival rate decreases throughout life. The relationship between the survival curve and the hazard function is graphically shown in Figures 5.1(a) and 5.1(b). Events occur almost uniformly over time for those patients in the first group (top survival curve) and the corresponding hazard function is constant over time (bottom hazard function). In contrast events occur quickly over the first four years in the third group (bottom survival function) and more constantly after 4. The corresponding hazard function (top hazard function) sharply declines until about year 4 and then remains relatively constant.

Survival curves are generally estimated using a nonparametric method developed by Kaplan and Meier. This methodology does not depend on assumptions about the shape of the survival curve or hazard function. Typically, a statistical comparison between patient groups defined by a single prognostic factor would use the log-rank statistic, a statistical test where the null hypothesis assumes that all of the subgroup-specific survival curves were the same and the alternative hypothesis assumes that at least two of the survival curves are different. When the p-value associated with this statistical test is <0.05 we conclude that there is evidence of at least one difference among the groups. In prognostic studies that involve a number of prognostic factors multivariable regression models are used that are similar to those used in multivariable logistic regression analysis.

The most widely used regression model used for survival analysis is the proportional hazard regression model.[2] The proportional hazards regression model is defined in terms of a baseline hazard function, $h_0(t)$, that depends on time but does not depend on any prognostic factors and the function, $\exp [b_1X_1 + b_2X_2 + b_3X_3]$ that depends on the prognostic factors but is not a function of time. This model is given by

$$h(t \mid X_1, X_2, X_3) = h_0(t) \exp [b_1X_1 + b_2X_2 + b_3X_3] \tag{3}$$

and the baseline hazard equals the hazard function when all of the prognostic factors are equal to 0. Note that if the baseline hazard is constant over time ($h_0(t) = c_0$), the hazard functions for

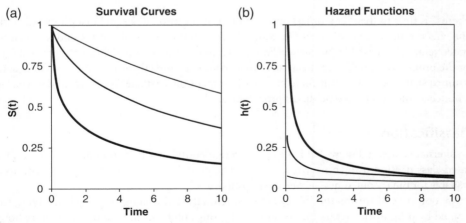

Figure 5.1 Survival curves and corresponding hazard functions. The hazard function for the survival curve with best prognosis (Figure 5.1(a) top curve) has a flat hazard function (Figure 5.1(b) bottom curve) and the hazard function for the survival curve with poorest prognosis (Figure 5.1(a) bottom curve) has a sharply decreasing hazard function (Figure 5.1(b) top curve).

all groups defined by the prognostic variables (X_1, X_2, X_3) will each be constant over time with intercepts determined by c_0 times $\exp [b_1X_1 + b_2X_2 + b_3X_3]$. This model can also be written in terms of the log of the hazard ratio (left-hand side of [3′]) and a prognostic index (right-hand side of [3′]).

$$\log [h(t \mid X_1, X_2, X_3) / h_0(t)] = b_1X_1 + b_2X_2 + b_3X_3 \qquad [3′]$$

Note that this prognostic index does not have an intercept term as it does in logistic regression analysis (see [2]). This model is used to estimate adjusted hazard ratios. In this model, the hazard ratio is a risk ratio that compares the hazard (the instantaneous probability of the event) for a group of patients with prognostic factors (X_1, X_2, X_3) to the hazard in the baseline group where $(X_1 = 0, X_2 = 0, X_3 = 0)$. However, since the proportional hazards regression model is relative, defined for the log hazard ratio, one cannot directly compute the survival rates at landmark times from the estimated regression equation from this analysis. To compute survival rates one would need to estimate the baseline hazard function or its corresponding survival curve. Unfortunately, information on the baseline hazard or survival curve is seldom included in published prognostic studies based on proportional hazard models.

The proportional hazards models can be extended to allow for different baseline hazard functions in different strata with a common prognostic index across the strata. This extended model is useful when a prognostic factor does not satisfy the proportional hazards assumption. The proportional hazards model can also be extended to include time-dependent prognostic factors that change over time. Examples of time dependent prognostic factors in a survival analysis would be the occurrence of a metastasis (the time varying among patients) or the longitudinal values of a biomarker for disease recurrence at different times after treatment.

Parametric survival models, though less commonly used, are an alternative to the proportional hazards models.[2] However, these methods require some assumptions about the general shape of the survival curve for the event of interest. The Weibull distribution has been frequently used to characterize the survival curves related to cancer outcomes. For this distribution the accelerated failure time model is appropriate and the regression model is given by:

$$\log [T] = b_0 + b_1X_1 + b_2X_2 + b_3X_3 \qquad [4]$$

where T is time to the event, or last observation time if censored is equal to a prognostic index. The effect of the prognostic factor is multiplicative on the time scale and is said to accelerate, or decelerate, the survival time. Survival rates at landmark times for patients with specified values for the prognostic variables in the model can be computed directly from the regression equation assumed shape of the survival curve. Standard errors of the coefficients can be used to compute confidence intervals for the predicted probabilities.

Classification

An alternative methodology that has been used to identify important prognostic factors is tree-based classification using binary recursive partitioning. Recursive partitioning algorithms are available for binary outcomes[3] as well as survival times.[4]

The objective of this methodology is to sequentially define subgroups by identifying rules defined by prognostic factors that produce subgroups that continue to be come more homogeneous with respect to the event of interest. At each step all possible splits for all prognostic factors are considered and each is ranked according to its ability to define two groups that are more homogeneous than the original group. Once the best split is identified, two groups are formed and the process repeats within each of the two groups. The process stops when there can be no further improvement in homogeneity or if the node has too few cases. At each step a splitting rule is defined with a cut-point for either a continuous or ordinal prognostic factor, or the best separation of categories without preserving order for a polychotomous prognostic factor. Prognostic factors that define the terminal nodes then define patients groups with differential risk. Predicted probabilities and rates from survival curves estimated within terminal nodes can be used for prognosis.

One of the concerns regarding tree-based methods is their stability. Multilevel trees involve higher-way interactions among the prognostic factors which are intrinsically difficult to estimate. However, the first few branches involve groups defined by one, two or three prognostic factors, similar to a linear model with two and three way interactions. Depending on the strength of the association of the prognostic factors, the sample size and the number of events the prognostic tree may be quite reproducible. The quality of a prognostic tree can be evaluated using resampling methods such as cross-validation or bootstrapping methods.[5]

Evaluation of a prognostic model

Evaluation of prognostic models

Prognostic studies can either be exploratory or confirmatory.[6] Exploratory studies are preliminary investigations of prognostic factors and one or more clinical end points, sometimes involving analyses of many different patient subsets. More importantly, they have no specific statistical hypotheses that are to be tested. Rather, their focus is on development including preliminary analyses to identify optimal cut-points for prognostic factors, investigations to select a subset or transform prognostic factors to reduce their number, and evaluation of alternative regression models for the prognostic index. The p-values and statistical significance reported in these studies do not have the same meaning that they do with a statistical test of a null hypothesis.[7] It is important that these exploratory studies are validated in well-designed confirmatory studies involving appropriate hypothesis tests.

A confirmatory study examines a specific hypothesis involving a small number of prognostic factors using a prospective study design. The study protocol might include a patient sample that is a consecutive series of patients rather than an ad hoc sample that may be subject to selection bias. All prognostic factors to be studied are well-defined prospectively and any cut-points established before data collection begins. This approach minimizes statistical errors due to multiple hypothesis testing of data-identified hypotheses that can be generated in exploratory studies.

In contrast to clinical trials, standards for evaluating prognostic factors are just being to be considered. Pepe and her colleagues have published five phases for developing new biomarkers as screening tests for early detection.[8] While some new screening tests are potentially useful for prognosis, new diagnostic procedures and tests also have the potential to provide prognostic information. Table 5.1 presents five phases relevant to the development of new prognostic factors. Exploratory studies would focus on the identification of informative prognostic markers (Phase I), the development of protocols related to measurement of the biomarker and determination of cut-points for continuous prognostic factors (Phase II). Once these methods have been developed, prognostic factors need to be evaluated using a case–control study to establish its ability to predict the clinical event of interest (Phase III). This is followed by a prospective study where the new prognostic factor is evaluated along with previously established prognostic factors

Table 5.1 Five phases in the development of a prognostic model

Phase I	Exploratory studies
Phase II	Development of measurement tools, assays, instruments, other definitions
Phase III	Establish the association with clinical end points
Phase IV	Prospective study including new and established prognostic factors
Phase V	Multi-site prospective studies

(Phase IV). Prognostic factors that are significant independent predictors need then to be validated in multi-site studies (Phase V).

Reliability of prognostic models

When a prognostic model is developed using data from one sample to estimate the coefficients in the prognostic index and the estimated prognostic index is used in a second independent sample to obtain predicted probabilities or rates, typically for the new sample the low predictions will be too low and the high predictions will be too high as a result of regression to the mean, all other things being equal. This is likely to occur when a model is 'overfit' with too many prognostic factors relative to the amount of variability in the clinical outcome. Prognostic models will generally be more reliable when the number of prognostic factors included in the model is less than m/10 or m/20 where m is the number of patients with the event (or the number without the event if it is smaller) for binary outcomes, and is the number of failures for failure (survival) times.[7]

Accuracy and generalizability of prognostic models

Two important aspects of a prognostic model are its accuracy in similar patient samples and its generalizability to different patient samples.[9] The accuracy of a prognostic model is the degree to which the predicted probability or rate agrees with the observed proportion of patients with the event of interest in a group of patients with the same prognostic factors. The predicted probabilities may be too high or two low in the second sample compared to the first (i.e. not well calibrated) and/or the predicted probabilities may not distinguish well among those who had the event and those who did not in the second sample (i.e. unable to discriminate). While not routinely done, calibration can be assessed by comparing predicted rates from a prognostic model to the rates observed in a reference population.[10] With binary events the area under the receiver operating curve (AUC) is used to assess discrimination using the predicted probabilities. The AUC ranges from 0.5 (no discrimination) to 1.0 (perfect discrimination). With survival times discrimination among the survival curves for groups defined by the prognostic factors in the model can be assessed by variability of the associated survival rates at landmark times.

Table 5.2 Validation studies for prognostic models

Internal validation
Prospective validation
Multi-site validation
Multiple independent validations
Multiple independent validation with varying follow-up periods

While accuracy of a prognostic model is important, it also needs to generalizable beyond the original sample it was developed on. This evaluation requires a new sample of patients. There are many different ways that a new sample may differ from the original sample: a different time period, a different geographical area, using different measurement techniques, a different case-mix of disease, or different lengths of follow up. Justice and colleagues[9] suggest a five-level hierarchy of external validation for prognostic models including

1. internal validation which tests for accuracy within sample used to develop the model
2. prospective validation where the accuracy is tested in data collected after the model is developed
3. multi-site validation where the prognostic model is evaluated at several geographic sites
4. multiple independent validations where the prognostic model is evaluated by independent investigators, and
5. multiple independent validations with varying follow-up periods.

Using a prognostic model

Braitman and Davidoff identify five key questions to consider before using a prognostic model for prognosis for a particular patient (see Table 5.3). First, the use of a prognostic model is limited to patients with characteristics similar to those of the sample patients (question 1). Exclusions of patients in the development of the prognostic model should be reviewed carefully; patients excluded should not characterize your patient. Second, as we have seen different statistical methods are used for different clinical outcomes. The definition of the clinical event of interest is important in identifying a model to compute a predicted probability (question 2). In addition, prognostic factors need to be available to you and easily translated into a predicted probability at the time you are interested in making a prognosis (question 3). Note that you may need to check that your patient's value for a prognostic factor was included in the range of values for that prognostic factor in the patient sample used to develop the prognostic model. Fourth, consider how you plan to use the prediction from the prognostic model (question 4). Prognosis can be used to identify those who need further treatment (high probability of the event) as well as those who may be spared further treatment (low probability of event). Finally, a prognostic model produces estimates of probabilities and it is important to know what the variability associated with the prediction (question 5). It is important to review the standard errors or confidence intervals for the predicted probabilities that you use.

Table 5.3. Five questions to consider before using a prognostic model*

1. Would your patient have been eligible for the study that led to the model?
2. Does the outcome variable in the prognostic model reflect the clinical outcome you want to predict?
3. Are values of all prognostic factors available for your patients where and when you need to use the model?
4. Will the predicted probability help in prognosis, choice of treatment, or other aspect of patient care?
5. Is the uncertainty in the predicted probability small enough for that estimate to aid in making a specific prognosis?

*Adapted from Braitman and Davidoff.[11]

References

1. Hosmer DW and Lemeshow S. *Applied logistic regression analysis*, 2nd edn. New York: John Wiley & Sons, Inc., 2000

2. Hosmer DW and Lemeshow S. *Applied survival analysis*. New York: John Wiley & Sons, Inc. 1999.

3. Breiman L, Friedman JH, Ohlsen RA, Stone J. *Classification and regression trees*. Belmont, CA: Wadsworth, Inc. 1984.

4. Segal MR. Regression trees for censored data. *Biometrics* 1988; 4:35–47.

5. Gimotty PA, Guerry D, Ming ME, Elenitsas R, Xu X, Czerniecki B, Spitz F, Schuchter L, Elder D. Thin primary cutaneous malignant melanoma: a prognostic tree for 10-year metastasis is more accurate than American Joint Committee on Cancer staging. *J Clin Oncol* 2004; 22(18): 3668–76.

6. Simon R, Altman DG. Statistical aspects of prognostic factor studies in oncology. *Br J Cancer* 1994; 69(6):979–85.

7. Harrell FE. *Regression modelling strategies*. New York: Springer-Verlag Inc., 2001.

8. Pepe MS, Etzioni R, Feng Z, Potter JD, Thompson ML, Thornquist M, Winget M, Yasui Y. Phases of Biomarker Development for Early Detection of Cancer. *J Natl Cancer Inst* 2001; 93:1054–61.

9. Justice AC, Covinsky KE, Berlin JA. Assessing the generalizability of prognostic information. *Ann Intern Med* 1999; 130:515–24.

10. Gimotty PA, Botbyl J, Soong S, Guerry D. A population-based validation for the AJCC staging system for melanoma staging. *JCO* 2005; 23(31):8065–75.

11. Braitman LE, Davidoff F. Predicting clinical states in individual patients. *Ann Intern Med* 1996; 125:406–12.

6

Evidence-based medicine

Paul Glare, Marco Maltoni, and Cinzia Brunelli

Introduction

Consider the following clinical situation, as presented in the article 'Doc, How much time do I have?' published in the *Journal of Clinical Oncology* a few years ago.[1] 'Mary Smith', a 42-year-old woman, has pancreatic cancer with liver metastases. Despite chemotherapy for 2 months, a repeat CT scan shows progressive disease. Her oncologist tells her that no further chemotherapy is indicated. There is a pause, and then she asks 'How much time do I have?'

The oncologist has several options for responding to this question. One would be to avoid answering – given the choice, the option preferred by many physicians[2] – and reply 'it's not possible for me to answer that question'. If the oncologist was prepared to offer a prognosis, this could be done in one of three ways:

1. By quoting the median survival
2. Formulating a prognosis in one's head using subjective judgement, or
3. By using a prognostic score, as described elsewhere in this book.

A fourth alternative for the oncologist would be to make explicit and systematic use of evidence-based medicine (EBM), to find and use an article on the prognosis of advanced pancreatic cancer. The renewed interest in research on prognosis and the growing number of physicians with EBM skills means that tracking down published evidence, using critical appraisal skills to judge the scientific validity and clinical utility of that evidence, and then applying it to the patient is now a reality for answering this question. The aim of this chapter is to briefly discuss these three steps. For a comprehensive description of this approach, the reader should consult other sources.[3, 4]

Prognosis and EBM

Along with questions of harm/aetiology, diagnosis and treatment/intervention, questions of prognosis are one of the four fundamental types of clinical question answerable by EBM. Methods for appraising prognosis studies have been developed over the past decade.[5] Generally speaking, prognosis studies address questions about the relative probabilities of the various outcomes of a patient's likely course.[6] They address issues such as 'what proportion of children with febrile seizures will develop epilepsy as adults?' or 'are patients with an hemorrhagic stroke more likely to die in the first 24 hours than patients with an embolic stroke?' as well as survival in advanced cancer.[7] The best feasible study design to answer such questions is a cohort study or case–control study. Search strategies for finding these studies in the medical literature are well established and criteria for determining their validity and usefulness are proposed.[5]

As the database of primary prognostic studies expands, the need for systematic reviews and meta-analyses becomes increasingly important. These methods provide powerful instruments for reorganizing and synthesizing the evidence and are particularly useful when the evidence from individual primary studies appears to be contradictory (notwithstanding the problems with the critical appraisal of the methodological quality of the primary studies included in the review).[8] Over the past 15 years, many papers have examined a variety of prognostic factors in advanced cancer: biological factors, symptoms and clinical and psychosocial variables, clinical prediction, prognostic scores. Only recently have systematic reviews, which try to organize the evidence, begun to be published.[9]

Importantly, 'background' questions relating to prognosis are not amenable to answering with EBM. These include questions about the basic biological processes of the terminal phase of cancer, which are best answered by standard textbooks (on paper or online). On the other hand, EBM is useful for answering the questions that are relevant to clinical decision-making in individual patients. These relate to questions about etiology/harm – does drinking coffee cause pancreas cancer? – diagnosis – is an elevated CA 19–9 diagnostic of pancreas cancer? – treatment – does adjuvant chemotherapy improve survival after a Whipple's procedure for pancreas cancer? – and prognosis – what is the median survival of a patients with advanced pancreatic cancer?

Different types of studies addressing questions concerning prognosis

The classic prognostic study is an observational study that aims to identify the factors that modify the natural history of a disease. Researchers conducting prognostic studies identify patients in the at-risk group – here we are concerned with patients with advanced cancer – with or without factors that may modify their prognosis, such as clinical features or psychosocial status, and then follow the patient over time to see when they develop the outcome of interest. In the case of death from advanced cancer, the outcome may be expressed in absolute terms (e.g. duration of median survival) or the percentage alive at a certain time point, such as one month or one year. In the case of the patient with pancreatic cancer, we would be looking for an observational study of patients with inoperable pancreatic cancer who have failed to respond to treatment, to see if issues such as age or comorbidities modify the generic prognosis of pancreatic carcinoma.

Within the broader field of prognostication and predicting survival, there are a number of other types of studies that are relevant, which use different study designs. These may need to be appraised by different criteria to the standard observational study. These include:

- Systematic reviews of prognostic factors
- Studies of the accuracy of physicians' subjective judgements of survival compared to actual survival – which are more like evaluating a clinical manifestation of disease or a diagnostic test evaluation,
- Studies of the utility of prognostic tools as clinical decision rules, and
- Qualitative studies of communication of prognostic information to patients.

These studies are often cohort studies, but could be designed as cross-sectional surveys or be part of a larger randomized controlled trial (RCT).[10] The usual classification of studies based on the study design (systematic review, RCT, cohort study) used for therapy/prevention studies[11] is not applicable to the prognosis field. Nevertheless, different evidence levels may be attributed to different types of studies depending upon their exploratory rather than confirmatory nature,[12,13] as presented in Table 6.1. Because of multiple testing, spurious associations can emerge, mostly

Table 6.1 Study type classification and levels of evidence

Meta-analysis of impact studies or cohort studies. Level 1A or B
Randomized controlled trials of the clinical benefit of implementing a prognostic score as an aid to clinical decision-making. Level II or I
Confirmative cohort studies. The main aim is to evaluate the agreement between actual survival and predicted survival by the prospective application of indexes and/or to test if a prognostic model still maintains its strength in a different sample of patients. Level IIIA
Explorative cohort studies. The main aim is to examine how the predictive power of a new prognostic factor relates to those already available and/or to estimate the magnitude of its effect. Level IIIB
Investigative cohort studies. The main aim is to investigate the association of putative new factors with survival. Level IIIC
Non-analytic studies (case reports/case series). Level IV

from studies examining a large number of prognostic factors, so the results of an investigative cohort study are much weaker than the same results from a confirmatory one and they should also be interpreted in a different way. For this reason, the recognition of the confirmatory nature of a study, even if not always easy because of a low quality of reporting, is crucial in the attribution of strength of the results examined.

The 'well-built clinical question' in prognostication

Faced with the young woman with advanced pancreatic cancer, how could EBM be used to answer her question? The initial query 'how much time do I have?' gives the oncologist little direction as to where to look in the literature for an answer. To locate suitable studies, the physician must be able to break the scenario down into individual concepts that can be searched for separately and then recombined to retrieve information on the topic. The evidence base of prognostication is much less well developed for prognosis than it is for intervention studies but is expanding with the revival of interest in care of incurables, the growing number of publications in this area and the number of healthcare professionals with skills in literature searching and critical appraisal of articles increases.

A useful approach to breaking the concept down is to turn the clinical scenario into a 'well-built clinical question' (WBCQ)[14] which frames the initial question 'Doc, how long do I have?' in a form that makes it both searchable and answerable. The WBCQ consists of four parts, the mnemonic PICO being a simple way of remembering the 'anatomy' of the WBCQ.

- A **P**opulation with a clinical problem
- An **I**ntervention or exposure
- The **C**omparator intervention or exposure
- The **O**utcome of interest.

In the case of the 42-year-old woman with pancreatic cancer, her age would intuitively appear to be relevant and her prognostic enquiry can be reframed as 'in patients with inoperable pancreatic cancer (population) who are under 50 (intervention/exposure), compared to those who are over 50 (comparator) what proportion have died after 3 months (outcome)? It is important to emphasize that depending on the aspect of the case that the clinician thinks relevant the

WCBQ could be framed differently, for example as an intervention-type WBCQ: 'In patients with inoperable pancreatic cancer (population), what is the median survival (outcome) of those receiving chemotherapy gemcitabine (exposure) compared to those who did not (comparator)?'

With experience in framing WBCQ, the key search terms are easy to identify and it is usually not necessary to rephrase the question as explicitly as has been illustrated here. Clearly, in the clinical interaction described in the scenario, the 42-year-old woman is likely to ask many other clinical questions for which EBM is appropriate. Some examples could include: Will screening prevent my children getting it? Are any second line treatments effective? Are tumour markers reliable for monitoring progress in pancreas cancer? and so on. Each could be framed and searched in a similar way to the question of prognosis.

Levels of evidence in prognostication

Having reframed the clinical interaction into a WBCQ, the oncologist is ready to search for suitable papers reporting clinical evidence to answer the question. Once such publications have been located, the oncologist will have to decide three fundamental issues before applying the results to the problem of the patient before him:

- ◆ Are the results real (valid)?
- ◆ Is the size of the effect clinically important?
- ◆ Is the evidence relevant to the clinical scenario?

The first issue is crucial, because unless the results are valid, there is no point in addressing the other two. The chance of the results being a true reflection of reality and free from bias depends on the study design. The term 'level of evidence' is used to indicate the degree to which bias has been eliminated from the study design. A hierarchy of evidence for studies of prognostic factors is shown in Table 6.1. Demonstrating that every reasonable attempt has been made to eliminate bias is the main factor that ensures results are valid.

The best way to eliminate bias is to perform an RCT which, along with meta-analyses of RCTs, has the highest place on the hierarchy, and is typically referred to as Level I or II evidence, depending on the classification system and whether or not there was a control group.[11] Of course, the RCT is only suitable for answering certain types of study question, notably those of therapy/intervention, and is not applicable to the types of study design that are feasible for answering most other types of clinical questions, especially prognosis (but also harm/aetiology and diagnosis). The types of study design that are necessary for conducting these type of studies – cohort studies, case control studies, and cross-sectional surveys – are all prone to bias that limits the validity of their results in comparison to an RCT, and they are usually labelled Level III or IV evidence.

Finding the studies: searching literature for studies on prognosis in advanced cancer

Electronic literature

As with other EBM activities, an electronic literature search is the starting point for locating articles on prognostication. Having identified which type of prognostication question one is interested in (prognostic factors, prognostic tools, accuracy of predictions), the best type of study to answer the question (observational study vs randomized trial), and the appropriate search terms using PICO, one is in a position to undertake an electronic search. There are a large number of ways to perform an electronic search and the choice of which method to use depends on the time available, the thoroughness required and the electronic resources that can be utilized. In general terms, the most time-efficient search method for the busy clinician is to use a pre-filtered medical information resource, such as Best Evidence (www.acponline.org/catalog/electronic/best_evidence.htm). The Cochrane Library is another pre-filtered information source that is widely used, but it is only useful for finding systematic reviews of intervention studies and will not contain the observational studies that make up the bulk of the literature on prognostic studies.(www.uptodate-software.com/cochrane/cochrane-frame.html). A very simple way for the busy clinician on the run to do quick, simple searches is to use Google Scholar.

For comprehensive electronic searching of the medical literature on prognosis, especially for the purposes of conducting a systematic review, the best approach is to perform a search of the two large electronic medical databases, Medline and EmBase. The size and complexity of these databases makes searching more difficult and time-consuming.[15] There are other electronic health science databases, such as CINAHL and PsychInfo, which can identify informative articles of a general type from bodies of literature other than the mainstream medical literature,[16, 17] but they are unlikely to contain many studies of prognostic factors. A number of other databases are available and potentially useful but generally not searched (Citation Indexes, Cancer LIT, Oncolink).

The most widely available way to access Medline is through PubMed. It and EmBase can also be accessed through OVID. To be able to use Medline successfully requires an understanding of the following:

◆ how the database is structured,

◆ how the articles are indexed,

◆ the difference between Medical Subject Headings (MeSH) and text words

◆ advanced features such as exploding terms, filtering and Boolean operators.

Textbooks and articles that explain these features are available, while academic medical librarians will provide tutorials for readers who are not familiar with these topics.

To illustrate the utilization of Medline to find articles on prognostic factors in advanced cancer, the output of the by a Working Group of the European Association of Palliative Care (EAPC), which recently performed a collaborative systematic review of this literature.[18] Because the studies were mostly observational, this review was conducted outside the framework of the Cochrane Library. This working group developed search strategies for four prognostic factor areas: physicians' subjective predictions, clinical factors (signs, symptoms and psychosocial variables), biological factors and predictive scores. It employed separate and combined Medline searches mapped to Medical Subject Headings (MeSH) terms and using text words. The search strategies used are presented in Table 6.2. Finding an article using Medline is akin to a driver locating a road in a street directory and the driver generally uses the index of street names rather than scanning the maps. To find the right road the driver needs to understand how the roads are indexed in the directory. The same applies to Medline, except that there are two indexing systems by which articles are grouped:

◆ One uses the controlled vocabulary of MeSH headings that are chosen by the indexing staff at the US National Library of Medicine and is usually applied first, as the articles are in a sense pre-filtered by the indexers.

◆ The other type, the keyword/text word search, looks for the exact word in the title or abstract. This search eliminates the classification made by the indexers, but depends on the choice of language of the authors.

Table 6.2 Literature search strategy

Line of search	Aim	Typical terms
1	Strategy for finding papers on advanced cancer patients	**Oncological terms AND palliative care terms:** neoplasms* OR cancer[†] OR tumor OR tumour OR oncolog$[†] AND terminal care* OR terminally ill* OR palliative care* OR hospices*
2	Strategy for searching papers on prognosis	**Prognosis terms:** Incidence* OR mortality* OR follow-up studies* OR prognos$[†] OR predict[†] OR course[†]
3	Strategy for searching papers on the specific topic of interest in advanced cancer prognosis	Prediction*,[†] Symptoms*,[†] Performance status[†] Biological factors*,[†] Prognostic score[†] OR prognostic index[†]
4	Combine the three steps to find the relevant citation	# 1 AND # 2 AND # 3
5	Limit search	e.g. human studies, English language

* MeSH heading;[†] text word.

- To overcome this problem, filters such as wild cards have been created, and is particularly useful when looking for very specific terms or phrases for which there is no good mapped term.
- In the case of prognosis, using the wild card ($) with a root text word like *prognos* (to produce *prognos$.tw*), it is possible to search simultaneously for all the articles using the words prognosis, prognoses, prognostic and prognostication in the text or abstract.

Screening out irrelevant articles is the big challenge for electronic searching that is not pre-filtered. This is particularly the case for searching on far-advanced cancer, including its prognostication. MeSH terms like *neoplasms* and *prognosis* are very widely used in oncological studies and the number of irrelevant studies retrieved is huge. As an example, a recent Cochrane review of supportive care for patients with gastrointestinal cancer had to screen some 1800 citations to find 14 that met their inclusion criteria.[19] The 'limit' function helps to exclude some irrelevant articles, with filters for humans, English language and publication types also helpful depending on the nature of the question being searched. The adjacency function available with text word searching, e.g. cancer adj5 prog$, is particularly helpful for narrowing a search.

By using the WBCQ approach, the correct framing of the clinical question type guides the best feasible primary study design and the right search strategy to perform. In this example, framing it as a question of prognosis, the best type of study to answer this type of question is a cohort study.[20] If the issue of prognosis was to be framed as an intervention type of question, the key terms for the search strategy become clear: pancreas cancer, survival, and chemotherapy. The best type of study to answer this type of question is a RCT.[21]

After scanning for the potentially important citations by their titles, the next task is to read the abstracts to confirm their relevance, and inclusion/exclusion criteria need to be set for this purpose. In the case of the EAPC Working Group's search, the following criteria were used to include/exclude studies:

- patients with cancer
- median survival of less than 90 days

- full paper available (not just abstract)
- published in English language prior to 31/12/2003.

Reviews and other papers not based on original data, unless formal meta-analyses, were excluded.

Grey literature and hand searching

'Grey' literature sources such as online repositories of theses and dissertations are also available, but intended for those undertaking formal reviews rather than busy clinicians. No results for prognostication and palliative care were obtained when several such sites were searched, even though some such works have been undertaken.[22–24] National research registers exist but are also unlikely to be useful for prognostication. Caresearch is a useful Australian website dedicated to the grey literature in palliative care (www.caresearch.org.au).

Hand-searching articles is particularly important in the field of prognostication in advanced cancer, as anecdotal experience indicates that even very thorough searches will not identify many articles in this field. Some palliative care journals, or at least their early volumes, were not indexed by Medline. Letters to the editor and published conference abstracts are not included on Medline as a rule and may contain this information. Occasional other articles that meet inclusion criteria are sometimes omitted for inexplicable reasons. The MeSH headings and text words used to classify these studies can be very variable. One approach to hand-searching is to scan the References section of any electronically identified articles; the other is to hand-search textbooks and major journals in the palliative care and oncology filed. Contacting experts in the field is also important.

Are the results true? Assessing the quality of prognosis studies

When speaking about the quality of a study, one refers to various aspects including the study design, data gathering, analysis procedures, and quality of reporting.[25] As mentioned previously, it is particularly important to evaluate the validity of the study – defined as the extent to which the results of a study are correct for the circumstances being studied by being free from bias. Validity can also be thought of in terms of the extent to which the results of a study provide a correct basis for generalization to other circumstances or to individual patients.[25] These two types of validity are sometimes referred to as internal and external validity. The first one is by far the most important because unless the results are believable, there is no point in considering them further.

In the case of intervention studies, which would be a more unusual way of evaluating prognostic factors, the best feasible study design is the RCT, and the criteria for valid results that make bias unlikely include:

- concealment of treatment allocation during randomization
- analysing results on an intention-to-treat basis
- blinding of the investigators
- low rates of participant drop-out rates from each treatment arm.[26]

The main aspect of validity of a systematic review is that an exhaustive search has been completed so that the risk of *publication bias* has been reduced.

In the case of prognosis studies that evaluate whether or not a particular clinical or biological factor is a predictor of an outcome, the best feasible design is a cohort study. The sources of bias in a cohort study are different to those in an RCT. The following section introduces some methodological aspects which need to be focused on in order to understand what is relevant for quality evaluation in studies about prognosis in advanced cancer: some are generic to all study types while others are specific to the type of study design (prognostic factors, prognostic scores as clinical decision rules and accuracy of predictions)

Generic issues

Prospective and retrospective studies

The best design for a study of a prognostic factors is a cohort study, which involves empanelling a cohort of patients and prospectively following them for an adequate time span until sufficient events (the outcome of interest) occur. In the case of survival prediction, death is the outcome and it can be measured as either a binary outcome (alive or not), a proportion or a time (from enrolment to death). Death can be measured in the whole cohort, or used to compare differences between groups of patients with different values of the prognostic factor or score at enrolment. Retrospective studies, involving data gathered from stored files, are inferior to prospective ones. While they have the advantage of gathering data more quickly when long follow-up periods are needed, they have the disadvantage that clinical data retrospectively gathered are likely of lower quality due to either higher percentages of unrecoverable missing data due to unavailability of the data on the stored charts or else the heterogeneous methods of measurements used to gather the data from the charts. Consequently, they are more prone to *measurement bias*. Retrospective studies tend to be uncommon amongst the studies of prognosis in far advanced cancer and palliative care because the follow-up time needed to measure the outcome is rather short, with median survivals typically only a month or two.[27, 28] Much of the evidence on prognostication in advanced cancer is still based on such data.

Target population

A representative sample The patient sample in which the prognostic factor is studied should not be systematically different from the underlying population. In some illnesses only the most difficult or rare cases get referred to a hospital or specialist, but this is generally not the case with cancer. In the case of patients with far advanced cancer, many of the patient samples studied have been referred to hospice or palliative care services. Depending on the locale, only 20–60 per cent cases are referred to hospice/palliative care so may be systematically different to other patients dying of cancer. Even within hospice/palliative care, the criteria for referral vary.

That this is capable of introducing a spectrum bias into such studies is shown by the example of pain, which is well known to become more prevalent and severe as cancer progresses, but has not been found to be a survival predictor in many palliative care/hospice studies. This is because pain is more likely to trigger an earlier referral to hospice/palliative care, introducing a bias that could be classified as either a *lead-time bias* or *spectrum bias*.

The subjects were homogeneous for prognostic risk Generally speaking, prognostic studies should involve a well-defined cohort of patients at a common point in the course of their disease, the so-called 'inception cohort'.[29] This is a problem for patients with far advanced cancer as there are no standard criteria to define this phase at this time. The 'common point' in advanced cancer is difficult to define as what patients undergoing palliative care have in common is the end and not the inception. Some authors have attempted to deal with this problem by giving more or less detailed, but not homogeneous, definitions of the clinical characteristics of the patients or of the care programmes they had to undergo to be defined as 'advanced cancer patients' (e.g. extent of disease, performance status) but this is still unlikely to overcome this problem. Again, referral to hospice depends on local health service delivery policy and does not provide a common point in the course of the disease. A more useful approach may be to use 'the time at which standard anti-cancer treatment options have been exhausted'.[30, 31] Other approaches could include the onset of decreased functional level that typically represents the beginning of the terminal phase for patients with advanced cancer,[32] or the onset of elevated serum C-reactive protein or other markers of systemic inflammation, which indicate the genesis of the cancer–cachexia syndrome that is the final common pathway for many patients dying from cancer.[33]

In its systematic review, the EAPC Working Group took the approach of using median survival as an inclusion criterion, accepting only those studies in which the median survival of the sample is lower than a given cut-off.[18] As many studies have shown that the median survival in populations of advanced cancer patients undergoing palliative care is around 90 days,[34, 35] it is reasonable to choose this cut-off. This approach is clearly not possible with a primary study conducted prospectively.

Sample size

The sample size needs to be large enough to provide precise estimates. This issue is as important for prognostic studies as it is for clinical trials, but it is an issue that is not given enough consideration in the planning of prognostic studies. Sample size is strictly related to the precision of the estimates obtained but does not of itself improve the validity of the study results. Nevertheless, it assumes a particular relevance in confirmatory studies in which failure to include a sufficient number of patients–events will result in low power to confirm the prognostic value of a single factor or of a set of factors.[12] Sample size calculation for survival data can be rather complex but for studies bases on regression models a practical rule has been suggested: the number of events (deaths in the case of survival data) should be at least ten times the number of prognostic variables investigated.[12]

Missing data

At least 80 per cent of patients should be accounted for. In prognosis studies generally, this raises the issue of *length of follow-up*: too long a follow-up is difficult and costly to provide, while too short a follow-up requires an increase of sample size to obtain an in increase in the number of events registered, because in survival analysis it is the number of events, not the number of patients, which give power to the study. Because the survival time is short in advanced cancer, the duration of follow-up is not the problem as the event is usually registered for a high percentage of the patients enrolled, with the consequence that number of events and number of patients are almost the same. However, studies conducted by hospital-based palliative care teams are more likely to have missing data than hospice teams. The main potential consequence of missing data on the results of a study is a post-hoc *selection bias*.

Quality of measurement

Both the prognostic and the outcome variables ought to be clearly defined, measured with valid and reliable instruments and be available for all or a high proportion of patients.[29] As regards the outcome variable – length of survival from a defined starting point – although most of the patients in advanced cancer studies are enrolled in palliative care programmes and as such are followed until death by the staff, the event (death) should ideally be documented by death certificates or an equivalent document. Cause of death may also be relevant in patients with major comorbidities. More problems arise with prognostic variables for which the definition is not always clear and the measurement method chosen is not well validated. This is particularly the case for patient reported subjective measurements, such as quality of life (QOL) scores.

A summary of the quality criteria for studies of prognostic factors is shown in Table 6.3.

Table 6.3 Checklist of quality criteria for study evaluation

Prospective study design

Well-defined cohort of patients assembled at a common point in the course of their disease

Random patient selection

Percentage of patients lost to follow-up ≤ 20%

Ratio between the number of events (death) and the number of potential predictors ≥10

Prognostic variables fully defined, accurately measured and available for all or a high proportion of patients

Reliable measurement of outcome (date of death)

Specific issues with other types of prognostic studies

Studies of prognostic factors

Studies of prognosis take mainly two forms: some investigate the prognostic value of a particular variable (typically studies on tumour markers) while others investigate many variables simultaneously with the aim of evaluating which of them show a strong independent prognostic value, so as to develop a prognostic model to make prognoses on individual patients.

The multifactorial nature of confirmatory and exploratory studies raises many problems of heterogeneity of the data, as the range of prognostic factors examined is very wide and often constituted by subjective variables for which a standard for measurement that is widely accepted does not yet exist. A clear example can be found when examining the prognostic value of QOL measured by patients' self-evaluation, for which many different questionnaires investigating different domains of QOL with different questions and different response scales are available: how does one deal with different and sometimes contradictory results about the prognostic predictiveness of a specific domain?

Furthermore different studies show a wide variability in the analytical methods applied for variable selection in model building, for handling of continuous variables and for adjustment for different confounders. This variability, together with the heterogeneity in the set of factors examined together makes it very difficult to compare and synthesize the results from different studies and often prevents the possibility of performing a quantitative meta-analysis.

Finally, the fact that a prognostic factor is significantly associated with the outcome of interest does not necessarily mean it is clinically relevant. Statistical significance simply indicates the strength of the evidence against the hypothesis of no effect, while clinical importance depends upon the degree to which the knowledge of the factor can reduce the uncertainty about prognosis. Thus when examining a single prognostic factor the hazard ratio (HR) can help in evaluating its prognostic strength, preferably when it is adjusted for known prognostic factors; on the contrary, when dealing with a set of factors all included in a model, an indication of the variability explained by the model (namely the reduction in the uncertainty of the outcome) is given by the goodness-of-fit index,[36] which is unfortunately seldom presented in papers about prognosis.

Studies of the accuracy of clinical prediction of survival and prognostic scores

In addition to the general issues there are a number of others that are relevant to studies of the accuracy of clinical predictions of survival and prognostic scores.

The first is 'when the clock was started'. Many of the studies do not clearly state in the methodology section when the physician made the prediction in relation to the commencement of the observation period. Ideally it should be made before the observation period commences and if not as soon as possible afterwards (within the first 24 hours).

A second issue is whether the clinician making the prediction should be in charge of the care of the patient. While no ethical physician would consciously decide to alter treatment so that their survival predictions became more accurate, it is possible that formulating a specific prognosis for research purposes might subconsciously alter decision-making about treatment. This issue creates a potential methodological problem, as some studies indicate the nature of the physician–patient relationship impacts on the accuracy of clinical predictions.[37]

Evaluating the accuracy of survival predictions (whether subjective, or actuarial based on scores) is akin to evaluating diagnosis rather than prognosis. Like other studies of the clinical manifestations of disease, which evaluate the usefulness of symptoms and signs in determining the diagnosis,[38] the question here is 'Using clinical acumen, can I determine how long this dying patient has to live?'

To date one prognostic study has been published that was conducted like a standard diagnostic test evaluation, using the clinical prediction of survival (CPS) as the gold standard to compare a prognostic score.[39] In evaluating the validity of such a study, one needs to ask:

- *Did the clinician face diagnostic uncertainty?*: given the established inaccuracy of clinical predictions, this clearly applies!

- Was there a blind comparison with an independent gold standard applied similarly to the treatment group and the control group? CPS was used as the gold standard to which was compared a prognostic score.

- Did the results of the test being evaluated influence the decision to perform the reference standard? This situation which is referred to as verification bias or workup bias is more of a problem in situations where the reference standard is invasive (e.g. comparing ventilation/perfusion scans with pulmonary angiography in patients with suspected pulmonary emboli) and is less likely to be an issue with this population.

What is the effect size and how precise is it?

As with any study, once we are statisfed that the results are valid, we want to know how big the effect size of the exposure/study factor is, whether that is a therapeutic intervention or a prognostic factor. An effect should be not only statistically significant but also clinically important. In the case of prognostic studies the effect of interest is either the likelihood of an event over time (or in the case of advanced cancer, the likelihood of death by a certain time) or else the relative risk or hazard ratio associated with the prognostic factor of interest. As the HR determined in a study is an estimate of the true HR for that factor in the whole population, we also are interested in the precision of that estimate, so that the 95 per cent confidence intervals (95 per cent CIs) should be reported, and ideally the confidence intervals will be narrow.

For example, the ISIS-2 in patients hospitalized with a myocardial infarction reported almost 20 years ago showed that treatment with streptokinase and aspirin compared to placebo reduced the odds of vascular death over the next five weeks by 42 per cent, clearly very imporant clincially as well as highly significant statistically.[40] This estimate of the effect was precise, the 95 per cent CI being narrow (34–50 per cent). In older oncology studies, a survival difference between treatments is often reported as a percentage rather than as a HR. As Martin reports in Chapter 9 of this volume in his discussion on prognosis of advanced lung cancer, the additon of cisplatin to vinorelbine improves the survival of lung cancer patients from 31 weeks to 40 weeks, these 9 weeks being not only statsitically significant (p < 0.01) but clincially significant.[41] No HR or 95 per cent CI for this difference were given. More recent studies address this. For example, propohylactic cranial irradiation for patients with small cell lung cancer produces a clincially and staistically significant 5.4 per cent increase in the rate of survival at three years (15.3 per cent in the control group vs 20.7 per cent in the treatment group) and this repsresents a the relative risk of death in the treatment group as compared with the control group was 0.84 (95 per cent confidence interval, 0.73 to 0.97; p = 0.01).[42] As a final example, also reports a US study showing blacks have a statistically significantly worse survival than whites (p = 0.046). However, the effect size is small (HR 1.17) and the 95 per cent CI relatively wide (1.00–1.37).[43]

Applying the findings to the patient

Having decided the study is valid, the effect size is suffciently large to be clinically important and is precisely estimated, the final step in the process is to decide if the results can applied to the care of the patient concerned. The first thing to look at is whether or not the patient would have met the inclusion criteria for the study. If not, the question to ask is whether they are sufficiently different that it would make the results unapplicable. Other factors to consider are whether all the clinically important outcomes have been considered in the study (e.g. QOL as well as survival) and whether the benefits are worth the costs and risks, if an intervention or other controllable exposure is involved. The latter trade-off should involve some input from the patient

Putting it into practice: the case of Mary Smith

When Mary Smith, the 42-year-old woman with advanced pancreatic cancer, asks you 'Doc, how long do I have?' you decide to take an evidence-based medicine approach to answering this question. You formulate the WBCQ using PICO: in patients with advanced pancreatic cancer (population) after 6 months time (exposure), what proportion of patients are still alive (outcome). You carry out a literature using PubMed (http://www.ncbi.nlm.nih.gov/entrez/) and type in the terms: *pancreatic cancer* and *survival analysis* and *cohort study*.

Nearly 50 citations are selected. By scanning the titles you find that most of them are irrelevant. You find number 88, an article published in *Digestive Diseases* in 2001, entitled *Prognostic parameters determining survival in pancreatic carcinoma and, in particular, after palliative treatment.*[20] You read the abstract and it seems to be relevant, and you know your local medical library holds this journal.

You obtain a copy of the article and appraise it using the quality criteria mentioned above. In particular you notice that the methods section is extremely brief, < 100 words in length:

- Prospective or retrospective study?: This is a *prospective study* conducted at a university hospital in Germany.
- Target population: Patients seen during a 7-year period were included although it is not stated what years this period included, nor is it stated whether these were all the cases seen at the hospital, or whether they are representative of other patients with pancreas cancer. It is implied, but again not clearly stated, that the patients were included in the study from the time of diagnosis.
- Sample size: almost 200 patients were included, which is a relatively large number, although more than 100 factors were evaluated, which could raise a power issue.
- Follow-up was very complete, survival duration being known in > 99 per cent cases.
- Quality of measurement: it does not say how the date of death was established.

From this appraisal, you conclude that it is difficult to be certain that the study is not at a risk of bias because details are lacking about many of the aspects you would like to know more about, particularly the representativeness of the sample. Nevertheless you are prepared to accept these limitations at this stage, and decide to look at the results.

The results indicate that amongst the patients having only palliative treatment, the median survival was 6.8 months (95 per cent CI 4.6–7.4 months), and that the maximum survival was just over 3 years: 10 of the 112 factors were significant on univariate analysis, but only three were relevant on multivariate analysis: prior chemotherapy, tumour stage and anorexia. The Kaplan Meier curves indicate that patients have a median survival of approximately 3 or 9 months from diagnosis, depending on which of these risk factors they have. The KM curves do indicate that even in the poor prognostic group, patients have a 10 per cent chance of being alive in 18 months.

You try to apply these results to your patient but as there are no inclusion or exclusion criteria for the study and data on patient characteristics, you find this difficult. You can tell her that you know of a German study and that patients with inoperable pancreatic cancer participating in it typically lived for 6 months, 10 per cent of them were still alive in 18 months to 2 years but nobody lived for 5 years, and that patients who had chemotherapy did best ... however, it is impossible to know if the study participants were like her because insufficient details were given and you really should try to look for another study.

This goes to show that a study that fails the initial criteria probably isn't worth appraising further. So you seek another article, and find one called *Palliative treatment of advanced pancreatic carcinoma in community-based oncology group practices*,[44] and start the process over again.

References

1. Loprinzi CL. Johnson ME. Steer G. Doc, how much time do I have? *J Clin Oncol* 2000; 18:699–701.
2. Christakis N. *Death foretold*, pp. 84–106. Chicago, IL: University of Chicago Press, 1999.
3. McKibbon A. *Evidence-based medicine: principles and practice.* NY: Dekker, 1999.
4. Guyatt G, Rennie D (eds) *Users' guides to the medical literature. A manual for evidence-based practice.* Chicago, IL: AMA Press, 2002.
5. Laupacis A, Wells G, Richardson WS, Tugwell P. Users' guides to the medical literature. V. How to use an article about prognosis. Evidence-Based Medicine Working Group. *JAMA* 1994; 272(3):234–7.
6. Sackett SL, Haynes RB, Guyatt GH *et al. Clinical epidemiology. A basic science for clinical medicine*, 2nd edn, pp. 173–86. Boston, MA: Little, Brown, 1991.
7. Craig JC, Irwig LM, Stockler MR. Evidence-based medicine: useful tools for decision making. *Med J Aust* 2001; 174:248–53.
8. Moja LP, Telaro E, D'Amico R, Moschetti I, Coe L, Liberati A. Assessment of methodological quality of primary studies by systematic reviews: results of the metaquality cross sectional study. *BMJ* 2005; 330(7499):1053.
9. Vigano A, Bruera E, Jhangri GS, Newman SC, Fields AL, Suarez-Almazor ME. Clinical survival predictors in patients with advanced cancer. *Arch Intern Med* 2000; 160(6):861–8.
10. Anker SD, Negassa A, Coats AJ, Afzal R, Poole-Wilson PA, Cohn JN, Yusuf S. Prognostic importance of weight loss in chronic heart failure and the effect of treatment with angiotensin-converting-enzyme inhibitors: an observational study. *Lancet* 2003; 361(9363):1077–83.
11. National Health and Medical Research Council. *How to use the evidence: assessment and application of scientific evidence.* Commonwealth of Australia 2000:8.
12. Altman DG, Lyman GH. Methodological challenges in the evaluation of prognostic factors in breast cancer. *Breast Cancer Res Treat* 1998; 52(1–3):289–303.
13. Drew PJ, Ilstrup DM, Kerin MJ, Monson JR. Prognostic factors: guidelines for investigation design and state of the art analytical methods. *Surg Oncol* 1999; 7(1–2):71–6.

14. Richardson WS, Wilson MC, Nishikawa J. *et al*. The well-built clinical question: a key to evidence-based decisions. *ACP Journal Club* 1995; Nov/Dec:A12–13.

15. Greenhalgh T. How to read a paper: the Medline database. *BMJ* 1997; 315:180–3.

16. Matzo ML. Palliative care: prognostication and the chronically ill: methods you need to know as chronic disease progresses in older adults. *Am J Nurs* 2004; 104(9): 40–50.

17. Sulmasy DP, Sood JR. Factors associated with the time nurses spend at the bedside of seriously ill patients with poor prognoses. *Med Care* 2003; 41:458–66.

18. Maltoni M, Caraceni A, Brunelli C. *et al*. Prognostic factors in advanced cancer patients: Evidence-based clinical recommendations. *J Clin Oncol* 2005; 23: 6240–8.

19. Ahmed N, Ahmedzai S, Vora V, Hillam S, Paz S. *Supportive care for patients with gastrointestinal cancer*. The Cochrane Library (Oxford) 2005; 1: ID#CD003445

20. Ridwelski K, Meyer F, Ebert M. *et al*. Prognostic parameters determining survival in pancreatic carcinoma and, in particular, after palliative treatment. *Digest Dis* 2001; 19(1):85–92.

21. Louvet C, Labianca R, Hammel P. *et al*. Gemcitabine in combination with oxaliplatin compared with gemcitabine alone in locally advanced or metastatic pancreatic cancer: results of a GERCOR and GISCAD phase III trial. *J Clin Oncol* 2005; 23(15):3509–16.

22. Glare P. Performance status and symptoms: clinical predictors of survival in patients with terminal cancer. Master of Medicine treatise, University of Sydney, 2004.

23. Chow E. A predictive model for survival in metastatic cancer patients attending an out-patient palliative radiotherapy clinic microform. Ottawa: National Library of Canada (Bibliothèque nationale du Canada), 2002. Available at The National Library of Canada. http://www.nlc-bnc.ca/thesescanada/

24. Vigano A. Survival predictors in advanced cancer, Master of Science thesis: University of Alberta, 1998.

25. Juni P, Altman DG, Egger M. Assessing the quality of randomized controlled trials. In M Egger, G Davey Smith, DG Altman (eds) *Systematic reviews in health care. Meta-analysis in the context*, 2nd edn, pp. 87–108. London: BMJ Books, 2001.

26. Begg CB, Cho MK, Eastwood S. *et al*. Improving the quality of reporting randomized controlled trials. The CONSORT statement. *JAMA* 1996; 276:237–9.

27. Pirovano M, Maltoni M, Nanni O. *et al*. for the Italian Mulitcenter and Study Group on Palliative Care. A new palliative prognostic score: a first step for the staging of terminally ill cancer patients. *J Pain Symp Manage* 1999; 17:231–9.

28. Glare P, Virik K. independent validation of palliative prognostic score in terminally ill cancer patients in the acute care setting in Australia. *J Pain Symp Manage* 2001; 22: 891–8.

29. Altman DG. Systematic reviews of evaluations of prognostic variables. *BMJ* 2001; 323:224–8.

30. Llobera J, Esteva M, Rifa J. *et al*. Terminal cancer. duration and prediction of survival time. *Eur J Cancer* 2000; 36:2036–43.

31. Faris M. Clinical estimation of survival and impact of other prognostic factors on terminally ill cancer patients in Oman. *Supp Care Cancer* 2003; 30–4.

32. Lunney JR, Lynn J, Foley DJ. *et al*. Patterns of functional decline at the end of life. *JAMA* 2003; 289:2387–92.

33. Walsh D, Mahmoud F, Barna B. Assessment of nutritional status and prognosis in advanced cancer: interleukin-6, C-reactive protein, and the prognostic and inflammatory nutritional index. *Supp Care Cancer* 2003; 11(1):60–2.

34. Glare P, Christakis N. Predicting survival in patients with advanced disease. In D Doyle, G Hanks, N Cherny, K Calman (eds) *Oxford textbook of palliative medicine*, 3rd edn, pp. 29–42. Oxford: Oxford University Press, 2004.

35. Glare P, Eychmuller S, McMahon P. Diagnostic accuracy of the Palliative Prognostic (PaP) score in hospitalized patients with advanced cancer. *J Clin Oncol* 2004; 22: 4823–8.

36. Hosmer DW, Lemeshow S. *Applied logistic regression*, 2nd edn. New York: Wiley-Interscience. 2000

37. Christakis NA, Lamont EB. Extent and determinants of error in doctors' prognoses in terminally ill patients: prospective cohort study. *BMJ* 2000; 320:469–72.

Chunilal SD, Eikelboom JW, Attia J. *et al*. Does this patient have pulmonary embolism?. *JAMA* 2003; 290:2849–58.

38. Morita T, Tsunoda J, Inoue S. *et al*. Improved accuracy of physicians' survival prediction for terminally ill cancer patients using the Palliative Prognostic Index. *Palliat Med* 2001; 15:419–24.

39. ISIS-2 (Second International Study of Infarct Survival) Collaborative Group Randomised trial of intra-venous streptokinase, oral aspirin, both, or neither among 17,187 cases of suspected acute myocardial infarction: ISIS-2. *Lancet* 1988; 2(8607):349–60.

40. Le Chevalier T, Brisgand D, Douillard JY, Pujol JL, Alberola V, Monnier A, Riviere A, Lianes P, Chomy P, Cigolari S. *et al*. Randomized study of vinorelbine and cisplatin versus vindesine and cisplatin versus vinorelbine alone in advanced non-small-cell lung cancer: results of a European multicenter trial including 612 patients. *J Clin Oncol* 1994; 12(2):360–7.

41. Auperin A, Arriagada R, Pignon JP, Le Pechoux C, Gregor A, Stephens RJ, Kristjansen PE, Johnson BE, Ueoka H, Wagner H, Aisner J. Prophylactic cranial irradiation for patients with small-cell lung cancer in complete remission. Prophylactic Cranial Irradiation Overview Collaborative Group. *New Engl J Med* 1999; 341(7):476–84.

42. CM, Neslund-Dudas C, Simoff M. *et al*. In lung cancer patients, age, race-ethnicity, gender and smoking predict adverse comorbidity, which in turn predicts treatment and survival. *J Clin Epidemiol* 2004; 57(6):597–609.

43. Koeppler H, Duru M, Grundheber M. *et al*. Palliative treatment of advanced pancreatic carcinoma in community-based oncology group practices. *J Supp Oncol* 2004; 2:159–63.

7

Tools for formulating prognosis

Jay F. Piccirillo and Anna Vlahiotis

Appropriate treatment methods and accurate prognosis become especially important in the palliative care of patients with advanced or terminal cancer, where clinical factors related to the tumour seem less important than those factors related to the individual with the disease. Doctors attempt to determine a so-called 'cancer death trajectory'[1] by coupling individual factors such as quality of life and presence or severity of comorbid ailments with biological measures to facilitate more comprehensive prognostication. Much research has examined the individual prognostic importance of a host of clinical, biological, psychosocial and quality of life parameters,[2, 3] and has attempted to integrate significant factors into more inclusive prognostic measures. More inclusive prognostic tools are designed to improve decision-making and to enhance prediction of clinical outcomes, not only to benefit patients and families who want to maximize remaining time but to benefit medical professionals aiming to plan supportive services and allocate resources.[4] The design of a clinically valuable and methodologically sound prognostic model or index requires near perfect discrimination – the ability to distinguish between survival and death as measured by the area under the Receiver Operating Characteristic – and calibration – the ability to accurately predict the probability of death (prediction vs observation).[5] Unfortunately, because of the lack of consistency amongst prognostic factors between cancer patients, and because of variation in the accuracy of physicians' judgements or clinical predictions of survival (CPS), no single prognostic index has been universally successful in predicting outcomes across patient populations. Multiple models and prognostic indices have been developed and applied in the past two decades in the quest for accurate prediction. This chapter discusses some of the more widely recognized prognostic tools that have been researched and validated statistically in various patient populations.

SUPPORT model

One of the earliest prognostic indices used in the prediction of outcomes in advanced cancer patients was the SUPPORT Prognostic Model (Study to Understand Prognoses and Preferences for Outcomes and Risks of Treatments).[6] The model was developed in two phases at several academic hospitals across the United States as the result of a prospective cohort study of 8,329 'seriously-ill', though not necessarily terminally ill, cancer patients who were hospitalized between 1989 to 1994. The prediction of survival using the SUPPORT model was based on readily obtainable patient factors and physiologic indicators. In order to determine the influence of each potential prognostic factor, the authors analyzed a Cox proportional hazards regression model – after bivariate screening of individual variables and calculation of restricted cubic splines of the biological factors and risk of death – to determine which variables had significant and independent effects upon survival. The final SUPPORT model included as prognostic factors patient age, disease category, severity of disease, long-term health status, cancer presence, and length of hospital stay. To validate the index, Knaus *et al.* applied the model to 4,028 patients analysed in the second phase of the study. Calibration charts that measured the goodness of fit revealed closely calibrated curves, and measurement of ROC curve areas yielded a result of 0.78, which is indicative of very good discrimination.

The model confirmed previous reports that physiologic variables were the most important prognostic factors, but that other measures such as age or length of hospital stay also had independent value. From the results of statistical analyses using restricted cubic splines to weight factors and their relationships to outcome, the authors concluded that 'the SUPPORT prognostic model provides a new, accurate, and flexible empiric method for estimating a patient's risk of death over time'.

Palliative Performance Scale

Anderson *et al.* developed a prognostic tool for use in decision-making in palliative care as a modification of the Karnofsky Performance Scale.[7] Though the Palliative Performance Scale (PPS) was intended to measure other aspects of physical status, it had prognostic value as well. This index used an objective structured rating to gauge a patient's general health from 0 (death) to 100 (normal – considering circumstances). The authors assessed a total of 332 patients (both at home and upon admission to a hospice unit), and preliminary results revealed the correctly hypothesized positive relationship between PPS score and survival – those patients with lower scores had shorter survival times, and only two patients with PPS ratings greater than 60 died in hospice care. To further test this prognostic model, researchers in Asia prospectively analysed 245 terminally ill cancer patients admitted to the palliative care unit of a hospital in Shizuoka, Japan between September 1996 and August 1997 and October 1997 and April 1998.[8] The patients were analysed according to sex, age, tumour site, and PPS score, and were followed up for periods as long as 6 months. Kaplan–Meier survival curves revealed results similar to the initial PPS inception study: patients with PPS ratings between 10 and 20 survived for the least amount of time, PPS scores of 30–50 survived significantly longer than the first cohort of patients, and patients with scores of 60 or greater survived longer than all other patients. The authors felt that the PPS was a valid tool for rating patient health status as a correlate of survival, though the distinctions between categories were not prominent.

In an effort to correct for limited tests of reliability and validity, a team of researchers employed the PPS between 1 February and 31 July of 2001 to a cohort of palliative care patients in Sydney, Australia.[9] Using a score determined by palliative care specialists, 153 patients were scored upon admission and followed to determine length of stay and post-admission survival. The results of the study showed that mortality decreased from more than 90 per cent of patients with a PPS score of 10 to virtually no deaths in patients with a PPS score of 70. The graphic representation of the findings implies that survival was greater with each increase in PPS score category, suggesting that the PPS score has the power to predict outcomes in such populations.

Palliative Prognostic Index

Another response to the lack of clinical methods for use in the accurate prediction of survival in palliative care was the development of the Palliative Prognostic Index (PPI). This tool is an extension of the PPS, and was developed by the same Japanese research team that utilized the tool in predicting how long a patient is likely to live.[10] A retrospective cohort study processed the assessments of 245 patients across two different intake groups using a training–testing procedure. This method employed an original cohort of patients for model development (patient characteristics and clinical symptoms used in multivariate analyses) and the second set of patients served as the validation cohort in which the predictive values garnered from multivariate analyses were applied and evaluated for accuracy. The patients were divided into three groups according to their PPI scores, which ranged from 0 to 15 with higher scores indicating decreased overall health. The index was validated in the second set of patients, where 3- and 6-week survival was predicted with a significant degree of accuracy groups. In this analysis, both the positive value and negative predictive values behaved in expected ways, leading the authors to conclude that their methods were suitable in predicting short-term survival of terminally ill cancer patients.

Palliative Prognostic score

In order to address the need to identify the clinical and biological prognostic factors associated with terminally ill cancer patients, several Italian doctors completed a prospective multi-centre study of 519 hospice home care patients with a median survival of 32 days. From this research, they developed and assessed the usefulness and accuracy of the Palliative Prognostic (PaP) Score.[11] From October 1992 until November 1993, patients with advanced solid tumours no longer suitable for primary treatment were screened for personal data (age and sex), performance status, state of illness and present symptoms, biological parameters and data relative to the terminal phase of their disease or clinical predictors of survival (CPS). The PaP score was constructed by integrating the statistically significant results from individual multivariate analyses based on clinical parameters and on biological variables into a separate regression model. The model included as factors predictive of mortality anorexia, CPS, dyspnea, KPS score, lymphocyte percentage, and total white blood count. The added score, based on the subdivision of regression coefficients per each parameter by the smallest coefficient, ranged from 0 to 17.5. Patients were classified into one of three groups (A – 30-day survival greater than 70 per cent; B – survival between 30–70 per cent, and C – survival less than 30 per cent). The comparison of Kaplan–Meier survival curves revealed that patients in Group A (those with lower PaP scores) had increased survival as compared to patients with higher PaP scores in Groups B and C.

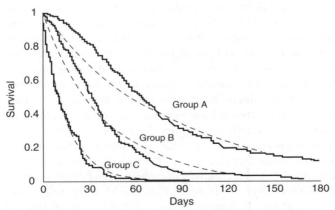

Figure 7.1 Reprinted from *Journal of Pain and Symptom Management* 17; Pirovano M, Maltoni M, Nanni O. *et al*. A new palliative prognostic score: a first step for the staging of terminally ill cancer patients. Italian Multicenter and Study Group on Palliative Care, 231–239; 1999, with permission from The US Cancer Pain Relief Committee.

Thus the authors inferred that the PaP score would be clinically useful in predicting survival among prognostically homogenous classes of patients.

The same research team[12] engaged in a successful validation of the PaP score. By evaluating the accuracy of prediction in the application of the score on a different population of 451 patients being cared for in palliative care units in Italy, the researchers were able to validate the prognostic value of the index in order to prepare it for clinical use. Verification of the prognostic capability of the PaP score was accomplished by applying the same previously used scoring system to a new series of analytic cases: a baseline grade was recorded based on each patient's prognostic factors, and the sum of the scores was calculated in order to classify each patient into one of three groups according to 30-day survival. As expected, the designated survival time probability for the first group was greater than 70 per cent, between 30–70 per cent for the second set of patients, and less than 30 per cent for the last group.

As part of the process of predictive model validation, Australians Glare and Virik[13] attempted to determine the applicability of the PaP score by employing the method with an independent sample of patients different from that in which the model was originally developed and validated. They conducted a prospective study of 100 terminally ill cancer patients receiving palliative care in a single Australian centre. To validate the PaP score, they employed the same scoring method as originally devised by the Italians, and divided the patients in the same fashion (according to the probability of 30-day survival). A highly significant difference in Kaplan–Meier survival curves revealed that survival probability decreased as Pap score increased, thus validating the predictive model. 'The concordance in the ability of these different data sets to differentiate groups of patients suggests that the PaP Score for prognostication in terminally ill patients possesses wide applicability, irrespective of the setting.' [13] There were, however, differences in the patient population in this study as compared to the patient sets in the original training–testing analyses. The differences, such as lower KPS scores and generalized inferior health of the Australian patients, served to reinforce the already-evidenced predictive power of the PaP Score by providing model validation across clinical differences, as well.

Survival Prediction Score

In response to the need for validation of a predictive model for survival in a greater variety of settings, Canadian researchers[14] initiated the analysis of survival for metastatic cancer patients at an outpatient palliative radiotherapy clinic in Toronto, Canada. The authors collected demographic data, patient-rated level of distress (according to degree of certain symptoms), analgesic consumption, primary tumour site, KPS, time since first diagnosis, weight loss, and date of death/last follow-up for 395 patients with advanced cancer at the Toronto-Sunnybrook Regional Cancer Centre. Each covariate was evaluated for its association with survival, and covariates achieving statistical significance in bivariate screening were entered into Cox proportional hazards models to test for individual goodness of fit (with and without each variable in the model) in order to decipher which measures had predictive value. The final model, which contained primary tumour site, site of metastases, fatigue, appetite, shortness of breath, and KPS, was then assessed for predictive accuracy by measuring the overall calibration and discrimination. The model provided Survival Prediction Scores (SPS) ranging from 0 to 32, and patients were stratified by risk of mortality into three groups. Patients in Group A (SPS ≥ 13) had the lowest risk of mortality, Group B (SPS 14 to 19) patients had intermediate risk, and patients in Group C (SPS ≥ 20) had the highest risk. An assessment of predicted survival using the Cox regression model vs actual survival established by Kaplan–Meier survival curves revealed a close fit between the models.

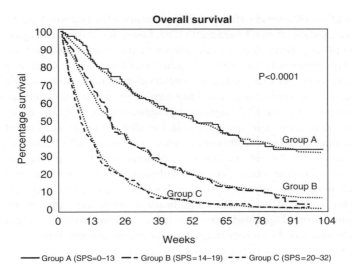

Figure 7.2 Reprinted from *International Journal of Radiation Oncology, Biology, Physics*, 53, Chow E, Fung K, Panzarella T, Bezjak A, Danjoux C, Tannock I. A predictive model for survival in metastatic cancer patients attending an outpatient palliative radiotherapy clinic; 1291–1302, 2002 with permission from Elsevier.

Good/Bad/Uncertain Index

A stratification-based prognostic tool titled the Good/Bad/Uncertain Index was developed by a research team in order to build on the established Eastern Cooperative Oncology Group (ECOG) performance status measure by identifying a set of indicators that collectively reflected the extent of disease and degree of suffering experienced by advanced cancer patients.[15] The team first developed and pilot tested a comparative questionnaire on almost 200 patients by asking them about their disease and expectations for subsequent health status. A model building process based on the responses of 1500 patients to a revised questionnaire revealed several prognostically important factors to be assessed on an ordinal scale: physician estimates of survival, patient-rated KPS score, and appetite measurement. Regression coefficients derived from Cox proportional hazards models were weighted according to severity and classified into risk groups of positive, neutral, or negative, and were associated with prognosis based on whether a patient 'experienced' two, three, or four of the classified variables. Positive and negative implications influenced prognosis according the number of classified variables experienced. For example, a patient experiencing three of four negative indicators would receive a negative prognosis. Validation was completed by assessing prognostic power according to survival curves of 729 patients involved in clinical trials for advanced cancer care. The separation of survival curves according to patients having a good prognosis, uncertain prognosis, or bad prognosis indicated substantive predictive power of the index.

Other stratification-based predictive models

Other development-validation analyses have established successful prognostic tools applicable to specific patient populations. Taiwanese researchers conducted a prospective development-validation testing study of terminally ill cancer patients in the palliative care facility associated with National Taiwan University Hospital.[16] To determine the relationships between survival and demographic data, clinical parameters, performance status, and symptom severity, 356 development set patients and 184 validation set patients were analysed using Cox regression and Kaplan–Meier survival curves. In addition to predicting survival on the basis of symptom parameter presence or absence, the authors also attempted to measure the relationship between severity of decompensation and the time of presentation of certain symptoms or parameters. The predictive model determined a prognostic score where the values of corresponding regression coefficients were divided in half, rounded to the nearest decimal, and summed for a final score ranging from 0 (no altered variables) to 8.5 (maximal alteration for all variables). When scores were < 3.5, 2-week survival was predicted with 0.72 and 0.61 accuracy for the development and validation sets, respectively. With scores < 6.0, 1-week survival was predicted with 0.72 and 0.66 accuracy, respectively. The authors inferred that certain symptoms affecting a patient's survival appeared at an earlier stage in the dying process, whereas other symptoms and signs affecting survival appeared at a relatively late stage in the process. The death trajectory could be thus be stratified by severity stages according to the presentation of certain symptoms or signs.

The Prognostigram

The Prognostigram is a new interactive multimedia patient-specific prognostic tool developed at Washington University School of Medicine for predicting survival in adult cancer patients. It is a web-based program which creates individualized survival curves based on the Cox proportional hazards model of survival data from the hospital-based tumour registry at Barnes-Jewish Hospital (St. Louis, Missouri, USA) and the population-based SEER Program (National Cancer Institute, USA). Adjusted survival curves are generated, taking into account the impact of comorbid health information, and are presented on the same graphical figure as the survival curve for age, gender, and race-matched peers.

The project was completed in three distinct phases. The first stage of the project consisted of the analysis of the relationship between baseline demographic, clinical, comorbid, and tumour information and survival for the more than 35,000 adult patients in the Barnes-Jewish Hospital Oncology Data Services (ODS) tumour registry. From this analysis, unique survival curves were generated based on the cogent predictive factors. In the second phase of the project, baseline demographic, clinical, and tumour information from the nation-wide population-based Surveillance, Epidemiology, and End Results (SEER) Cancer Incidence and Survival Monograph (1973–1996)[17] dataset was used to generate unique survival curves. Comorbidity information is not contained within the SEER dataset, but the prognostic impact of comorbidity was added based on the observed impact of comorbidity within the Barnes-Jewish dataset. The third, and final, phase of the project focused on creating the web page to display the prognostigrams.

The data for this prognostic component comes from a review of the medical records of 36,372 new adult patients presenting to Barnes-Jewish Hospital for initial treatment of cancer between 1 January, 1995 and 29 December, 2003. Data analysis of the BJH dataset began with a description of the population, including age, gender, race, comorbidity severity, anatomic site of the tumour, and morphologic extent. Description of survival, including mean, median, and mode for each tumour site and stage was performed. Bivariable analyses, including t-tests and chi-square analyses, were performed. For these statistical comparisons, the impact of each covariate was related to overall survival. Cox proportional hazards multivariable analysis was then performed to identify the significant independent predictor variables for each anatomic site. Predictor variables which had a significance level of p < 0.01 or less in bivariable analysis were added to the multivariable model. Life survival curves were generated for each combination of significant independent predictor variables. Ninety-five per cent confidence bands were generated around the survival curve estimates. The adjusted hazard ratios for comorbidity were determined so that these weights could be added to the SEER dataset that only contains baseline prognostic information including, age, gender, race, anatomic site (ICD-O code[18]), and extent of disease, but not comorbid health status. Bivariable analyses were performed on this dataset, also, for each anatomic site, to identify the prognostic factors for survival. Multivariable analysis was again performed to determine the independent prognostic factors.

Life survival curves are generated for patients at the time of diagnosis and for patients who have survived any number of years after diagnosis. A comparison of survival for the patients contained in the Barnes-Jewish Hospital ODS dataset and SEER dataset was performed as a check for approximate equality of the two populations. The curves were similar in all cancer sites except for Kaposi's sarcoma, where there were no observations. For all other sites, the survival curves were similar and so we then applied the hazard ratios for comorbidity obtained from BJH ODS dataset to the SEER dataset. In this way, the impact of comorbidity was added to the SEER-derived prognostigrams. Survival information, based on the SEER data, is displayed in a fashion similar to that described for the Barnes-Jewish ODS dataset.

Patient-unique survival curves generated by the Prognostigram program are displayed in a most straightforward format and are intended for patients, families, healthcare providers, and other professionals. The format for the survival curve plots are such that 'Percentage (of clinically similar newly diagnosed patients) surviving' is the y-axis and 'Survival duration in months' (after initial therapy) is on the x-axis. Overlaid onto the survival curves is a second plot, demonstrating the natural mortality of a cohort of age-, gender-, and race-matched peers without head and neck cancer. This natural mortality data was obtained from the National Center for Health Statistics Vital Statistics Mortality Data, Multiple Cause of Death, as incorporated into a table by R. R. Monson, Ph.D. of the Department of Epidemiology, Harvard School of Public Health, Boston, MA.

In Figure 7.3 (see overleaf), we show a survival curve for white men between the ages of 70 and 74 with metastatic lung cancer from the *Prognostigram* program.

In Figure 7.4 (see overleaf), we show the same two survival curves as above but the cancer patient survival curve is adjusted for the impact of severe comorbidity (third curve). As can be seen, the new solid line demonstrates a worse survival as a result of severe comorbidity. The 1-year survival rate goes from 15 per cent to 10 per cent and 2-year survival goes from 4 per cent to 2 per cent, in each case a 50 per cent reduction!

Conclusion

Prognostic tools are designed to improve decision-making and to enhance prediction of clinical outcomes. This should lead to benefits for patients and their families who want to maximize remaining time. In addition, improved prognostication should benefit medical professionals who must plan supportive services and are often called upon to manage and allocate scarce resources. In this chapter we have presented some of the more widely recognized prognostic tools that have been researched and statistically validated in various patient populations. Additional prognostic tools, including those using neural networks, will surely be developed and validated. The real challenge will be to identify the best ways to incorporate these prognostic tools into clinical decision-making.

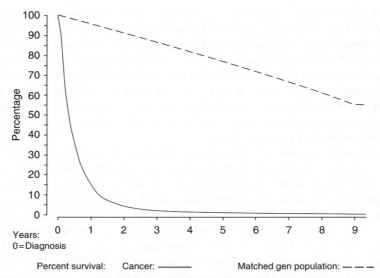

Figure 7.3 The dashed line represents the survival for age, gender, race-matched peers and the solid line represents the survival for 6,193 men with distant spread of lung cancer. The 1-year survival rate for the cancer patients is 15 per cent and the 2-year survival rate is 4 per cent.

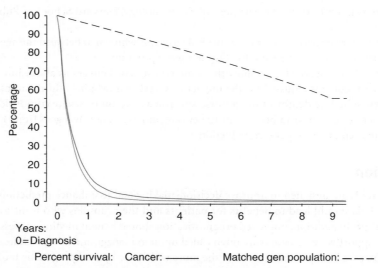

Figure 7.4 The same two curves as in Figure 7.3, but the cancer patient survival curve is adjusted for the impact of severe comorbidity.

References

1. Institute of Medicine. *Approaching death: improving care at the end of life*, Washington, DC: National Academy Press, 1997.

2. Maltoni M, Amadori D. Prognosis in advanced cancer. *Hematology – Oncology Clinics of North America* 2002; 16:715–29.

3. Vigano A, Donaldson N, Higginson IJ, Bruera E, Mahmud S, Suarez-Almazor M. Quality of life and survival prediction in terminal cancer patients: a multicenter study. *Cancer* 2004; 101:1090–8.

4. Chow E, Harth T, Hruby G, Finkelstein J, Wu J, Danjoux C. How accurate are physicians' clinical predictions of survival and the available prognostic tools in estimating survival times in terminally ill cancer patients? A systematic review. *Clinical Oncology (Royal College of Radiologists)* 2001; 13:209–18.

5. Altman DG, Royston P. What do we mean by validating a prognostic model? *Statistics in Medicine* 2000; 19:453–73.

6. Knaus WA, Harrell FE, Lynn J. *et al.*, The SUPPORT prognostic model. Objective estimates of survival for seriously ill hospitalized adults. Study to understand prognoses and preferences for outcomes and risks of treatments. *Ann Intern Med* 1995; 122:191–203.

7. Anderson F, Downing GM, Hill J, Casorso L, Lerch N. Palliative performance scale (PPS): a new tool. *Journal of Palliative Care* 1996; 12:5–11.

8. Morita T, Tsunoda J, Inoue S, Chihara S. Validity of the palliative performance scale from a survival perspective. *Journal of Pain and Symptom Management* 1999; 18:2–3.

9. Virik K, Glare P. Validation of the palliative performance scale for inpatients admitted to a palliative care unit in Sydney, Australia. *Journal of Pain and Symptom Management* 2002; 23:455–7.

10. Morita T, Tsunoda J, Inoue S, Chihara S. Improved accuracy of physicians' survival prediction for terminally ill cancer patients using the Palliative Prognostic Index. *Palliative Medicine* 2001; 15:419–24.

11. Pirovano M, Maltoni M, Nanni O. *et al.* A new palliative prognostic score: a first step for the staging of terminally ill cancer patients. Italian Multicenter and Study Group on Palliative Care. *Journal of Pain and Symptom Management* 1999; 17:231–9.

12. Maltoni M, Nanni O, Pirovano M, *et al.* Successful validation of the palliative prognostic score in terminally ill cancer patients. *Journal of Pain and Symptom Management* 1999; 17:240–7.

13. Glare P, Virik K. Independent prospective validation of the PaP score in terminally ill patients referred to a hospital-based palliative medicine consultation service. *Journal of Pain and Symptom Management* 2001; 22:891–8.

14. Chow E, Fung K, Panzarella T, Bezjak A, Danjoux C, Tannock I. A predictive model for survival in metastatic cancer patients attending an outpatient palliative radiotherapy clinic. *International Journal of Radiation Oncology, Biology, Physics* 2002; 53:1291–302.

15. Sloan JA, Loprinzi CL, Laurine JA, *et al.* A simple stratification factor prognostic for survival in advanced cancer: the good/bad/uncertain index. *Journal of Clinical Oncology* 2001; 19:3539–46.

16. Chuang RB, Hu WY, Chiu TY, Chen CY. Prediction of survival in terminal cancer patients in Taiwan: constructing a prognostic scale. *Journal of Pain and Symptom Management* 2004; 28:115–22.

17. Ries LAG, Young JL, Keel GE *et al.* (editors). SEER Survival Monograph: Cancer Survival Among Adults: US SEER Program, 1988–2001, Patient and Tumor Characteristics. National Cancer Institute, SEER Program, NIH Pub No. 07-6215, Bethesda, MD, 2007.

18. Fritz A, Percy C, Jack A. *et al. International Classification of Diseases for Oncology*, Geneva: World Health Organization, 2000.

Ethical perspectives

Bert Broeckaert and Paul Glare

Introduction

Recently, the European Association of Palliative Care (EAPC) promulgated guidelines on the role of prognostication and prognostic factors in palliative care.[1] Attention to ethical aspects of prognostication were evident throughout these guidelines. From the beginning the international expert working group that prepared these guidelines had taken an interdisciplinary approach, drawing on and bringing together the wide-ranging expertise (medicine, nursing, statistics, social sciences, ethics) of its members.

When developing guidelines on prognostication, it is indeed crucial not to separate the ethical discussion from the medical discussion. Doing so would give the ethical aspects of prognostication only a secondary status and deny the inevitable ethical impact of each and every medical guideline that is given.

This chapter intends to offer a short introduction to the ethical dimensions of prognostication. In our view prognostication raises important ethical issues. On the other hand it seems that it is predominantly the classical bioethical themes that are at stake here: informed consent, patient's interest, confidentiality, etc. In what follows we try to highlight the way these themes ermerge and are of importance here. A detailed discussion of the important ethical principles involved falls outside the scope of this chapter.

We first briefly examine the ethical aspects of doing research on prognostic factors, thus taking a research ethics perspective. In the second part we discuss the ethical aspects of prognostic factors in clinical practice, thus moving to the field of clinical ethics. At the end of this chapter we briefly explore the relationship between ethics and guidelines on prognostication (research).

Ethical aspects of research on prognostic factors

As in any other type of research involving patients, in research on prognostic factors too the *informed consent* of the patients involved is of crucial importance. The principe of informed consent implies (1) that the (competent) patient freely consents to the treatment, examination … that is proposed (2) that, in order to be able to make an informed decision, all relevant information has been provided to him/her.

It is clear that when the research involves extra examinations, (informed) consent must be sought and given. The main prognostic factors that have been examined to date have involved performance status and symptoms, so that extra examinations have not been an issue. However, there is now increasing interest in quality of life and biochemical markers, including laboratory parameters that are not routinely collected such as cytokines, making extra assessments involving batteries of questionaires and multiple blood tests part of the burden for participants. Though all this may still be simpler than in the study of prognostic factors in early cancer which may involve other issues such as genetics and tissue banking, obtaining the (informed) consent of the patients involved remains an important ethical obligation.

Often times, research on survival/prognosis is done as a subanalysis of data collected for a randomized controlled trial (RCT). Though the original study has been approved by an institutional review board (IRB), it is unclear if particpants have understood that prognostic aspects will be looked at and valid (informed) consent was obtained for this (new) study. Uncertainty and disputes can be avoided by integrating the prognosis study right from the beginning in the study design and the informed consent procedure.

In order to be able to make an *informed* decision, participants in research on prognostic factors in advanced cancer need to be given adequate information that explains for them why the research is being done, who is doing it, what it involves, the burdens and risks, as well as issues of dissemination of the results, confidentiality and withdrawal.

As with all palliative care research, studying prognostic factors raises the issue of research on vulnerable patients. When undertaking research on this population one always needs to keep in mind whether there will be any benefits and/or burdens for the patient. The burdens of prognostic research for the individual patient will often be limited. As for the benefits, there will usually be hardly any direct benefit for the patient participating in the research. In our experience, however, palliative patients are often very sensitive to the potential benefits for future patients and thus remarkably altruistic in their concerns. It is of course immoral to press or manipulate vulnerable palliative patients in any way in order to get them to participate in a study, but paternalistically denying these patients the opportunity to unselfishly help others seems equally problematic.

Finally, a peculiar aspect of studying prognostic factors is that this type of research can potentially be very confronting for the patient and their family. While palliative care concerns itself with patients who are approaching death, the reality is that many patients try to maintain some hope by operating in a certain degree of denial. These patients may find research on prognostic factors very confronting. The way and the time when the study is introduced are therefore extremely important. Of equal importance is the careful wording of the Participant Information Statement (PIS). Researchers are advised to negotiate the language used in the PIS with their local IRB.

Clinical aspects of prognosis

The clinical skill of prognosis

The clinical act of prognosis can be broken down into three component parts, each of which has its own ethical concerns. They are:

- ◆ Establishing the prognosis
- ◆ Using the prognosis
- ◆ Communicating the prognosis.

Establishing prognosis

Because predicting length of survival is a very difficult and hazardous undertaking, physicians often feel uncomfortable when formulating prognoses and even try to avoid prognostication. Several arguments can be given, however, that clearly demonstrate that in most cases prognostication is both necessary and inevitable, and that poor prognostication or a refusal to prognosticate can have dire consequences.

First there is the fact that treatment decisions in advanced cancer patients are often partly dependent upon prognostic estimations. Will the patient benefit from the effect of any chemotherapy (symptom relief, improved quality of life)? Is there enough time left to benefit from other long-term treatments? In order to be able to answer questions in this vein in a responsible way, prognostic information that is as reliable as possible is of vital importance. Such information is clearly in the patient's best interests, enables both physician and patient to make an informed decision and avoids in vulnerable patients any additional harm or discomfort resulting from inappropriate therapies. In treatment decisions in which prognostic estimations do play a role, whether they are explicitly formulated or not, it is far preferable to depend upon conscious and evidence-based prognostication than upon implicit assumptions about survival that are not substantiated and often highly questionable.

Reliable prognostic information is not only important for treatment decisions in the strict sense. A lot of more general but equally crucial decisions taken by patients, families, caregivers and others can not but take the estimated length of survival into account. Should I urgently put my affairs in order and make provisions for my wife and children? Is it the time yet to discuss hospice care? Has the time come to sit up with our dying relative? Is this patient eligible for our palliative care service? When deciding in these matters, it is clearly far preferable to base these decisions on adequate prognostic information, thus decreasing the number of bad deaths and tragic regrets (had I only known…). Adequate prognostication is in the best interests of all involved and is certainly in the patient's best interests. Seen from this perspective, it is not a surprise to find out that patients have a moral right, often recognized by law, to be informed about their prognosis, which in itself constitutes an extra argument to demonstrate the professional and moral duty of physicians to prognosticate.

Having recognized that the clinical act of prognostication is ethically justified, the next ethical concern is the matter of *informed consent*. As with research on prognosis, informed consent is needed by the clinician if extra examinations, manipulations, or assessment by experts are involved. The right to physical integrity is a basic human right. This means that a physician too needs, when possible, to seek the informed consent of the patient involved before 'touching' (examining, treating,…) him or her. When a (competent) patient does not consent, this refusal must be respected. Here too the idea of informed consent implies the provision of the relevant information to the patient. As this information might be quite confronting, it is crucial to give adequate attention to the way and the time it is presented to the patient.

A third ethical concern regarding establishing prognosis is the problem of *accuracy and bias*. The inaccuracy of survival predictions in advanced cancer is well documented. As an ethical principle, it can be stated that prognosis should be as accurate as possible and necessary, but with the important caveat that it should not create disproportionate burden to the patient. A common approach used in specialist palliative care practice aimed at upholding this principle is to give the prognosis within a range that is broad enough to include the predicted survival yet narrow enough to be meaningful to the patient and family to help them set their goals and priorities, such as hours, days to weeks, weeks to months, months to years. Although there is no hard empirical evidence to support this stance, it is believed that by not giving a specific prognosis such as 2 weeks or 6 months, the burden of being given a death sentence is minimized and disappointment and/or anger resulting from prognostic inaccuracy are avoided as much as possible.

An important corollary is that bias should be avoided. Reviews of physicians' survival predictions revealed that physicians are accurate only 10–30 per cent of the time and that they tend to overestimate the survival by a factor of two to five. The psychology of prognostication and the reason for this inherent optimism has been extensively studied,[2] and is largely tied up with wanting to maintain a dimension of hope. Physicians need to be aware of this tendency to be overly optimistic in their predictions and try to adjust for it. Other research has shown that prognostic accuracy is inversely proportional to the duration of the physician–patient relationship, so that if an accurate, unbiased prognosis is required an experienced, dispassionate expert should be consulted.[3]

Using prognosis

While prognosis is often only discussed the medical literature in terms of its narrow sense of how the phsycian responds to the question 'how long do I have?'[4] the epidemiological definition of prognosis is; the relative probability of the various outcomes of the natural history of a disease.[5] When considered in this broad way, it is apparent that physicians are prognosticating all the time and are using their prognoses to make clinical decisions. From an ethical point of view therefore, physicians need to be aware of the fact that their predictions have an inherent inaccuracy and are prone to bias. While reliable clinical prediction rules have been developed in some areas of medicine,[6] this is not the case with prognosis in advanced cancer. Treatment decisions are and should be based on a number of variables, including prognosis and all these variables should receive and continue to receive due attention. This means that treatment decisions can and should not be taken on the basis of prognosis alone. The fact that prognostic information is per definition probabilistic and that even the very best prognostication will be dramatically inaccurate in a significant number of cases, provides an additional reason for never losing sight of the individual patient and their individual trajectory and for always keeping an open mind. An intense assessment of the personal history, wishes and concerns of the individual remains of crucial importance. Prognostication should always be deeply embedded in a dialogical approach that is both flexible and patient-centred.

Communicating prognosis

The third component of prognostication is the *communication* of the clinician's formulated prognosis. While communication was discussed at length in Chapter 4, the ethical issues involved need to be discussed here. It is in the transfer of prognostic information from the physician to the patient or others that ethical issues are most apparent.

According to the 'classical' Western bioethical discourse, the ethics of communicating prognosis is mainly determined by the patient's individual autonomy: patients have a right to be informed, not only about their diagnosis and about the therapy options, but also about their prognosis. Given greater demands for patient involvement in medical decision-making in the classical Western bioethical discourse, the disclosure of terminal prognosis at the request of the patient is seen as ethically justified because it upholds the principle of self-determination and enables patients to make treatment decisions consistent with their life goals.

However, *cultural and legal differences* do play a role here and should be taken into account. There are for instance significant cultural differences regarding the place of the family, the patient/nurse/physician relationships in general and the tendency towards medical paternalism or patient autonomy in particular. For example, a recent survey of palliative care physicians from Canada, Europe and South America found that they all agreed that cancer patients should be informed of their diagnosis and the terminal nature of their illness. They all agreed that 'do not resuscitate' orders should be present and these should be discussed with the patient in all cases. However, while 93 per cent of Canadian physicians stated that at least 60 per cent of their patients wanted to know about the terminal stage of their illness, only 26 per cent of European physicians and 18 per cent of South American believed this to be the case.[7]

As well as cultural differences there are also legal differences between different jurisdictions in which physicians operate. In a number of countries specific patient rights explicitly state the right of the patient to be informed about their medical condition and its evolution. At this stage interest is starting to be shown in the disclosure of prognosis to terminally ill patients as a medico–legal issue.[8]

The western stress on a patient's individual autonomy, on knowing the truth, knowing what's going on and what is going to happen, might give the impression that patients not only have the right, but even have a *duty to be informed*. It is important to make clear that whereas there is no doubt about a patient's *right* to be informed, there is no such thing as a *duty* to be informed. On the contrary, patients do have the right (sometimes explicitly recognized by law) to refuse to be informed about prognosis or any other aspect of their diagnosis or treatment. Though a physician can regret this attitude and its consequences when death is near, nobody can or should be forced to opt for the kind of 'conscious' dying process the physician or other caregivers consider to be a good death.

How to communicate prognosis? What to communicate? When prognosis is communicated, cultural and psychological considerations are most relevant in order to avoid additional harm to the patient. We should refer here to the often paradoxical nature of the wish to be informed: patients often give the impression that they want to hear the truth, the whole truth and nothing but the truth, the physician responds to this request, tells the bad news and is, to their surprise, confronted with a patient who reacts in a dismissive or angry way. To avoid tragic situations like this, it is of paramount importance for a physician to balance as well as possible the level of information asked and the level of information given, and to make sure the patient understands the information the way it was intended. In any case, without excellent communication skills and without adequate support to patient, family and caregivers, communicating prognosis is an ethical minefield.

Confidentiality is the final ethical issue we want to consider here. Apart from the physician and the patient, who should know? Usually the team of caregivers will and should be informed about the prognosis, as this prognostic information is important for their work. As with other areas of medicine, confidentiality is a concern here. What about the family and their questions? In palliative care practice families will often want to know the prognosis in order to make their plans for caring for the patient in the time remaining, and often such information will be requested in the patient's absence. This can be particularly relevant in the case of imminently dying patients, when families want to know if other members should be called back from out of town. As a general rule it is the patient who decides who will be informed and who will not. It is therefore both necessary and important to obtain, when possible, the patient's permission to discuss their illness (involving the prognosis as well as the diagnosis and treatment) with (specific members of) the family.

What about other individuals? For instance, an interesting related issue to the medico–legal aspects of prognostication is that law enforcement agencies and attorneys may also ask palliative care physicians to provide specific prognoses for terminally ill patients facing criminal charges.

Guidelines on prognosis and ethics

The development and promulgation of guidelines on prognosis raise some ethical issues of their own. Given the importance and necessity of prognostication on the one hand and the fact that in clinical reality prognostic accuracy seems to be the exception rather than the rule on the other, it is clear that both guidelines on prognostication research and guidelines on the use of prognostic factors in clinical practice can be very useful. There is, of course, nothing wrong with the composing and disseminating of guidelines that start from a thorough and sound review of the available literature and also take the ethical aspects of prognostication very seriously. However, one should be aware of the fact that even those guidelines that have been written by the best international specialists and with the very best intentions, can sometimes have an adverse impact.

Guidelines just as these on prognostication in advanced cancer are usually not written for palliative care experts, but rather for physicians that have only a limited knowledge of palliative care. Physicians in search for and using guidelines may lack palliative care experience and skills, and also may not share the palliative care ethos that the palliative care specialists that have drafted the guidelines take for granted.

There is a risk that guidelines will fail to open the eyes of the physician to the delicate issues involved, tending instead to close them: the combination of a huge workload and the appeal of quick and neat procedures could cause physicians to loose sight of the individual patient and their personal needs and wishes, reducing them to 'just a case of …'. These few remarks do not question the importance of guidelines at all, on the contary. We are simply arguing that guidelines should be screened for possible unintended adverse side-effects and should include an explicit warning that at all times the individual patient should be at the centre of attention.

Conclusion

In this short chapter we have tried to give a concise overview of the ethical issues prognostication involves. Though of course the professional importance of diagnostical and therapeutical skills cannot be denied, the ability of physicians to prognosticate should receive more attention than it usually gets. Prognostication is indeed both necessary and inevitable. Adequate prognostication is in the best interests of all involved and is therefore a moral duty for the physician, but establishing an adequate prognosis is not enough. Attention should also be given to the appropriate use and communication of prognostic information. Prognostication, state-of-the art though it may be, that is not deeply embedded in an open, flexible, patient-centred and dialogical approach can be very problematic.

References

1. Maltoni M, Caraceni A, Brunelli C. *et al*. Prognostic factors in advanced cancer patients: evidence-based clinical recommendations – a study by the Steering Committee of the European Association for Palliative Care. *J Clin Oncol* 2005; 23(25):6240–8.

2. Lamont EB, Christakis NA. Some elements of prognosis in terminal cancer. *Oncology* 1999; 13(8):1165–70.

3. Christakis N, Lamont EB. Extent and determinants of error in doctors' prognoses in terminally ill patients: prospective cohort study. *BMJ* 2000; 320:469–72.

4. Loprinzi CL, Johnson ME, Steer G. Doc,how much time do I have? *J Clin Oncol* 2000; 18(3):699–701.

5. Sackett DL, Haynes RB, Guyatt GH, Tugwell P. *Clinical epidemiology, a basic science for clinical medicine*, 2nd edn. Boston, MA: Little, Brown and Company, 1991.

6. Stiell IG, Greenberg GH, McKnight RD, Nair RC, McDowell I, Worthington JR. A study to develop clinical decision rules for the use of radiography in acute ankle injuries. *Ann Emerg Med* 1992; 21(4):384–90.

7. Bruera E, Neumann CM, Mazzocato C, Stiefel F, Sala R. Attitudes and beliefs of palliative care physicians regarding communication with terminally ill cancer patients. *Palliat Med* 2000; 14(4):287–98.

8. Rich BA. Prognostication in clinical medicine: prophecy or professional responsibility? *J Leg Med* 2002; 23(3):297–358.

Part II

Prognostication in specific cancers

9

Lung cancer

C. Martin Tammemagi

Introduction

Lung cancers, although having common anatomic and cellular origins, are a clinically and biologically heterogeneous group of diseases. Recent studies using gene expression and proteomic profiling have demonstrated that even within specific histologic categories, considerable molecular heterogeneity exists. Regardless of this heterogeneity, overall, long-term (5 year) survival for all stages of lung cancer is poor and when considering advanced lung cancer is even more disheartening. In spite of these generalizations, the clinician and patient need appreciate that even for advanced stage disease, some individuals do experience long-term survival and that within the short term (< 5 years) there is considerable heterogeneity regarding length of survival. Many methodologic pitfalls have hampered development of a valid and complete understanding of prognostic factors in advanced lung cancer. Thus, prognostication remains a daunting task. Nevertheless, we currently do have enough knowledge to make moderately good predictions, and future studies are expected to improve our prognostic capabilities.

In this chapter, advanced lung cancer refers to disease that is not surgically resectable with curative intent, that is, stage IIIb (any T, N3, M0, or T4, any N, M0) and stage IV (any T, any N, M1) non-small cell lung cancer (NSCLC) and extensive stage small cell lung cancer (SCLC). However, many prognostic studies pool stage IIIa, IIIb and IV NSCLC and limited and extensive SCLC. Data from some such studies are included here, as the number of IIIa NSCLC and limited SCLC are usually relatively small, and there is little evidence to suggest that many prognostic factors act differently by these staging levels.

The author of this chapter led the Lung Cancer Comorbidity Study (LCCS), which provides results and examples pertinent to this discussion. The LCCS was a historical cohort study that investigated factors affecting survival in 1154 lung cancer patients diagnosed in the Henry Ford Health System in Detroit between 1995 and 1998. Sociodemographic, exposure, clinicopathologic, treatment and survival data were collected from the institutional Tumour Registry and by direct detailed abstraction of medical records. Of this cohort 767 individuals had stage III or IV NSCLC or SCLC (many tumour registries follow regulations which require assignment of American Joint Committee on Cancer [AJCC] stage to SCLC). In the following discussion, selected results are presented from the LCCS when they are thought to be representative and generalizable to other populations.

Statistical and methodologic issues

Although methodologic and statistical issues are discussed in detail elsewhere in this book, some concepts are reiterated here as they have particular relevance and are exemplified in this chapter. Complete evaluation of a prognostic factor should address a number of questions:

1. What is the *strength of association* between prognostic factor and survival, assessed by magnitude of hazard ratio or relative risk, confidence intervals (CI) and p-value, in univariate and adjusted analysis (adjusted for other relevant predictors of survival)?

2. What is the *distribution/frequency* of the factor in the study population and in the target population in which the prognostic factor will be applied?

3. What is the *predictive ability* of the factor in the study population?

4. *Has the prognostic factor been validated*, and what are the parameters described in questions 1–3 in the validation population(s)?

Unfortunately, the majority of studies address questions 1 and 2, but not 3 and 4. Common limitations in studies of prognostic factor in lung cancer include the following:

1. Assessments are univariate or if multivariate, are incompletely adjusted.

2. Predictive value of prognostic factors and prognostic models are not evaluated.

3. Potential prognostic factors are not validated in separate populations.

4. Study samples are not representative of the cancer population they purport to be studying.

Most prognostic studies determine the importance of prognostic factors based on p-values and/or confidence intervals. However, a highly significant p-value does not ensure that a prognostic factor explains survival variation or is highly predictive of survival, and often fails to do so. A useful statistic that provides a sense of the predictive ability of Cox proportional hazards models is the *c statistic*, which can be thought of as follows: considering all possible pairs of individuals under study with differing survival times, the c statistic represents the proportion for which the regression model/prognostic factor(s) correctly predicts the survival order.[1] The c statistic is analogous to the receiver operator characteristic area under the curve (ROC AUC), a test statistic considered to be optimal for evaluating the classification of dichotomous outcomes. Consider this example taken form the LCCS: the hazard ratio for advanced versus local/regional disease is 4.12 (95 per cent CI 3.41–4.97: $p < 0.001$) and the c statistic is 0.63. Although the hazard ratio is large and the p-value is highly significant, this variable can predict the longer survivor in each informative pairing in the study cohort only 13 per cent better than chance. Few past prognostic studies have reported the c statistic.

Accurate prognostication in advanced lung cancer is further made difficult due to the nature of the data and analysis. Cox models, on which the vast majority of prognostic models are based, are semi-parametric, that is, follow-up times are placed in rank order and ranks are analysed as opposed to actual follow-up times. Cox models do not readily allow prediction of specific individual survival times. When survival times for a study cohort are spaced over a prolonged period, as might occur with breast or prostate cancer patients, small alterations in follow-up times that result from measurement error or because of the influence of unmeasured factors, are not expected to cause large changes in the ranks of survival times. In advanced lung cancer, usually over 50 per cent of patients die within a year of diagnosis and approximately 85 per cent die within two years. Survival events are compressed together and events are separated by relatively small periods. Under these conditions, uncontrolled factors distorting survival times are expected to have greater impact on rank survival order, leading to bias estimates of association between prognostic factor and survival. In most circumstances, it is expected that resultant changes to rank survival orders would be random, adding 'noise' to the data, and leading to estimates biased towards the null, in other words, hiding associations.

Descriptive epidemiology

Lung cancer is a major public health concern. Globally, lung cancer is the leading cause of cancer death, and lung cancer is estimated to cause over 1.3 million deaths annually. In the United States in 2005, it was estimated that there would be 172,570 new cases of lung cancer and 163,510 deaths due to lung cancer[2] Although lung cancer incidence usually ranks second to prostate cancer in men and second to breast cancer in women, lung cancer is the leading cause of cancer death in both men and women. In the US in 2005, it is estimated that in men, prostate and lung cancers represent 33 and 13 per cent of all new cases of cancer, but represent 10 and 31 per cent of all cancer deaths, respectively.[2] In women, breast and lung cancers represent 32 and 12 per cent of new cancer cases and 15 and 27 per cent of cancer deaths.

Overall lung cancer survival is poor: even in developed countries 5-year survival rates are approximately 13–15 per cent and have improved little over the last 30 years. The high mortality statistics for lung cancer are attributed to its aggressive nature and to the majority of cases being diagnosed at an advanced stage when surgery with curative intent is no longer possible. US 1995–2000 data indicate that 16, 37 and 39 per cent of patients are diagnosed with local, regional and distant disease, respectively[2], and 5-year survival proportions for these groups were 49, 16 and 2 per cent. The 3- and 5-year survival of NSCLC patients with clinical stage cIIIA (n = 511) disease were 18 and 13 per cent, with stage cIIIB disease (n = 1030) were 7 and 5 per cent, and with stage cIV (n = 1427) disease were 2 and 1 per cent, respectively.[3]

Natural history

Approximately 85–90 per cent of lung cancers can be attributed to smoking and smoking is by far the most important cause of all histologic types of bronchogenic lung cancers. Additional aetiologic factors include occupational or environmental exposures to arsenic, cobalt, radon, uranium, cadmium, and organic chemicals, such as benzene; and occupational, medical, or environmental exposures to radiation. Chronic obstructive pulmonary disease is a smoking-independent risk factor for lung cancer. Prolonged exposures to second-hand smoke or to air pollution are thought to increase lung cancer risk by approximately 1.25-fold.

That family history of lung cancer appears to be an independent predictor of lung cancer risk, suggests that genetically determined susceptibilities exist. Although numerous polymorphisms in carcinogen-activating genes, detoxifying genes, and DNA repair genes have been evaluated, a complete picture has not emerged, as most past studies have evaluated only one or a few gene polymorphisms in isolation. In the future, single nucleotide polymorphism (SNP) association studies evaluating the entire genome or relevant pathways are expected to provide a more complete understanding of inherited susceptibility.

It has been estimated that lung carcinogenesis results from genetic alterations to between 10 and 20 tumour suppressor genes or oncogenes, and that additional epigenetic events are involved (e.g., transcriptional silencing of *p16* gene by hypermethylation). Also, most lung cancer cells have complex cytogenetic/karyotypic changes, some of which occur in non-random chromosomal locations, possibly indicating loci of tumour suppressor genes.

Some genetic alterations occur in lung tumours with regularity and are thought to play important roles in lung carcinogenesis and/or progression. TP53 tumour suppressor gene mutations are the most frequent genetic alteration occurring in lung cancer, occurring in 80–100 per cent of SCLC and 50–80 NSCLC. *RB1* (retinoblastoma tumour suppressor gene) mutations occur in 80–90 per cent of SCLC and 20–30 per cent of NSCLC. CDKN2a (P16INK4A) abnormalities are seen in 60 per cent of NSCLC and < 10 per cent of SCLC. Mutations/deletions in *FHIT* (fragile histidine triad gene) at chromosomal location 3p14.2 occur in about 75 per cent of SCLC and NSCLC. Upregulation of telomerase is seen in most lung cancers, including up to 98 per cent of SCLC. Other genes implicated in lung carcinogenesis include *MYCN, KRAS, TP73, MADH2, MADH4, PPP2R1B* and *PTEN*. Understanding of critical genetic alterations involved in lung carcinogenesis is hoped to lead to corrective therapeutic interventions. To date, gene therapies, for example, reintroduction of wild-type *p53* gene function using adenovirus gene-vectors, have not lead to improved survival.

Factors affecting prognosis (Table 9.1)

Host-related innate factors

Age is a powerful predictor of survival in localized and advanced lung cancer and is associated with important predictors of reduced survival, including loss of functional status and comorbidity. However, age is predictive of survival independently of these factors, and this

Table 9.1 Prognostic factors having strong, moderate and weak associations* with survival in advanced lung cancer, classified by the strength of evidence†

Strength of association Strength of evidence	Strong effects	Moderate effect	Weak or primarily univariate effects
Strong evidence/ established effect (consistent effects in multiple studies with multivariate analyses)	Stage, T, N, M, III vs IV Number of metastatic sites Performance/functional status Adverse symptoms Weight loss Neurologic symptoms Anaemia Adverse comorbidity	Age	Gender (male vs female)
Some substantial (based on more than one study or a large well-designed study with multivariate analyses)	Malignant pleural effusions Illicit drug use	SCLC vs NSCLC Quality of life Peri- and post-diagnosis smoking Lactate dehydrogenase (LDH) Tissue polypeptide antigen	Marital status Tissue polypeptide antigen Aneuploidy CYFRA 21-1 p53
Some weak or uncertain evidence (based on isolated or small or poorly designed studies)	Liver metastasis	Albumin Coagulation factors Proteinuria Hypercalcaemia	Depressed mood Neuron-specific enolase Tumour microvessel density (angiogenesis) Replication errors on 2p and 3p Ki-67 Bcl-2, K-ras/p21 protein overexpression c-erbB-I

* Strength of association here reflects the effect size, that is the size of the hazard ratio, and not how much survival variation is explained as might be measured by pseudo-R^2 statistic or how well the variable predicts survival in a population, as might be done with the c statistic. Although the effect size is based on the average effect for the exposed group compared to the unexposed group, it gives the best estimate which to apply to any single future lung cancer patient. In contrast, R^2 statistic and the c statistic incorporate into their statistic how common the exposure is in the population in which they are computed. Consider the following illustration: in the LCCS, in adjusted analysis, *illicit drug use* had a hazard ratio of 1.8, but occurred only in about 2 per cent of the study population. Of value to the clinician is the knowledge that a patient who is an illicit drug user is at about twice the risk of dying. Yet, because of the rarity of illicit drug use, this prognostic factor was a poor predictor for the study population as a whole (c statistic = 0.504).

† This classification system was designed to provide a sense of how important and credible selected prognostic factors are. They are based on the research experience and review of literature, but have not been compiled using a quantitative analyses and must be consider to an extent subjective.

in part is attributable to age-related decline in organ function, and increased probability of competing causes of death.

Gender

Many studies have found that male compared to female lung cancer patients have shorter survival. Generally, this effect is strongest when all stages are considered and analysis is univariate. Male gender is often associated with other prognostic factors, such as advanced stage, current smoking at diagnosis, and greater frequency of adverse symptoms. As a consequence, the prognostic impact of gender declines and sometimes disappears in multivariate analysis when other relevant covariates are considered in analysis.

Race

Overall in the US, African Americans have shorter lung cancer survival than their white counterparts. Some of this disparity is explained by African Americans being diagnosed at a more advanced stage. However, survival differences remain following adjustment or stratification by stage. For lung cancer patients with local, regional and distant lung cancer the 5-year survival proportions were 44, 15, and 1 per cent for African Americans and were 50, 16 and 2 per cent for Caucasians (Surveillance Epidemiology and End Results [SEER] data for individuals diagnosed between 1995-2000 and followed through 2001).[4] Some multivariate studies have failed to explain all of the African American disparity in lung cancer survival, and this has led to the hypothesizing that African Americans had a biologically more aggressive cancer. The LCCS found that African Americans patients had worse survival in advance lung cancer ($HR_{black\ vs\ white}$ = 1.17, 95 per cent CI 1.00–1.37; p = 0.046) and had worse distributions of most prognostic factors measured, and adjustment for the factors listed in Table 9.2 explained away all of the disparity in survival, negating the need for a biologic hypothesis.[5, 6]

Table 9.2 Multivariate Cox proportional hazards model hazard ratios for predictors of all causes survival in advanced lung cancer (Lung Cancer Comorbidity Study data (9); N = 648; c statistic = 0.733).

Predictor Variable	Distribution	Hazard ratio (95 per cent CI; p-value)
Age (per 10 years)	mean = 66.4 (SD = 10.6)	1.14 (1.04–1.25; p = 0.005)
Smoking (current smoker at diagnosis)	49.1 per cent	1.28 (1.07–1.52; p = 0.006)
Illicit drug use (yes vs no)	2.3 per cent	1.79 (1.08–2.96; p = 0.02)
Stage (IV vs III and unstaged)	51.9 per cent	2.00 (1.67–2.40; p = < 0.001)
Histology (adenocarcinoma vs squamous cell)	32.6 per cent	1.26 (0.99–1.59; p = 0.06)
Histology (bronchioloalveolar vs squamous cell)	0.8 per cent	0.64 (0.24–1.76; p = 0.39)
Histology (not otherwise specified vs squamous cell)	26.5 per cent	1.30 (1.02–1.67; p = 0.04)
Histology (SCLC vs squamous cell)	15.7 per cent	1.62 (1.22–2.16; p = 0.001)
Adverse symptoms (trilevel: 0, 1, ≥2)	20.2, 39.8, 40.0 per cent	1.40 (1.25–1.58; p = < 0.001)
Adverse comorbidity (trilevel: 0, 1, ≥2)	40.7, 34.9, 24.4 per cent	1.25 (1.11–1.41; p = < 0.001)
Surgery (yes vs no)	12.3 per cent	0.62 (0.46–0.85; p = 0.003)
Chemotherapy (yes vs no)	52.9 per cent	0.42 (0.34–0.50; p= < 0.001)
Radiation therapy (yes vs no)	49.4 per cent	0.90 (0.76–1.07; p = 0.23)

Germline polymorphisms

Many germline polymorphisms have been studied as susceptibility factors increasing risk of lung cancer, and some have been studied as prognostic factors. To date few have been demonstrated unequivocally to be associated with cancer prognosis.[7]

Host-related acquired factors – sociodemographic and exposure factors

Socioeconomic status (SES) and marital status (being spouseless) are often found to be associated with survival in univariate analysis when all stages of lung cancer are included in analysis. However, the impact of SES and marital status are mediated by other prognostic factors, in particular stage and treatment. When analysis of SES and marital status are restricted to advanced disease and are adjusted for receipt of treatment, their effects are usually modest and not significant. This was the case in the LCCS.

Peri- and post-diagnosis smoking

A growing body of research has found that current smoking at diagnosis and/or continued smoking following diagnosis is independently associated with reduced lung cancer survival. In the LCCS in advanced lung cancer, adjusted from important covariates (Table 9.2), the hazard ratio for current smoking was 1.28 (95 per cent CI 1.07–1.52; p = 0.006).[8] The mechanism explaining this association is unclear, but appears to involve biological processes.

Illicit drug use

In the LCCS in advanced cases, adjusted for important covariates (Table 9.2), illicit drug use had a hazard ratio of 1.79 (95 per cent CI 1.08–2.96; p = 0.02). No illicit drug user with advanced lung cancer lived past 16.6 months, whereas 22.8 per cent of non-illicit drug users were alive at this follow-up time.

Clinical factors

Comorbidity is the occurrence of disease other than the index cancer under consideration and is present pre- or peri-diagnosis and is unrelated to cancer treatment. Some feel that the impact of advanced lung cancer is so devastating that it overrides the effects of comorbidity. Multivariate analyses have found that this is not the case. Comorbidity may act directly to reduce survival, may act to impede receipt of cancer treatment or aggressiveness of treatment, and additionally may combine with the effects of lung cancer to shorten survival. The LCCS evaluated the impact of 56 comorbidities on lung cancer survival.[5, 9] Eighteen comorbidities were independently associated with reduced survival. When analysis was restricted to advanced disease (stage III and IV NSCLC and SCLC), all 18 demonstrated elevated hazard ratios. Ten of eighteen adverse comorbidities had significantly elevated hazard ratios and four demonstrated trends to significance. Predictive comorbidities included HIV/AIDS, tuberculosis, previous metastatic cancer, thyroid/glandular disease, electrolyte/mineral imbalance, anaemia, blood disorder, dementia, neurologic disease, congestive heart failure, chronic obstructive pulmonary disease, asthma, pulmonary fibrosis/interstitial disease, liver disease, gastrointestinal bleeding, renal disease, connective tissue/musculoskeletal disease, and osteoporosis. For lung cancer patients with advanced disease, the median survivals for patients with 0, 1 or ≥ 2 adverse comorbidities were 9.97, 6.30, and 4.37 months, respectively. Adjusted for the covariates listed in Table 9.1, adverse comorbidity as a tri-level variable (0, 1, and ≥2) had a hazard ratio of 1.25 (95 per cent CI 1.11–1.41; p < 0.001). Comorbidity is a powerful predictor of survival.

Functional/performance status at time of cancer diagnosis is a summary metric that captures effects due to a number of prognostic factors, including age-related decline, comorbid conditions, and cancer-related loss of function, as well as additional difficult to measure factors. Functional status can be measured using a number of scales, including the Karnofsky score, and the Eastern Cooperative Oncology Group Performance Status Scale (ECOG PS), and is built into many quality of life instruments, including the lung cancer-specific European Organization for the Research and Treatment of Cancer Quality of Life Questionnaire and Lung Cancer Module (QLQ-LC13) and the Functional Assessment of Chronic Illness Therapy – Lung (FACIT-L). Regardless of scale used, functional status has been found in multiple studies to be an important, usually independent, predictor of survival.

Quality of life (QOL) is a measure that usually incorporates functional status, but assesses additional constructs, including psychological and social well-being. A number of studies have found that QOL is a significant, independent predictor of survival in cancer patients[10] and in advanced lung cancer patients.[11] It is unclear as to how important the non-performance status components of QOL are, in particular after adjustment for age, comorbidity and variables reflecting extent of cancer.

Clinical factors – cancer-associated

Stage

AAJC/International Union Against Cancer (IUCC) TNM staging measures anatomic extent of disease and is the single most important predictor of lung cancer survival. Even within advanced lung cancers, staging is an important independent predictor of disease, and this includes comparisons of stage III vs IV; IIIA vs IIIB[12]); levels of T and N.[13] In addition, location and increasing number of metastatic sites involved[14–16] and liver metastases[17] were associated with reduced survival. Malignant pleural effusion is a negative prognostic factor.[18, 19]

Symptoms

Cancer-related pretreatment symptoms are a pathophysiologic measure of extent of cancer. As a measure of extent of cancer, they generally correlate with stage, but in addition are an independent predictor of lung cancer survival.[20] In the LCCS, hoarseness, hemoptysis, dyspnoea, non-cardiac chest pain, extrathoracic pain, neurologic symptom, weight loss, and weakness/fatigue were significantly associated with higher stage and/or shorter survival. In advanced lung cancer, adjusted for important covariates (Table 9.2), having one or more of these adverse symptoms versus none had a hazard ratio of 1.68 (95 per cent CI 1.35–2.10; $p < 0.001$).

Histology (advanced NSCLC vs extensive SCLC).

Extensive stage SCLC appears to have worse prognosis than advanced stage NSCLC. In the LCCS, adjusted for covariates (Table 9.2), the hazard ratio for SCLC compared to other histologic types pooled was 1.38 (95 per cent CI 1.08–1.75; $p = 0.01$).

Clinicopathologic laboratory findings

Numerous clinical laboratory findings have been reported to be associated with reduced survival, including hypercalcaemia, anaemia, low haemoglobin, abnormal serum lactate dehydrogenase levels, low albumin, perturbations in coagulation factors and proteinuria (for references see Brundage et al.[21]). Although numerous studies have found that laboratory results are prognostic, Watine concluded that the biomedical literature does not support routine use of laboratory variables as prognostic factors.[22]

Tumour-associated alterations/biomarkers

With the remarkable development of molecular biology and accompanying technology in the 1980s and 1990s, a plethora of genetic alterations and other biomarkers have been evaluated for their prognostic potential in lung cancer patients. A large number of them appear to be isolated, exploratory findings that have yet to be validated. For many of the more common genetic alterations occurring in lung cancer, enough study data has accumulated in recent years to enable systematic review and meta-analysis to provide a more reliable insight into their true prognostic potential. Isolated individual findings are too numerous and of too little practical value to list here. The results of selected meta-analyses are presented.

Ki-67 is a nuclear protein involved in cell proliferation. Meta-analysis concluded that Ki-67 expression was a significant associated with reduced lung cancer survival.[23] No assessment was presented for advanced disease alone.

In lung cancer cells, aneuploidy or DNA content abnormalities, which are thought to reflect high genomic instability, are common. Meta-analysis assessing the survival effect of aneuploidy on the survival of patients with resected lung cancers found a significant deleterious effect.[24]

CYFRA 21-1 is a cytokeratin 19 fragment. Meta-analysis found that elevated pretreatment serum CYFRA 21-1 levels were a significant predictor of reduced survival in NSCLC patients[25] This meta-analysis used individual updated data (n = 2063) and adjusted for the effects of important covariates, including age, stage and performance status. In addition, CYFRA 21-1 was significantly predictive of reduced survival in non-resected cases (HR = 1.78, 95 per cent CI 1.54–2.07; p < 0.0001).

Tumour microvessel density putatively reflects tumour angiogenesis, which is required for tumour growth. Meta-analysis found microvessel density was significantly associated with reduced survival in surgically resected NSCLC.[26] Data was not available to draw conclusions regarding associations in advanced disease.

The *p53* tumour suppressor gene product is involved with cell cycle regulation, apoptosis and stabilization of the genome. Meta-analysis concluded that *p53* alterations were associated with reduced lung cancer survival overall and in stage III-IV NSCLC (HR = 1.48, 95 per cent CI 21.29–1.70).[27]

Meta-analysis found that Bcl-2, an anti-apoptotic protein, overexpression was associated with improved NSCLC survival.[28] These findings did not apply to SCLC, nor were advanced cancers evaluated separately.

The RAS proto-oncogene is involved in signal transduction and cell proliferation. Meta-analysis found that KRAS2 mutations or overexpression of the RAS gene product, p21 protein, was associated with significantly worse survival in NSCLC (HR 1.35, 95 per cent CI 1.16–1.56).[29] Results were not available for advanced disease.

The *HER-2/neu* gene codes for a receptor-type tyrosine protein kinase (c-erbB-2), which is involved in regulation of normal cell growth and differentiation. Amplification of the *HER-2* gene and overexpression of the protein receptor is observed in a spectrum of cancers. Meta-analysis of c-erbB-2 (*HER2neu*) expression found that overexpression was associated with reduced survival but the investigators concluded that this finding could be due to bias.[30]

Epithelial growth factor receptor (EGF-R) is a cell surface receptor that is known to heterodimerize with HER2 receptor, and EGF-R overexpression is involved in local tumour growth. Meta-analysis of EGF-R expression did not indicate an association with survival in lung cancer.[31]

The findings of these meta-analyses must be interpreted with caution, as several limitations apply. When aggregate data are pooled, there is inadequate control of confounding variables. For example, associations exist between *p53* alterations and higher stage, T, and N, which are powerful predictors of survival, and inadequate adjustment for stage is expected to lead to residual confounding.[32] Most studies fail altogether to adjust for important prognostic factors, such as comorbidity, symptoms, and smoking history. Stratification of models by levels of a potential confounder often leads to small uninformative strata. Most often only one or a few biomarkers are assessed at a time so a complete picture is not attained. Of particular concern in this discussion is that high-quality resected tumour samples are frequently unavailable for patients with advanced disease. Consequently, associations in advanced disease have been less well studied. It is thought that the genetic alterations impact survival in early stage disease by fostering tumour progression. However, in advanced disease progression has already occurred and it is unclear whether biomarkers act additionally on further steps, such as metastases from metastases, which might explain biomarker association with reduced survival in advanced disease. One cannot assume that biomarkers that are predictive of survival in early disease have similar effects in advanced lung cancer.

Results of meta-analyses suggest that relationships may exist between Ki-67, tumour microvessel density (angiogenesis), Bcl-2, KRAS2 mutations/p21 protein overexpression, aneuploidy, CYFRA 21-1, and *p53* and lung cancer survival and for the latter three an association may exist in advanced disease. However, these biomarkers, as with other molecular biomarkers, have not been validated and developed to the point where they have widespread utility in clinical practice. Recent work relating tumour gene expression and tumour proteomic profiles to lung cancer survival has produced potentially exciting results. Again, refinement, validation and generalizability of findings have not advanced to the point where they can be usefully applied in clinical practice.

Therapies affecting prognosis

Therapy for advanced NSCLC and extensive SCLC differ and are discussed separately.

Advanced NSCLC

For patients with advanced NSCLC that are free of significant systemic manifestations or comorbidities, chemotherapy has been shown to improve median survival time when compared to best supportive care alone.[33]

Non-resectable stage III NSCLC

Many randomized studies of patients with non-resectable stage III NSCLC show that treatment with neoadjuvant or concurrent cisplatin-based chemotherapy and chest irradiation is associated with improved survival compared with radiation treatment alone. A meta-analysis of patient data from 11 randomized clinical trials showed that cisplatin-based combinations plus radiation therapy resulted in a 13 per cent reduction in risk of death compared to radiation therapy alone.[33]

Stage IV NSCLC

Randomized trials have found that cisplatin-based chemotherapy provides modest benefits in short-term survival compared with supportive care alone in patients with inoperable stage IIIB or IV disease,[33] see Figure 9.1. Cisplatin-based chemotherapy appears superior to alternative therapeutic agents. In a randomized trial of 612 patients, the median survival for the vinorelbine and cisplatin treatment arm was 40 weeks compared to 31 weeks for the vinorelbine alone arm (p = 0.01).[34] Although side-effects may vary, generally outcomes have been similar with most platinum-based therapies. A prospective randomized trial compared four platinum-based chemotherapy regimens for advanced NSCLC (cisplatin + paclitaxel, cisplatin + gemcitabine, cisplatin + docetaxel, and carboplatin + paclitaxel). No significant differences in survival were found, with the median survival being

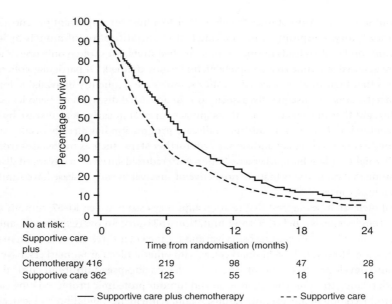

Figure 9.1 Survival in trials of supportive care versus supportive care plus chemotherapy (only trials using regimens based on cisplatin).[33] Non-small Cell Lung Cancer Collaboration Group. Chemotherapy in non-small cell lung cancer: a meta-analysis using updated data on individual patients from 52 randomised clinical trials. *BMJ* 1995; 311(7010):899–999.

7.9 months.[35] At this time no platinum-based chemotherapy combination can be regarded as standard therapy. Response and survival are greater in patients with good performance status and a limited number of metastatic sites.

In older patients who have age-related reduction in functional reserves of many organs, with or without significant comorbidity, cisplatin-based combination chemotherapy may be contraindicated. Alternative therapies have been effective. In a randomized trial of patients > 70 years with advanced NSCLC, single-agent vinorelbine yielded superior survival when compared with supportive care alone (28 vs 21 weeks).[36] In patients with contraindications to platinum-based regimens, evidence indicates that single-agent vinorelbine or single-agent gemcitabine work as effectively as nonplatinum combinations.

Extensive SCLC

Combination chemotherapy, containing two or more drugs, is the cornerstone treatment of extensive SCLC, and optimal response often requires treatment with at least moderate toxicity, when possible. Comparably effective combination chemotherapy regimens are presented at the US National Cancer Institute website: www.cancer.gov/cancertopics/pdq/treatment/small-cell-lung/healthprofessional. Optimal combinations of agents are still under investigation. A phase III Japanese study found that irinotecan plus cisplatin significantly improved survival compared to etoposide plus cisplatin. The median survival and proportion surviving two years were 12.8 months and 19.5 per cent in the irinotecan plus cisplatin arm compared to 9.4 months and 5.2 per cent in the etoposide plus cisplatin arm.[37]

Duration of chemotherapy longer than six months or instituting maintenance chemotherapy has not been associated with prolonged survival. Radiation therapy plays an important role in palliation of symptoms related to primary tumour and metastatic disease, but chest irradiation combined with chemotherapy has not been shown to improve survival when compared to chemotherapy alone. Patients who have achieved complete remission following treatment can be considered for prophylactic cranial irradiation (PCI). Approximately 60 per cent of patients whose SCLC have been controlled develop SCLC brain metastasis within two years post treatment. A meta-analysis (N = 987) found that the PCI treated patients survived longer than the control arm: 3-year survival proportions 20.7 vs 15.3 per cent (HR = 0.84; 95 per cent CI 0.73–0.97; p = 0.01).[38]

Data from clinical trials in advanced lung cancer generally indicate that increased survival due to treatment can be measured in weeks or a limited number of months and generally median survival seldom exceeds one year. It should be noted that these figures may represent the upper limit at the current time, because clinical trials often are restricted to healthier patients who have the potential to respond if a treatment regimen works. Clinical trials frequently exclude subjects who are too old, who have significant comorbidity burdens or who have impaired performance status.

Short-term prognosis

Generally, over 50 per cent of patients have died within 1 year, 85 per cent within 2 years and 3-year survival proportions ranges from 2–7 per cent.

Long-term prognosis

The long-term prognosis for patient with advanced lung cancer is grave, with 5-year survival proportions being 5 and 1 per cent, for stage IIIB and IV disease, respectively.

References

1. Harrell FE, Jr., Lee KL, Mark DB. Multivariable prognostic models: issues in developing models, evaluating assumptions and adequacy, and measuring and reducing errors. *Stat Med* 1996; 15(4):361–87.

2. Jemal A, Murray T, Ward E, Samuels A, Tiwari RC, Ghafoor A, *et al.* Cancer statistics, 2005. *CA Cancer J Clin* 2005; 55(1):10–30.

3. Mountain CF. Revisions in the international system for staging lung cancer [see comments]. *Chest* 1997; 111(6):1710–7.

4. American Cancer Society. *Cancer facts and figures 2005*. Atlanta, GA: American Cancer Society, 2005.

5. Tammemagi CM, Neslund-Dudas C, Simoff M, Kvale P. In lung cancer patients, age, gender, race-ethnicity and smoking predict adverse comorbidity, which in turn predicts lung cancer treatment and survival. *Journal of Clinical Epidemiology* 2004; 57(6):597–609.

6. Tammemagi CM, Neslund-Dudas C, Simoff M, Kvale P. Lung carcinoma symptoms – an independent predictor of survival and an important mediator of African-American disparity in survival. *Cancer* 2004; 101(7):1655–63.

7. Erichsen HC, Chanock SJ. SNPs in cancer research and treatment. *Br J Cancer* 2004; 90(4):747–51.

8. Tammemagi CM, Neslund-Dudas C, Simoff M, Kvale P. Smoking and lung cancer survival – the role of comorbidity and treatment. *Chest* 2004; 125(1):27–37.

9. Tammemagi CM, Neslund-Dudas C, Simoff M, Kvale P. Impact of comorbidity on lung cancer survival. *Int J Cancer* 2003; 103(6):792–802.

10. Dancey J, Zee B, Osoba D, Whitehead M, Lu F, Kaizer L. *et al.* Quality of life scores: an independent prognostic variable in a general population of cancer patients receiving chemotherapy. The National Cancer Institute of Canada Clinical Trials Group. *Qual Life Res* 1997; 6(2):151–8.

11. Ganz PA, Lee JJ, Siau J. Quality of life assessment. An independent prognostic variable for survival in lung cancer. *Cancer* 1991; 67(12):3131–5.

12. Kreisman H, Lisbona A, Olson L, Propert KJ, Modeas C, Dillman RO. *et al.* Effect of radiologic stage III substage on nonsurgical therapy of non-small cell lung cancer. *Cancer* 1993; 72(5):1588–96.

13. Mountain CF. New prognostic factors in lung cancer. Biologic prophets of cancer cell aggression. *Chest* 1995; 108(1):246–54.

14. Albain KS, Crowley JJ, LeBlanc M, Livingston RB. Survival determinants in extensive-stage non-small-cell lung cancer: the Southwest Oncology Group experience. *J Clin Oncol* 1991; 9(9):1618–26.

15. Thorogood J, Bulman AS, Collins T, Ash D. The use of discriminant analysis to guide palliative treatment for lung cancer patients. *Clin Oncol (R Coll Radiol)* 1992; 4(1):22–6.

16. Thomas M, Rube C, Semik M, von Eiff M, Klinke F, Macha HN. *et al.* Trimodality therapy in stage III non-small cell lung cancer: prediction of recurrence by assessment of p185neu. *Eur Respir J* 1999; 13(2):424–9.

17. Hilsenbeck SG, Raub WA, Jr., Sridhar KS. Prognostic factors in lung cancer based on multivariate analysis. *Am J Clin Oncol* 1993; 16(4):301–9.

18. Naito T, Satoh H, Ishikawa H, Yamashita YT, Kamma H, Takahashi H. *et al.* Pleural effusion as a significant prognostic factor in non-small cell lung cancer. *Anticancer Res* 1997; 17(6D):4743–6.

19. Sugiura S, Ando Y, Minami H, Ando M, Sakai S, Shimokata K. Prognostic value of pleural effusion in patients with non-small cell lung cancer. *Clin Cancer Res* 1997; 3(1):47–50.

20. Feinstein AR, Wells CK. A clinical-severity staging system for patients with lung cancer. *Medicine (Baltimore)* 1990; 69(1):1–33.

21. Brundage MD, Davies D, Mackillop WJ. Prognostic factors in non-small cell lung cancer: a decade of progress. *Chest* 2002; 122(3):1037–57.

22. Watine J. Managing patients with lung cancer. Biomedical literature does not support routine use of laboratory variables as prognostic factors. *BMJ* 2000; 320(7231):379–80.

23. Martin B, Paesmans M, Mascaux C, Berghmans T, Lothaire P, Meert AP. *et al.* Ki-67 expression and patients survival in lung cancer: systematic review of the literature with meta-analysis. *Br J Cancer* 2004; 91(12):2018–25.

24. Choma D, Daures JP, Quantin X, Pujol JL. Aneuploidy and prognosis of non-small-cell lung cancer: a meta-analysis of published data. *Br J Cancer* 2001; 85(1):14–22.

25. Pujol JL, Molinier O, Ebert W, Daures JP, Barlesi F, Buccheri G. *et al.* CYFRA 21-1 is a prognostic determinant in non-small cell lung cancer: results of a meta-analysis in 2063 patients. *Br J Cancer* 2004; 90(11):2097–105.

26. Meert AP, Paesmans M, Martin B, Delmotte P, Berghmans T, Verdebout JM. *et al.* The role of microvessel density on the survival of patients with lung cancer: a systematic review of the literature with meta-analysis. *Br J Cancer* 2002; 87(7):694–701.

27. Steels E, Paesmans M, Berghmans T, Branle F, Lemaitre F, Mascaux C. *et al.* Role of p53 as a prognostic factor for survival in lung cancer: a systematic review of the literature with a meta-analysis. *Eur Respir J* 2001; 18(4):705–19.

28. Martin B, Paesmans M, Berghmans T, Branle F, Ghisdal L, Mascaux C. *et al.* Role of Bcl-2 as a prognostic factor for survival in lung cancer: a systematic review of the literature with meta-analysis. *Br J Cancer* 2003; 89(1):55–64.

29. Mascaux C, Iannino N, Martin B, Paesmans M, Berghmans T, Dusart M. *et al.* The role of RAS oncogene in survival of patients with lung cancer: a systematic review of the literature with meta-analysis. *Br J Cancer* 2005; 92(1):131–9.

30. Meert AP, Martin B, Paesmans M, Berghmans T, Mascaux C, Verdebout JM. *et al.* The role of HER-2/neu expression on the survival of patients with lung cancer: a systematic review of the literature. *Br J Cancer* 2003; 89(6):959–65.

31. Meert AP, Martin B, Delmotte P, Berghmans T, Lafitte JJ, Mascaux C. *et al.* The role of EGF-R expression on patient survival in lung cancer: a systematic review with meta-analysis. *Eur Respir J* 2002; 20(4):975–81.

32. Tammemagi MC, McLaughlin JR, Bull SB. Meta-analyses of p53 tumour suppressor gene alterations and clinicopathological features in resected lung cancers. *Cancer Epidemiol Biomarkers Prev* 1999; 8(7):625–34.

33. Non-small Cell Lung Cancer Collaborative Group Chemotherapy in non-small cell lung cancer: a meta-analysis using updated data on individual patients from 52 randomised clinical trials. *BMJ* 1995; 311(7010):899–909.

34. Le Chevalier T, Brisgand D, Douillard JY, Pujol JL, Alberola V, Monnier A. *et al.* Randomized study of vinorelbine and cisplatin versus vindesine and cisplatin versus vinorelbine alone in advanced non-small-cell lung cancer: results of a European multicenter trial including 612 patients. *J Clin Oncol* 1994; 12(2):360–7.

35. Schiller JH, Harrington D, Belani CP, Langer C, Sandler A, Krook J. *et al.* Comparison of four chemotherapy regimens for advanced non-small cell lung cancer. *N Engl J Med* 2002; 346(2):92–8.

36. Effects of vinorelbine on quality of life and survival of elderly patients with advanced non-small-cell lung cancer. The Elderly Lung Cancer Vinorelbine Italian Study Group. *J Natl Cancer Inst* 1999; 91(1):66–72.

37. Noda K, Nishiwaki Y, Kawahara M, Negoro S, Sugiura T, Yokoyama A. *et al.* Irinotecan plus cisplatin compared with etoposide plus cisplatin for extensive small cell lung cancer. *N Engl J Med* 2002; 346(2):85–91.

38. Auperin A, Arriagada R, Pignon JP, Le Pechoux C, Gregor A, Stephens RJ. *et al.* Prophylactic cranial irradiation for patients with small-cell lung cancer in complete remission. Prophylactic Cranial Irradiation Overview Collaborative Group. *N Engl J Med* 1999; 341(7):476–84.

10

Colorectal cancer

Tony Geoghegan and Michael J. Lee

Introduction

In less than a decade, metastatic cancer of the colon or rectum has changed from being primarily a surgically palliated disease to one in which there has been increasing success with combination chemotherapy and molecular targeted therapy.

Colon cancer

Colon cancer is the third commonest malignancy in both sexes. Risk factors for the development of the disease include advanced age, cigarette smoking, inflammatory bowel disease and a genetic predisposition, namely, the hereditary and non-hereditary polyposis syndromes.

Factors affecting prognosis

The prognosis of colon cancer is determined by the depth of penetration of the tumour through the bowel wall, nodal involvement and the presence or absence of metastatic disease. The adverse prognostic indicators associated with colonic carcinoma include bowel obstruction and perforation.[1] An elevated pre-treatment level of carcinoembryonic antigen is associated with a poor prognosis.[2] Postoperative carcinoembryonic antigen is only of benefit in patients who are candidates for resection of pulmonary or hepatic metastases. The number of lymph nodes examined may also impact on patients' survival.

Evaluation of the patient for prognosis

Radiology

Plain film radiography retains an important role in evaluating the prognosis in patients with colorectal cancer as pulmonary or bone metastasis may be identified. Computed tomography (CT) plays a central role in the diagnosis and evlaution of recurrent disease. Fluoro-18-deoxyglucose-positron emission tomography (FDG-PET) has developed as an important imaging technique in patients with colorectal cancer. Advances in whole-body imaging with FDG-PET play an important role in determining prognosis by establishing which patients are suitable for further curative resection with recurrent hepatic disease. Positron emission tomography computed tomography (PET/CT) is superior to contrast-enhanced CT alone in the detection of recurrent disease following hepatectomy, extrahepatic metastases and local recurrence.[3] FDG-PET provides important prognostic information when equivocal findings arise with conventional imaging modalities.The sensitivity of FDG-PET may be reduced in the detection of recurrent colorectal metastases in patients undergoing cytotoxic therapy as chemotherapy may reduce the cellular uptake of FDG-PET.[4]

PET-CT influences clinical management and guides further intervention, namely biopsy, surgery, radiotherapy and excludes the requirement for further procedures influencing therapy and prognosis. Endorectal ultrasound plays a central role in the evaluation of the depth of invasion of rectal cancers, the detection of local lymph node enlargement, invasion of local structures and determining local recurrence following surgery.

Pre-operative magnetic resonance (MR) imaging with endorectal coils has a beneficial effect on patient outcome in rectal cancer by allowing patients with more advanced disease to undergo more radical surgery.

An aggressive surgical approach offers patients with pelvic recurrence from rectal and colon cancer the best potential for survival. The presence of hydronephrosis indicates a lower chance for complete surgical resection of the recurrence, but local control and improved survival may still be achieved.[5] Central pelvic recurrence is associated with better survival and is more resectable than pelvic side wall disease.

The utility of MR imaging in evaluating the prognostic factors for local recurrence of rectal cancer following curative resection have been studied. The presence of peri-rectal spiculate nodules and perivascular encasement on the pre-operative MR images are significant predictors of a local recurrence after curative surgery for a rectal carcinoma.[6] This suggests that pre-operative MR imaging can provide useful information to help in the planning of pre-operative adjuvant therapy. MRI can delineate tumour involvement of circumferential resection margin as this is predictive of curative resection margins(CRM)/R0 feasibility. Positive CRM on MRI imaging is an absolute indication for neo-adjuvant chemo-radiotherapy.

Interventional radiologists play an increasingly important role in the management of patients with non-operable colorectal cancer by placing colorectal stents in patients with malignant strictures of the bowel.

Pathology

Lymph node involvement is the most important prognostic factor in colorectal cancers, highlighting the importance of specimen examination. Incomplete lymph node evaluation can downstage the tumour and exclude the patient from adjuvant therapy, with detrimental effect on outcome.[7] Patients found to have lymph node metastasis after curative resection for CRC form a large and prognostically diverse group. Newland *et al.* have identified six pathological variables which act independently in determining the survival of patients with CRC and lymph node metastasis. The most potent variable was apical lymph node involvement, spread involving a free serosal surface, invasion beyond the muscularis propria, location in the rectum, venous invasion and high tumour grade.[8] In patients undergoing hepatectomy, infiltrative growth pattern of hepatic tumour is strongly correlated with a poor prognosis after hepatectomy.[9] Mucinous and signet-ring cell subtypes are stable and increasing, respectively. Importantly, it seems that the signet-ring cell subtype has worse outcomes, whereas survival rates for mucinous tumours are similar to adenocarcinomas.

Poorer survival among African-American patients in the United States with adenocarcinomas of the colon may not be attributable to an advanced pathologic stage of disease at diagnosis, but instead may be due to aggressive biologic features like high tumour grades. Recent studies have reported poor prognosis in colorectal carcinomas with non-polypoid growth pattern.[10] Colorectal carcinomas with non-polypoid growth pattern tend to show more malignant characteristics than those with polypoid growth pattern, explaining their poorer outcome.

The intensity of tumour budding at the invasive margin is suggested to be a significant pathologic index, indicating higher malignancy potential and an adverse prognostic indicator in patients with colon carcinoma.[11] Immature neo-vascularization is observed in poorly differentiated tumours and is correlated with metastasis, resulting in a poorer prognosis.[12]

Liver and pulmonary metastasis

Liver metastases are the major cause of death in colorectal resection for cancer. Metastatic disease to the liver will occur in approximately 50 per cent of patients with colon cancer. For patients with unresectable liver metastases radiofrequency ablation has developed as a safe technique associated with low morbidity and mortality rates. For patients considered suitable for liver resection for metatstatic disease, a negative resection margin has resulted in a 5-year survival rate of 25 per cent to 40 per cent.[13] In selected patients with coexisting limited pulmonary metastases and hepatic metastases, resection can be considered.

Colorectal liver metastases are unique because of the potential for cure. Presently surgical resection is the gold standard of treatment. Hepatic resection offers the best hope of survival for patients with CRC metastatic to the liver. Recurrences are observed in up to 60 per cent of patients after curative hepatic resection. The prime limitations in planning liver resection, beside the objective of a CRM/R0 situation, are safety aspects regarding comorbidity and acceptable extent of parenchyma loss are the most important features.[14] Shirabe et al. have recommended a surgical margin of more than 10 mm due to the risk of occult intrahepatic invasion.[15] Intrahepatic spread from liver metastases of colorectal cancer is well described. Its prognostic value after hepatectomy has been examined by Sasaki et al. In their study of 67 consecutive patients who underwent hepatectomy for metastasis from colorectal cancer, intrahepatic lymphatic invasion was shown to be an independent predictor of recurrence and death in this group of patients.[16] Adjuvant chemotherapy following hepatic resection has been shown to significantly improve survival and disease-free survival. However, no decrease in the recurrence rate in the remnant liver has been observed.[17] Assershon et al. studied the influence of the metastatic site as an additional predictor for response and outcome in advanced colorectal carcinoma.[18] The presence of liver metastasis was a better predictor of overall response to chemotherapy than either performance status or number of metastatic sites on presentation. The probability of response was significantly reduced by a raised carcino-embryonic antigen (CEA) and the presence of peritoneal metastases. In liver metastases, a normal serum albumin was as significant a predictor for response as good performance status. The most important factor for survival was initial performance status. The number of metastatic sites on presentation had no influence on survival. The site of metastasis can predict response to 5-FU-based chemotherapy. Patients with stage IV disease selected for elective palliative resection of asymptomatic colorectal cancers have substantial postoperative survival that was significantly better than those never having resection. Limited metastatic tumour burden and less extensive liver involvement were associated with better survival and a higher likelihood of benefit from elective bowel resection. Yamada et al. have shown that recurrence after hepatectomy is influenced by factors associated with the primary colorectal cancer rather than factors surrounding the first liver metastasis. In their study, venous invasion was the most important predictable factor for hepatic-only second recurrence.[19] Weber et al. have shown that the proliferation index of cancer cells is a reliable prognostic factor after hepatectomy in patients with CRC metastasis.[20] Development of an anastomotic leak is associated with worse long-term survival after potentially curative resection for colorectal cancer. Needle-track deposits are common after biopsy of suspected colorectal liver metastases. Biopsy of metastases confers poorer long-term survival on patients after liver resection and cannot be justified in patients with potentially resectable disease.[21] In the regional management of isolated colorectal metastases, staging laparoscopy with intra-operative ultrasound avoids unnecessary laparotomy and influences definitive surgical intervention.

Over the years there have been extensive efforts in devising new modalities of treatment for this disease. These include methods to increase the resectability such as portal vein embolization and two-stage surgery, with newer drugs and methods such chronotherapy and hepatic artery infusion chemotherapy, newer methods of radiotherapy, local ablative therapies such as cryoablation, radiofrequency ablation, microwave ablation and laser interstitial thermal therapy, and biological therapy. In patients with unresectable colorectal metastases, cryosurgery and radiofrequency ablation can be used in isolation or as an effective adjunct to resection in achieving complete clearance of the liver. Both the median overall survival and 5-year survival rates seem to be improved.

Age

While colorectal cancer is predominantly a disease of the elderly population, the prognosis in patients under the age of 40 has been controversial. A distal location of the tumour and advanced stage are considered poor prognostic indicators for overall survival.[22] Young age is not a poor prognostic marker in colorectal cancer. In addition to radical surgery, venous invasion and tumour grade are predictors of poor survival in patients under 50 years of age.[23]

Laboratory markers

Pre-operative CEA levels are less likely to be elevated in patients with poorly differentiated colorectal cancers. The value of monitoring CEA levels after initial surgery lies in determining which group of patients may benefit from additional surgery with curative intent. The expression of multiple tissue antigens is associated with shorter disease-free survival.

Serum carbohydrate antigen CA19–9 has been reported as the most significant prognostic indicator of metastatic colorectal cancer. Kohne *et al.* performed a multivariate analysis to identify factors which may allow prediction of outcome in patients treated with 5-fluorouracil (5-FU)-based therapy. Variables associated with a worse prognostic outcome included platelet count in excess of 400×10^9, alkaline phosphatase > 300 IU/l, white blood cell count $> 10 \times 10^9$/l and haemoglobin $< 11 \times 10^9$/l. Negative predictors also included a number of tumour sites – more than one or more than two, presence of liver metastasis or peritoneal carcinomatosis and the presence of lung metastasis. The authors recommend that patients may be divided into three risk groups – low, intermediate and high – depending on four baseline clinical parameters: performance status, WBC count, alkaline phosphatase and the number of metastatic sites.[24] Yuste *et al.* performed a retrospective review of 91 patients with colorectal metastasis treated with bolus 5-fluorouracil-based chemotherapy. They confirmed the prognostic value of performance status for both time to progression and survival. Alkaline phosphatase levels were significantly related to time to progression. Additional factors influencing survival time included elevated tumour marker levels and the presence of liver metastasis.[25] The largest prognostic study of each tumour marker in advanced colorectal cancer has been performed by Webb *et al.*[26] Serum AFP and immunohistochemical stains beta HCG, CA 125 and C-erb B2 have no prognostic significance. Serums CEA, beta HCG and CA 125 in advanced colorectal cancer prior to chemotherapy convey an independent poor prognosis which may reflect not just tumour burden but aggressive biology. Deleted colon cancer protein expression in colorectal cancer metastasis has been studied in predicting outcome to palliative fluorouracil-based chemotherapy. Ascelle *et al.* showed that the expression of DCC protein in CRC metastasis is similar to that observed in the corresponding primary tumours and represents a dominant predictor of survival in patients with unresectable advanced CRC who are undergoing palliative FU-based chemotherapy.[27]

A series of biochemical and genetic markers are under evaluation as independent prognostic indicators of disease survival. CD24 is a cell adhesion molecule that has been implicated in metastatic tumour progression of various solid tumours. CD24 is commonly upregulated in colorectal cancer and is a new independent prognostic marker which corroborates the importance of CD24 in tumour progression of this disease.[28] Thrombospondin-1 is a negative prognostic factor for survival in resected colorectal liver metastases.[29] Elevated tumour vascular endothelial growth factor content may discriminate between early and late stages of colorectal cancer and may be used as an independent prognostic parameter in the management of these patients.[30] Pre-operative neutrophil-to-lymphocyte ratio may represent a simple method of identifying colorectal cancer patients with a poor prognosis pre-operatively.[31] Galectin-3 is a beta-galactoside-binding protein whose expression has been correlated with progression and metastasis in colon cancer. It is expressed at elevated levels in a variety of neoplastic cells and is an independent factor for prognosis in colorectal cancer.[32] Placenta growth factor expression correlates with disease progression and patient survival and may be used as a prognostic indicator for colorectal cancer.[33] The evaluation of molecular staging to discriminate good from poor prognosis patients, with the potential to direct adjuvant therapy, continues. Bcl-2 is a model apoptosis suppressor postulated to promote tumourigenesis. Recently, it has been reported that Bcl-2 undergoes phosphoregulation of its Ser70 to substantially alter its molecular function. Previous studies further suggest that such phospho-Bcl-2 regulation may influence tumour progression in colorectal and other cancers; however, phosphorylation status of the Ser70 of Bcl-2 (pSer70) *in vivo* in tumours remains obscure. Loss of pSer70 Bcl-2 expression is closely linked to biological aggressiveness in colorectal tumours and represents a statistically significant molecular index for prognosis of patients with these cancers.[34]

Therapies affecting prognosis

Surgery

The standard treatment for colon cancer is resection of the primary tumour and lymph nodes for local disease. No difference in survival has been identified between open and laparascopic techniques.[35] Surgery is curative in 25–40 per cent of highly selected patients who develop resectable metastases in the liver and lung. Improved surgical techniques and the advances in pre-operative imaging have allowed for better patient selection for resection.

Radiation therpay

In contrast to rectal cancer, the role of adjuvant radiation therapy for patients with colon cancer is not well defined.

Chemotherapy

The use of irinotecan and oxaliplatin have been extended from the treatment of recurrent or stage IV disease to local disease. Improved response rates and prolonged overall survival are achieved with irinotecan combined with 5-FU-leucovorin when compared to 5-FU-leucovorin alone.[36]

Patients with unresectable metastatic disease are treated with systemic chemotherapy. Surgical resection can be offered to patients with local disease and liver or pulmonary metastatic disease. Chemotherapy trials in patients with locally advanced, unresectable, or metastatic disease, typically with 5-FU-based regimens, demonstrate partial responses and prolongation of the time to progression of disease[37] in addition to improved survival and quality of life for patients receiving chemotherapy, compared to best supportive care.[38] Irinotecan combined with 5-FU-leucovorin has demonstrated improved survival in patients with advanced or metastatic disease compared with

5-FU-leucovorin alone, albeit with increased, yet controllable, toxic effects.[39] Newer colorectal cancer chemotherapy schemas are serving as the platform on which combined novel targeted agents such as inhibitors of the epidermal growth factor receptor and vascular endothelial growth factor are based.

Accepted first-line regimens are either irinotecan-based (IFL, FOLFIRI, AIO) or oxaliplatin-based (FOLFOX4, FOLFOX6). Second line chemotherapy is based on the choice of first line chemotherapy treatment. Patients who had been treated with a FOLFOX-based regimen as part of their first-line regimen should receive irinotecan-based chemotherapy for second-line treatment.

Rectal cancer

The prognosis of rectal cancer is determined by the extent of penetration of the tumour through the bowel wall and the presence of lymph node involvement. The TNM system is the internationally accepted standard for the staging of all solid cancers including cancer of the rectum and colon. Importantly, the TNM system does not provide information in relation to prognosis. The TNM classification is outlined in Box 10.1.

Box 10.1 The TNM tumour staging system

Primary tumour (T)

TX – Primary tumour cannot be assessed or depth of penetration not specified

T0 – No evidence of primary tumour

Tis – Carcinoma *in situ* (mucosal); intraepithelial or invasion of the lamina propria

T1 – Tumour invades submucosa

T2 – Tumour invades muscularis propria

T3 – Tumour invades through the muscularis propria into the subserosa or into non-peritonealized pericolic or perirectal tissue

T4 – Tumour perforates the visceral peritoneum or directly invades other organs or structures

Regional lymph nodes (N)

NX – Regional lymph nodes cannot be assessed

N0 – No regional lymph node metastasis

N1 – Metastasis in 1–3 pericolic or perirectal lymph nodes

N2 – Metastasis in four or more pericolic or perirectal lymph nodes

N3 – Metastasis in any lymph node along the course of a named vascular trunk

Distant metastasis (M)

MX – Presence of metastasis cannot be assessed

M0 – No distant metastasis

M1 – Distant metastasis

High-risk groups for rectal cancer include those with hereditary conditions including hereditary non-polyposis colon cancer (HNPPC), Lynch syndrome type I and II, familial polyposis and inflammatory bowel disease,[40, 41] a first-degree relative with colorectal cancer or adenomas, a personal history of colorectal, endometrial, breast or orvarian cancer.[42, 43]

Evaluation for prognosis

The accurate staging of rectal cancer influences treatment and prognosis by determining which patients are suitable for local excision or which patients require more extensive surgical management in addition to determining which patients require pre-operative radiotherapy or chemotherapy. The pre-operative staging of rectal cancer is based on clinical examination, CT, MRI and endoscopic ultrasound and biopsy.[44] Endoscopic ultrasound plays a central role in determing tumour stage and the status of perirectal nodes with accuracy of 95 per cent and 74 per cent respectively. The American Joint Committe on Cancer recommend a minimum of 12 lymph nodes for analysis to exclude the presence of nodal involvement by tumour[45–47] as the number of lymph nodes examined may influence prognosis.[48] Microsatellite instability has been associated with improved survival independent of tumour stage in a population-based study of 607 patients less than 50 years of age with colorectal carcinoma.[49]

Therapies affecting prognosis

Surgery

Surgical resection of the primary tumour and regional lymph nodes is the treatment for rectal cancer. Transanal resection is peformed for patients with superficial lesions, stage 0 and stage I rectal cancers with a T1 lesion. T1 and Tis lesions of the lower one-third of the rectal wall are amenable to transrectal excision. The presence of positive resection margins or local lymph node involvement necessitates definitive resection of the tumour.[50] The technique of resection may impact on local recurrence and failure rates between 4–8 per cent following rectal resection with appropriate mesorectal excision have been reported.[51] Total mesorectal excision with a colorectal or coloanal anastamosis avoids the need for abdominoperoneal resection and stoma formation.

Patients with Stage II and Stage III disease are at increased risk of local and systemic recurrence. Pre- and postoperative radiotherapy decrease local recurrence but have not been demonstrated to improve prognosis,[52] with the exception of a single trial which demonstrated a survival benefit from pre-operative radiotherapy in comparison to surgery.[53]

Radiation therapy and chemotherapy

Postoperative treatment regimens relate to the integration of chemotherapy and radiotherapy. The efficacy of postoperative radiotherapy and 5-FU chemotherapy in patients with stage ii and stage III rectal cancer has been established by a series of prospective randomized controlled trials,[54] demonstrating an increase in the disease free-interval and overall survival when chemotherapy is combined with radiotherapy postoperatively.

In patients with advanced disease, palliation may be achieved in 10–20 per cent of patients with 5-FU.[55] Several studies suggest an advantage when leucovorin is added to 5-FU in terms of response rate and palliation of symptoms but not always in terms of survival.[56] Irinotecan (CPT-11) has been approved by the US Food and Drug Administration for the treatment of patients whose tumours are refractory to 5-FU.[57] Oxaliplatin, alone or combined with 5-FU and leucovorin, has also shown activity in 5-FU refractory patients.[58]

Stage IV rectal cancer

Stage IV rectal cancer denotes distant metastatic spread of disease. Metastatic disease to the liver can be managed by hepatic resection, intra-arterial chemotherapy, cryotherapy, interstitial radiation and embolisation. Liver resection may be considered for patients with less than three hepatic metastases. The 5-year survival rates post-resection are between 20–40 per cent.[59]

For patients not suitable for liver resection, cryotherapy is associated with long-term tumour control.[60] The favourable prognostic indicators are a low level of the serum glycoprotein carcino-embryonic antigen level, no extrahepatic disease, lymph node negative primary tumour and clear resection margins. Resection of pulmonary and liver metastases may be considered in selected patients. The role of additional systemic therapy after potentially curative resection of liver metastases is uncertain. A trial of hepatic arterial floxuridine plus systemic fluorouracil (5-FU) plus leucovorin was shown to result in improved 2-year disease-free and overall survival (86 per cent versus 72 per cent, P = 0.03), but did not show a significant statistical difference in medial survival, compared to systemic 5-FU therapy alone.[61] Intra-arterial chemotherapy for liver metastases with floxuridine provides no survival benefit when combined with systemic chemotherapy.[62] 5-FU is considered to be the standard therapy for palliation in stage IV rectal cancer.[63] For patients who do not respond to 5-FU, irinotecan (CPT-11), a topoisomerase 1 inhibitor, is now considered to be standard therapy.[64]

For patients with local recurrence alone following initial attempted curative resection, aggressive local therapy with repeat low anterior resection and coloanal anastomosis, abdominoperineal resection, or posterior or total pelvic exenteration can lead to long-term disease-free survival.[65] Chemoradiotherapy may increase resectability for patients with advanced pelvic recurrence.[66] The presence of hydronephrosis is a contraindication to resection with curative intent.[67] Reflecting stage IV disease, in patients with recurrent rectal cancer, chemotherapy has been used for palliation with fluorouracil (5-FU)-based treatment and is considered to be standard therapy.[68] Similarly, irinotecan is now considered standard therapy for patients with stage IV disease who do not respond to or progress on 5-FU.[69] Raltitrexed (Tomudex) is a specific thymidylate synthase inhibitor which has demonstrated activity similar to that of bolus 5-FU and leucovorin.[70] Oxaliplatin, alone or combined with 5-FU and leucovorin, has shown promising activity in previously treated and untreated patients with metastatic colorectal cancer and in patients with 5-FU refractory disease.[71]

Short and long-term prognosis

Metastases from colorectal cancer are most often confined to the liver or lungs, in which 20–25 per cent may be resected with curative intent. Without treatment, no patients are alive after 4 years, whereas 30 per cent are alive 4 years after radical resection. Early use of chemotherapy increases survival, and about 20 per cent of patients may thus become suited for local therapy. The prognostigram curve for the survival of more than 23,000 cases of Stage IV colorectal cancer cases is shown in Figure 10.1.

After the primary operation, surveillance is recommended, with measurement of carcinoembryonal antigen every 3–6 months for 3 years, then every 6–12 months from years 3 to 5, plus ultrasound or CT scan every 6 months for 3 years, then yearly for up to 5 years. Clinical staging is the most important prognostic indicator.

A prognostic model to predict survival of patients presenting with metastatic colorectal carcinoma has recently been developed by a German group.[72] In asymptomatic patients not needing surgery, just 3 of 13 factors investigated proved to be independent predictors of survival: performance status, CEA level, and chemotherapy. In patients with symptomatic primary tumours

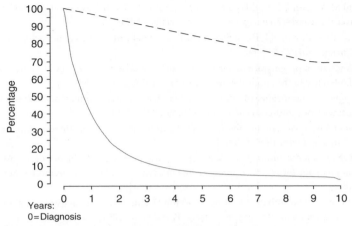

Figure 10.1 Prognostigram curve for survival of 23,676 cases of stage IV colorectal cancer cases

requiring palliative resection, three additional factors are significant: ASA-class, metastatic load, and extent of primary tumour.

References

1. Steinberg SM, Barkin JS, Kaplan RS. *et al.* Prognostic indicators of colon tumours. The Gastrointestinal Tumour Study Group experience. *Cancer* 1986; 57: 1866–70.

2. Filella X, Molina R, Grau JJ. *et al.* Prognostic value of CA 19.9 levels in colorectal cancer. *Ann Surg* 1992; 216: 55–9.

3. Wiering B *et al.* The impact of fluor-18-deoxyglucose-positron emission tomography in the management of colorectal metastases. *Cancer* 2005; 15:2658–70.

4. Akhurst T *et al.* Recent chemotherapy reduces the sensitivity of [18F] fluorodeoxyglucose positron emission tomography in the detection of colorectal metastases. *J Clin Oncol* 2005; 23:8713–16.

5. Larsen SG, Wiig JN, Giercksky KE. Hydronephrosis as a prognostic factor in pelvic recurrence from rectal and colon carcinomas. *Am J Surg* 2005; 190:55–60.

6. Oh YT *et al.* Assessment of the prognostic factors for a local recurrence of rectal cancer: the utility of preoperative MR imaging. *Korean J Radiol* 2005; 6:8–16.

7. Ratto C *et al.* Accurate lymph node detection in colorectal specimens resected for cancer is of prognostic significance. *Dis Colon Rectum* 1999; 42:143–54.

8. Newland RC *et al.* Pathological determinants of survival associated with colorectal cancer with lymph node metastases. A multivariate analysis of 579 patients. *Cancer* 1999; 73:2076–82.

9. Nagashima I, Oka T, Hamada C, Naruse K, Osada T, Muto T. Histopathological prognostic factors influencing long-term prognosis after surgical resection for hepatic metastases from colorectal cancer. *Am J Gastroeneterol* 1999; 94:739–43.

10. Labropoulou EP *et al.* Colorectal carcinoma: contribution of growth pattern on prognosis. *Tech Coloproctol* 2004; 8:208–10.

11. Park KJ. Intensity of tumor budding and its prognostic implications in invasive colon carcinoma. *Dis Colon Rectum* 2005; 48:1597–602.

12. Yonenaga Y *et al.* Absence of smooth muscle actin-positive pericyte coverage of tumor vessels correlates with hematogenous metastasis and prognosis of colorectal cancer patients. *Oncology* 2005; 69:159–66.

13. Jain S, Sacchi M, Vrachnos P, Lygidakis NJ, Andriopoulou E. Recent advances in the treatment of colorectal liver metastases. *Hepatogastroenterology* 2005; 52:1567–4.

14. Scheele J *et al.* Resection of colorectal liver metastases. What prognostic factors determine patient selection? *Chirurg* 2001; 72:547–60.

15. Shirabe K. Analysis of prognostic risk factors in hepatic resection for metastatic colorectal carcinoma with special reference to the surgical margin. *Br J Surg* 1997; 84:1077–80.

16. Sasaki A. Prognostic significance of intrahepatic lymphatic invasion in patients with hepatic resection due to metastases from colorectal carcinoma. *Cancer* 2002; 95:105–11.

17. Kokudo N *et al.* Effects of systemic and regional chemotherapy after hepatic resection for colorectal metastases. *Ann Surg Oncol* 1998; 5:706–12.

18. Assersohn L, Norman A, Cunningham D, Benepal T, Ross PJ, Oates J. Influence of metastatic site as an additional predictor for response and outcome in advanced colorectal carcinoma. *Br J Cancer* 1999; 79:1800–5.

19. Yamada H, Kondo S, Okushiba S, Morikawa T, Katoh H. Analysis of predictive factors for recurrence after hepatectomy for colorectal liver metastases. *World J Surg* 2001; 25:1129–33.

20. Weber JC. Is a proliferative index of cancer cells a reliable prognostic factor after hepatectomy in patients with colorectal liver metastases? *Am J Surg* 2001; 182:81–8.

21. Jones OM, Rees M, John TG, Bygrave S, Plant G. Biopsy of resectable colorectal liver metastases causes tumor dissemination and adversely affects survival after liver resection. *Br J Surg* 2005; 92:1165–8.

22. Alici S. Colorectal cancer in young patients: characteristics and outcome. *Tohoku J Exp Med* 2003; 199:85–93.

23. Makela J. Kiviniemi H, Laitinen S. Prognsotic factors after surgery in patients younger than 50 years old with colorectal adenocarcinoma. *Hepatogastroenterology* 2002; 49:971–5.

24. Kohne CH *et al.* Clinical determinants of survival in patients with 5-fluorouracil-based treatment for metastatic colorectal cancer: results of a multivariate analysis of 3825 patients. *Ann Oncol* 2002; 13:308–17.

25. Yuste AL. Analysis of clinical prognostic factors for survival and time to progression in patients with metastatic colorectal cancer treated with 5-fluorouracil-based chemotherapy. *Clin Colorectal Cancer* 2003; 2:231–4.

26. Webb A *et al.* The prognostic value of CEA, beta HCG, AFP, CA125, CA19–9 and C-erb B-2, beta HCG immunohistochemistry in advanced colorectal cancer. *Ann Oncol* 1995; 6:581–7.

27. Aschele C. Deleted in colon cancer protein expression in colorectal cancer metastases: a major predictor of survival in patients with unresectable metastatic disease receiving palliative fluorouracil-based chemotherapy. *J Clin Oncol* 2004; 22:3758–65.

28. Weichert W. Cytoplasmic CD24 expression in colorectal cancer independently correlates with shortened patient survival. *Clin Cancer Res* 2005; 11:6574–81.

29. Sutton CD. Expression of thrombospondin-1 in resected colorectal cancer predicts poor prognosis. *Clin Cancer Res* 2005; 11:6567–73.

30. Ferroni P. Prognostic value of vascular endothelial growth factor tumour tissue content of colorectal cancer. *Oncology* 2005; 69:145–53.

31. Walsh SR. Neutrophil-lymphocyte ratio as a prognostic factor in colorectal cancer. *J Surg Oncol* 2005; 91:181–4.

32. Endo K. Galectin-3 expression is a potent prognostic marker in colorectal cancer. *Anticancer Res* 2005; 25:3117–21.

33. Wei SC. Placenta growth factor expression is correlated with survival of patients with colorectal cancer. *Gut* 2005; 54:666–72.

34. Kondo E. Expression of phosphorylated Ser 70 of Bcl-2 correlates with malignancy in human colorectal neoplasms. *Clin Cancer Res* 2005; 11:7255–63.

35. Clinical Outcomes of Surgical Therapy Study Group. A comparison of laparoscopically assisted and open colectomy for colon cancer. *N Engl J Med* 2004; 350:2050–9.

36. Saltz LB, Cox JV, Blanke C. *et al*. Irinotecan plus fluorouracil and leucovorin for metastatic colorectal cancer. Irinotecan Study Group. *N Engl J Med* 2000; 343: 905–14.

37. Petrelli N, Herrera L, Rustum Y. *et al*. A prospective randomized trial of 5-fluorouracil versus 5-fluorouracil and high-dose leucovorin versus 5-fluorouracil and methotrexate in previously untreated patients with advanced colorectal carcinoma. *J Clin Oncol* 1987; 5:1559–65.

38. Scheithauer W, Rosen H, Kornek GV. *et al*. Randomised comparison of combination chemotherapy plus supportive care with supportive care alone in patients with metastatic colorectal cancer. *BMJ* 1993; 306:752–5.

39. Rothenberg ML, Eckardt JR, Kuhn JG. *et al*. Phase II trial of irinotecan in patients with progressive or rapidly recurrent colorectal cancer. *J Clin Oncol* 1996;14:1128–35.

40. Thorson AG, Knezetic JA, Lynch HT. A century of progress in hereditary nonpolyposis colorectal cancer (Lynch syndrome). *Dis Colon Rectum* 1999; 42:1–9.

41. Smith RA, von Eschenbach AC, Wender R. *et al*. American Cancer Society guidelines for the early detection of cancer: update of early detection guidelines for prostate, colorectal, and endometrial cancers. *Cancer J Clin* 2001; 51:38–75.

42. Ransohoff DF, Lang CA. Screening for colorectal cancer. *N Engl J Med* 1991; 325:37–41.

43. Fuchs CS, Giovannucci EL, Colditz GA. *et al*. A prospective study of family history and the risk of colorectal cancer. *N Engl J Med* 1994; 331:1669–74.

44. Snady H, Merrick MA. Improving the treatment of colorectal cancer: the role of EUS. *Cancer Invest* 1998; 16:572–81.

45. Colon and rectum. In American Joint Committee on Cancer, *AJCC cancer staging manual,* 6th edn, pp. 113–24. New York: Springer, 2002.

46. Compton CC, Greene FL. The staging of colorectal cancer: 2004 and beyond. *CA Cancer J Clin* 54; 2004:295–308.

47. Nelson H, Petrelli N, Carlin A. *et al*. Guidelines 2000 for colon and rectal cancer surgery. *J Natl Cancer Inst* 2001; 93:583–96.

48. Swanson RS, Compton CC, Stewart AK. *et al*. The prognosis of T3N0 colon cancer is dependent on the number of lymph nodes examined. *Ann Surg Oncol* 2003; 10:65–71.

49. Gryfe R, Kim H, Hsieh ET. *et al*. Tumour micro satellite instability and clinical outcome in young patients with colorectal cancer. *N Engl J Med* 2000; 342:69–77.

50. Lopez-Kostner F, Lavery IC, Hool GR. *et al*. Total mesorectal excision is not necessary for cancers of the upper rectum. *Surgery* 1998; 24:612–7.

51. MacFarlane JK, Ryall RD, Heald RJ. Mesorectal excision for rectal cancer. *Lancet* 1993; 341:457–60.

52. Medical Research Council Rectal Cancer Working Party. Randomised trial of surgery alone versus radiotherapy followed by surgery for potentially operable locally advanced rectal cancer. *Lancet* 1996; 348:1605–10.

53. Martling A, Holm T, Johansson H. *et al*. The Stockholm II trial on preoperative radiotherapy in rectal carcinoma: long-term follow-up of a population-based study. *Cancer* 2001; 92:896–902.

54. Thomas PR, Lindblad AS. Adjuvant postoperative radiotherapy and chemotherapy in rectal carcinoma: a review of the Gastrointestinal Tumour Study Group experience. *Radiother Oncol* 1988; 13:245–52.

55. Erlichman C, Fine S, Wong A. *et al*. A randomized trial of fluorouracil and folinic acid in patients with metastatic colorectal carcinoma. *J Clin Oncol* 1988;6:469–75.

56. Doroshow JH, Multhauf P, Leong L. *et al*. Prospective randomized comparison of fluorouracil versus fluorouracil and high-dose continuous infusion leucovorin calcium for the treatment of advanced measurable colorectal cancer in patients previously unexposed to chemotherapy. *J Clin Oncol* 1990; 8:491–501.

57. Conti JA, Kemeny NE, Saltz LB. *et al.* Irinotecan is an active agent in untreated patients with metastatic colorectal cancer. *J Clin Oncol* 1996; 14:709–15.

58. de Gramont A, Vignoud J, Tournigand C. *et al.* Oxaliplatin with high-dose leucovorin and 5-fluorouracil 48-hour continuous infusion in pre-treated metastatic colorectal cancer. *Eur J Cancer* 1997; 33:214–9.

59. Scheele J, Stangl R, Altendorf-Hofmann A. *et al.* Indicators of prognosis after hepatic resection for colorectal secondaries. *Surgery* 1991; 110:13–29.

60. Ravikumar TS, Kaleya R, Kishinevsky A. Surgical ablative therapy of liver tumours. *Cancer: Principles and Practice of Oncology Updates* 2000; 14:1–12.

61. Kemeny N, Huang Y, Cohen AM. *et al.* Hepatic arterial infusion of chemotherapy after resection of hepatic metastases from colorectal cancer. *N Engl J Med* 1999; 341:2039–48.

62. Wagman LD, Kemeny MM, Leong L. *et al.* A prospective, randomized evaluation of the treatment of colorectal cancer metastatic to the liver. *J Clin Oncol* 1990; 8:1885–93.

63. Moertel CG: Chemotherapy for colorectal cancer. *N Engl J Med* 1994; 330:1136–42.

64. Cunningham D, Pyrhonen S, James RD. *et al.* A phase III multicenter randomized study of CPT-11 versus supportive care (SC) alone in patients (Pts) with 5FU-resistant metastatic colorectal cancer (MCRC). *Proceedings of the American Society of Clinical Oncology* 1998; 17:A-1, 1a.

65. Ogunbiyi OA, McKenna K, Birnbaum EH. *et al.* Aggressive surgical management of recurrent rectal cancer – is it worthwhile? *Dis Colon Rectum* 1997; 40:150–5.

66. Lowy AM, Rich TA, Skibber JM. *et al.* Preoperative infusional chemoradiation, selective intraoperative radiation, and resection for locally advanced pelvic recurrence of colorectal adenocarcinoma. *Ann Surg* 1996; 223:177–85.

67. Rodriguez-Bigas MA, Herrera L, Petrelli NJ. Surgery for recurrent rectal adenocarcinoma in the presence of hydronephrosis. *Am J Surg* 1992; 164:18–21.

68. Moertel CG: Chemotherapy for colorectal cancer. *N Engl J Med* 1994; 330:1136–42.

69. Rothenberg ML, Eckardt JR, Kuhn JG. *et al.* Phase II trial of irinotecan in patients with progressive or rapidly recurrent colorectal cancer. *J Clin Oncol* 1996; 14:1128–35.

70. Cunningham D. Mature results from three large controlled studies with raltitrexed (Tomudex). *Br J Cancer* 1998; 77:15–21.

71. Cvitkovic E, Bekradda M. Oxaliplatin: a new therapeutic option in colorectal cancer. *Semin Oncol* 1999; 26:647–62.

72. Stelzner S, Hellmich G, Koch R, Ludwig K. Factors predicting survival in stage IV colorectal carcinoma patients after palliative treatment: a multivariate analysis. *J Surg Oncol* 2005; 89(4):211–7.

11

Breast cancer

Fabio Efficace and Laura Biganzoli

Introduction

Breast cancer ranks first amongst cancers affecting women throughout the world. More than 1,050,000 new breast cancer cases occur worldwide annually, with nearly 580,000 occurring in developed countries. In most developed countries, 5-year survival rates are higher than 70 per cent.[1] A greater percentage of patients are being diagnosed when curative approaches are still possible. However, approximately 10 per cent of newly diagnosed patients will present with metastatic disease and an additional 50–75 per cent will eventually relapse.[2] The treatment for metastatic disease, in spite of clinical responses to the various standard therapies (hormonal, chemotherapeutic, biological agents or their combination), is generally palliative and median survival is approximately 2 years.

Natural history of the condition

This represents the behaviour of the disease in breast cancer patients who have not been treated from the time of diagnosis until death. The main strength of these data is that they can provide the basis to compare the efficacy of a given treatment modality over the natural course of the disease. Nevertheless, it is difficult to rely on recent evidence regarding the natural course of the disease as the majority of breast cancer patients, regardless of the stage, are commonly treated.

Natural history data suggests that advanced breast cancer patients consist of a heterogeneous population whose prognoses depend on a number of host and tumour-related variables. Some patients with advanced disease might achieve prolonged survival coexisting with their disease, while others die rapidly after presentation. One of the most representative and accurate studies in this area was described by Bloom and colleagues[3] and examined the natural history of 250 untreated advanced breast cancer patients. In this study, 95 per cent of patients died with distant metastasis or extensive local cancer, whilst only 5 per cent of patients died of other non-cancer-related causes. Clinical staging was performed according to the Manchester system and 23.2 per cent and 74.4 per cent of patients were stage 3 and 4 respectively. Overall 97.6 per cent of these patients were characterized by clinical features that would result in a T3 or T4 classification according to the TNM staging system. As the majority of the patients were clinically staged as Manchester stage 4, it is likely that most of these had distant metastasis. The patients were observed at the Middlesex Hospital in London from 1805 to 1933 and survival was measured from the time of onset of symptoms until death. The median survival time was 2.7 years. In this study, the shortest duration of survival was 2 months (three cases) and the longest was 18 years and 3 months (one case). Survival rates at years 3, 5 and 10 were 44 per cent, 18 per cent and 4 per cent respectively. Less than 1 per cent of the patients survived 15 years. This research is also representative, as the survival figures are very similar to other published reports of untreated breast cancer patients. In the proportion of patients for which tumour grade was available

(86 out of 250 patients), Bloom and colleagues[3] also showed that survival was correlated to tumour grade. At 5 years 22 per cent of patients with grade I and II were still alive, whilst all those with grade III had died. The longest survival for patients with grade I was 166 months, whilst no patient with grade III survived for more than 53 months.

As for the pattern of spread, it is important to mention that breast cancer does metastasize broadly and lung, liver, and bones represent the most common sites of distant metastasis. The prognoses of patients who developed recurrent disease is also closely related to the site of relapse. Generally, patients with locoregional or bone only recurrences have more favourable prognoses than patients who relapse with visceral metastases.

Overall, the natural history literature on advanced disease also highlights that patients' quality of life (QOL) can be seriously compromised. Particularly, the final stages of life of these patients can be associated with suffering due to metastatic disease and patients may also experience a painful death. This evidence has also crucial implications when prioritizing treatment goals for metastatic breast cancer (MBC) patients. Thus, QOL represent a key issue to consider when deciding between various treatment options.

Factors affecting prognosis

The literature on the identification of prognostic factors for clinical outcomes in breast cancer is extensive, much of it focused on the investigation of variables associated with risk of relapse and factors predicting treatment response in early breast cancer. Relatively little interest has been paid to the investigation of prognostic factors for overall survival in MBC patients.

Studies in this area vary considerably with respect to a number of methodological issues, including the selection of patients, the availability of baseline clinical parameters, sample size and definition of outcome variables. Owing to this, it is difficult to compare findings among different researchers and identify a clear set of prognostic variables. Results are also contradictory in a number of studies and the prognostic impact of some factors is still under discussion. Whilst taking this into account, this paragraph provides an overview of some key variables that have been shown to independently predict survival in MBC patients in several multivariate analyses.

As an example of the variability of the studies in this area, it is worthy of note that the information about metastatic involvement is not uniform. Some studies have investigated the prognostic value of the specific location of the metastatic site, whilst others, for example, have classified the site of metastases into larger categories (visceral dominant sites, bone and soft tissue dominant sites). It is clear that the latter studies have made difficult a clear understanding of the prognostic role from a specific metastatic location and also a direct comparison with other findings. Nevertheless, the metastatic site has been shown to be an independent key prognostic factor for survival in MBC. Visceral involvement (mainly, liver, lung, brain and pleura) has been shown to predict worse prognosis.[4–8] In particular, metastases to the liver were found to be a strong prognostic factor for shorter survival in several multivariate analyses.[4, 5, 6, 8–10]

Dunphy and colleagues[8] found that in stage IV oestrogen receptor (ER) negative or ER positive hormone refractory patients, those with a liver-site tumour were three times more likely to die than those without. The prognostic importance of liver involvement for survival was also confirmed by those studies where this variable was validated on an independent dataset.[4, 9] Whilst the metastatic location is an important prognostic factor, the prognostic value of the number of metastatic sites is not clear as it failed to demonstrate an independent role in a number of multivariate analyses where this variable was investigated.

Another important prognostic factor is the hormone receptor status. Several studies identified ER negative status as an independent variable predicting poor survival.[5, 6, 9–11, 13] Interestingly, a close relationship has also been shown between ER status and metastatic recurrence.

Clark and colleagues[6] confirmed this evidence by analysing a large sample of 1015 relapsed patients from the time of initial recurrence. The authors showed that ER negative patients had significantly more recurrences in visceral sites (including liver and lung) than ER positive patients. On the contrary, for example, ER positive tumours were more likely to recur in bone. Median survival for ER negative patients was 25, 16 and 10 months respectively for soft tissue, bone and visceral sites. Median survival for ER positive patients was 47, 24 and 16 months for soft tissue, bone and visceral sites respectively. Within a metastatic site, ER status affected median survival. No matter what the site of recurrence, ER negative patients had worse prognoses for survival than ER positive patients.[6]

Disease-free interval (DFI) is also an important prognostic factor and was shown to be associated with duration of survival in several studies. Patients with a shorter DFI have been shown to have a poorer prognosis than those with a longer DFI.[4, 6, 10, 11, 13, 14] Rizzieri and colleagues[10] analysed 425 MBC patients undergoing induction therapy with doxorubicin, fluorouracil and methotrexate and showed that a shorter DFI from initial diagnosis to diagnosis of metastases ($\leq$ 2 years) independently predicted worse prognosis not only for overall survival but also for progression-free survival. However, when interpreting the value of this variable from different studies, attention has to be paid to patient selection criteria. Some prognostic factor analyses also include patients with primary advanced disease, while others omit these patients in the analysis of DFI. Previous adjuvant chemotherapy is also a relevant independent prognostic factor for survival, as it has been identified in a number of studies. Generally, patients who have received prior adjuvant chemotherapy have shown a poor prognosis for survival.[4, 8–10]

Serum lactate dehydrogenase (LDH) was also found to be an important prognostic factor in a number of studies and was also included in two recent prognostic indices for survival in MBC patients[4, 5] Abnormal levels of LDH have been found to be independently associated with a shorter duration of survival, however different cut-off levels were used, thus making a direct comparisons of the results among studies difficult.[4, 5, 7] Also, performance status has been found to be an independent prognostic factor and generally, patients with a poor performance status are likely to have worse prognoses.[5, 7, 11, 12] Table 11.1 reports a summary of some of the most relevant independent prognostic factors for survival identified in the multivariate analyses discussed in this section. These factors, apart from LDH values that are not 'monitored' in clinical practice for breast cancer, represent essential information for the medical oncologist to decide the optimal treatment, i.e. chemotherapy versus endocrine therapy, to prescribe to a patient with metastatic breast cancer. The endocrine receptors status is always determined on the primary tumour and usually is not re-tested on the metastatic site. Information on the other prognostic factors reported in Table 11.1 are easily collected from patient's anamnesis (prior adjuvant

Table 11.1 Relevant prognosis factors for survival in metastatic breast cancer patients

Prognostic factor	Worse prognosis	References*
Oestrogen receptor status	With negative status	5, 6, 9, 10, 11, 13
Liver metastasis	With such involvement	4, 5, 6, 8, 9, 10
Prior adjuvant chemotherapy	With such therapy	4, 8, 9, 10
Disease-free interval	With shorter interval	4, 6, 10, 11, 13, 14
Serum lactic dehydrogenase (LDH)	With abnormal levels	4, 5, 7
Performance status	With poor scores	5, 7, 11, 12

* Studies where the variable was identified in the multivariate analysis.

chemotherapy, disease-free interval) and clinical/radiological evaluation (liver metastasis, performance status). For more in-depth knowledge of the full models predicting survival in these studies, the reader should refer to the reference list reported in the table.

When discussing prognostic factors for survival in MBC patients, it is important to mention that in addition to the traditional clinical variables, pre-treatment patients' self-reported QOL parameters also play a key role. Over the recent years a growing body of evidence has demonstrated that patient's QOL is an independent and strong prognostic factor for survival in a wide range of metastatic cancer disease sites. This evidence has also been clearly demonstrated in MBC patients;[12, 14, 15, 16] however, this has not been replicated in earlier stages of the disease.[16, 17] As an example, physical well-being, pain and appetite loss (as reported by patients themselves), have been shown to be independent prognostic factors for survival in MBC patients beyond a number of key biomedical variables such as metastatic site, ER receptor status, DFI and performance status.[12, 14, 15] The studies in this area vary in terms of sample sizes, QOL questionnaires used and number of clinical variables controlled in the analyses. Nonetheless, it is noteworthy that all the studies in this area conducted in MBC patients have identified at least one QOL parameter independently predicting survival. At present, the reason underlying the mechanism of the association between survival and QOL is not yet entirely clear. However, it would seem that patients with advanced disease are better judges of their own underlying health status than a number of traditional clinical parameters. This accurate perception could then be reflected in reported QOL scores, so that patients with worse underlying disease (and consequently worse expected prognosis) would report worse QOL scores.[16] At present, this non-causative relationship between QOL and survival in MBC patients seems to be the most reasonable explanation, which would also best account for the contradictory findings of the prognostic value of QOL parameters for survival in breast cancer patients with and without distant metastases.[18] Further research is needed to clarify how to implement this information in routine clinical practice. Nevertheless, the remarkable and robust link between patients' QOL parameters and duration of survival in MBC patients provides additional arguments for a more patient-centred approach in the clinical decision-making process.

Therapies affecting prognosis

Advanced breast cancer is essentially incurable and almost all the women diagnosed with this disease will eventually die from it. Therefore, important goals in current therapy are disease and symptoms control and prolongation of survival, provided that the QOL is not compromised.

Disease control is essentially evaluated by measuring objective responses (RR) and time to progression (TTP) or progression-free survival (PFS). In patients receiving an endocrine treatment, clinical benefit (CB), defined as RR plus long-lasting stable disease, is considered an important index of treatment efficacy. Despite the fact that research on surrogate end points has substantially intensified in the past decade,[19] currently there is not evidence that RR/CB and/or TTP/PFS could be considered as surrogate markers of survival in advanced breast cancer.

In the last few years the introduction of new agents/combinations in the treatment of advanced breast cancer has generated a clear positive impact on short-term prognosis while a clear impact on survival rate is rarely observed.

Endocrine therapy

The anti-aromatase agents have challenged the role of the anti-oestrogen tamoxifen as first-line treatment for metastatic breast cancer. The results of four randomized trials are summarized in Table 11.2.[20–23] No differences were seen in terms of overall survival.

Table 11.2 Randomized phase III studies of anti-aromatase agents vs tamoxifen as initial therapy of metastatic breast cancer

	Anastrozole	Anastrozole	Letrozole	Exemestane
No. patients	170 vs 182	340 vs 328	453 vs 454	182 vs 189
RR, %	21 vs 17	33 vs 33	30 vs 20*	46 vs 31*
CB, %	59 vs 46*	56 vs 56	49 vs 38*	66 vs 49*
Median PFS, (months)	11 vs 6*	8 vs 8	9 vs 6*	10 vs 6*

RR, objective response; CB, clinical benefit; PFS, progression free survival.

* Statistically significant.

Chemotherapy

Taxanes are amongst the most effective agents in breast cancer. The combination of this class of drugs with anthracyclines and other cytotoxic agents have been widely investigated. More than 3,000 patients have been randomized in phase III trials comparing a standard anthracycline-based regimen with a taxane-anthracycline based regimen as first-line chemotherapy for metastatic breast cancer. Interestingly, all but two trials (n < 500 randomized patients) failed to show a statistically significant survival increase in favour of the anthracycline-taxane arm, although benefits in terms of response rate, and in some cases in terms of TTP, were observed. However, it should be noted that, due to the small sample size, all trials were underpowered and could not show a reasonable and clinically meaningful increase in survival: therefore only a meta-analysis of all trials would be appropriate to address the question of the reliability of the above-mentioned trials.[24] In addition, in the larger of the two trials that showed a survival advantage in favour of the taxane-based combination, less than 30 per cent of the patients who progressed after having been treated in the standard arm did subsequently receive a taxane. This low cross-over rate in the investigational agent at the moment of disease progression was observed in two other chemotherapy trials that showed a survival advantage in favour of the experimental arm.[25, 26] This attitude does not reflect clinical practice and represents a strong bias in the interpretation of the survival data. The impact of the cross-over rate on survival is well illustrated by a recently reported trial in which tamoxifen and letrozole were compared as first-line treatment in metastatic breast cancer patients. Although letrozole proved to be more effective than tamoxifen in terms of RR and TTP, no difference was observed in terms of overall survival. However, when the survival analysis was carried out by censoring those women who crossed over to the other study drug at the time of disease progression, a survival benefit in favour of letrozole was observed.[22]

Biological agents

A different outcome was observed by treating patients with metastatic breast cancer that overexpressed HER-2 (human epidermal growth factor receptor) with chemotherapy plus trastuzumab.[27, 28] The combination resulted in being better than chemotherapy alone in terms of RR, median TTP, and also median survival despite the fact that a relevant proportion of patients (48–67 per cent) who were initially assigned to receive chemotherapy alone received, after disease progression, trastuzumab alone or with chemotherapy. To date these trials represent the only clear evidence of a treatment affecting survival in patients with advanced breast cancer. In addition, a QOL improvement was also observed[29] in favour of the combined treatment in the study by Slamon et al.[27]

There are two possible explanations for the observed survival advantage of trastuzumab plus chemotherapy over chemotherapy alone although in presence of extensive cross-over: (a) a targeted compound such as trastuzumab is more effective when administered in the earliest phase of metastatic breast cancer; (b) in both trials, in the combination arm, trastuzumab was given in combination with drugs highly synergistic with the antibody. It is possible that patients treated with trastuzumab after the failure of chemotherapy alone received this compound either as a single agent or in combination with less 'synergistic' cytotoxic agents and therefore a less effective treatment than the per protocol combined regimen.

The introduction of new agents in the treatment of metastatic breast cancer has positively affected the prognosis of these patients. The difficulty in detecting a clear impact on survival is partially due to the inadequate sample size of clinical trials to detect small yet clinically relevant differences. Cautiousness is needed while reading the reports of trials showing a survival advantage in favour of a specific treatment over another regimen, i.e. cross-over rates and the adequacy of the control arm should be carefully evaluated.

Short-term prognosis

Once metastases are detected, the median survival generally ranges from 18 to 24 months. However, prognosis also depends on a given prognostic profile of the patient. Although the identification of a single prognostic factor is helpful, more comprehensive and clinically useful information can be obtained by using them in combination, so as to provide a prognostic index.

Yamamoto and colleagues[4] conducted a prognostic factor analysis for survival on 233 MBC patients randomized to compare hormonal agents (tamoxifen versus medroxyprogesterone acetate) in combination with doxorubicin and cyclophosphamide. At the time of analysis the median follow up time was 25.1 months. The authors devised a prognostic index, identifying three risk groups; in addition they also validated the prognostic index on an independent dataset of 279 MBC patients. The study took into account a large number of candidate predictor variables for survival, including age, menopausal status, performance status, hormone receptor status and several laboratory parameters, including white blood cell count, haemoglobin level and serum albumin. The final multivariate model retained the following five variables: adjuvant chemotherapy (ADJCT); liver metastasis (HEP); distant lymph node metastasis (DLNs); serum lactic dehydrogenase (LDH) and disease-free interval (DFI). DLNs was defined as any lymph node involvement other than regional lymph node metastasis (ipsilateral axillary, interpectoral, supraclavicular, and internal mammary). Based on these variables they constructed a prognostic index ranging from 0 to 6: the higher the score the poorer the prognostic profile of the patient. The value of this simple validated index lies in its practical use for routine clinical practice. The prognostic index score is calculated by summing the weights of each prognostic variable as follows. ADJCT: 0 (if patients have not received ADJCT following surgery) or 1 (if patients have received ADJCT following surgery); DLNs: 0 (if patients present no DLNs) or 1 (if patients present DLNs); HEP: 0 (if patients present no HEP) or 1 (if patients present HEP); LDH: 0 (if serum LDH ≤ one times normal) or 1 (if serum LDH more than one times normal); DFI: 0 (if DFI ≥24 months) or 2 (if DFI < 24 months). Based on this prognostic index, they identified three risk groups: low risk (with a prognostic index score ≤ 1), intermediate risk (with a prognostic index score of 2 or 3) and high risk (with a prognostic index score of ≥4). The high risk group (16 per cent of the sample) had a median survival of 10.6 months (95 per cent CI 2.9–18.2) and a poor short-term prognosis, with a 1-year survival rate of 45 per cent. This figure was also confirmed in the validation dataset where the high-risk group showed a median survival of 10 months and a 1-year survival of 41 per cent. However, patients with better prognostic profiles could achieve better short-term prognoses. The intermediate-risk group (47 per cent of the sample) and the low-risk group (37 per cent of the sample) in the original dataset had a 1-year survival rate of 82 per cent and 88 per cent respectively. Similarly, the intermediate- and low-risk groups, in the validation dataset, had a 1 year survival of 80 per cent and 96 per cent respectively.

Ryberg and colleagues[5] conducted a prognostic factor analysis on 469 MBC patients treated with epirubicin-based chemotherapy. The median survival time for these patients was 14.7 months with a median follow up time of 76.3 months. In this study, the following variables independently predicted duration of survival: location of metastases (soft tissue, lung, liver, pleura and bone), performance status, age, LDH and ER status. Based on these variables the authors devised a prognostic index. Each prognostic factor was assigned a score defined as the rounded off value of the Cox regression coefficient ×10. Based on this, the authors identified four risk groups: good, intermediate I, intermediate II, and poor. Given this index was not validated, details on how to calculate the prognostic index score are not reported here (the reader can refer to the original article). The authors also applied the prognostic index to a new series of 116 patients and found similar median survival figures in the good and the poor risk groups. However, the survival data for the intermediate groups I and II differed considerably compared to the previous series of patients (old series). For descriptive purposes, the survival figures for the four risk groups identified in this study in the original dataset (old series) and in the new series of 116 patients are reported in Table 11.3 and shown in Figure 11.1. Although the applicability of this index is limited, it is worthy of note the remarkable differences in terms of median survival between the good and the poor risk patients. The poor risk group had a median survival of 7 months and a 1 year survival rate of 19 per cent. On the contrary, the short term prognosis for the group with the most favourable prognostic profile was much better with 87 per cent of the patients surviving 1 year (Table 11.3).

Long-term prognosis

Patients with none or very few negative prognostic factors can achieve substantially longer survival than patients with an unfavourable prognostic profile. Such information is important, as patients with very good prognostic profiles could achieve longer median survival than usually expected in MBC patients treated with conventional chemotherapy. As an example, according to the prognostic index reported by Yamamoto and colleagues,[4] a patient belonging to the low-risk group,

Table 11.3 Distribution of 585 patients with metastatic breast cancer into risk groups and their corresponding PI, median, one-, two-, and five-year survival. Reproduced with the permission of Springer Science and Business media.

Risk groups	PI score*	Series	Number of patients (%)	Median survival (months)	One-year survival (%)	Two-year survival (%)	Five-year survival (%)
Good	0–10	Old	113 (29)	34	87	63	26
		New	21 (19)	32	90	67	23
Intermediate I	11–15	Old	95 (25)	19	68	34	6
		New	38 (34)	28	76	52	22
Intermediate II	16–22	Old	86 (22)	12	51	17	0
		New	38 (33)	18	71	35	5
Poor	> 22	Old	95 (24)	7.0	19	4	1
		New	16 (14)	5.7	31	13	0

* PI score: the individual prognostic sum score (details on how to calculate the PI score are reported in Ryberg et al.[5])

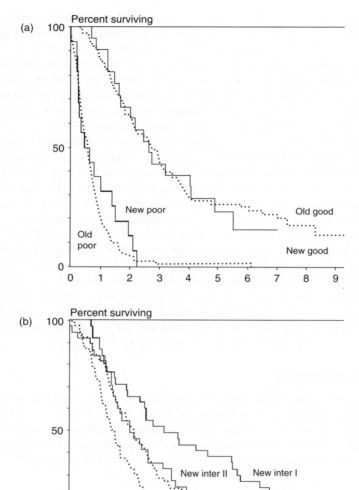

Figure 11.1 (a) Kaplan–Meier survival plot. The survival for both series in the good and the poor groups, x axis percentage of patients alive, y axis survival in years, ---- the old series, ___ the new series. (b) Kaplan–Meier survival plot. The survival for both series in the intermediate I + II groups, x axis percentage of patients alive, y axis survival in years, ---- the old series intermediate I and intermediate II, ___ the new series intermediate I and intermediate II. From Ryberg M, Nielsen D, Osterlind K, Skovsgaard T, Dombernowsky P. Prognostic factors and long-term survival in 585 patients with metastic breast cancer treated with epirubicin-based chemotherapy. *Annals of Oncology* 2001; 12:81–7. Reproduced with the permission of Springer Science and Business Media.

that is with a DFI ≥24 months and with no more than one of the following negative factors: prior ADJCT, presence of DLNs, liver metastasis, and serum LDH more than one times normal, could achieve a median survival of 45.5 months (95 per cent CI, 38.8–52.3) and a 2- and 5-year survival rate of 70 per cent and 41 per cent respectively. The high-risk group patients had a significantly worse long term prognosis with a 2- and 5-year survival rate of 7 per cent and 0 per cent respectively. Similar long-term survival figures were highlighted by Ryberg and colleagues.[5] In their study, patients with the most favourable prognostic profile had a median survival of 34 months and a 2- and 5-year survival rate of 63 per cent and 26 per cent respectively. However, patients receiving the same treatment but classified in the poor risk group had a 2- and 5-year survival rate of 4 per cent and 1 per cent, respectively. Long-term survival figures were considerably different between the good and the poor risk patients (Table 11.3).

References

1. Stewart BW, Kleihues P. *World Health Organization. World cancer report*. Lyon: IARC Press, 2003.
2. Overmoyer BA. Chemotherapeutic palliative approaches in the treatment of breast cancer. *Semin Oncol* 1995; 22(Suppl 3):2–9.
3. Bloom HJ, Richardson WW, Harries EJ. Natural history of untreated breast cancer (1805–1933). Comparison of untreated and treated cases according to histological grade of malignancy. *Br Med J* 1962; 5299:213–21.
4. Yamamoto N, Watanabe T, Katsumata N. *et al*. Construction and validation of a practical prognostic index for patients with metastatic breast cancer. *J Clin Oncol* 1998; 16:2401–8.
5. Ryberg M, Nielsen D, Osterlind K, Skovsgaard T, Dombernowsky P. Prognostic factors and long-term survival in 585 patients with metastatic breast cancer treated with epirubicin-based chemotherapy. *Ann Oncol* 2001; 12:81–7.
6. Clark GM, Sledge GW Jr, Osborne CK, McGuire WL. Survival from first recurrence: relative importance of prognostic factors in 1,015 breast cancer patients. *J Clin Oncol* 1987; 5:55–61.
7. Hortobagyi GN, Smith TL, Legha SS, *et al*. Multivariate analysis of prognostic factors in metastatic breast cancer. *J Clin Oncol* 1983; 1:776–86.
8. Dunphy FR, Spitzer G, Fornoff JE, *et al*. Factors predicting long-term survival for metastatic breast cancer patients treated with high-dose chemotherapy and bone marrow support. *Cancer* 1994; 73:2157–67.
9. Falkson G, Gelman R, Falkson CI, Glick J, Harris J. Factors predicting for response, time to treatment failure, and survival in women with metastatic breast cancer treated with DAVTH: a prospective Eastern Cooperative Oncology Group study. *J Clin Oncol* 1991; 9:2153–61.
10. Rizzieri DA, Vredenburgh JJ, Jones R. *et al*. Prognostic and predictive factors for patients with metastatic breast cancer undergoing aggressive induction therapy followed by high-dose chemotherapy with autologous stem-cell support. *J Clin Oncol* 1999; 17:3064–74.
11. Tampellini M, Berruti A, Gerbino A. *et al*. Relationship between CA 15–3 serum levels and disease extent in predicting overall survival of breast cancer patients with newly diagnosed metastatic disease. *Br J Cancer* 1997; 75:698–702.
12. Efficace F, Biganzoli L, Piccart M. *et al*. Baseline health-related quality-of-life data as prognostic factors in a phase III multicentre study of women with metastatic breast cancer. *Eur J Cancer* 2004; 40:1021–30.
13. Robertson JF, Dixon AR, Nicholson RI, Ellis IO, Elston CW, Blamey RW Confirmation of a prognostic index for patients with metastatic breast cancer treated by endocrine therapy. *Breast Cancer Res Treat* 1992; 22:221–7.
14. Kramer JA, Curran D, Piccart M. *et al*. Identification and interpretation of clinical and quality of life prognostic factors for survival and response to treatment in first-line chemotherapy in advanced breast cancer. *Eur J Cancer* 2000; 36:1498–506.
15. Coates A, Gebski V, Signorini D. *et al*. Prognostic value of quality-of-life scores during chemotherapy for advanced breast cancer. Australian New Zealand Breast Cancer Trials Group. *J Clin Oncol* 1992; 10:1833–38.

16. Coates AS, Hurny C, Peterson HF. *et al.* Quality-of-life scores predict outcome in metastatic but not early breast cancer. *J Clin Oncol* 2000; 18:3768–74.

17. Efficace F, Therasse P, Piccart MJ. *et al.* Health-related quality of life parameters as prognostic factors in a nonmetastatic breast cancer population: an international multicenter study. *J Clin Oncol* 2004; 22:3381–8.

18. Efficace F, Bottomley A. Toward a clearer understanding of the prognostic value of health-related quality of life (HRQOL) parameters in breast cancer. *J Clin Oncol* 2005; 23:1335–6.

19. Buyse M, Thirion P, Carlson RW, Burzykowski T, Molenberghs G, Piedbois P, for the Meta-Analysis Group In Cancer. Tumour response to first line chemotherapy improves the survival of patients with advanced colorectal cancer. *Lancet* 2000; 356:373–8.

20. Nabholtz JM, Buzdar A, Pollak M. *et al.* Anastrozole is superior to tamoxifen as first-line therapy for advanced breast cancer in postmenopausal women: results of a North American multicenter randomized trial. *J Clin Oncol* 2000; 18:3758–67.

21. Bonneterre J, Thurlimann B, Robertson JF. *et al.* Anastrozole versus tamoxifen as first-line therapy for advanced breast cancer in 668 postmenopausal women: results of the Tamoxifen or Arimidex Randomized Group Efficacy and Tolerability Study. *J Clin Oncol* 2000; 18:3748–57.

22. Mouridsen H, Gershanovich M, Sun Y. *et al.* Phase III study of letrozole versus tamoxifen as first-line therapy of advanced breast cancer in postmenopausal women: analysis of survival and update of efficacy from the International Letrozole Breast Cancer Group. *J Clin Oncol* 2003; 21:2101–9.

23. Paridaens R, Therasse P, Dirix L. *et al.* First line hormonal treatment (HT) for metastatic breast cancer (MBC) with exemestane (E) or tamoxifen (T) in postmenopausal patients (pts) – A randomized phase III trial of the EORTC Breast Group. *J Clin Oncol* 2004; 22 (14S *Proc Am Soc Clin Oncol*) 6s (abs. 515).

24. Di Leo A, Bleiberg H, Buyse M Overall survival is not a realistic end point for clinical trials of new drugs in advanced solid tumors: a critical assessment based on recently reported phase III trials in colorectal and breast cancer. *J Clin Oncol* 2003; 21:2045–7.

25. Albain KS, Nag S, Calderillo-Ruiz G. *et al.* Global phase III study of gemcitabine plus paclitaxel (GT) vs. paclitaxel (T) as frontline therapy for metastatic breast cancer (MBC): First report of overall survival. *J Clin Oncol* 2004; 22(14S *Proc Am Soc Clin Oncol*) 5s (abs. 510).

26. O'Shaughnessy J, Miles D, Vukelja S. *et al.* Superior survival with capecitabine plus docetaxel combination therapy in anthracycline-pretreated patients with advanced breast cancer: phase III trial results. *J Clin Oncol* 2002; 20:2812–23.

27. Slamon DJ, Leyland-Jones B, Shak S. *et al.* Use of chemotherapy plus a monoclonal antibody against HER2 for metastatic breast cancer that overexpress HER2. *N Engl J Med* 2001; 344:783–92.

28. Extra JM, Cognetti F, Maraninchi D. *et al.* Trastuzumab (Herceptin) plus docetaxel versus docetaxel alone as first-line treatment of HER2 positive metastatic breast cancer (MBC): results of a randomised multicentre trial. *Eur J Cancer* 2004; 2(Suppl. 4th European Breast Cancer Conference), 125, (abs. 239).

29. Osoba D, Slamon DJ, Burchmore M, Murphy M. Effects on quality of life of combined trastuzumab and chemotherapy in women with metastatic breast cancer. *J Clin Oncol* 2002; 20:3106–13.

12

Bladder cancer

Luigi Schips and Richard Zigeuner

Introduction

Bladder cancer is one of the most frequently diagnosed cancers in humans, the fourth most common cancer in males and the eighth most common cancer in females, which translates into male-to-female ratio of approximately 2.5:1.[1] Histologically, the majority (more than 90 per cent) of cases are transitional cell carcinomas (TCCs). Rare cases include squamous cell carcinoma, especially caused by schistosomiasis in endemic regions and indwelling catheters, as well as adenocarcinomas, and urachal carcinoma. The main risk factor for bladder TCC development is smoking, which increases cancer risk about fourfold compared to non-smokers[2]. Further risk factors include analgesic abuse, chronic and recurrent urinary tract infections, especially caused by long-term indwelling catheters or bladder calculi, and occupational exposure to aromatic amines, which can be observed in workers in textile, rubber, chemical and leather industries, as well as hairdressers.[3]

While advanced cancer at diagnosis is an exception in TCCs, all other histologic types of bladder cancer are predominantly advanced at diagnosis. A clear distinction between superficial and advanced stages is mandatory because treatment of advanced bladder cancer requires radical surgery including cystectomy and urinary diversion in case of muscle-invasive, non-metastatic cancer, and systemic chemotherapy in metastatic disease. Approximately 50 per cent of patients presenting with invasive cancer harbour occult metastases at diagnosis. Presence of distant metastases significantly compromises prognosis: metastatic bladder cancer has to be regarded an incurable disease at present.

Natural history

The most frequent first sign of bladder cancer is painless haematuria, either gross or microscopic, affecting approximately 80 per cent of patients. Further symptoms include irritative voiding complaints, like frequency, urgency and dysuria, especially when carcinoma *in situ* is present. In selected cases, predominantly those with advanced cancer, symptoms of the upper urinary tract like flank pain due to hydronephrosis are found, caused by invasive bladder cancer involving the ureteral orifice. In advanced cases, imaging like ultrasound, computed tomography (CT) or magnetic resonance imaging (MRI) may show an intravesical mass. In the case of metastatic disease, symptoms caused by distant metastases may be the first manifestation of the disease, dependent on their location (most commonly pain or pathologic fractures from bone metastases). The diagnostic procedure of choice for bladder cancer is cystoscopy. In the majority of cases, the endoscopic presentation of bladder cancer is a papillary, exophytic tumour, often pedunculated. Since bladder cancer represents a field change disease involving the whole bladder mucosa, multifocal tumours are common. Advanced cancers usually are of solid appearance, the surface is often covered by necrosis or even calcifications. In contrast, carcinoma *in situ* is a flat lesion in the level of the bladder mucosa and cannot be reliably diagnosed by conventional cystoscopy.

The suspected diagnosis of bladder cancer after cystoscopy may be confirmed by cytology and/or biopsy. Urinary and bladder wash cytology are routine tools in diagnosis and follow-up of bladder cancer. In high-grade tumours, cytology yields excellent specificity and good sensitivity (70–80 per cent), whereas sensitivity in low-grade cancers is poor. However, when bladder cancer is suspected, the first line treatment is transurethral resection of the bladder (TURB). This procedure is curative in superficial cancers, in invasive tumours the role of TURB is only diagnostic.

The histological classification of bladder cancer is listed in Table 12.1. Grossly, bladder cancer is subdivided in superficial stages, which include stages pTa, pT1 and carcinoma *in situ* (CIS) on the one hand, and invasive stages consisting of stages pT2–4. At diagnosis, 70–80 per cent of bladder cancers are superficial. However, if early diagnosis is missed and patients ignore episodes of recurrent gross haematuria, advanced cancer is diagnosed more frequently, especially in older populations (unpublished data from our institution).

Tumour grade has been traditionally assessed in a three grade system according to the World Health Organization (WHO) as grade 1, grade 2, and grade 3. In the recent version of the WHO classification, a two grade system including only low grade (LG) and high grade (HG) has been implemented. At diagnosis, 60 per cent of tumours are low grade. Invasive cancers are almost uniformly high grade.

The true natural history of bladder cancer is unknown, since almost no patient remains untreated due to the typical signs and symptoms. However, based on the hypothesis that all bladder cancers begin as superficial tumours, one can assume that progression to invasive and high-grade cancer occurs when early diagnosis had been missed. After TURB of superficial tumours, the majority of patients will have tumour recurrence. Early recurrence within

Table 12.1 TNM staging system for bladder cancer

pT-category	Extension
pTis	Carcinoma in situ: limited to mucosa, flat lesion, high grade
pTa	Papillary exophytic tumour, limited to mucosa, not invading lamina propria
pT1	Tumour invading lamina propria
pT2a	Tumour invading inner half of the detrusor muscle
pT2b	Tumour invading the outer half of the detrusor muscle
pT3a	Tumour invading perivesical fat microscopically
pT3b	Tumour invading perivesical fat macroscopically
pT4a	Tumour invading prostate stroma, or vagina, uterus
pT4a	Tumour invading pelvic or abdominal wall
Nx	Lymph node status not assessed
N0	No nodal metastases
N1	Single nodal metastasis < 2cm
N2	Multiple nodal metastases < 5cm
N3	Multiple nodal metastases > 5cm
Mx	Distant metastases not assessed
M0	No distant metastases
M1	Distant metastases

3–6 months mainly results from incomplete resection and/or implantation metastases, whereas later recurrences reflect the character of transitional cell carcinoma as a field change disease. Most of these cases are of the same stage and grade. However, progression to higher grade can be observed in up to 25 per cent[4] and to invasive or even metastatic stages in up to 10 per cent.[5] High-grade tumours have an even higher recurrence rate (up to 80 per cent), progression to muscle invasive cancer occurs in up to 50 per cent without adjuvant treatment[6]. In patients with pT-1 high-grade cancer, up to one third will progress to muscle invasive cancer even after histologically confirmed complete resection and adjuvant Bacille Calmette-Guérin (BCG) therapy.

In case of invasive cancer diagnosed by TURB, further staging has to be performed to exclude or confirm metastatic disease. Standard staging procedures include chest X-ray, abdominal and pelvic contrast enhanced computerized tomography (CT) to evaluate the nodal status as well as local tumour extension and a bone scan to exclude bone metastases, especially in patients with bone pain or elevated levels or serum alkaline phosphatase. If a CT scan cannot be performed because of a contraindication for administration of contrast agents, such as renal failure or allergy, MRI is the alternative staging procedure.

Elderly patients with severe age-related comorbidities presenting with advanced bladder cancer represent an often unsolvable problem. To this group of patients, neither radical surgery nor chemotherapy can be offered. At our own institution, 65 per cent of patients presenting with newly diagnosed muscle-invasive bladder cancer are older than 75 years and 45 per cent are older than 80 years. Treatment with curative intent cannot be offered to the vast majority of patients. Thus our treatment options are limited to supportive care from first diagnosis in these cases. Patients with incurable invasive bladder cancer frequently return to the emergency room because of recurrent severe bleeding, which results in considerable blood loss and painful blood clot retention and requires bladder drainage and irrigation with large size indwelling catheters of 20–22 Fr. Palliative treatment options include repeated TURB with the intention of haemostasis but no impact on survival. Patients presenting with symptomatic hydronephrosis, renal failure or pyonephrosis may be aided with insertion of a percutaneous nephrostomy tube, which drains the upper urinary tract and bypasses the affected bladder. However, indication of nephrostomy in end-stage cancer patients presenting with uraemia or septicaemia has been repeatedly questioned. The majority of patients die within 6 months after drainage, have trouble handling the nephrostomy and thus frequently return to hospital care. Impact of nephrostomy on quality of life in these patients has never been systematically evaluated and is therefore unknown. Thus, universally valid recommendations cannot be given – the decision has to be made on an individual basis with the patient. The indication for nephrostomy must be balanced between relief of complaints and gaining quality of life on the one hand and unethical prolongation of suffering on the other. One major goal in any case of advanced cancer has to be adequate pain management on an interdisciplinary basis between urologists, medical oncologists, anaesthesiologists and supportive care experts. Today, continuous percutaneous administration of opiods in combination with non steroidal anti-inflammatory drugs are widely used. Metastasis-related bone pain is usually treated with bisphosphonates, out of which zoledronic acid applied intravenously every 3–4 weeks seems to be the most effective drug.

Factors affecting prognosis

Tumour-related

In superficial bladder cancer, the most important prognostic parameters for tumour recurrence are grade, stage, and associated carcinoma *in situ*. Additional indicators include tumour size (smaller or larger than 3 cm), multifocality, lymphovascular invasion, papillary or solid cystoscopic appearance, and frequency of prior tumour recurrences. As a consequence, three distinct risk groups of superficial bladder cancer have been defined:

1. Low risk: single tumour, newly diagnosed, stage pT-a, low grade, less than 3 cm in diameter

2. High risk: Any pT-a/pT-1 high grade, any carcinoma *in situ*

3. Intermediate risk: All other tumours pT-a/pT-1 low grade, recurrent tumours, multifocal tumours, and tumours larger than 3 cm.

Because of the high risk of recurrence, close surveillance by cystoscopy is mandatory. The standard recommendation is cystoscopy at 3-month intervals for at least the first year, every 6 months for the second to third year, and once a year thereafter. In case of tumour recurrence and repeat TURB, the surveillance schedule starts again from the beginning.

In advanced bladder cancer, prognosis is essentially dependent on T-stage and nodal status.[7] Grade does not have a major impact on prognosis, since almost all cases of advanced bladder cancer are high grade. The likelihood of lymph node metastases increases with tumour stage. Patients with stage pT2 are at risk for pelvic lymph node metastases of 10–30 per cent, whereas this likelihood increases to 30–65 per cent in stage pT3. When lymph node involvement is present, prognosis is dependent on extent of node metastases as well as the appropriate surgical procedure. Up to 30 per cent of patients with microscopic lymph node metastases (pN-1) can survive several years after extended lymph node dissection. However, when grossly enlarged nodes are present, surgery alone does not impact on prognosis.

Presence of distant metastases significantly compromises prognosis. Presently metastatic bladder cancer has to be regarded an incurable disease. Approximately 50 per cent of patients presenting with invasive cancer harbour occult metastases at diagnosis.

Patient-related factors

Poor prognostic factors include anaemia, poor performance status, dilation of the upper urinary tract and renal failure.

Therapies affecting prognosis

Surgery

The first step in the treatment of a newly diagnosed bladder tumour is TURB, even if advanced bladder cancer is clinically suspected from the beginning. TURB is an approach with curative intent in superficial cancer only, whereas in the case of muscle-invasive bladder tumours it yields valuable information regarding the level of invasion. If performed properly, TURB has to be carried out in separate steps:

1. Resection of the exophytic parts of the tumour;

2. Separate resection of the superficial margins of the tumour bed;

3. Separate resection of the deep portion of the tumour bed.

This latter specimen must contain smooth muscle tissue to enable a correct histological diagnosis. The quality of the TURB specimen is essential, since fulguration artefacts and/or too superficial resection may result in understaging of the resected tumour, which in fact is an invasive cancer. If there is any doubt regarding the histological diagnosis, a second TURB within 4–6 weeks has to be performed. This results in upstaging of a tumour originally classified as superficial to muscle invasive in a significant number (up to 20 per cent) of cases.[8]

After muscle invasive cancer has been confirmed histologically, absence of distant metastases has to be documented. After exclusion of distant metastases, the standard approach to treat muscle-invasive and locally advanced bladder cancer (stages T2–4, N0–2, M0), is radical cystoprostatectomy in males and anterior pelvic exenteration in females, both combined with pelvic lymph node dissection and followed by urinary diversion. An essential pre-requisite before performing a cystectomy is an adequate performance status of the patient. Regarding urinary diversion, a large number of different procedures have been described. Briefly, urinary diversion can be performed in continent or non-continent fashion. For non-continent diversion, the most widely used is the ileal conduit, developed by Bricker in 1950.[9] A segment of ileum, approximately 20–30 cm long, is isolated by maintaining its blood support. The ureters are implanted into the oral part, while the aboral end is implanted into the right abdominal wall as a stoma, draining the urine in a urinary bag. Alternatively, a colon conduit can be used.

For continent diversion, a variety of different versions has been developed. Today, the most popular versions are orthotopic bladder substitutions, called neobladder. The principle is to isolate a bowel segment of 40–60 cm, mostly ileum. The bowel segment is detubularized by antimesenteric longitudinal incision. Subsequently, a T-, S-, or W-shaped plate is formed using running sutures, and closed to form a reservoir. The ureters are implanted in the proximal part of the neobladder, while the most distal part is anastomosed to the urethra. This neobladder enables the patients to void in an almost natural way. Orthotopic bladder substitution can only be performed if urethral involvement is ruled out. Today, this is usually done by urethroscopy prior to operation and intraoperative frozen sections of the urethral surgical margin. If presence of tumour can be excluded, orthotopic substitution can be safely performed.

In the case of urethral involvement, urethrectomy has to be carried out. Continent urinary diversion in these cases can be constructed either as an ileal or ileocaecal pouch with continent stoma via the umbilicus, which is drained by intermittent self-catheterization, or less frequently by ureterosigmoideostomy.

Postoperative complications after cystectomy have been reported in up to 30 per cent of cases, including major complications in up to 10 per cent and a perioperative mortality in most contemporary series of 1–3 per cent.[7] In patients with locally advanced bladder cancer, perioperative chemotherapy, either as a neoadjuvant or adjuvant treatment, may be performed.

Radiotherapy

In carefully selected patients, bladder sparing treatments such as partial resection or radiotherapy, either alone or combined with chemotherapy, may be an option. Results of radiotherapy are dependent on the extent of tumour. In these patients, a second TURB, which is usually reserved for high-risk superficial cancer patients, reduces tumour burden and may be helpful as an additional therapeutic tool for patients who are not candidates for radical surgery. Best results for radiotherapy or radio-chemotherapy can be achieved if a macroscopically complete TURB is possible. Complete response rates of 50–75 per cent have been shown.[10] Currently there are no randomized trials comparing surgery and radiotherapy. However, some matched controls analyses have shown to provide results for radiotherapy, either alone or combined with chemotherapy, comparable to radical cystectomy series, although results are flawed by selection biases and definitive conclusions cannot be drawn.

Local failures of radiotherapy or radio-chemotherapy can be treated by salvage cystectomy, if the patient is an appropriate candidate for major surgery.

Chemotherapy

In patients with established metastatic disease, systemic chemotherapy is usually administered. Since single agent chemotherapy yields disappointing results, cisplatin-based combination chemotherapies are widely used. The most popular combination is methotrexate, vinblastine, adriamycin and cisplatin (M-VAC), developed by Sternberg.[11] Treatment toxicity is high with therapy-associated mortality rates of approximately 3–5 per cent. Alternative treatment regimens have been developed by replacement of adriamycin by epirubicin (M-VEC), or a triple-drug therapy of cisplatin, methotrexate and vinblastine (CMV). More recently, the combination of cisplatin with gemcitabine has been shown to reduce treatment related morbidity significantly with comparable response rates. Paclitaxel and docetaxel have been used in clinical trials of patients with advanced bladder cancer. Response rates ranging from 25 to 80 per cent have been reported. Further trials are ongoing.

In summary, impact of bladder cancer treatment on survival cannot be determined in absence of data on that topic. Prospective randomized trials between treated and untreated populations are not available and can hardly be carried out for ethical reasons. Patients with advanced bladder cancer are left untreated only in case of high age, severe comorbities, poor performance status, extensive metastatic disease, or a combination of two or more adverse factors. Thus, these patients cannot be compared with a population undergoing treatment with curative intent.

Short-term prognosis

Outcome of cystectomy is strongly dependent on stage and grade.[7] In patients with node-positive cancer, early relapse and death from tumour will occur in the majority of patients. However, especially in patients with stage pN-1, long-term survival may be achieved by extended lymph node dissection. Approximately 50 per cent of patients with invasive cancer harbour occult metastases at presentation. The majority of these patients develop clinically evident metastatic disease within one year.[12] Neo-adjuvant cisplatin-based chemotherapy has been shown to provide a 7 per cent survival benefit in patients with locally advanced disease in a meta-analysis.[13] In patients with pN-1 disease after surgery, adjuvant chemotherapy has shown an increase of median survival of one year with 30 per cent of patients achieving long-term survival of several years.

In patients with metastatic disease, systemic chemotherapy is administered. While the partial response rate is about 50 per cent, in the initial reports even 70 per cent, complete remissions can be observed in only 20 per cent of patients, with no proven impact on survival. Median survival of these patients ranges from 9–14 months (Figure 12.1).[14]

Long-term prognosis

In long-term follow-up, approximately one-third of patients with low-grade pTa tumours demonstrate progression in stage and/or grade. Although the majority of these patients show just a grade shift, 3–11 per cent of patients with pTa tumours develop muscle-invasive cancer within seven years.[15,16] In one series of 20 patients who had been free of recurrence for more than 5 years, seven developed muscle-invasive cancer.[17]

Since transitional cell carcinoma represents a field change disease found most commonly in the bladder, all other organs containing urothelium may be involved by cancer. Recurrences in the upper urinary tract have been reported at an overall incidence of 2–4 per cent after treatment

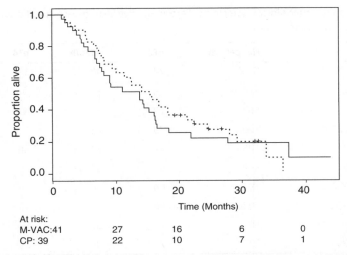

At risk:

M-VAC:41	27	16	6	0
CP: 39	22	10	7	1

- - - - M-VAC (median, 15.4months) ——— CP (median, 13.8 months) Log-rank, P=0.65

Figure 12.1 Overall survival of patients with metastatic TCC of the bladder, according to the two treatment arms. M-VAC, methotrexate, vinblastine, doxorubicin, cisplatin; CP, carboplatin, paclitaxel. From Dreicer R, Manola J, Roth BJ *et al*. Phase III trial of methotrexat, vinblastine, doxorubicin and cisplatin versus carboplatin and paclitaxel in patients with advanced carcinoma of the urothelium. *Cancer* 2004; 100:1639–645.Reproduced with permission from John Wiley and Sons Inc.

of superficial bladder cancer. Most upper tract recurrences occur within the first 5 years. However, in a population of long-term surviving patients with high-risk superficial bladder cancer treated with BCG, the risk of upper tract recurrence has been reported between 13–38 per cent over a follow-up period of 15 years. Although the risk of recurrence is highest within the first 5 years, it persists over at least 15 years. Annual upper tract surveillance by intravenous urography had been traditionally performed for many years, yet has been widely abandoned, since the majority of recurrences are diagnosed by clinical presentation like bleeding and blood clot-induced flank pain rather than imaging. Outcome of upper tract recurrence is frequently lethal with a tumour-associated mortality of 40–70 per cent dependent on stage and grade.

After cystectomy, overall 5 year survival rates averaged over all stages and grades are 50 per cent. However, considerable differences exist between different stages. If cystectomy is performed in stage pT-1 and/or carcinoma *in situ*, especially after failed BCG therapy, 10-year cancer-specific survival rates range from 60–90 per cent, dependent on grade and p53 status. Five and ten-year progression-free survival rates in patients with stage pT2N0 are in a range of 60–80 per cent, and 30–60 per cent in stage pT3 N0. In patients with node positive disease, survival rates after 5 and 10 years decrease to about 15–30 per cent, dependent on the number of lymph nodes involved. Grade has no major impact on survival, since almost all cases of invasive bladder cancer are high grade. Since transitional cell carcinoma is an aggressive, rapidly progressing tumour with a median time to metastasis of 1 year, differences between 5 and 10 year survival rates are moderate, since most metastases are diagnosed within 3 years from surgery and development of metastases after more than 5 years is rare. A selection of studies showing 5-year progression-free survival rates after cystectomy related to pathological T-stages and note status is listed in Table 12.2.

Table 12.2 Prognosis after radical cystectomy: Percentage five year disease-specific survival by pathologic stage in selected series

Author	No. patients	pT2	pT3a/b	pT4	N+
Takahashi *et al.* 2004	518	74	47	38	30
May *et al.* 2004	230	74	50	NA	21
Madersbacher *et al.* 2003	507	73	56	NA	33
Vallencien *et al.* 2002	100	73	63	NA	8
Stein *et al.* 2000	1054	89	62–78	50	35
Bassi *et al.* 1999	369	63	33–53	28	15
Skinner *et al.* 1997	197	64	44	36	44
Ghoneim *et al.* 1997	1026	66	31	19	23
Schoenberg *et al.* 1996	101	84	56	NA	48
Waehre *et al.* 1993	227	79	36	29	22

NA, not assessed.

As mentioned before, adjuvant chemotherapy can provide long-term survival in a subset of patients with node positive cancer, especially pN-1, provided that a cisplatinum-based combination therapy is used, whereas monotherapies fail to yield a survival advantage. In established metastatic disease treated by systemic chemotherapy, median survival of patients is 1 year, long-term survival can be achieved only in a small subset of patients.

Favourable prognostic factors include only node or soft tissue metastases, these patients can achieve 10–15 per cent prolonged survival of 6 years, whereas outcome of patients with visceral and/or bone metastases is even poorer. A selection of clinical trials is listed in Table 12.3.

Table 12.3 Remission rates and median survival (months) in patients after systemic chemotherapy for metastatic bladder cancer. Selection of phase II/III trials.

Author	No. patients	Agents	% OR	Median survival
Dreicer *et al.* 2004	85 (phase III)	M-VAC vs CP	36 vs 28	8.7 vs 5.2
Neri *et al.* 2002	31 (phase II)	GE	57	
Von der Maase *et al.* 2001	405 (phase III)	GC vs M-VAC	49 vs 46	
Pycha *et al.* 1999	32 (phase II)	CP	72	7
Zielinski *et al.* 1998	20 (phase II)	CP	65	8.5
Vaughn et al, 1998	33 (phase II)	CP	50	
Logothetis *et al.* 1990	110 (phase III)	M-VAC vs CISCA	65 vs 46	12 vs 9
Sternberg *et al.*	25 (phase II)	M-VAC	71	9.5

OR: overall response; M-VAC: methotrexate, vinblastine, adriamycin, cisplatin; CP: carboplatin+paclitaxel; GC: gemcitabine+cisplatin; GE: gemcitabine+epirubicin; CISCA: cisplatin, cyclophosphamide, adriamycin.

References

1. Greenlee RT, Murray T, Bolden S, Wings PA. Cancer statistics. *CA Cancer J Clin* 2000; 50:7–33.

2. Morrison AS. Advances in the etiology of urothelial cancer. *Urol Clin North Am* 1984; 11:557–66.

3. Chapman JW, Connolly JG, Rosenbaum L. Occupational bladder cancer: a case-control study. In Connolly JG (ed.) *Carcinoma of the bladder*, New York: Raven Press, 1981, p. 45.

4. Prout GR, Barton BA, Griffin PP, Friedell G. Treated history of non-invasive grade I transitional cell carcinoma. *J Urol* 1992; 148:1413–19.

5. Lutzeyer W, Rubben H, Dahm H. Prognostic parameters in superficial bladder cancer: an analysis of 315 cases. *J Urol* 1982; 127:250–2.

6. Messing EM, Young TB, Hunt VB. *et al.* Comparison of bladder cancer outcome in men undergoing hematuria home screening versus those with standard clinical presentations. *Urology* 1995; 45:387–96.

7. Stein JP, Lieskovsky G, Cote R. *et al.* Radical cystectomy in the treatment of invasive bladder cancer: long-term results in 1,054 patients. *J Clin Oncol* 2001; 19:666–75.

8. Schips L, Augustin H, Zigeuner R. *et al.* Is a second transurethral resection (TUR) justified in patients with newly diagnosed superficial bladder cancer? *Urology* 2002; 59:220–3.

9. Bricker EM. Bladder substitution after pelvic evisceration. *Surg Clin N Amer* 1950; 30:1511–21.

10. Kaufman DS, Shipley WU, Griffin PP. *et al.* Selective bladder preservation by combination treatment of invasive bladder cancer. *N Engl J Med.* 1993; 329:1377–82.

11. Sternberg CN, Yagoda A, Scher HI. *et al.* Preliminary results of M-VAC (methotrexate, vinblastine, doxorubicin and cisplatin) for transitional cell carcinoma of the urothelium. *J Urol* 1985;133: 403–7.

12. Babaian RJ, Johnson DE, Llamas L, Ayala AG. Metastases from transitional cell carcinoma of urinary bladder. *Urology* 1980; 16:142–4.

13. Winquist E, Kirchner TS, Segal R, Chin J, Lukka H, Genitourinary Cancer Disease Site Group, Cancer Care Ontario Program in Evidence-based Care Practice Guidelines Initiative. Neoadjuvant chemotherapy for transitional cell carcinoma of the bladder: a systematic review and meta-analysis. *J Urol* 2004; 171:561–9.

14. Dreicer R, Manola J, Roth BJ. *et al.* Phase III trial of methotrexate, vinblastine, doxorubicin and cisplatin versuscarboplatin and paclitaxel in patients with advanced carcinoma of the urothelium. *Cancer* 2004; 100:1639–45.

15. LeBlanc B, Duclos AJ, Bernard F. *et al.* Long-term follow-up of initial Ta grade 1 transitional cell carcinoma of the bladder. *J Urol* 1999; 162:1946–50.

16. Zieger K, Wolf H, Olsen PR, Hojgaard K. Long-term follow-up of non-invasive bladder tumours (stage Ta): Recurrence and progression. *BJU Int* 2000; 85:824–8.

17. Thompson RA, Campbell EW, Kramer HC, Jacobs SC, Naslund MJ. Late invasive recurrence despite long-term surveillance for superficial bladder cancer. *J Urol* 1993; 149:1010–1.

13

Prostate cancer

Timothy Gilligan

Introduction

Prostate cancer presents a unique challenge for the prognostician. It kills more men in the United States than any other malignancy except lung cancer but its 5-year relative survival rate of 99.5 per cent is the highest of any common malignancy other than non-melanoma skin cancer.[1] In other words, for every 1000 men diagnosed with prostate cancer, there are only five more deaths in the five years after diagnosis compared to what would have been expected without a diagnosis of prostate cancer. Yet we lose nearly 30,000 men annually in the US to this disease. There are three central truths about prostate cancer that explain these apparently conflicting facts. First, screening for prostate cancer by measuring serum levels of prostate specific antigen (PSA) has led to extremely early diagnosis of disease so that even very aggressive tumours are usually diagnosed long before they cause death. In the years 1996–2002, over 90 per cent of prostate cancers were diagnosed at the localized or regional stage while only 5 per cent were metastatic and 4 per cent were unstaged. Moreover, most cancers diagnosed today are not only localized/regional but non-palpable on digital rectal examination (clinical stage T1). Second, prostate cancer is a relatively slow-growing cancer so that even metastatic disease can be controlled for years with hormonal chemotherapy. The median time from radiographically detectable metastasis to death is as long as 5 years in some contemporary series. Third, while some prostate cancers are aggressive and potentially deadly, most are indolent. The incidence of indolent prostate cancer has been shown most clearly in the Prostate Cancer Prevention Trial, which demonstrated that prostate cancer can be detected by biopsy in 24 per cent of men over the age of 55 years.

The development of ways to distinguish aggressive and potentially life-threatening prostate cancers from harmless prostate cancers thus represents a high priority goal in prostate cancer research. Only then will it be possible to focus aggressive treatment on the cancers that need to be treated while allowing the majority of prostate cancer patients who have indolent tumours to be spared the side-effects of unneeded treatment. The cardinal feature of dangerous prostate cancers is the capacity to metastasize and thus the central challenge in prognosticating localized tumours is predicting which tumours will spread to other parts of the body. In advanced stage disease, metastasis has already occurred and, thus, all metastatic cancers are life-threatening. This chapter will discuss the current state of our knowledge about the prognosis of men with metastatic prostate cancer.

The natural history of advanced stage prostate cancer

The dependence of the vast majority of prostate cancers on androgen-receptor stimulation represents a signal characteristic of the disease. The finding in the mid-twentieth century that androgen deprivation resulted in remission in most men with advanced stage prostate cancer was rewarded with a Nobel Prize and androgen deprivation remains the most effective treatment for men with metastatic disease. However, over time, prostate cancers almost always develop the ability to grow in the setting of castrate serum testosterone levels. Metastatic prostate cancer is thus divided into two broad categories: androgen-dependent and androgen-independent (also referred to as hormone-refractory or hormonal-therapy-refractory) disease. This terminology, however, is now thought to be misleading because even so-called androgen-independent prostate cancer cells continue to be responsive to androgen-receptor stimulation. It appears that these tumours are not androgen independent but rather have developed the capacity to undergo androgen stimulation in the setting of extremely low androgen levels as a result of such mechanisms as increased expression of androgen receptors. A more accurate terminology would thus appear to be castration-sensitive versus castration-refractory prostate cancer.

Median overall survival for men with metastatic prostate cancer who have not yet received hormonal therapy or chemotherapy is 3–4 years in most multicentre randomized trials. Men with disease limited to lymph nodes and the axial skeleton appear to live longer, with a median survival of 4–5 years while men with more extensive disease have reported overall survival of less than 30 months.[2] Over the past decade, largely due to extensive use of PSA testing both before and after the diagnosis of prostate cancer, there has been a strong trend toward diagnosing men with prostate cancer generally, and with metastatic prostate cancer in particular, at earlier and earlier points in the course of their disease. As the population of prostate cancer patients under study has a smaller and smaller disease burden, the duration of time from diagnosis to death becomes longer. It is thus not surprising that some recent single-centre studies have reported longer survival figures.

On average, metastatic prostate cancers treated with androgen deprivation respond to this treatment for about 18–22 months before progressing. However, there is substantial variation from man to man, and some men respond to androgen deprivation for years. In the one study with over 1000 subjects, more than 20 per cent were progression-free at 5 years. Prognostic factors have been identified. For example, in men with disease limited to lymph nodes and the axial skeleton, median progression-free survival has been as long as 4 years in multicentre trials.[2]

There is considerably less variation in survival among men with metastatic castration-refractory prostate cancer. Even in the selected population of men participating in a randomized trial investigating what is now considered the most effective chemotherapy, 3-year survival was 17 per cent, and fewer than 5 per cent of men were alive at 6 years. The median survival of men with castration-refractory metastatic disease is about 18 months in contemporary multicentre studies of chemotherapy, but this may be an underestimate because men may show evidence of progression during androgen deprivation long before their oncologist believes there is an indication for chemotherapy. Nonetheless, as noted above, overall survival for metastatic prostate cancer patients has been consistently reported as 3–4 years from the time that androgen deprivation is *initiated*. Some recent single-centre studies have reported median survival in castration-refractory metastatic prostate cancer of over 4 years, but such figures most likely reflect patient populations with more minimal disease burdens, who have long been known to survive longer.[3]

While there is some heterogeneity among men with metastatic prostate cancer, the prognosis of men with a rising PSA after definitive local treatment but no radiographically detectable metastases is much more widely variable. Some of these men never develop any other evidence of disease beside the elevated PSA and require no treatment. Others have disease with local relapse only, which can sometimes be cured with salvage local therapy. It must be emphasized that determining which men have local-only relapse and which men have distant micrometastatic disease remains beyond our capabilities. Similarly, we remain unable to determine which men with apparently local-only relapse stand to benefit from treatment (i.e. would progress to symptomatic or terminal disease without treatment and will avoid or delay such outcomes with treatment), which need no treatment due to indolent disease, and which will fail to benefit from treatment due to treatment failure.

Most men with rising PSAs after local therapy are destined to develop metastatic disease, but they may need to survive other competing causes of death for many years before metastases become apparent. One study of 379 men who developed a rising PSA after undergoing radical prostatectomy at Johns Hopkins reported that prostate-cancer-specific survival at 5, 10, and 15 years was 93, 73 and 55 per cent, respectively.[4]

Prognostic factors in advanced disease

PSA-only relapse after local treatment

These are men who have undergone radical prostatectomy, external-beam radiation or brachytherapy (radioactive seed implantation) for clinically localized prostate cancer who then develop a rising serum PSA in the absence of any radiographic evidence of metastatic cancer. As noted above, this is a heterogeneous population: some have indolent cancer that will not affect survival, others have local only relapse amenable to cure with salvage local therapy, and others have micrometastatic disease destined to progress and become terminal. The challenge is figuring out who's who. Within this heterogeneous group of men, high- and low-risk groups can be identified: the shorter the interval between local treatment and biochemical relapse, the shorter the PSA doubling time, and the higher the Gleason sum, the shorter the predicted survival. It is essential to keep in mind that some studies of "metastatic" prostate cancer will use an elevated PSA following local therapy as evidence of micrometastatic disease in setting of normal radiological imaging; such men clearly have a superior prognosis compared to men with radiographically detectable metastases.

Hormonal-therapy-naive metastatic prostate cancer

Numerous prognostic factors associated with survival have been identified in men with metastatic prostate cancer. In men who have not yet undergone androgen deprivation, numerous factors correlate with shorter survival, including more extensive metastases, poorer performance status, young age at diagnosis, anaemia, pain, elevated serum alkaline phosphatase, and elevated erythrocyte sedimentation rate. Although shorter PSA doubling time predicts shorter survival in men with biochemical failure after local treatment who have normal radiographic imaging, it is not clear how significant PSA doubling time is for men with radiologically imageable metastatic prostate cancer who have not yet received androgen deprivation. A lower PSA nadir (e.g. < 4.0 ng/mL) during androgen deprivation therapy predicts a longer time before disease progression. Surprisingly, the Gleason sum has not been clearly shown to be associated with survival in hormonal-therapy-naive patients with imageable metastatic disease.

Castration-refractory metastatic prostate cancer

Halabi and colleagues analysed data from six Cancer and Leukemia Group B (CALGB) trials that cumulatively enrolled 1101 men with metastatic, castration-refractory prostate cancer.[5] Factors associated with shorter survival in a 760-subject learning set included higher Gleason sum, higher Eastern Cooperative Oncology Group (ECOG) performance status, lower haemoglobin level, and higher serum levels of lactate dehydrogenase (LDH), PSA, and alkaline phosphatase. Increased levels of serum interleukin-6 have also been associated with shorter survival in a few studies but this variable has not yet been incorporated into commonly used prognostic tools. A subsequent study determined that quality of life measures such as insomnia and appetite loss were also independent predictors of survival, but models using these variables are not more accurate than models excluding them.[6] Anorexia and weight loss also appear to be poor prognostic signs in multiple studies and, conversely, overweight and obesity are associated with a more favourable prognosis.[7] It is unclear whether age is associated with outcomes in advanced disease. A recent re-analysis of the dataset of CALGB trials for men with metastatic, castration-refractory disease reported that men aged 50–59 and men aged 80–89 had shorter prostate cancer-specific survival than men aged 70–79.[8] This analysis and others have also reported that higher serum testosterone was associated with shorter survival.

More recently, shorter survival has been associated with each of the following: a shorter prostate specific antigen doubling time either before or after androgren deprivation, a higher PSA nadir during androgen deprivation therapy, a higher PSA value at the initiation of androgen deprivation therapy, a shorter interval between the initiation of androgen deprivation therapy and the emergence of castration-refractory disease, and a higher PSA velocity (i.e. rate of rise, or ng/ml/year).[3, 9, 10] A recent analysis of 129 men treated at a single institution reported that PSA doubling time and the time to progression during androgen deprivation therapy were the most significant variables in a multivariable analysis.[3] Most of these variables function on a continuum and the cut-offs identified in studies have more to do with the specific population of patients being evaluated and the duration of follow-up rather than any clear threshold effect. Nonetheless, with regard to PSA doubling times, a value of less than 3 months appears to be particularly concerning while values longer than 12 months are associated with relatively indolent disease.

Impact of therapy on prognosis in advanced disease

Hormonal therapy for metastatic or unresectable disease

Androgen deprivation therapy was demonstrated to be active against prostate cancer in two 1941 publications and it remains the most effective therapy for metastatic prostate cancer. Early reports demonstrated that castration resulted in a temporary remission of the cancer as well as the resolution or reduction of some of the complications of cancer such as pain, lower urinary tract obstruction, and neurologic deficits due to spinal cord compression. Because of the dramatic benefit with regard to symptoms, hormonal therapy became the mainstay of treatment for metastatic prostate cancer, even in the absence of clear evidence of a survival benefit. Indeed, early controlled trials failed to show a survival benefit. Several more recent studies comparing earlier androgen ablation to delayed androgen ablation have reported a modest survival benefit from early treatment, with a meta-analysis indicating an absolute improvement in overall survival at 10 years of about 6 per cent.[11] The optimal time to initiate androgen deprivation remains undefined, but it is clear that this treatment can substantially improve quality of life in men with symptomatic disease.

Secondary hormonal therapy using agents such as estrogens or ketoconazole (which inhibits adrenal androgen and other corticosteroid hormone synthesis) is sometimes used in men whose cancer progresses despite castrate serum testosterone levels. While such treatment sometimes lowers the serum PSA, it has never been shown convincingly to prolong survival or improve quality of life.

Chemotherapy

Two chemotherapeutic agents have demonstrated a benefit against prostate cancer: mitoxantrone and docetaxel. Mitoxantrone was tested in two large randomized controlled trials that compared mitoxantrone plus prednisone to prednisone alone. There was no survival difference but mitoxantrone was shown to improve quality of life by reducing pain. Mitoxantrone was then compared to docetaxel in two large randomized trials and, in both trials, median survival was about 2 months longer with docetaxel (about 18 months compared to about 16 months). Similar improvements in quality of life and reductions in pain were observed with the two chemotherapy agents.

Prognosis of advanced prostate cancer

PSA-only relapse after local treatment

Limited data is available on prognostic factors for men experiencing biochemical failure after definitive local therapy. PSA doubling time was found to be a surrogate end point for prostate-cancer-specific mortality in an analysis of two multi-institutional databases.[10] Ten-year cancer-specific survival was less than 30 per cent in men with a PSA doubling time of less than three months compared to over 80 per cent in men with a doubling time of three months or longer. In the Johns Hopkins study cited above, men with biochemical relapse after radical prostatectomy could be divided into different risk groups based on the following factors: PSA doubling time, tumour grade and interval between surgery and relapse.[4] Men who experienced a rise in PSA 3 years or less after radical prostatectomy, had a PSA doubling time of less than 3 months, and a Gleason sum of 8, 9 or 10 had a median survival of only 3 years whereas men with a PSA doubling time of at least 9 months had a 15-year survival rate of 75 per cent.[4] The prognostic implications of a rising PSA after definitive local therapy are thus highly contextual.

Hormone-therapy-naive metastatic prostate cancer

Estimating the survival of hormone-therapy-naive patients with metastatic disease is challenging. On average, men respond to androgen ablation for about 18–22 months before progressing and overall survival is about 3 to 4 years, but those figures are increasing as men receive androgen deprivation for smaller and smaller disease burdens. Historical studies may thus underestimate survival not only because of marginal improvements in treatment but also, and more importantly, because extensive use of PSA testing has allowed us to detect minimal disease states and start the survival clock running sooner. There are no validated nomograms for the prognosis of men with metastatic prostate cancer who have not yet developed castration-refractory disease.

Castration-refractory metastatic prostate cancer

Median survival for men with metastatic, castration-refractory prostate cancer is about 19 months (see Figure 13.1). Analysing the CALGB dataset discussed above, Halabi and colleagues developed

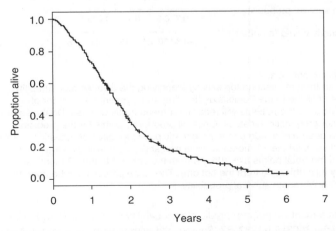

Figure 13.1 Overall survival of men with castration-refractory metastatic prostate cancer treated with docetaxel chemotherapy.

a nomogram for survival that uses the following variables: Gleason sum, Eastern Cooperative Oncology Group (ECOG) performance status, hemoglobin level, the presence of extra-osseous visceral metastases and the serum levels of lactate dehydrogenase (LDH), PSA, and alkaline phosphatase (see Figure 13.2).[5] The area under the receiver operating characteristic (ROC) curve was 0.68. An independent 341-subject validation set was then divided into quartiles by predicted survival and the predicted vs observed survival for these four groups was compared with the following results: 8.8 vs 7.5 months, 13.4 vs 13.4 months, 17.4 vs 18.9 months, and 22.8 vs 27.2 months. Other nomograms have been published, but Halabi's is based on the largest sample, is multi-institutional and was validated on an independent group of patients rather than depending on bootstrapping techniques.[3, 6, 12] However, because the nomogram is based entirely on patients who were participating in clinical trials, men with poor performance status were excluded and the prognostic implications of performance status could not be assessed. In the future, it appears highly probable that PSA doubling time, PSA nadir during androgen deprivation therapy and duration of response to androgen deprivation will all be validated as important variables in multivariable analyses. Other variables that have been shown to be associated with survival are pain

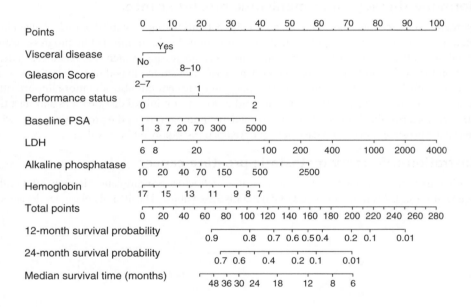

Instructions to physicians:
Please start from the second top axis by identifying the disease measurability. Draw a vertical line to the Points axis (top line) to represent the number of prognostic points the patients will receive for measurable disease. Do the same for the other prognostic variables. Once all prognostic points for the predictors have been determined, add up the prognostic points for each prognostic variable. You can determine the 12-month survival probability by drawing a vertical line down from the "total points axix" (fourth from the bottom) to the 12-month survival probability axis (third line from the bottom). The same process can be done to estimate the 24-month survival probability.

Figure 13.2 Pretreatment nomogram predicting probability of survival. From Halabi S. *et al. Journal of Clinical Oncology* 2003; 21:1232–37. Reproduced with permission from the American Society of Clinical Oncology.

scores and body mass index, most likely because they relate to the patient's overall metastatic burden. In the most recent anlaysis of the CALGB trials dataset, median survival times were 11.5 months for men with normal body mass index, 16.1 months for overweight men and 16.9 months for obese men.[7] Further in the future, molecular genetic markers and various cytokine levels will also likely be incorporated into prognostic tools.

End-stage prostate cancer

When prostate cancer spreads, the metastases most often grow in the bones and lymph nodes. Involvement of the lungs, liver, brain and other organs is much less common. Partly as a result of this, end-stage prostate cancer typically manifests as a wasting syndrome characterized by fatigue, weight loss, declining performance status and increasing bone pain. Renal failure may occur due to urinary tract obstruction from either malignant retroperitoneal adenopathy or from the primary tumour itself. Prostate cancer is also associated with thromboembolic complications. But the function of other non-osseous organs is rarely compromised by the cancer. The decline of the patient's quality of life and functional status is thus often the clearest sign of late stage disease progression and may not be accompanied by dramatic radiographic changes.

Conclusion

Early stage prostate cancer carries a highly favourable prognosis; most of these tumours are never destined to cause illness except as a result of complications from overtreatment. Metastatic prostate cancer, on the other hand, is a highly deadly disease but takes longer to kill the patient than most other metastatic solid tumours. The exquisite, albeit temporary, sensitivity to androgen deprivation results in the ability to control metastatic prostate cancer for 18 months to 2 years with a generally well tolerated therapy, while the use of chemotherapy can extend survival a little further. Prognosticating survival in prostate cancer patients is challenging because of the heterogeneity of the disease and, even more so, because of the trend toward diagnosing all stages of prostate cancer at lower and lower levels of disease burden. Nonetheless, numerous large studies of prostate cancer outcomes have been completed and tools exist for predicting an individual's survival. In contemplating the prognosis of a prostate cancer patient, it is important to remember that metastatic, castration-refractory disease is the deadly version of prostate cancer with a median survival of less than 2 years.

References

1. Ries LAG, Harkins D, Krapcho M. *et al. SEER cancer statistics review, 1975–2003*. Bethesda, MD: National Cancer Institute, 2006.
2. Eisenberger MA, Blumenstein BA, Crawford ED. *et al.* Bilateral orchidectomy with or without flutamide for metastatic prostate cancer. *N Engl J Med* 1998; 339:1036–42.
3. Svatek R, Karakiewicz PI, Shulman M. *et al.* Pre-treatment nomogram for disease-specific survival of patients with chemotherapy-naive androgen independent prostate cancer. *Eur Urol* 2006; 49:666–74.
4. Freedland SJ, Humphreys EB, Mangold LA. *et al.* Risk of prostate cancer-specific mortality following biochemical recurrence after radical prostatectomy. *JAMA* 2005; 294:433–9.
5. Halabi S, Small EJ, Kantoff PW. *et al.* Prognostic model for predicting survival in men with hormone-refractory metastatic prostate cancer. *J Clin Oncol* 2003; 21:1232–7.
6. Collette L, van Andel G, Bottomley A. *et al.* Is baseline quality of life useful for predicting survival with hormone-refractory prostate cancer? A pooled analysis of three studies of the European Organisation for Research and Treatment of Cancer Genitourinary Group. *J Clin Oncol* 2004; 22:3877–85.

7. Halabi S, Ou SS, Vogelzang NJ. *et al.* Inverse relationship between body mass index and clinical outcomes in men with advanced castration-recurrent prostate cancer. *Cancer* 2007; 110:1478–84.

8. Halabi S, Vogelzang NJ, Ou SS. *et al.* Clinical outcomes by age in men with hormone refractory prostate cancer: a pooled analysis of 8 Cancer and Leukemia Group B (CALGB) studies. *J Urol* 2006; 176:81–6.

9. D'Amico AV, Moul J, Carroll PR. *et al.* Surrogate end point for prostate cancer specific mortality in patients with nonmetastatic hormone refractory prostate cancer. *J Urol* 2005; 173:1572–6.

10. D'Amico AV, Moul JW, Carroll PR. *et al.* Surrogate end point for prostate cancer-specific mortality after radical prostatectomy or radiation therapy. *J Natl Cancer Inst* 2003; 95:1376–83.

11. Nair B, Wilt T, MacDonald R. *et al. Early versus deferred androgen suppression in the treatment of advanced prostatic cancer.* Cochrane Database Syst Rev: CD003506, 2002.

12. Smaletz O, Scher HI, Small EJ. *et al.* Nomogram for overall survival of patients with progressive metastatic prostate cancer after castration. *J Clin Oncol* 2002; 20:3972–82.

14

Pancreatic cancer

Moritz Koch, Jürgen Weitz, and Markus W. Büchler

Introduction

Pancreatic cancer is the fourth most common type of cancer in the USA and usually occurs at the age of 65 to 75 years, but younger patients can also be affected by this disease. Ductal adenocarcinoma is the predominant histopathologic tumour type and accounts for more than 85 per cent of all malignant tumours of the pancreas. Pancreatic ductal cancer has the poorest prognosis among all gastrointestinal cancers. The often late clinical presentation and the very aggressive tumour biology are mainly responsible for the poor outcome. At the time of diagnosis, more than 80 per cent of pancreatic cancer patients present with an advanced tumour stage due to local invasive infiltration or distant metastasis. Therefore, the overall 5-year survival rate in pancreatic cancer is less than 5 per cent.[1] Due to the poor survival, the incidence and mortality are almost equivalent; in 2003 the estimated number of new patients in the USA was 30,700 with 30,000 patients dying from the disease. Epidemiological data from Europe show over 60,000 newly diagnosed patients with pancreatic cancer and almost the same number of deaths per year.[2] The majority of pancreatic cancers are sporadic tumours occurring without a hereditary origin; a familial background is found in 5–10 per cent of patients with pancreatic cancer. Among other etiological factors (e.g. smoking and obesity) chronic pancreatitis plays an important role with a 15 to 25-fold increased risk for developing pancreatic cancer.[1]

Despite recent advancements in multimodal treatment regimens (e.g. radiotherapy and chemotherapy) surgery remains the only curative therapy for patients with resectable pancreatic cancer.[2] In advanced pancreatic cancer only palliative treatment options are available as there is no therapy which results in long-term survival of the patients. This chapter will focus on different aspects in the treatment and prognosis of patients with advanced pancreatic cancer.

Natural history of the condition

Carcinoma of the pancreas has a very poor prognosis.[1] Early local spread into peripancreatic tissue with subsequent peritoneal dissemination and often distant metastasis (predominantly in liver and lungs) are the main factors for a poor outcome. Furthermore, pancreatic carcinoma is a highly aggressive tumour which is often diagnosed late because of the absence of early symptoms, especially in tumours of the body and tail. Therefore, the majority of patients present with an advanced pancreatic cancer at the time of diagnosis. The median survival of patients with advanced pancreatic cancer is 4–6 months and less than 10 per cent of patients live beyond a year. Although there are no clinical signs clearly identifying patients with advanced tumour stage, symptoms, such as persistent back pain, marked and rapid weight loss, obstructive jaundice, gastric outlet obstruction and abdominal mass with ascites usually indicate an unresectable tumour.

Local invasion in pancreatic cancer takes place predominantly in the retroperitoneum beyond the pancreas.[3] This dorsal extension is the most frequent reason for locally incomplete tumour resections. The tumour can extend in any direction in the retroperitoneal tissue and may invade great vessels, for example the portal vein, the superior mesenteric vessels, and the coeliac artery. Anterior extension may lead to tumour spread in the visceral peritoneum of the bursa omentalis with subsequent tumour cell dissemination in the peritoneal cavity and later development of peritoneal carcinomatosis (Figure 14.1). Peritoneal carcinomatosis in patients with advanced pancreatic cancer is frequently associated with ascites. A common finding in advanced pancreatic cancer is the invasion of intrapancreatic perineural spaces and further extension into the extrapancreatic retroperitoneal nerve plexus which is responsible for severe back pain. Lymphatic spread is a further type of tumour extension and is frequently observed, even in small pancreatic tumours. The liver and subsequently the lungs are preferred sites of hematogenous metastasis in pancreatic cancer (Figure 14.2).

In conclusion, untreated advanced pancreatic cancer is a rapidly progressing and always lethal disease that is characterized by symptoms such as pain, cachexia, gastric outlet obstruction, obstructive jaundice, ascites, thromboembolic events and sudden decrease in the performance status of the patients.

Factors affecting prognosis

Prognostic factors are used for several reasons: to understand the natural course of the disease, to compare and to predict the results of therapeutic interventions, to identify subgroups of patients with poor outcome and to predict the outcome for an individual patient. Several molecular and clinical factors are known in pancreatic cancer that might influence and contribute to the poor prognosis of this disease. Prognostic factors can be divided into tumour-related, patient-related and treatment-related factors. The classical tumour-related staging system is the TNM classification (Table 14.1).[4] Although the TNM staging system for pancreatic cancer was frequently changed over the last 15 years it remains the strongest predictor for prognosis in exocrine pancreatic cancer.[5] Several studies have defined prognostic factors in pancreatic cancer, but most of these parameters have been identified in patients with potentially resectable tumours. There are only a few studies evaluating prognostic parameters in advanced and unresectable pancreatic cancer.

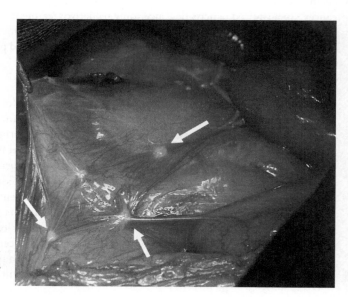

Figure 14.1 Intraoperative finding of peritoneal carcinomatosis from pancreatic cancer.

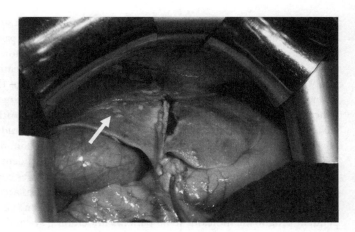

Figure 14.2 Liver metastases from pancreatic cancer (intraoperative situs).

On the genetic level, pancreatic cancer has been extensively researched and well characterized in the last decade but the molecular mechanisms responsible for the aggressive nature of this disease remain poorly understood. Typical genetic changes found in pancreatic cancer are mutated and activated oncogenes (e.g. K-*ras*, HER2/neu) and inactivated tumour-suppressor genes (e.g. *p*16, TP53, MADH4).1 Furthermore, many growth factors and their receptors are overexpressed in human pancreatic cancer.[6] For many of these factors a prognostic significance has only been shown in univariate analysis and therefore, they have to be further validated in larger studies with multivariate analysis including other known prognostic factors. Tumour-related prognostic factors are generally not available in clinical routine and therefore not helpful for patients with

Table 14.1 TNM clinical classification of pancreatic cancer (according to Sobin *et al.*[4])

T – primary tumour	
T1	Tumour limited to pancreas, 2 cm or less in greatest dimension
T2	Tumour limited to pancreas, more than 2 cm in greatest dimension
T3	Tumour extends beyond pancreas, but without involvement of coeliac axis or superior mesenteric artery
T4	Tumour involves coeliac axis or superior mesenteric artery
N – regional lymph nodes	
NX	Regional lymph nodes cannot be assessed
N0	No regional lymph node metastasis
N1	Regional lymph node metastasis
M – distant metastasis	
MX	Distant metastasis cannot be assessed
M0	No distant metastasis
M1	Distant metastasis
Stage grouping	
Stage IA	T1N0M0
Stage IB	T2N0M0
Stage IIA	T3N0M0
Stage IIB	T1, T2, T3 N1 M0
Stage III	T4, any N, M0
Stage IV	Any T, any N, M1

advanced and unresectable pancreatic cancer. However, a Swedish study assessed cytologic material obtained by fine needle aspiration from patients with unresectable pancreatic carcinoma and showed that nuclear morphometry and DNA ploidy are prognostic indicators for short term survival.[7]

Patient-related prognostic factors are very helpful for the treating oncologist, as they can be easily assessed for every patient in clinical practice. As most of these factors have been solely defined in patients undergoing surgery for pancreatic cancer there are only few data in advanced pancreatic cancer. A Spanish study dealt specifically with prognostic parameters in patients with advanced pancreatic cancer. In this retrospective single-centre study, including 134 patients with advanced pancreatic cancer not suitable for surgical resection, multivariate analysis revealed baseline performance status and distant metastases as independent significant prognostic factors for a decreased survival.[8] Furthermore, a prognostic index was constructed in this study which allows the classification of patients into three different groups according to their relative risk of death. The serum tumour marker carcinoembryonic antigen (CEA) was shown to be an independent prognostic indicator in 65 patients undergoing systemic chemotherapy for advanced pancreatic cancer in a Japanese study. In this study, performance status and distant metastasis were also confirmed as independent prognostic factors. Another study analysed prognostic factors in 287 patients with pancreatic cancer of which 193 patients had advanced disease undergoing only palliative treatment. In these 193 patients, multivariate analysis defined chemotherapy, UICC tumour stage and loss of appetite as significant factors showing an impact on patient survival.[9] As appetite belongs to the physical condition of the patient, this study also confirmed that the physical condition or performance status of the patient is one of the most important prognostic factors in advanced pancreatic cancer.

Onset symptoms in patients and tumour location in pancreatic cancer have also been demonstrated to be closely correlated with prognosis, as patients with initial jaundice and a pancreatic head cancer are referred more quickly to first medical treatment. They therefore have a better prognosis than, for example, patients presenting with unspecific back pain and a pancreatic cancer in the tail. Table 14.2 summarizes relevant prognostic factors in advanced pancreatic cancer.

Therapies affecting prognosis

Surgery

As surgery remains the only potentially curative therapy providing long-term survival it is the strongest prognostic factor in pancreatic cancer. Although less than 20 per cent of patients with pancreatic cancer can be curatively resected, 5-year survival rates of up to 20 per cent after resection have been reported by experienced groups.[10] Survival analysis of patients undergoing surgery for pancreatic cancer indicated that curative (R0) resection is the most powerful independent predictor of long-term survival (Figure 14.3).[10] Multivariate analysis from large medical databases

Table 14.2 Factors influencing prognosis in patients with advanced pancreatic cancer

Tumour-related factors	UICC tumour stage
	Serum tumour marker CEA
	Tumour location (head, body, tail)
Patient-related factors	Performance status
	Loss of appetite
	Distant metastasis
	Onset symptoms
Treatment-related factors	Chemotherapy

revealed curative resection with negative resection margins (R0), lymph node status, tumour size and absence of perineural and vascular invasion as the most powerful independent predictors of long-term survival.[2]

Moreover, it has become increasingly evident in the last decade that prognosis of cancer patients also depends strongly on surgical volume and specialization.[11] Many studies showed that a higher case-load and specialization in a surgical centre results in an improved outcome of pancreatic cancer patients.[11] Mortality rates have fallen to below 4 per cent in high-volume centres with special experience in pancreatic surgery.[1]

Therefore, patients in good physical condition who have no radiological signs of distant metastasis are recommended to undergo surgical exploration in a specialized high-volume centre. Randomized studies comparing the standard Kausch–Whipple operation with the pylorus-preserving pancreatoduodenectomy have shown that both procedures are comparable with regard to prognosis and outcome of the patients. Extended lymph node dissection and portal vein resection have been performed by several surgeons in an attempt to further improve the prognosis of patients with pancreatic cancer, but there is no evidence in the literature that these procedures improve long-term survival. There is now an increased use of adjuvant chemotherapy in pancreatic cancer because the ESPAC-1 trial demonstrated a survival benefit of patients receiving chemotherapy (5-FU with folinic acid) after resection of pancreatic cancer.

The majority of patients with pancreatic cancer are in an advanced stage at the time of diagnosis and therefore have no chance of curative therapy. Thus treatment strategies are predominantly

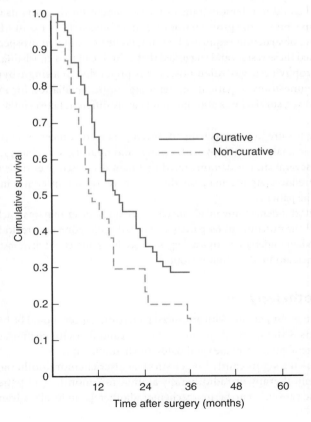

Figure 14.3 Kaplan–Meier survival curves for patients who had curative or non-curative resection; p < 0.001. From Wagner M, Redaelli C, Lietz M, Seiler CA, Friess H, Büchler MW, Curative resection is the single most important factor in determining outcome in patients with pancreatic adenocarcinoma. *Br J Surg*, 91, 586–594 (2004). Copyright British Journal of Surgery Society. Reproduced with permission. Permission is granted by John Wiley and Sons Ltd on behalf of the BJSS Ltd.

palliative and aim to improve quality of life and to prolong survival. Therapy options in advanced pancreatic cancer can be divided into surgical palliative procedures – surgical bypass, palliative resection – and in non-surgical palliative treatments – endoscopic stenting, systemic chemotherapy.

The main symptoms associated with advanced pancreatic cancer are gastric outlet obstruction with concomitant weight loss, obstructive jaundice and pain. Controversy remains regarding whether these symptoms should be treated surgically or non-surgically. The major symptom requiring intervention is obstructive jaundice. Several randomized trials compared operative bypass procedures with biliary stenting and demonstrated that surgical bypass is associated with higher early morbidity and initial mortality rate but shows very good long-term results, whereas endoscopic stenting has a low initial morbidity and mortality but often bears the risk of reinterventions and late biliary complications with additional hospital stays for the patients. Recurrent jaundice and cholangitis are common problems of stenting due to stent occlusion or migration, although the the risk of stent obstruction has been reduced significantly in recent years due to development of new self-expandable metal stents. However, median survival or procedure-related deaths do not differ significantly when comparing surgical bypass to endoscopic stenting procedures.

Symptomatic gastric outlet obstruction can either be treated surgically with a gastrojejunostomy or endoscopically with a stent. Approximately 3–20 per cent of patients with advanced pancreatic cancer will develop mechanical gastric outlet obstruction: thus it remains debatable whether a prophylactic gastrojejunostomy during surgical exploration of an unresectable pancreatic cancer should be performed. A prospective randomized trial from the Johns Hopkins hospital examined this question and could not demonstrate a survival benefit for the patients with prophylactic gastrojejunostomy, but in the group without gastric bypass 19 per cent of the patients developed gastric outlet obstruction requiring later intervention. A Dutch prospective randomized trial study confirmed these results and suggested that a double bypass consisting of a hepaticojejunostomy and a prophylactic gastrojejunostomy is preferable to a single bypass consisting of only a hepaticojejunostomy in patients undergoing surgical palliation for unresectable pancreatic cancer. However, survival was also not significantly different between the two treatment groups in this study.

Pain is a common presenting feature in patients with advanced pancreatic cancer and several treatment options (e.g. systemic analgetic therapy with opiates and neurolytic coeliac plexus block) are available. Although several studies demonstrated that pain decreased over time after coeliac plexus blockade compared to systemic analgesic therapy, there was no difference in the quality of life or in survival of the patients.

The role of palliative pancreatoduodenectomy in advanced pancreatic cancer remains unclear. A retrospective study compared the outcome of 64 patients who had undergone pancreatoduodenectomy with 62 patients who had undergone surgical bypass procedures and could demonstrate an improved survival in the pancreatoduodenectomy group.[2]

Chemotherapy or radiotherapy

The selection of systemic treatment for patients with advanced pancreatic cancer should be based on the extent of disease. Patients with locally advanced disease are candidates for chemoradiotherapy, whereas those with visceral metastases are candidates for chemotherapy.

Several small trials have shown a significantly longer survival after chemoradiotherapy – 10 months – compared to chemotherapy or radiotherapy alone – 6–7 months – in patients with locally advanced pancreatic cancer.[12] Furthermore, chemoradiotherapy in locally advanced unresectable pancreatic cancer has been demonstrated to result in downstaging of the tumour in 15–30 per cent of patient.13 Approximately 50 per cent of the downstaged patients are then resectable and will therefore have a significant survival benefit (with a median survival between 15 and 32 months) compared to unresectable patients.[13] However, larger randomized phase III trials are needed to better define the exact role of chemoradiotherapy in these cases.

Systemic chemotherapy has been demonstrated to improve survival and quality of life in advanced pancreatic cancer.[14] Gemcitabine is the reference drug for first line treatment in advanced pancreatic cancer as it is the first agent that has shown an improvement of disease-related symptoms and survival. A randomized phase III trial compared gemcitabine with 5-FU in 126 patients with advanced pancreatic cancer and showed a significantly better clinical benefit response and survival for the gemcitabine group.[12] Recent phase II studies examined several combinations of gemcitabine with new cytotoxic agents and with novel targeted agents. Most of these studies showed promising results that have yet to be confirmed in larger phase III studies before drawing further clinical conclusions. However, there is still a need for new molecular targets to further improve the poor outcome of patients with advanced pancreatic cancer.

Short-term prognosis

The definition of short-term prognosis in advanced pancreatic cancer is still a challenging topic for every oncologist. Although it is known that patients with advanced pancreatic cancer have a very poor prognosis with no chance of a cure, it is difficult for the treating clinician to predict the short-term prognosis of the individual patient accurately. From cancer statistics and several trials it is known that the median survival in advanced pancreatic cancer is 4–6 months and the 1-year survival rate is below 10 per cent. These numbers may help in the communication between physician and patient, but if the patient with an advanced pancreatic cancer asks for his individual prognosis there is often no definitive answer to this question. Prognostic scores have been become more and more attractive in the last years to better predict the individual prognosis of patients with advanced tumours. There is no general prognostic scoring system available for advanced pancreatic cancer, although some studies calculated clinical scores to classify patients with advanced pancreatic cancer into different prognostic groups. Most of these trials showed that the performance status of the patient and more recently (since the era of gemcitabine) the use of chemotherapy are the main factors which influence the short-term prognosis of patients with this condition. The Spanish study mentioned above identified prognostic factors in 134 patients with advanced pancreatic cancer and proposed a score based on two prognostic parameters, baseline performance status and absence of metastases, allowing the classification of these patients into three groups according to their relative risk of death. This and other prognostic scores might help to identify patients with an extremely poor prognosis who should not be enrolled in any further therapeutic intervention.

The general effectiveness of palliative therapy regarding improvement of short-term prognosis was examined in a large retrospective cohort study from the US which included 1,696 patients with locally advanced pancreatic cancer.[14] In this study, the adjusted median survival in the group of patients with chemoradiotherapy was 47 weeks, in the group with radiation 29 weeks, in the group with chemotherapy 27 weeks and in the group without treatment 15 weeks (Figure 14.4). However, only 44 per cent of patients in this population-based cohort received any form of palliative treatment. Although there are some therapeutic possibilities available with the potential to improve short-term prognosis of patients with advanced pancreatic cancer, the use of such therapies outside of clinical trials is still scarce.

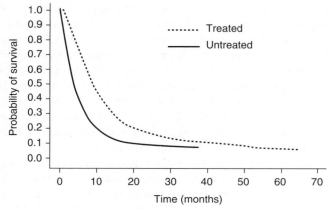

Figure 14.4 Survival adjusted for age, sex, and comorbidity for patients receiving treatment versus untreated patients. From Krzyzanowska, J Clin Oncol 21(18), September 15, 2003, 3409–14. Reproduced with permission from the American Society of Clinical Oncology.

Long-term prognosis

Long-term survival in patients with advanced pancreatic cancer (e.g. 5-year survivors) is practically never observed: long-term prognosis in this context should be defined as survival for more than 1 year. For patients with untreated advanced pancreatic cancer the 1-year survival rate is below 5 per cent. With the use of chemotherapy (gemcitabine) this can be improved by up to 18 per cent.[12] Trials combining chemotherapy and radiation reported 1-year survival rates of over 30 per cent, however the 2-year survival rates were only 2 per cent, demonstrating that there is no long-term prognosis in advanced pancreatic cancer despite use of effective treatment modalities.

As patients with pancreatic cancer have a very high probability of ultimately dying from their disease, it is important to know whether a specific patient will survive a defined period of time rather than have knowledge about median survival of all patients. Therefore, predictive nomograms are increasingly used to better define and predict outcome of patients with cancer. The only prognostic nomogram available for patients with pancreatic cancer was recently developed by Brennan *et al.* in patients who had undergone resection for pancreatic cancer.[15] The nomogram includes several prognostic and clinical variables and predicts the probability that a patient will survive for 1, 2 and 3 years from the time of resection.[15]

Table 14.3 summarizes known factors influencing short- and long-term prognosis of patients with advanced pancreatic cancer. In conclusion, improved prognostic scores are needed to better define and predict outcome of patients with advanced pancreatic cancer.

Table 14.3 Factors influencing short-term and long-term prognosis of patients with advanced pancreatic cancer

Short-term prognosis (< 12 months)	Performance status
	Distant metastasis
	No chemotherapy
Long-term prognosis (> 12 months)	Performance status
	Absence of distant metastasis
	Chemotherapy
	Radiotherapy

References

1. Li D, Xie K, Wolff R, Abbruzzese JL. Pancreatic cancer. Lancet 2004; 363:1049–57.

2. Alexakis N, Halloran C, Raraty M, Ghaneh P, Sutton R, Neoptolemos JP. Current standards of surgery for pancreatic cancer. Br J Surg 2004; 91:1410–27.

3. Hermanek P. Pathology and biology of pancreatic ductal adenocarcinoma. Langenbeck's Arch Surg 1998; 383:116–20.

4. Sobin LH, Wittekind C (eds). TNM classification of malignant tumors, 6th edn. New York: John Wiley and Sons, 2002.

5. Merkel S, Mansmann U, Meyer T, Papadopoulos T, Hohenberger W, Hermanek P. Confusion by frequent changes in staging of exocrine pancreatic carcinoma. Pancreas 2004; 29:171–8.

6. Shi X, Friess H, Kleeff J, Ozawa F, Büchler MW. Pancreatic cancer: factors regulating tumor development, maintenance and metastasis. Pancreatology 2004; 1:517–24.

7. Linder S, Lindholm J, Falkmer U, Blasjo M, Sundelin P, von Rosen A. Combined use of nuclear morphometry and DNA ploidy as prognostic indicators in nonresectable adenocarcinoma of the pancreas. Int J Pancreatol 1995; 18:241–8.

8. Cubiella J, Castells A, Fondevila C, Sans M, Sabater L, Navarro S, Fernandez-Cruz L. Prognostic factors in nonresectable pancreatic adenocarcinoma: a rationale to design therapeutic trials. Am J Gastroenterol 1999; 94:1271–8.

9. Ridwelski K, Meyer F, Ebert M, Malfertheiner P, Lippert H. Prognostic parameters determining survival in pancreatic carcinoma and, in particular, after palliative treatment. Dig Dis 2004; 19:85–92.

10. Wagner M, Redaelli C, Lietz M, Seiler CA, Friess H, Büchler MW. Curative resection is the single most important factor determining outcome in patients with pancreatic adenocarcinoma. Br J Surg 2004; 91:586–94.

11. Weitz J, Koch M, Friess H, Büchler MW. Impact of volume and specialization for cancer surgery. Dig Surg 2004; 21:253–61.

12. van Cutsem E, Aerts R, Haustermans K, Topal B, van Steenbergen W, Verslype C. Systemic treatment of pancreatic cancer. Eur J Gastroenterol Hepatol 2004; 16:265–74.

13. Beger HG, Rau B, Gansauge F, Poch B, Link KH. Treatment of pancreatic cancer: challenge of the facts. World J Surg 2003; 27:1075–84.

14. Krzyzanowska MK, Weeks JC, Earle CC. Treatment of locally advanced pancreatic cancer in the real world: population-based practices and effectiveness. J Clin Oncol 2003; 21:3409–14.

15. Brennan MF, Kattan MW, Klimstra D, Conlon K. Prognostic nomogram for patients undergoing resection for adenocarcinoma of the pancreas. Ann Surg 2004; 240:293–8.

15

Hepatoma

Kelvin K. Ng and Ronnie T. Poon

Introduction

Hepatoma, also known as hepatocellular carcinoma (HCC), is a common malignant disease in the world with a fulminant disease course, low resectability rate, high recurrence after hepatic resection and liver transplantation, poor response to systemic treatment and hence grave prognosis (Figure 15.1). It is the most common primary liver malignancy and ranks fifth in the overall frequency of malignancies in the world, with a global annual incidence of about one million new patients. Regions with a high incidence of HCC include South-East Asia, some of the western Pacific Islands and most parts of sub-Saharan Africa. In fact, 70 per cent of all new HCC cases occur in Asia, where chronic hepatitis B viral infection is common. The incidence of HCC in Western countries is also rising because of the high prevalence of hepatitis C viral infection. The average age of presentation of this tumour is in the early to middle 60s. Patients with hepatitis B virus-induced HCC are generally younger than those with hepatitis C virus-induced tumours, and HCC occurs more frequently in males than females, with an overall ratio of 3:1.

In general, the long-term survival of HCC patients still remains dismal. Hepatic resection and liver transplantation have been regarded as the curative treatments of choice for this tumour. However, these treatment options are limited by the low resectability rate (20–30 per cent) and shortage of liver grafts around the world. Furthermore, high incidence of intrahepatic and/or extrahepatic recurrence after surgical treatment is a main cause of late death of patients and remains a major obstacle to improving the prognosis of HCC patients. In fact, most patients present with advanced HCC that cannot be treated surgically.

A number of factors have been proven to have a prognostic value for HCC, including tumour pathologic, tumour biologic, host and treatment factors. Each of these factors exerts its effect not only on the aggressiveness of the tumour, but also on the risk of recurrence after treatment, thus influencing the overall prognosis of this deadly tumour. In recent years, tremendous efforts have been devoted to both clinical and basic science research on the risk factors for tumour recurrence, the use of adjuvant therapy to prevent recurrence, and management of recurrence after treatment. However, controversy remains in such areas as the relative importance of different risk factors, the value of adjuvant therapy and the roles of various different treatment modalities for recurrence. Updated knowledge on the potential prognostic factors for HCC is essential to direct the appropriate strategy to improve the long-term prognosis of HCC patients.

Natural history of HCC

The natural history of HCC varies among global regions because of different aetiologic or carcinogenic factors, among which hepatitis B virus, hepatitis C virus and aflatoxin are the most

(a)

(b)

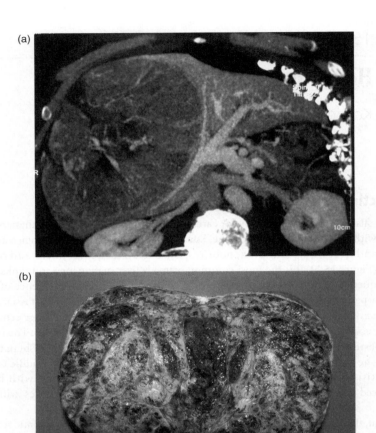

Figure 15.1 (a) Computed tomography appearance of large hepatocellular carcinoma shows a typical arterial enhancing pattern with central tumour necrosis. (b) Heterogeneous tumour features of hepatocellular carcinoma on gross examination.

important areas of interest. Hepatitis virus-induced HCC accounts for the majority of HCC patients in Asia and some Western countries, whereas aflatoxin-induced HCC most often occurs in southern Africa, particularly in Mozambique. Patients with aflatoxin-induced HCC usually die within one to two months after clinical onset of the disease, when the tumour mass reaches a huge size within a relatively normal liver. This tumour is often poorly differentiated and grows quickly. In contrast, hepatitis virus-induced HCC is more commonly well differentiated and grows slowly within a fibrous capsule in the background of a cirrhotic liver. Apart from tumour dissemination, patients with virus-associated HCC frequently die from hepatic failure. The estimated 1-year survival rates of untreated HCC patients in Japan and United States are 25.9 and 22.6 per cent, respectively.[1]

In the modern management of HCC patients, a multidisciplinary approach has been widely practiced. To evaluate the efficacy of various treatment options and to assess the patients' prognosis precisely, understanding the natural history of untreated HCC patients is mandatory. Over the past 10 years, the survival of untreated HCC patients has shown a trend of improvement for two reasons. First, the widespread use of screening ultrasonography in patients with chronic liver disease has enabled diagnosis of early stage HCC. Thus, the survival of patients appears to have prolonged because of the lead-time bias. Second, the improved management of variceal bleeding, the use of potent antibiotics to treat severe infection and the advanced technology in liver support systems have enhanced the quality of care for patients with decompensated cirrhosis. In a recent study of 102 cirrhotic patients with untreated HCC,[2] the median survival was 17 months (range 1–60 months). The overall actuarial survival rates at 1, 2 and 3 years were 54, 40 and 28 per cent, respectively: 77 percent of the patients had died at the time of analysis and the most common causes of death were tumour progression, variceal bleeding, hepatic failure and severe infection. The actuarial probability of developing complications from liver decompensation at 1, 2 and 3 years was 47, 70 and 80 per cent, respectively. The most frequent complications encountered were intractable ascites, hepatic encephalopathy, systemic infection and variceal bleeding. Concerning the deterioration of liver function reserve, the actuarial probability at 1, 2 and 3 years was 43, 58 and 76 per cent, respectively. The actuarial probability of tumour growth at 6, 12 and 24 months was 50, 71 and 83 per cent, respectively. Moreover, the actuarial probability of developing vascular invasion by tumour and extrahepatic tumour spread at 1, 2 and 3 years was 21, 29, 46, 9, 11 and 22 per cent, respectively. Subgroup analysis showed that life expectancy of untreated HCC patients depended on the presence of cancer-related symptoms (constitutional syndrome, abdominal pain and ascites), and the identification of the invasive phenotype of the tumour (vascular invasion and extrahepatic spread). Hence, the 1-, 2- and 3-year actuarial survival rates of asymptomatic patients without invasive tumour pattern were 80, 65 and 50 per cent, respectively. On the contrary, the corresponding survival rates of those patients with either one adverse factor were significantly worse: 29, 16 and 8 per cent, respectively.

Factors affecting prognosis

The significant prognostic factors for HCC patients have been extensively studied and they can be classified as host and tumour factors.[3,4] Many of these carry a significant value in long-term prognosis of hepatoma (Table 15.1).

Tumour factors

Pathologic factors

There are extensive studies on the prognostic effects of conventional pathologic factors on the risk of recurrence and long-term survival of HCC patients. These include tumour size, number of tumour nodules, presence of satellite nodules, venous invasion, capsule state and histologic differentiation.

Large tumour size, especially > 5 cm in diameter, is invariably an independent prognostic factor and has a significantly high risk of recurrence. Studies have demonstrated both longer 5-year overall survival and disease-free survival rates of small HCC of < 5 cm in diameter, compared with large HCC of > 5 cm in diameter. The influence of large tumour size is attributed to increased tumour invasiveness, as demonstrated by a high incidence of intrahepatic metastasis and portal venous invasion. Multiple tumour nodules and presence of satellite nodules around the main tumour are associated with poor prognosis in terms of poor survival and a high recurrence rate. Multiple tumours could be caused by either intrahepatic metastasis or multicentric

Table 15.1 Significant long-term prognostic factors for patients with hepatoma

Prognostic factors	Value favouring good prognosis
Host factors	
Sex	Female
Associated hepatitis status	Inactive hepatitis B/C infection
Cirrhosis	Absence
Tumour factors	
Tumour size	Size < 5 cm
Number of tumour nodules	Solitary
Satellite nodules	Absence
Microscopic/macroscopic venous invasion	Absence
Serum AFP concentration	Low
Serum AFP mRNA	Negative
Serum AFP-L3	Negative
PCNA index	Low
Telomerase activity	Low
Tumour microvessel density	Low
Intercellular adhesive molecules	Normal expression

occurrence, whereas satellite nodules are considered to arise from intrahepatic metastasis. Both of these factors indicate the invasiveness of the tumour.

HCC is characterized by its high propensity for vascular invasion. The presence of microscopic venous invasion is the most consistently reported risk factor for recurrence after resection or transplantation, and is also an independent factor for poor prognosis. In some studies, it is the single most important factor for recurrence. Likewise, macroscopic portal vein involvement by the tumour in the form of portal vein thrombi is also regarded as a poor prognostic factor. It is widely accepted that intrahepatic metastasis by the portal venous system is an important mechanism for intrahepatic recurrence after resection.

The pathologic tumour–node–metastasis (pTNM) staging system fashioned by the Union Internacional Contra la Cancrum (UICC) incorporates tumour size, number of tumour nodules, and vascular invasion into its tumour (T) classification[5] (Table 15.2). Conceivably, it is useful in stratifying patients according to the risk of recurrence, and it shows good correlation between the staging group and patient outcome. In recent reports, pTNM staging has been shown to provide an accurate prognostic classification of long-term survival after resection of HCC.

The effects of other tumour pathologic features such as tumour encapsulation and histologic differentiation on the risk of recurrence and long-term prognosis are less conclusive. The presence of tumour capsule has been associated with a lower incidence of recurrence in some studies, probably because of a reduced incidence of local venous invasion and direct invasion into the surrounding liver. Paradoxically, in other studies, tumour encapsulation was a strong predictor of portal venous invasion, owing to a high incidence of tumour invasion into blood vessels in the tumour capsule. Well-encapsulated and non-necrotic HCC has a significantly

Table 15.2 Pathologic tumour-node-metastasis (pTNM) staging system

T1	Solitary tumour without vascular invasion
T2	Solitary tumour with vascular invasion, or multiple tumours, none > 5 cm
T3	Multiple tumours > 5 cm, or tumour involving a major branch of the portal or hepatic vein(s)
T4	Tumour(s) with direct invasion of adjacent organs other than the gallbladder or with perforation of visceral peritoneum
N0	No regional lymph node metastasis
N1	Regional lymph node metastasis
M0	No distant metastasis
M1	Distant metastasis
Stage I	T1 N0 M0
Stage II	T2 N0 M0
Stage IIIA	T3 N0 M0
Stage IIIB	T4 N0 M0
Stage IIIC	Any T N1 M0
Stage IV	Any T Any N M1

higher tumour pressure and greater pressure gradient, and both of these factors are found to associate with venous invasion and intrahepatic metastasis. The prognostic significance of histologic differentiation of HCC on the risk of recurrence has also been debated and the results from various studies are inconsistent.

Biologic factors

Several tumour biologic factors related to tumour growth and invasiveness of HCC have been evaluated in recent years as new prognostic factors for HCC. Serum alpha-fetoprotein (AFP) concentration is useful not only for diagnosis of HCC, but also as a prognostic indicator for HCC patients. Patients with high serum AFP levels at diagnosis tend to have large tumour size, bilobar involvement, massive or diffuse types HCC, and venous invasion by tumour. High serum AFP level is associated with significantly shorter median survival. AFP mRNA in the peripheral blood has been proposed as a predictive marker of dissemination of tumour cells into the systemic circulation, and is therefore considered a prognostic factor for early intrahepatic and distant metastases of HCC. Patients with positive serum AFP mRNA are found to have a higher possibility of metastasis and worse overall and disease-free survival than those in the negative group. Lens culinaris agglutinin A-reactive fraction of AFP (AFP-L3) is another useful marker of distant metastasis and poor prognosis for HCC patients. Patients with positive AFP-L3 have worse liver function and a more advanced tumour with poor tumour histology, compared with the negative group.

It is known that the malignant potential of various tumours can be reflected by the nuclear DNA content of the tumour cells. The association between DNA aneuploidy and the risk of tumour recurrence has been illustrated by some studies using flow cytometric analysis. However, other authors could not demonstrate a correlation between DNA ploidy and the risk of recurrence and survival. The proliferative activity of tumour cells is directly related to tumour growth and is a potential prognostic indicator. It can lead to the development of clonal sub-populations with an increased capacity for invasion and metastasis. Proliferating cell nuclear antigen (PCNA) is an auxiliary protein for DNA polymerase-delta. Its expression is related to DNA synthesis and cell proliferation, and it is a marker for G1/S phase in the cell cycle. This marker can be detected by immunohistochemical study and is a commonly used index of tumour proliferative activity. A high PCNA index has been shown to be an independent predictor of recurrence, especially for small HCC. It is also associated with a high incidence of venous invasion and direct liver invasion, suggesting that this marker is related not only to tumour growth but also to tumour invasiveness.

Telomerase is another nuclear protein that is associated with tumour cell proliferation. It is a ribonucleoprotein enzyme that stabilizes the ends of chromosomes, or telomeres. In normal dividing somatic cells, progressive shortening of the ends of the chromosomes has been observed and this eventually leads to cell senescence. A majority of malignant tumours have been found to express reactivated telomerase, which allows continued proliferation of the tumour cells. Recent studies have suggested that a high telomerase activity in HCC could be a predictor of early postoperative recurrence.

Expression of androgen receptor has also been proposed to be related to the growth of HCC. However, the significance of androgen receptor as a prognostic factor for recurrence is conflicting in different studies, and the exact mechanism of androgen receptor expression in HCC has not been clearly clarified. Similarly, conflicting results have been reported regarding the significance of mutation of the p53 gene, a tumour suppressor gene, on the risk of recurrence in HCC. This gene encodes a nuclear protein that controls cell cycle, apoptosis and cellular differentiation. Mutation of the p53 gene is commonly observed in various cancers. Nevertheless, its role in determining the recurrence risk of HCC remains to be further investigated.

Angiogenesis, the process by which tumours develop new blood vessels, is now recognized to play a crucial role in tumour growth and metastasis. HCC is a hypervascular tumour charac-terized by neovascularization, and its invasiveness is closely related to its angiogenic activity. Tumour expression of mediators of angiogenesis such as vascular endothelial growth factor and basic fibroblast growth factor has been associated with the invasive features of HCC, including portal vein infiltration and capsular tumour invasion. Recent evidence shows that a high tumour microvessel density, an index of angiogenic activity, is associated with an increased risk of recurrence and a shorter recurrence time after resection of HCC. Another new concept regarding cancer invasion and metastasis relates to the intercellular adhesiveness between tumour cells. Reduced expression of intercellular adhesion molecules such as cadherins has been found to be correlated with vascular or capsular invasion in HCC, and it might have partly contributed to early recurrence of HCC after resection.

Host factors

Sex and age

It has been reported that female HCC patients tend to develop well-encapsulated and less invasive tumours, and they have longer overall survival, lower recurrence rate and better pro-gnosis than male HCC patients. The oestrogen receptor (ER) is found to be closely related to the prognosis of HCC patients, in which ER-positive HCC has a less malignant biologic behaviour and higher percentages of early stage HCC than ER-negative HCC. The 5-year survival rates of ER-positive and ER-negative HCC patients are 24 and 10 per cent, respectively. In addition, the presence of variant ER transcripts in the tumour is a strong negative survival predictor in untreated HCC patients, when compared with those with wild-type ER. It is controversial whether the age of HCC patients has an independent influence on the overall prognosis. Some studies have shown that younger HCC patients often have more invasive tumours and worse prognosis than the older patients. However, other studies showed inconsistent findings.

Associated hepatitis status and liver cirrhosis

The active inflammatory activity in the non-tumourous liver, as indicated by the serum transaminase levels or histologic assessment of hepatitis activity, is closely associated with survival of HCC patients. It is also an independent risk factor for intrahepatic tumour recurrence after resection. Long-term disease-free survival has been observed in patients without active hepatitis, and suppression of coexisting hepatitis is therefore necessary to prevent tumour recurrence after treatment. It has been hypothesized that active hepatitis activity in the liver remnant might enhance the development of intrahepatic metastasis by upregulating the expression of vascular adhesion molecules. A high viral load is an independent risk factor for recurrence. The precore mutant-type hepatitis B virus and genotype 1b hepatitis C virus are associated with a high risk of ongoing hepatocarcinogenesis. Studies have shown that the recurrence rate of HCC in patients with hepatitis C virus infection was higher than that in patients with hepatitis B virus infection, and this could have contributed to a higher risk of multicentric tumour recurrence in chronic hepatitis C cirrhosis. In some cases, double infection with hepatitis B and C virus is associated with a high surgical complication rate and hospital mortality rate, together with early tumour recurrence after hepatic resection for HCC patients.

The effect of underlying cirrhosis on the risk of recurrence and hence long-term prognosis of HCC patients is an issue under debate. Cirrhosis was reported in some studies to be a significant risk factor for recurrence in the liver remnant, presumably as a result of a predisposition to multicentric hepatocarcinogenesis. However, this correlation was not indicated in other studies, and it has been suggested that the risk of developing new HCC is probably limited in early cirrhosis.

Hepatitis and cirrhosis not only affect the risk of hepatocarcinogenesis, but more importantly, affect the liver function and hence the treatment options of patients. In patients with Child–Pugh[6] class C cirrhosis, surgical resection is contraindicated even for small HCC, and in patients with Child–Pugh class B cirrhosis, any major hepatic resection is contraindicated. Functional reserve of the remnant cirrhotic liver is an independent prognostic predictor of long-term survival in HCC patients after liver resection. These liver functional indicators include alanine transaminase, gamma-glutamyl transpeptidase, serum bilirubin level, serum albumin level, prothrombin time, indocyanine green retention value and Child–Pugh classification. Even in patients with unresectable tumour, liver function is still an important prognostic factor because locoregional therapies may not be applicable in patients with very poor liver function.

Prognostic staging systems

There are several staging systems of prognostic value for HCC. Apart from providing reliable information about the natural history of the disease, some staging systems permit the categorization of patients into various treatment groups with variable associated prognosis. The previously mentioned pTNM staging system is useful in predicting long-term prognosis of HCC patients after surgical resection. In a cohort of 518 patients with hepatic resection in our centre, there were significant differences between stages I and II, between stages II and IIIA, and between stages II and IIIB (Figure 15.2). There are two widely adopted staging systems which are derived from a large number of cohort patients, namely, Cancer of the Liver Italian Programme (CLIP)

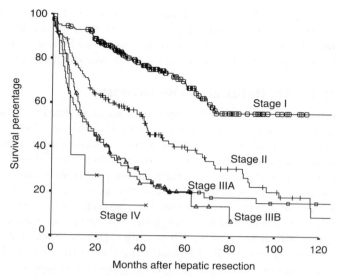

Figure 15.2 Survival curves of patients stratified according to pathologic tumour–node–metastasis (pTNM) staging system.

score[7] and Barcelona Clinic Liver Cancer (BCLC) staging classification,[8] which were designed to provide prognostic information for the full spectrum of HCC patients with resectable or unresectable disease.

Cancer of the Liver Italian Programme score

The CLIP score was derived from a retrospective analysis of 435 HCC patients in 1988 (Table 15.3). Unlike the pTNM staging system, a CLIP score is composed of several other parameters of prognostic value, including Child–Pugh stage, tumour morphology and extension, serum AFP level and presence of portal vein thrombosis. It has been shown that a CLIP score provides accurate prognostic information and a high predictive power for survival of HCC patients. The 1-year and 5-year overall survival rates of HCC patients were 84 and 65 per cent for patients with CLIP score of 0, 66 and 45 per cent for those with score of 1, 45 and 17 per cent for those with score of 2, 36 and 12 per cent for those with score of 3, and 9 and 0 per cent for those with scores of 4–6, respectively.

Barcelona Clinic Liver Cancer staging classification

The BCLC staging system was proposed in 1999, with the aim of defining prognosis and treatment strategies in patients with resectable or transplantable disease, or those undergoing locoregional therapies (Table 15.4). This system stratifies HCC patients into four risk groups, proposing different strategies for each group. Stage A HCC patients (early stage) are suitable for curative treatment modalities, including hepatic resection, liver transplantation and local ablation therapies such as percutaneous ethanol injection or radiofrequency ablation. Stages B and C HCC patients (intermediate and advanced stages) should qualify for palliative treatment such as transarterial chemoembolization (TACE) or some new agents in the setting of clinical trials. Lastly, stage D HCC patients (terminal stage) should only receive symptomatic

Table 15.3 Cancer of the Liver Italian Programme (CLIP) scoring system

	Score
Child–Pugh stage	
A	0
B	1
C	2
Tumour morphology	
Uninodular and extension < 50%	0
Multinodular and extension < 50%	1
Massive or extension > 50%	2
Alpha-fetoprotein (ng/ml)	
< 400	0
> 400	1
Portal vein thrombosis	
No	0
Yes	1

treatment because of their extremely grim prognosis despite any interventions. The overall survival rates at 1, 3 and 5 years in patients with stage A HCC were 85, 62 and 51 per cent, respectively (Figure 15.3). Within this group, the 3-year survival rate dropped to 35 per cent if patients developed unresolved portal hypertension as indicated by a preoperative hepatic venous pressure gradient of 10 mmHg or more. For patients with stages B and C HCC, the overall survival rates at 1, 3 and 5 years were 54, 28 and 7 per cent, respectively (Figure 15.4). Patients with stage D HCC had the poorest survival of only 10 per cent after both 1 and 3 years, and no patient was alive after 5 years.

Table 15.4 Barcelona Clinic Liver Cancer (BCLC) staging classification

	Performance status	Tumour stage	Liver function
Stage A Early HCC			
A1	0	Single, < 5 cm	No portal hypertension and normal bilirubin level
A2	0	Single, < 5 cm	Portal hypertension, normal bilirubin level
A3	0	Single, < 5 cm	Portal hypertension and abnormal bilirubin level
A4	0	< 3 tumours, all < 3 cm	Child–Pugh A–B
Stage B Intermediate HCC	0	Single, > 5 cm or > 3 tumours, > 3 cm	Child–Pugh A–B
Stage C Advanced HCC	1–2	Vascular invasion or extrahepatic spread	Child–Pugh A–B
Stage D Terminal HCC	3–4	Any	Child–Pugh C

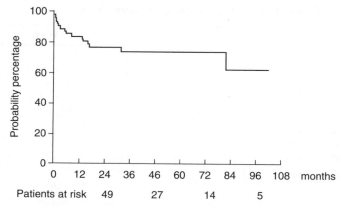

Figure 15.3 Overall survival of patients with early HCC treated by orthotopic liver transplantation.[8] From Llovet JM, Bru C, Bruix L. Prognosis of hepatocellular carcinoma: the BCLC staging classification. *Semin Liver Dis* 1999; 19:329–38. Reprinted with permission from Thieme.

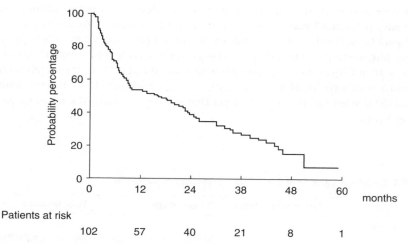

Figure 15.4 Overall survival of patients with untreated non-surgical HCC in the setting of RCT. [8] From Llovet JM, Bru C, Bruix L. Prognosis of hepatocellular carcinoma: the BCLC staging classification. *Semin Liver Dis* 1999; 19:329–38. Reprinted with permission from Thieme.

Impact of treatment on prognosis

With the application of different prognostic factors and staging systems, HCC patients could be stratified into different treatment groups according to their prognosis. Those patients with good prognosis should receive curative treatments such as hepatic resection, liver transplantation and ablation therapy. However, the proportion of such patients is small (< 30 per cent). On the other hand, patients with fair prognosis can be treated palliatively by TACE or some local ablation therapies. For patients with poor prognosis, symptomatic treatment is the only option. Each of these treatment modalities is associated with a different long-term prognosis[9] (Table 15.5).

Hepatic resection

Hepatic resection can effectively eliminate the cancer, but it is limited by its inability to eliminate the remaining portions of the liver carrying the risk of malignant transformation, as well as its not being able to improve hepatic function. Therefore, hepatic resection is generally recommended for patients with technically resectable HCC and well-preserved liver function. Unfortunately, the incidence of resectable HCC in noncirrhotic patients remains low, and the overall respectability rate of HCC patients is less than 20 per cent in most studies. Nevertheless, favourable results of hepatic resection have been obtained in selected groups of HCC patients. Large series of liver resection for HCC patients have reported 3- and 5-year survival rates between 38–65 per cent and 33–50 per cent, respectively. Despite these survival results, the incidence of tumour recurrence after resection exceeds 50 per cent, thus contributing to a low disease-free survival. The majority of recurrence occurs in the liver remnant, and aggressive treatment of recurrence by re-resection, local ablation or TACE can prolong patient survival.

Liver transplantation

Orthotopic liver transplantation is theoretically the best treatment for HCC patients as it involves the widest possible resection margins for cancer, removes the remnant liver at risk of malignant change, and restores hepatic function. This is a particular good treatment option for patients with early HCC, and hence a low metastatic potential, but advanced Child–Pugh class C cirrhosis. In such patients, other effective treatments cannot be offered because of poor liver function, and prognosis is dismal and determined by the cirrhosis rather than HCC without further treatment. However, the scarcity of liver grafts has made this treatment modality less effective and available to HCC patients, when compared with hepatic resection. Milan criteria[10] – solitary tumour < 5 cm or < 3 tumour nodules, each < 3 cm – are the most widely used criteria for inclusion of HCC patients for liver transplantation, based on which the 4-year survival rate of up to 75 per cent could be achieved. However, the overall survival benefit of liver transplantation has been limited by the long waiting time for liver grafts for HCC patients. An intention-to-treat analysis has revealed a decrease in survival from 84 to 54 per cent when the mean waiting time increased from 62 to 162 days.[11] Live donor liver transplantation is a solution to eliminate

Table 15.5 Long-term prognosis of HCC patients receiving different treatment modalities

Curative treatment	Survival rates
Hepatic resection	3-year, 38–65% 5-year, 33–50%
Liver transplantation	4-year, 75%
Radiofrequency ablation	3-year, 45–68% 5-year, 33–40%
Percutaneous ethanol injection	5-year, 24–40%
Palliative treatment Transarterial chemoembolization Systemic chemotherapy	3-year, 26–29% Median survival, 4 months

the limiting factor of long waiting time for liver grafts, and is theoretically a more preferred choice for HCC patients. However, the potential risk of donor hepatectomy needs to be considered in offering such treatment.

Local ablation therapy

Local ablation therapy has been practiced widely for unresectable HCC. It has the advantage of effective tumour destruction and preservation of maximal non-tumourous liver tissue at the same time. Among different local ablation therapies, percutaneous ethanol injection (PEI) and radiofrequency ablation (RFA) are the most popular techniques with associated impressive prognosis.

PEI induces tumour necrosis by cellular dehydration, protein denaturation, and thrombosis of small vessels. It can be performed as an outpatient procedure under local anaesthesia, with ultrasound or computed tomography (CT) guidance. Histopathologic studies have shown that PEI can induce complete tumour necrosis in about 70 per cent of patients with HCC < 3 cm. The reported 5-year survival rates after PEI in patients with HCC < 5 cm was in the range of 24–40 per cent. Some adverse prognostic factors have been identified to influence the efficacy of PEI. These include liver function status, tumour size, pretreatment AFP level and multiple tumour nodules.

RFA has gained much enthusiasm in modern management of unresectable malignant liver tumours. As a form of thermal ablation treatment, it relies on the interaction of high frequency alternating current (460–480 kHz) with living tissue to generate heat energy through ionic vibration. At lethal temperatures above 60°C, there is instantaneous protein coagulation with irreversible damage of key intracellular enzymes, which contributes to coagulative necrosis of the target lesion. In recent years, there are new models of RF electrodes (multitined expandable, internally cooled, perfusion and bipolar electrodes), which can produce larger coagulation necrosis to extend the limit of ablation volume for liver tumours. The complete ablation rate of RFA for HCC approaches 100 per cent in many series, while the local recurrence at the RFA treatment site ranges from 5.7–39 per cent. The reported 3- and 5-year survival rates of RFA for HCC patients were in the ranges of 45–68 per cent and 33–40 per cent, respectively.

Transarterial chemoembolization

TACE is a regional therapy widely used for unresectable HCC since the 1980s. During the procedure, iodized poppyseed oil (lipiodol) and chemotherapeutic agents (doxorubicin, cisplastin, or mitomycin C) are administered through the feeding artery of the tumour, followed by arterial embolization with gelatin sponge particles. The long-term survival benefit of TACE for HCC patients has been demonstrated by two recent randomized controlled studies, which suggested a beneficial effect of TACE (3-year survival rate of 26–29 per cent) compared with conservative management.[12, 13] A meta-analysis of all the randomized clinical trials available in the literature has shown that TACE provided short-term (2-year) survival benefit, odds ratio = 0.42, as compared with control.[14]

Systemic treatment

HCC is relatively resistant to systemic chemotherapeutic agents. Doxorubicin is the most commonly used agent, but the overall response rate is low (< 20 per cent) with poor median survival of patients (~ 4 months). Immunotherapy using high-dose recombinant interferon-α2 has been shown to be superior to systemic doxorubicin in some studies. However, flu-like symptoms and significant toxicities are associated with high drug dosage. Somatostatin receptors have been identified in HCC, and hence octreotide, a somatostatin analogue, is potentially effective for tumour clearance by exerting a suppressive effect on cell growth. The role of octreotide for patients with advanced HCC needs to be further clarified by a large-scale randomized study.

Short- and long-term prognosis

As described above, the prognosis of hepatocellular carcinoma depends a lot on the stage at diagnosis and the provision or not of treatment. In patients presenting late with advanced disease (CLIP score 4–6, or Barcelona Stage D) for whom no treatment options are available the outlook is grim, with a median survival in the vicinity of 3–4 months with only a 10 per cent chance of being alive in 12 months, and little chance of surviving 5 years (Figure 15.2).

Conclusion

HCC remains a major health problem with poor prognosis worldwide. Because of the advances in imaging techniques, more frequent diagnosis of HCC are being made, especially in the asymptomatic phase. A wide range of treatment modalities are available for HCC patients, depending on the stage of the disease as well as the liver function state. Meanwhile, various prognostic factors have been identified, influencing the tumour recurrence risk and long-term survival of patients. Hence, stratification of HCC patients according to the prognosis to different treatment groups is important so that curative treatment can be reserved for the subgroup of patients with relatively good prognosis. For patients with advanced malignancy localized to the liver, local ablation or TACE may offer effective symptomatic palliation and prolongation of patients' survival, but the prognosis is still poor. For patients with distant metastases, no effective therapy can be offered and symptomatic palliative care is the best option.

References

1. Okuda K. Natural history of hepatocellular carcinoma including fibrolamellar and hepato-cholangiocarcinoma variants. *J Gastroenterol Hepatol* 2002; 17:401–5.

2. Llovet JM, Bustamante J, Castells A. *et al*. Natural history of untreated nonsurgical hepatocellular carcinoma: rationale for the design and evaluation of therapeutic trials. *Hepatology* 1999; 29:62–7.

3. Qin LX, Tang ZY. The prognostic significance of clinical and pathological features in hepatocellular carcinoma. *World J Gastroenterol* 2002; 8:193–9.

4. Poon RT, Fan ST, Wong J. Risk factors, prevention, and management of postoperative recurrence after resection of hepatocellular carcinoma. *Ann Surg* 2000; 232:10–24.

5. Greene FL, Page DL, Fleming ID. Liver including intrahepatic bile ducts. In *American Joint Committee on Cancer staging manual*, pp. 131–44. Chicago, IL: Springer, 2002.

6. Pugh RN, Murray-Lyon IM, Dawson JL. Transection of the oesophagus for bleeding oesophageal varices. *Br J Surg* 1973; 60:646–9.

7. The Cancer of the Liver Italian Program (CLIP) investigators. A new prognostic system for hepatocellular carcinoma: a retrospective study of 435 patients. *Hepatology* 1998; 28:751–5.

8. Llovet JM, Bru C, Bruix J. Prognosis of hepatocellular carcinoma: the BCLC staging classification. *Semin Liver Dis* 1999; 19:329–38.

9. Befeler AS, Di Bisceglie AM. Hepatocellular carcinoma: diagnosis and treatment. *Gastroenterology* 2002; 122:1609–19.

10. Mazzaferro V, Regalia E, Doci R. *et al*. Liver transplantation for the treatment of small hepatocellular carcinomas in patients with cirrhosis. *N Engl J Med* 1996; 334:693–9.

11. Llovet JM, Fuster J, Bruix J. Intention-to-treat analysis of surgical treatment for early hepatocellular carcinoma: resection versus transplantation. *Hepatology* 1999; 30:1434–40.

12. Llovet JM, Real MI, Montana X. *et al.* Arterial embolisation or chemoembolisation versus symptomatic treatment in patients with unresectable hepatocellular carcinoma: a randomised controlled trial. *Lancet* 2002; 359:1734–9.

13. Lo CM, Ngan H, Tso WK. *et al.* Randomized controlled trial of transarterial lipiodol chemoembolization for unresectable hepatocellular carcinoma. *Hepatology* 2002; 35:1164–71.

14. Llovet JM, Bruix J. Systematic review of randomized trials for unresectable hepatocellular carcinoma: Chemoembolization improves survival. *Hepatology* 2003; 37:429–42.

16

Head and neck cancer

Ceri Hughes and Steven J. Thomas

Introduction

Head and neck cancer is a multi-step process that involves both environmental carcinogens and genetic susceptibility. Alcohol consumption and cigarette smoking account for disease development in the majority of cases of upper aerodigestive tract cancers in western and southern Europe and the US.

Although it is probable that smoking and alcohol act independently as risk factors for upper aerodigestive tract cancers, they also act synergistically. The attributable risk of oral cancer with daily exposure to tobacco smoke and alcohol exceeds 70 per cent. Oral cancer is not uncommon and is an important cause of morbidity and mortality, with 267,000 cases reported globally in 2000, two-thirds of them in men. There are marked international variations in reported incidence. Melanesia has the highest incidence in the world (36.3 per 10^5 in men and 23.6 per 10^5 in women). Rates are also high in South Asia (13.0 per 10^5 in men and 8.6 per 10^5 in women).[1] Although smoking has been consistently associated with increased risk of oral cancer, it does not adequately explain geographical variation of this cancer which may well be attributed to Betel quid.

A number of other factors may have a role in the aetiology of head and neck cancers – tobacco chewing is an important factor in some populations and lip cancer is related to solar radiation. Gastro-oesophageal reflux disease has been associated with laryngeal cancers and human papilloma virus infection may have a role in head and neck cancer, in particular squamous cell cancer of the palatine tonsil. Epstein–Barr virus is strongly associated with nasopharyngeal cancer in some populations. For men over 80 years, the incidence of oral cancer has halved since 1975. The incidence of oral cancer diagnosed in men in their 40s and 50s has doubled and an increasing incidence of tongue cancer in young and middle-aged men has been reported in Europe and the USA. See the Cancer Research UK website, http://info.cancerresearchuk.org/cancerstats/types/oral/incidence.

A number of medical and allied health specialties along with their support services must be involved in comprehensive management. Head and neck cancer affects several anatomical sub sites, and each has specific presenting features, treatment challenges and morbidities associated with treatment. Advanced disease at any of these sites carries a poor prognosis and management is complex.

We refer to head and neck cancers as a group as the overall management principles are similar. Individual sub sites are discussed when specific issues are relevant and mucosal squamous cell carcinoma forms the largest diagnostic group. Although cancer of the thyroid gland is within the head and neck region and managed by head and neck oncologists, it is not included as its behaviour and the treatment rationales involved differ.

In discussion, we have included the American Joint Committee on Cancer (AJCC) classified sites:

+ oral cavity (including lip)
+ oropharynx
+ hypopharynx
+ larynx
+ nasopharynx
+ salivary gland.

The TNM system developed by the AJCC is the classification most commonly used to define head and neck cancer stage. Prognosis is best predicted by stage at presentation. The basis of the classification is similar for all head and neck sites with increasing primary tumour size, advancing nodal spread and distant metastasis advancing the disease stage. There are specific differences for some sub sites:

1. Nodal status in nasopharyngeal cancer has a lesser impact on prognosis and the distribution of lymphadenopathy differs.
2. Tumour size (T stage) is consistent for oral cavity, lip and oropharynx but due to complicated local anatomy and the significant prognostic effect that tumour invasion has on these sites, the T stage differs for hypopharynx, larynx and nasopharynx.

As with all cancers, the gold standard for management should be multidisciplinary care and this is usually hospital based, with a number of professionals contributing to a central clinic. Head and neck multidisciplinary teams have a complex structure, which includes medical, dental, nursing, diagnostic and many other specialties. In advanced disease the role of palliative medicine, nutrition support, speech and language therapists and the family practitioner become more relevant. The patient's management may then become more community or hospice based.

In broad terms management options include surgery, radiotherapy and chemotherapy. In early disease (stage I/II) surgery or radiotherapy are usually utilized alone and this accounts overall for about 40 per cent of cases. In advanced disease (stage III/IV), which accounts for the remaining 60 per cent of cases, surgery plays a lesser role as the morbidity associated with extensive ablative surgery becomes disproportionate to survival benefit. The use of chemoradiotherapy in a concurrent role is becoming more widespread. It has been shown in two multi-centre randomized controlled trials to have a significant effect on disease free survival and in one study on survival.[2, 3]

Natural history

Head and neck cancer usually presents as an ulcer or mass lesion. It may also present as a result of features such as voice change, dysphagia, weight loss, cachexia and skin involvement or airway compromise due to tumour extension into other structures. Advanced disease is more likely to present with the latter features.

Presentation is influenced by the site of disease. Oral lesions, because of the relative ease of self-examination and self-awareness, more frequently present early. Advanced primary oral cancer is less common and late presentation may be due to poor access to routine health care and associated socio-economic factors. Conversely cancer of hypopharynx and nasopharynx may present late due to anatomical factors (the tumour is not seen by the patient) but as with oropharyngeal disease, access to healthcare and socio-economic factors play a role.

Advanced head and neck cancer may present as:

- First presentation of primary disease (resectable or unresectable)
- Second primary tumour
- Recurrent disease (at primary site, locoregional or distant metastasis)
- Occult primary disease with metastasis (approximately 10 per cent)
- Distant metastasis from an identified primary.

Extent of disease is usually classified using the TNM system and for simplicity is described as Early (stage I/II) and Advanced (stage III/IV). In general, the presence of limited primary tumour and absence of nodal spread amounts to early disease with a better prognosis. The presence of a large primary tumour and spread to nodal tissue, often with invasion of adjacent structures, suggests advanced disease. Metastatic disease in the case of head and neck cancer occurs uncommonly at presentation (less than 5 per cent of cases). Patients with cancer of the upper aerodigestive tract also have around a 15 per cent risk of a second primary cancer, the majority of which will be metachronous.

Advanced disease may present at a stage when supportive therapy is the only option, and this is more common with recurrent disease. Supportive therapy in the case of head and neck cancer has difficult challenges such as the relief of pain, management of airway compromise, nutrition and psychosocial issues. These issues are covered later.

Factors affecting prognosis

Prognosis may affected by a number of factors.

Patient factors

Medical comorbidities frequently accompany head and neck patients as the same aetiological agents are common to cardiovascular and respiratory disease. Documentation of comorbidity is commonly overlooked and should be recorded using validated performance scores such as the World Health Organisation (WHO) or Karnofsky scores. Medical comorbidity is an independent predictor of mortality in head and neck cancer and the omission of it in cancer registry data may lead to misleadingly bad prognosis being ascribed to the index cancer.

Social class also influences prognosis. Head and neck cancer more commonly affects people of lower socio-economic groups. These patients may have poor access to primary medical and dental care and in many countries poor access to the complex and expensive treatments which are frequently necessary in the management of advanced head and neck cancers.

Disease factors

Pathological

Several pathological features influence prognosis and may be useful for guiding therapy and predicting outcome. These features may be related to the site of the primary tumour or the extent of locoregional disease. The presence of lymph node metastasis alone reduces the prognosis of head and neck cancers by around 50 per cent, but specific microscopic features may be used in determination of prognosis.

It is probably useful for the clinician to think of these features as being of major or minor significance. Although there is not agreement on the precise importance of individual risk factors most clinicians do agree on major factors. The presence of any major feature or a combination of minor features could influence prognosis and thus the need for adjuvant therapies such as radiotherapy and chemotherapy. However, the importance of minor factors is not clear and their relationship to prognosis is complex.

Major factors:

1. Positive resection margins after primary surgery

2. Extracapsular extension in a lymph node following neck dissection or on radiological assessment.

Minor factors may include:

1. Close resection margins

2. Lymph node size greater than 3 cm

3. Multiple lymph nodes involved, especially at multiple levels

4. Lymphovascular or perineural invasion

5. Discohesive features of the tumour's advancing front (compared to a pushing less infiltrative margin)

6. Tumour thickness

7. A significant host response to the tumour.

A number of scoring systems have been suggested as a way of stratifying risk factors, which may affect prognosis and guide treatment.[4, 5] The scoring systems allocate weights for the major and minor risk factors. These systems usually utilize information from surgery and are thus mainly useful in establishing a need for postoperative radiotherapy. Extrapolation of this method to score for prognosis may be possible but is rarely used in a formal manner.

Molecular markers

There is increasing evidence for the importance of molecular markers and it is hoped that this will add further information on predicting prognosis and in dictating therapy. The importance of DNA ploidy, epithelial growth factor receptor expression (EGFR), P53 expression, cytokines and cell adhesion molecules has been investigated extensively but clinical application is currently limited

Institution and resource

There is variation in provision of healthcare worldwide, and healthcare systems differ as does access to care. Published results of treatment from individual hospital groups also vary within healthcare systems. Not all cancer management is evidence-based and variation in management protocols may well affect clinical outcomes. These factors combine to make the institution and resource important variables.

Therapies affecting prognosis

In advanced head and neck cancer the treatment objective is cure. This is still the case when disease is deemed unresectable at the outset and definitive treatment for cure may be affected by chemo-radiotherapy. Treatment of recurrent disease usually has a better outcome when treatment includes surgery. Metastatic disease is usually treated by chemo-radiotherapy and not surgery.

Surgery

The concept of what is surgically resectable depends on the surgical experience of a head and neck team and their ability to reconstruct. There is a strong argument for a centralized service to maximize experience of these difficult cases. Individual cases should be evaluated and unresectable implies that either local control is unlikely to be achieved or the morbidity caused by ablation of the tumour outweighs the disease control advantage of surgery. This may be the case if resection involves sacrifice of vital structures such as the cranial nerves, brachial plexus and carotid artery.

The extent of surgery is usually dictated by the staging of the patient pre-operatively and involves removal of the primary tumour with an adequate surgical margin to allow safe resection and minimum morbidity from damage to adjacent structures. Treatment of the neck is dictated by the presence of disease or by the potential risk of occult disease according to the site and T stage of the primary tumour. The extent of neck surgery is influenced by the site and T stage of primary tumour. In general for upper aerodigestive tract cancer the more posterior the cancer, the greater the nodal metastases risk. For larynx and pharynx tumours, the more lateral the tumour the greater the risk. This is especially relevant when considering tumours of the lateral tongue that have a high incidence of occult cervical node metastasis. These tumours, in keeping with other tumours of the oral cavity, have a low incidence of level V disease which means that selective neck dissection of levels I–IV may be sufficient based on probability of metastasis to level V being low. The inclusion of level V in a comprehensive neck dissection may be far more important when dealing with an oropharyngeal tumour or metastatic disease from skin cancer of the posterior scalp.

For clarity, neck dissections are classified as comprehensive if all five lymph node levels are dissected and selective if particular groups are dissected, as may be the case in oral cancer (levels I–IV) or laryngeal cancer (II–IV). The comprehensive dissection may be likened to a traditional radical neck dissection, with removal of all five lymph node levels and with the exception that the internal jugular vein, sternocleidomastoid muscle and accessory nerve are spared in various combinations according to disease extent.

Radiotherapy and chemotherapy

Radiotherapy may be used alone or as part of combined modality therapy. Radiotherapy can be used for early stage disease and may match treatment success rates for surgery at some sites. In patients treated with surgery that have significant risk factors for recurrence the use of adjuvant radiotherapy reduces the risk of treatment failure. Radiotherapy can be used when treatment by surgery or chemotherapy is not feasible and may be the only treatment available.

Success of radiotherapy is influenced by a number of factors; altered time–dose fractionation, the combination of cytotoxic or molecular targeted drugs and optimization of dose distribution.

Altered time and dose fractionation

Two variations have been utilized:

1. Hyperfractionation which typically involves decreased dose per fraction and multiple fractions per day,
2. Accelerated fractionation which typically involves a larger fraction size with multiple doses per day resulting in shorter treatment time.

Improvement in locoregional control has been demonstrated. Meta-analysis comparing both regimens with conventional radiotherapy regimens in 6515 patients over a 28-year period has shown an overall survival benefit of 3 per cent at 5 years in favour of altered fractionation.[6]

Dose distribution

Intensity modulated radiotherapy (IMRT) has been utilized for more than 10 years, although is not commonplace in many institutions. Its prognostic significance has not been fully investigated but its main advantage may be more in reduction in morbidity. IMRT offers non-uniform dose distribution, which means maximum dose to target and sparing of damage to adjacent tissues such as the major salivary glands and the spinal cord.

Cytotoxic and molecular mediated drugs

Use of chemo-radiotherapy is a natural progression, founded on the success of chemotherapy alone in advanced head and neck cancer. The detailed mechanism of action of combined modality treatment is still not clear, but combination is usually with platinum derived agents or 5-fluorouracil (5-FU). Two large randomized controlled trials by the RTOG and EORTC groups have demonstrated improved locoregional control and disease free survival with adjuvant chemo-radiation versus radiotherapy alone.[2, 3]

Molecular targeted agents may block specific receptors such as the epidermal growth factor receptor (EGFR), over-expression of which is known to be associated with poor prognosis and aggressive clinical behaviour. This may result in a significant survival benefit, particularly in advanced disease. As tumour hypoxia is a known disadvantage to conventional radiation treatment, the addition of specific hypoxic cell cytotoxins may also increase response rate without added morbidity.

A number of other agents are currently under evaluation: drugs such as the cyclooxygenase-2 (COX-2) inhibitors which may influence processes linked to carcinogenesis, the farnesyl transferase inhibitors which target ras oncogene mutations and drugs targeting vascular endothelial growth factors (VEGF) involved with angiogenesis.

Short-term prognosis

In early stage head and neck cancer, treatment morbidity is often limited following surgery and/or primary radiotherapy. In contrast, the patient with advanced head and neck cancer presents many challenges. Treatment may be destructive to local anatomy and functional morbidity can be high. This is unsurprising when the complexity of the upper aerodigestive tract and its pivotal role in our daily function is considered.

In the short term patients with advanced head and neck cancer will have altered basic physiological functions and have morbidity and complications which require intense input from many specialists.

Pain

Although not a problem in early disease, control of pain in advanced disease is an issue. Tumours frequently cause pain by direct invasion of structures and surgery may be used to relieve pain from advanced disease in regions such as the tongue and mandible. Neurogenic and referred pain are clearly not easily solved by surgery. Palliative care physicians and pain control specialists are expert at management of pain and all but the simplest of cases benefit from their opinion. Generally the WHO 'pain ladder' is implemented with structured analgesic regimens.[7] The difficulty with achieving safe oral intake can be a problem and introduction of some analgesic preparations into feeding tubes can cause tube blockage, which is best avoided by discussion with the local pharmacy for advice on preparations suited to feeding tube use. A range of opiate topical patch preparations avoid the problem for more significant pain and patient-controlled analgesia (PCA) may become necessary as symptoms advance to the terminal stages.

Speech and swallow

Speech and swallow may be profoundly affected both from surgery undertaken to laryngeal structures and the oral cavity, or due to the side-effects from radiotherapy.

Xerostomia, mucositis and pain may be a specific limitation to speech. The use of IMRT and pre-emptive treatment with parasympathomimetic drugs such as pilocarpine (5mg TDS) have been shown to reduce the extent of xerostomia following radiotherapy. Once established, the use of artificial saliva, which may be mucin, cellulose or xanthan gum-based is helpful, as is the use of a saliva stimulant such as chewing gum. All these agents should have neutral pH and should contain fluoride to prevent dental caries.

Mucositis is usually best treated by local measures such as benzydamine hydrochloride mouth-wash (an atypical non-steroidal anti-inflammatory drug with anaesthetic and antimicrobial action). Prevention of secondary colonization by bacterial or fungal organisms can help with pain relief.

Speech may be generated in the case of laryngectomy by artificial larynx vibrators or by insertion of one-way valves by tracheo-oesophageal puncture. If this is not possible, alternative forms of communication such dry wipe boards and pointer picture boards are helpful.

Airway

Frequently tracheostomy is used in advanced disease either to facilitate surgery or make the airway safe during treatment by chemo-radiotherapy. Emergency airway provision may have occurred prior to first contact with the head and neck team dealing with definitive care in advanced cases.

The use of fenestrated tracheostomy tubes which allow voice production is not considered safe as these patients often have significant risk of aspiration. These patients may require long-term cannulation and need an un-cuffed, non-fenestrated tracheostomy tube. Assessment by speech and language therapists is vital and specialist nurse input for ongoing tracheostomy care is essential. Avoidance of insertion in the first place is usually preferable as decannulation is often not an option.

In all cases of advanced disease in which there is significant risk of acute airway compromise a plan should be made for management should the airway suddenly be lost. This avoids confusion and inappropriate treatment, which can occur in an emergency by clinicians not familiar with the patient.

Trismus

Both surgery and radiotherapy may cause limitation of mouth opening. This is primarily due to scarring and fibrosis around the muscles of mastication and the temporomandibular joint. Removal of the tip of the mandibular coronoid process and the attached temporalis muscle tendon (coronoidectomy) at the time of initial surgery may help to reduce the effects. Exercises using either progressive wedging with tongue spatulas stacked horizontally between the incisor teeth to force the jaws apart or use of a dental orthopaedic device such as the Therabite may be necessary. This may be needed on an ongoing basis as relapse occurs quickly.

Trismus is also a problem if further surgery or insertion of endoscopically placed feeding tubes is necessary. Intubation for anaesthesia requires awake fibreoptic insertion and conventional endoscopy may be impossible, making radiological insertion or open gastrostomy the only option.

Pathological fracture

Fracture can occur due to disease or radiotherapy used to treat it. In the mandible the jaw may lose its mechanical strength due to the size of a tumour that has invaded it. Radiotherapy for advanced cancer affecting or near to the mandible may also result in osteoradionecrosis.

This is essentially hypoxic, hypocellular hypovascular tissues with poor capacity to heal and limited resistance to infection. In the mandible this may result in sufficiently compromised strength to allow the bone to fracture under normal physiological conditions. A pathological fracture is painful and whilst immobilization will reduce pain it may be very difficult in frail individuals with advanced comorbidity and limited life expectancy. Hyperbaric oxygen therapy, which would normally be used in non-cancer patients with these fractures, is contraindicated in patients with malignancy due to potential for accelerating tumour growth. Decisions in these cases are difficult and discussion with the patient and multidisciplinary team are encouraged.

Nutrition

Specialist nutrition advice is important in all cancer management but none more so than in head and neck cases: this is particularly the case in advanced disease where treatment may preclude normal feeding methods.[8] Prior to treatment patients require formal nutritional assessment and optimization of nutrition. Patients may be managed using oral liquid enteral nutritional supplements alone but may require temporary insertion of nasogastric tubes or insertion of percutaneous endoscopically placed gastrostomy tubes (PEG tubes). If endoscopic placement is not possible, open gastrostomy or jejunostomy may be required. In all cases regular review by the nutrition team is essential.

Dental care

In the presence of limited mouth opening and with xerostomia, routine oral hygiene and dental care become a major issue. The onset of dental caries and periodontal disease, even in patients with a limited lifespan, can become a problem and can cause life-threatening infection and debilitating pain at a difficult time in a patient's treatment pathway. Prevention is paramount. Before treatment in advanced disease a specialist dental practitioner should have assessed patients and this is particularly important if radiotherapy is to be undertaken. Dietary advice on low caries foods should be given. Oral hygiene instructions may need to be improvised with the disease in mind and access to dental hygienists should be facilitated. The use of fluoride and antiseptic mouthwashes (chlorhexidine 2 per cent) may prevent problems by reducing dental caries and slowing periodontal disease.

Wound breakdown and fungation

Pharyngocutaneous fistulae can occur in all upper aerodigestive tract cancer surgery. There are many factors contributing to fistulae.[9] Prevention of fistulae includes pre-operative recognition of risk, the use of prophylactic antibiotics, nutrition manipulation and gastro-oesophageal reflux prophylaxis. Early drainage and good wound care are paramount. A cuffed tracheostomy tube may be required to reduce aspiration. Salivary bypass tubes and diversion of the flow of pharyngeal secretions into a collection bag may help control. Fistulae are often associated with skin loss and may require reconstruction.

In some cases patients with advanced disease have disease which is progressive and untreatable. Fungation of local or locoregional disease may be unavoidable. The input of specialist nurses with experience in their management cannot be underestimated. From a social and cross-infection standpoint, fungating wounds need occlusive covering. Anatomical site and local tissue conditions such as salivary fistula and infection may make adhesive dressings difficult to apply and a degree of patience and ingenuity help. Fungating wounds frequently have anaerobic organism colonization and use of a topical metronidazole preparation is helpful to reduce odour.

Psychosocial

In all cases of advanced disease, psychosocial aspects must be addressed. The involvement of disease and treatment on physiological functions such as taste, eating and speaking have a profound affect on the patients psychological well-being and on their ability to function socially. These are social activities, which are shared by patients and their families and carers. The affect of our interventions on appearance is also marked and it is important particularly in advanced disease that respect is given to the patients desire to continue interacting with other individuals.

Quality of life

Medical intervention is intended to maintain or improve functioning and well being and consequently to improve patients' quality of life.[10] Quality of life has been defined by the World Health Organisation (WHO) as the individual's perception of their position in life in the context of the culture and value systems in which they live and in relation to their goals, expectations, standards and concerns.[7]

Head and neck cancers have a profound effect on an individual. Physiological functions such as speech, eating and breathing are affected. Cancer clinicians often overlook factors such as self-image and psychological well-being. The term health status describes the individual's emotional, physical and health capability and its limits. Performance and functional status are best thought of as a manifestation of their health status, i.e. how well is this individual able to put their health status into action, in performing daily tasks and activities? Quality of life, however, shifts the emphasis towards the 'value' that the patient attributes to these domains and is uniquely determined by the individual.

The importance of using validated questionnaires for assessment is well recognized.[11] Measurement of health-related quality of life should be quantified for head and neck cancer patients and is frequently carried out using questionnaires such as the University of Washington Quality of Life scale (UW-QOL) or the European Organisation for Research into Cancer Head and Neck module (EORTC HN-35).

Assessing quality of life from the patient's own perspective would seem of paramount importance. With this in mind, the Schedule for the Evaluation of Individual Quality of Life (SEIQoL) was developed as an interview-based instrument using judgement analysis of patient-generated concerns.[12] An abbreviated and less cumbersome form of the measure was developed: the SEIQoL-Direct Weighting (SEIQoL-DW).[13]

Long-term prognosis

With great variation in site-related behaviour, prediction of outcome overall is difficult. Some guidance for prognosis may be gained from Table 16.1, which relates to all sites by stage of presentation.

Data from the Prognostigram program (see Figure 16.1) indicate that more than 50 per cent of patients with advanced head and neck cancer will be expected to still be alive at 2 years, depending on the primary site and stage. In the case of patients with distant metastases, if the primary site is in the oral cavity (including lip), the median survival is approximately 15 months, some 55 per cent of patients being alive at one year; the subgroup with hypopharyngeal primaries have a worse prognosis. In the case of metastatic laryngeal cancer, the prognosis is slightly better, with 70 per cent of patients expected to be alive at 1 year and the median survival being around 2 years. Five year survivals for most head and neck cancer types are of the order of 20–33 per cent (10–15 per cent for hypopharynx).

Table 16.1 Cancer stage and survival in the south and west of England, 1999–2000[14]

Stage	Two-year survival, crude rate all sites (%)	Cancer site (% of cases at each stage at diagnosis)				
		Larynx n = 190	Oral n = 241	Pharynx n = 161	Salivary gland n = 56	Other n = 79
I early disease	89.7	34	21	6	13	12
II locally advanced	71.8	27	16	13	17	8
III tumour in lymph nodes	57.6	17	15	22	7	8
IV metastatic	48.6	15	34	50	28	47
Unknown	69.8	7	11	9	35	25

Terminal phase

Malnutrition and cancer cachexia syndrome

Nutritional support to alleviate malnutrition is important at all stages of cancer care. Feeding reverses mucosal atrophy induced by starvation and increases anastomotic collagen deposition and strength. Experimental data suggest that enteral nutrition is associated with an improvement in wound healing and enteral feeding may reduce septic morbidity. It has been suggested that patients with a weight loss of greater than 10 per cent of their normal weight should be considered for enteral tube feeding.[8]

Abnormal metabolism found in cancer cachexia syndrome is resistant to conventional nutritional support and affects the patient's quality of life profoundly.[8] The management requires

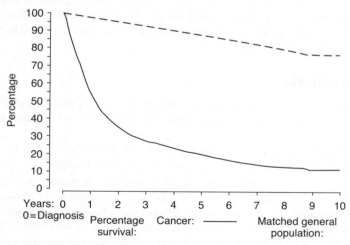

Figure 16.1 Prognostigram survival curve for patients with oral cavity and phayrynx cancers (all sites) presenting with distant disease.

an experienced team to deal with the psychological effects of this syndrome: this team should include nutrition specialists. Currently there are no established interventions to manage cancer cachexia effectively.

Carotid blowout syndrome

Patients with advanced cancer may enter a terminal phase and death usually results from a steady decline in their overall state rather than an acute event.[15]

Haemorrhage from carotid blowout is reported to occur in about 3–4 per cent of people undergoing neck dissection. Recently carotid blowout syndrome has been described and can be separated into threatened, impending and acute blowout. A treatment algorithm has been developed which includes interventional radiological techniques including stent occlusion and embolization. However, the initial management should be to secure the airway, apply pressure to control bleeding and initiate fluid resuscitation.[16]

Hospitals and hospices should have in place a plan for such eventualities.

In the case of catastrophic haemorrhage a sedative and analgesic combination such as morphine and midazolam should be given for relief of acute anxiety and pain, but this should be clearly prescribed.

A clear plan should be formulated in cases of advanced terminal disease for an event such as cardiac arrest. This plan should be documented in the patient's records and the decision should be discussed with team members that may be involved with care. If possible and considered appropriate, decisions such as resuscitation status should be frankly discussed with patients and their family.

References

1. Parkin DM. International variation. *Oncogene* 2004; 23(38):6329–40.

2. Bernier J, Domenge C, Ozsahin M. *et al*. Postoperative irradiation with or without concomitant chemotherapy for locally advanced head and neck cancer. *N Engl J Med* 2004; 350:1945–52.

3. Cooper JS, Pajak TF, Forastiere AA. *et al*. Postoperative concurrent radiotherapy and chemotherapy for high-risk squamous cell carcinoma of the head and neck. *N Engl J Med* 2004; 350:1937–44.

4. Martinez-Gimeno C, Moro Rodriguez E, Navarro Vila C, Lopez Varela, C. Squamous cell carcinoma of the oral cavity: a clinico–pathologic scoring system for evaluating risk of cervical lymph node metastasis. *Laryngoscope* 1995; 105:728–33.

5. Anneroth G, Hansen LS, Silverman S. Malignancy grading in oral squamous cell carcinoma.
   1. Squamous cell carcinoma of the tongue and floor of mouth: histologic grading in the clinical situation.
   J Oral Pathol 1986; 15:162–8.

6. Bourhis J, Audry H, Overgaard *et al*. Meta-analysis of conventional versus altered fractionated radiotherapy: in head and neck squamous cell carcinomas (HNSCC): final analysis. Int J Rad Oncol Biol Phys 2004; 60: 190–191

7. WHO. *Cancer pain relief and palliative care*. Geneva: World Helth Organisation, 1990.

8. Donaldson M, Bradley PJ. Current management of the nutrition needs of the head and neck cancer patient. *Curr Opin Otolaryngol Head Neck Surg* 2000; 8:107–12.

9. Makitie AA, Irish J, Gullane P J. Pharyngocutaneous fistula. *Curr Opin Otolaryngol Head Neck Surg* 2003; 11:78–84.

10. Schipper H. Quality of life: the final common pathway. *J Palliat Care* 1992; 8(3):5–7.

11. Rogers SN, Fisher SE, Woolgar JA. A review of quality of life assessment in oral cancer. *Int J Oral Maxillofac Surg* 1999; 28(2):99–117.

12. O'Boyle CA, Waldron D. Quality of life issues in palliative medicine. *J Neurol* 1997; 244(Suppl 4): S18–S25.

13. Hickey AM, Bury G, O'Boyle CA, Bradley F, O'Kelly FD, Shannon W. A new short form individual quality of life measure (SEIQoL-DW): application in a cohort of individuals with HIV/AIDS. *BMJ* 1996; 313(7048):29–33.

14. South West Cancer Intelligence Service. *Second head and neck audit report*. Bristol: South West Cancer Intelligence Service, 2001.

15. Forbes K. Palliative care in patients with cancer of the head and neck. *Clin Otolarygol* 1997; 22:117–22.

16. Cohen J, Rad I. Contemporary management of carotid blowout. *Curr Opin Otolaryngol Head Neck Surg* 2004; 12:110–15.

17

Gynaecological cancer

Jonathan Carter

Ovarian cancer

Introduction

Ovarian cancer unfortunately holds the dubious distinction as the most deadly of all the gynaecological cancers. More women die each year from ovarian cancer than from the more common corpus and cervical cancers combined. The main reason for this is that most patients are diagnosed with advanced stage disease. The most common histological variants include serous, mucinous, endometrioid, clear cell, Brenner, mixed and undifferentiated.

Natural history of disease

While 5–10 per cent of epithelial ovarian cancers have an hereditary component, the majority are sporadic. Spread patterns of ovarian cancer include local extension to adjacent pelvic structures along with transperitoneal spread of exfoliated cells. Lymphatic spread is more common than previously thought while haematogenous spread is less common. Risk factors for the development of ovarian cancer apart from family history include young age at menarche, not having conceived or having children, not breastfeeding and never having been on the oral contraceptive pill. The mechanism whereby these epidemiological derived factors exert their effect on the ovarian surface epithelium (OSE) relates to its repeated trauma with repeated or incessant ovulation. In those "susceptible" individuals the normal healing process of the OSE becomes disordered and malignancy develops. Thus the factors noted above that will reduce a woman's lifetime number of ovulations will reduce her risk of developing this disease.

Prognostic factors

Early stage ovarian cancer, i.e. International Federation of Gynecology and Obstetrics (FIGO) stage I and II, is uncommon. Recognized prognostic factors include the presence of ascites, firm adherence of the tumour in the pelvis and high tumour grade. Management of apparent early stage ovarian cancer involves resection of the involved ovary(s), usually with hysterectomy and surgical staging to define the extent of disease. Adjuvant therapy is usually prescribed for high-grade tumours or when both ovaries are involved, with or without surface involvement.

Unfortunately the majority of patients presenting with ovarian cancer present with advanced FIGO stage III or IV disease. By definition tumour has spread beyond the ovaries and pelvis to involve abdominal structures and retroperitoneal structures for stage III disease and more distant spread involving parenchymal liver spread in stage IV disease. Initial management involves aggressive surgical cytoreduction and combination chemotherapy, usually comprising a taxane and platinum compound. While the majority of patients can by rendered disease-free at the completion of treatment, unfortunately over the next 2–3 years the majority will indeed recur and ultimately most of these people will die of their disease.

Recognized prognostic factors for patients presenting with advanced disease include: advanced age, poor performance status, the presence of ascites, the amount of residual tumour left after primary surgery and finally response to chemotherapy.[1] Debate continues as to the effect of tumour biology versus ease of cytoreduction as a prognostic factor. All gynaecological oncologists are familiar with the scenario of patients being easily optimally cytoreduced with minimal effort, often with prolonged survival, in contrast to patients with apparently more biologically aggressive tumours which despite extended surgery succumb to disease progression early. Another controversial area is how important is resiudal tumour size or tumour volume after cytoreduction and how this is measured. In a recent meta-analysis of 6885 patients there was a positive correlation between percentage of cytoreduction and survival.[2] Older patients with bulky residual disease and gross ascites at presentation are less likely to do well than younger patients, optimally debulked and without ascites. The regression of the CA125 level has also been found to be of some prognostic significance in patients undergoing primary treatment. For example if the CA125 is elevated preoperatively, and there is a failure of normalization by the second or third cycle of chemotherapy, then the likelihood of attaining complete remission is low.

However, none of these factors is sufficiently sensitive enough to allow their use to dictate therapy. Having said this, the elderly patient with a poor performance status described above is more likely to be offered single agent neoadjuvant chemotherapy for three cycles prior to interval surgical exploration and cytoreduction. Commonly single agent carboplatin will be the chemotherapy of choice in such circumstances rather than dual agent therapy. Evidence indicates that such treatment does not adversely affect overall survival.

Therapies affecting prognosis

The surgical management of patients with ovarian cancer includes performing (1) surgical staging in apparent early ovarian cancer and where indicated (2) cytoreductive surgery in patients with advanced ovarian cancer.

Surgical staging in early ovarian cancer accurately determines the extent of disease, allowing for tailored postoperative therapy. Based on surgical staging data 20–30 per cent of apparent early staged cancers will be upstaged. Staging has been found to be inadequate when performed by either a general surgeon or general gynaecologist compared to a trained or certified gynaecologic oncologist. Subspecialists are also more likely to affect optimal cytoreduction and resultant survival advantage.[3]

Cyto-reductive or debulking surgery has been shown to:

1. Enhance immunologic competence of the patient,
2. Improve tumour perfusion and increased growth fraction,
3. Provide a physiological benefit for the patient by removing a large tumour mass, and
4. Increase survival if optimal debulking is performed.

There is no prospective data to support the theory that aggressive debulking affects survival. However, numerous retrospective studies and a large meta-analysis of 6,885 patients has confirmed a positive correlation between cytoreduction and survival. For each 10 per cent increase in maximal cytoreduction there is an associated increase in median survival of 5.5 per cent.[2]

If patients are unable to be optimally debulked for technical reasons, then they may be considered for "interval re-exploration" and "secondary debulking". The operation is generally performed after three cycles of chemotherapy and the disease has been found to be responsive to chemotherapy.

The performance of a second-look laparotomy (SLL) was commonplace after treatment for ovarian cancer. For those patients with no apparent clinical, biochemical or radiological evidence of disease such a procedure could provide prognostic information for the clinician and patient, but qas od no therapeutic benefit. Nowadays SLL is undertaken only in the context of a clinical trial where pathological response rates are required. No high-level data has shown a survival advantage from the procedure, indeed the procedure causes significant morbidity. Prognostic factors that may predict those patients that will have no evidence of disease at SLL include initial FIGO stage, tumour grade, the CA125 regression, the size of residual tumour after primary surgery, the size of largest metastatic disease at surgery and the number of lesions present prior to treatment.

The treatment of patients with recurrent ovarian cancer must be individualized. Often recurrence is manifest as an asymptomatic rise in the CA125 titre. Such patients can be managed conservatively with relatively non-toxic therapy such as tamoxifen. With development of symptoms or in patients requesting aggressive therapy, cytotoxic chemotherapy is reinstituted. If the treatment-free interval is greater than 6 months, the cancer is assumed to be still sensitive to initial chemotherapy and usually primary agents are reintroduced either singularly or in combination. The longer the treatment-free interval the greater the likelihood of attaining a secondary remission. It is unlikely however that patients can be cured once they have recurred.

The role for secondary surgery is limited to those patients with localized resectable disease. Advanced age, poor nutritional status, widespread tumour, the presence of ascites and previous failed chemo or irradiation therapy, especially if the treatment-free interval is less than 6 months, are all factors that have been found to portend a poorer outcome in patients undergoing palliative ovarian cancer surgery.[4]

Prognosis

Greater than 90–95 per cent of patients with early stage ovarian cancer will be cured of their disease with a combination of surgery and for patients with high-risk features adjuvant chemotherapy.

For patients with advanced disease, some 60–70 per cent can achieve clinical and biochemical remission with a combination of aggressive cytoreductive surgery and combination chemotherapy.

Despite a large number of patients being rendered disease-free after primary treatment, unfortunately almost half of these patients relapse some 18–24 months after completing therapy. While many of these can achieve secondary remission with further therapy, few if any are actually cured of their disease.

The terminal phase of the disease is often quite distressing with gross abdominal distension from ascites and small and/or large bowel obstruction that may be multifocal and not amenable to palliate surgery.

Cervical cancer

Introduction

With the development and implementation of national cervical cancer screening programmes, the incidence of cervical cancer in most developed countries is dramatically falling. Unfortunately in Third World countries cervical cancer remains a major health problem with over 500,000 new cases reported each year throughout the world, resulting in a significant mortality rate. Worldwide cervical cancer remains the most common cause of cancer related death in women.

Invasive cervical cancer is generally a disease of low socio-economic groups, with a mean age at diagnosis of 52 years. Many epidemiological risk factors have been implicated in its development and these include early age at coitarche, multiple sexual partners and smoking. Infection with human papilloma virus (HPV) has been strongly implicated as a causative agent.

Squamous cell carcinomas account for about 80 per cent of all invasive cervical cancers and adenocarcinomas and mixed tumours (adenosquamous) the bulk of the rest. Less frequently encountered cell types include small cell (neuroendocrine), adenoid basal, adenoid cystic, primary melanoma, sarcoma and primary lymphoma. Squamous and adenocarcinomas should be treated in a similar fashion.

Early lesions may be asymptomatic and are usually detected on routine pap testing. Common symptoms include post coital, intermenstrual or post-menopausal bleeding. Offensive vaginal discharge may also be present. Pain, bladder and bowel symptoms, weight loss and bone pain may occur in advanced disease.

Spread patterns include initial local spread, followed by lymphatic spread to regional pelvic nodes. Haematogenous and peritoneal spread occurs but is uncommon, particularly in early stage disease. Historically lymphangiograms were used to assess regional nodal spread. They have been found to have a false negative rate of 10–20 per cent. In more recent times computed tomography (CT) scans have been used to radiologically assess disease spread. Their limitations include missing small positive lymph nodes and overcalling nodes enlarged by inflammation. CT scans are more useful in evaluating para-aortic nodes (sensitivity 67 per cent) than pelvic nodes (sensitivity 25 per cent).

Natural history of disease

The natural history of cervical cancer corresponds to infection of the lower genital tract with the oncogenic genotypes of HPV. Infection of basal cells in the cervical mucosa and resultant incorporation into the host cell genome results in inhibition of tumour suppressor genes and resultant development of dysplasia and malignant change. Cervical cancer initially results in local or direct spread and local pelvic lymph node spread. In more advanced stages direct spread to the bladder and bowel will occur as well as distant spread, commonly manifest as distant lymphatic spread and supraclavicular lymphadenopathy.

Prognostic factors

In early stage disease, tumour is either limited to the cervix (stage I) or has just spread away from the cervix to involve the adjacent vaginal epithelium or lateral parametrial tissue (stage II). For early stage and small volume tumours, treatment is often surgical, involving radical resection of the cervix and uterine corpus after formal dissection of the ureter (radical hysterectomy). This allows wide resection of the parametrial tissue around the cervix, allowing a tumour-free margin. Pelvic lymphadenectomy completes the surgical staging to define the extent of disease and allow a rationale approach to prescription of adjuvant radiation therapy. Cases unsuitable for primary surgery are treated with pelvic irradiation with concurrent chemotherapy.

In patients with early cervical cancer, prognostic factors for a prolonged disease-free survival include small tumour size on clinical assessment, absence of lymph vascular space invasion (LVSI) by tumour, superficial invasion the tumour into the cervix, low tumour grade and negative or no parametrial spread of tumour. Both lesion size and the presence of LVSI were found to be independent factors on statistical analysis.[5]

The status of the pelvic and para-aortic lymph nodes has major prognostic significance. Assessment is either surgical or using imaging, likely CT scan. In those patients afforded the opportunity of a surgical staging procedure the following are deemed as poor prognostic factors: the presence of nodal disease particularly if multiple nodal groups are involved and bilateral spread to nodal basin. When trying to predict the likelihood of nodal involvement based on clinical features, the following factors have been found to be associated with microscopic pelvic node metastasis: depth of invasion, parametrial involvement, LVSI, tumour grade and gross versus occult primary tumour. Independent risk factors for pelvic node metastasis were LVSI, depth of invasion and parametrial involvement.[6]

Prognostic factors for recurrence in patients who are node negative after surgery include large tumour size, deep stromal invasion, the presence of LVSI, and extension of tumour into the lower uterine segment. A prognostic scoring system has been proposed in such circumstances,[6] but whether the addition of further therapy, usually radiation with or without chemotherapy will significantly reduce recurrence and prolong survival has not been adequately tested. Some argue that delivery of small field irradiation to such high-risk node negative patients is appropriate. Factors found to increase the risk of treatment failure after treatment with radiation therapy for locally advanced cervical cancer (after assessment of nodal status) include patient age, performance status, para-aortic lymph node status, tumour size and pelvic node status. When modelling for survival, all these factors and clinical stage and bilateral extension were significant.[7]

Patients with recurrent disease after radiation therapy, where disease is confined to the central pelvis, can still be salvaged with exenterative surgery. Such extended surgery should only be undertaken where the prospect for survival is high. Survival after exenteration is related to the tumour size, the interval from the initial treatment to recurrence, side wall fixation, margin status of the operative specimen, lymph node metastases and cell type, with adenocarcinomas performing more poorly than squamous cancers. Large recurrent tumours, having previously been irradiated, are more likely to be resected with close or positive margins and are more likely to have overt or occult spread, all indicating poor prognosis and in fact incurable disease. A longer disease-free interval from primary treatment to recurrence, often indicates a biologically less aggressive tumour. If it is able to be cleanly resected, there is a high likelihood of cure.

Therapies affecting prognosis

Where disease invades less then 3 mm into the cervical stroma, a cone biopsy may be adequate treatment. Lymph node involvement is rare.[8] With disease invading more than 3 mm, especially if there is LVSI further, treatment is usually recommended, as the risk of recurrence and lymph node involvement is significant. This would usually involve a modified radical hysterectomy and lymph node dissection.[9] There appears to be no difference in survival between a type II and type III radical hysterectomy.[10]

A strong argument exists for pre-treatment surgical staging and debulking enlarged positive lymph nodes. Such an approach may afford a survival benefit without affecting treatment-related morbidity or mortality. An extraperitoneal rather than transperitoneal approach will significantly reduce treatment related morbidity.[11]

Primary treatment of early stage cervical cancer can be either surgery or combination radiotherapy/chemotherapy. The results of treatment appear to be equivalent, though this is an area of continuing debate.[12] Factors to be considered when deciding upon treatment include the patient's general health, her informed decision about treatment options and her age. Surgery allows for the preservation of coital and ovarian function, tends to have lower morbidity than that associated with radiation therapy, and fewer long-term bladder and bowel complications. Surgery will also allow the debulking of enlarged lymph nodes, and allow full pathological staging.[13]

With squamous disease in younger patients, the ovaries may be conserved and transposed out of the pelvis. For postmenopausal patients with glandular tumours they should be removed. There are few reports of ovarian metastases in younger patients with glandular tumours and it is possible to conserve them in this group after discussion with the patient about possible risks.

There does not appear to be any contraindication to the use of hormone treatment when they are removed.

The debate to primarily operate or chemo-irradiate large bulky (stage IB2) cervical cancers remain unresolved. The proponents of the latter management plan would argue that large volume tumours are more likely to have lymph node spread, and if operated upon, more likely to be resected with close or compromised margins thus requiring further treatment. Unfortunately the addition of chemo-irradiaion in such circumstances results in a significant increase in morbidity. Small bowel is often adherent within the pelvis if a transperitoneal surgery has been undertaken and such fixed bowel loops receive high doses of radiation: subsequent damage and morbidity inflicted is much higher than if this treatment were used primarily. The opponents of this approach argue the recurrence rate is high if large volume tumours are not resected and these patients then require a post-irradiation "cleansing" hysterectomy anyway. In addition such patients have a high likelihood of having bulky pelvic or paraaortic lymph nodes that are unlikely to be sterilized with radiation doses used and pre-treatment surgical resection of such bulky nodes results in a survival advantage, that appears to be stage independent.[13]

The place of central cleansing hysterectomy after definitive chemoradiation is unclear but may be considered if there is any doubt about response to treatment. Prospective data would suggest a lower incidence of local relapse and progression-free survival.[14]

Prognosis

Patients with early stage disease and without nodal or extracervical spread have a good prognosis with an 85 per cent 5-year survival. With increasing tumour volume, increasing nodal spread and unresectable nodal disease, recurrence rates increase.

The terminal phase of patients with advanced and recurrent cervical cancer is often one of bleeding from pelvic recurrence, sciatic pain from pelvic nerve plexus involvement, and development of ureteric obstruction and uraemia. Progressive enlargement and local invasion of pelvic and para-aortic lymph nodes will often produce intractable bone pain requiring palliative irradiation for control of symptoms.

Corpus cancer

Introduction

Uterine corpus cancer is predominantly a disease of elderly obese women. The increased natural oestrogen derived from the peripheral conversion of androstenedione in the peripheral fat to oestrone results in unopposed stimulation on the endometrium. Rarely thin younger women develop endometrial cancer, unrelated to oestrogenic stimulation. Their endometrium is usually atrophic and the histological variants are either clear cell or of serous variety. With the increasing sedentary life style in most developed countries, ready access to fast food outlets, often with food high in fats and carbohydrates, our population is becoming increasingly obese. It is not unreasonable then to expect an increase in the incidence of corpus cancer. Endometrial cancer is the fourth most common cancer in women behind breast, bowel and lung, and the seventh leading cause of death from malignancy in females. The disease tends to affect affluent, obese women who are nulliparous or have low parity. Mean age at diagnosis is 61 years.

The majority of tumours are of endometrioid histology. Less commonly mucinous, serous, clear cell and squamous cancers can also occur – the latter three have a poorer prognosis than the endometrioid tumours. Tumours are graded by the amount of poorly differentiated or solid component present. Grade 1 tumours have less than 5 per cent, grade 2 have 5–50 per cent and grade 3 tumours have more than 50 per cent of undifferentiated tumour present.

Natural history of disease

Eighty per cent of endometrial cancers occur in postmenopausal women. The majority present with postmenopausal bleeding, less commonly vaginal discharge and rarely are they asymptomatic, diagnosed on ultrasound with a thickened endometrial stripe. Twenty per cent are found in premenopausal women and 5 per cent are under the age of 40 years. The latter women usually present with menorrhagia or heavy periods. It behoves the general gynaecologist to evaluate women with menorrhagia to exclude malignancy prior to undertaking definitive treatment of what was thought to be benign bleeding. Under normal circumstances the proliferative effects of oestrogen are counterbalanced by the stabilizing effects of progestogen. With unopposed oestrogen effects the endometrium thickens, becomes hyperplastic and atypia develops. Once there is the presence of atypia, the hyperplasia is considered premalignant.

Prognostic factors

The majority of patients with endometrial cancer present with early stage I or II disease where surgery alone is curative in most cases. In patients with advanced disease, tumour has spread to the regional nodes, or intra-abdominal spread. Surgical treatment alone is unlikely to be curative and a combination of radiation, hormonal treatment or chemotherapy may be utilized.

Nodal involvement in patients with apparent early uterine cancer varies with tumour grade and depth of myometrial invasion. Up to 34 per cent of apparent stage I patients with have nodal involvement if surgical staging is undertaken. Survival correlates with nodal involvement with a 50 per cent 5-year survival for positive pelvic nodes and 25 per cent for positive para-aortic nodes. Risk factors for nodal involvement in early corpus cancer based on surgico–pathologic data include

1. stage (Ia vs Ib)
2. histology (adenocarcinoma vs others: clear cell or papillary)
3. grade (1 vs 2 vs 3)
4. myometrial invasion
5. peritoneal cytology
6. location of tumour (fundus vs lower uterine segment)
7. adnexal involvement
8. other extrauterine spread and
9. LVSI.[15]

A substantial risk for lymph node metastasis exists if the surgical–pathologic study identifies superficial myometrial invasion by grade 3 cancer, intermediate myometrial invasion by grade 2 or 3 cancer, deep myometrial invasion by cancer of any grade, vascular space involvement, and extension of tumour to the cervix and/or adnexa.[16]

A strong correlation exits between histologic grade, myometrial invasion and prognosis. Lymph vascular space invasion has been suggested as an independent risk factor for recurrence and death, indeed after aortic node metastases, LVSI is the single most important adverse prognostic feature for recurrence.[17]

One of the most important prognostic factors is the presence of high-risk histology. These include papillary serous, clear-cell and squamous carcinomas, and all have a worse prognosis when compared to the endometrioid variety. Such histologies have been found to have significantly reduced survival, extrauterine spread at the time of staging laparotomy and recurrence outside the abdominal-pelvic cavity. In endometrial cancers with squamous differentiation (benign or malignant) the prognosis is affected by the grade and depth of invasion of the glandular component, not the squamous component, as well as the presence of LVSI.

While the presence of positive peritoneal cytology has been incorporated into the FIGO staging system and denotes stage IIIA disease, its significance remains controversial. Positive washings are common in patients with metastases to adnexa and pelvic or paraaortic nodes; hence there exists some correlation with histologic grade and depth of myometrial invasion. Gynecologic Oncology Group (GOG) data implicate malignant cytology as a serious adverse finding with respect to the risk for regional/distant and abdominal failure.[17] However, others have suggested it is not an independent poor prognostic factor. More often than not, patients with positive washings in absence of other risk factors are not given further treatment and suffer no ill effects, nor do they have a shortened survival.

Hormone receptor status has been suggested as a prognostic factor: hormone receptor-rich EC has a better prognosis than hormone-receptor poor endometrial cancer (EC), even after correcting for stage and grade. Hormone receptor levels are often inversely proportional to grade and PR appears to be a stronger predictor of survival than estrogen receptor positivity (ER).

Therapies affecting prognosis

The contemporary management of patients with endometrial cancer is to rationalize adjuvant treatment based upon confirmed extra uterine spread and risk factors for recurrence obtained from a formal surgical staging procedure. Reliance on the pre-operative grade and an intraoperative assessment of myoinvasion to determine the need for a pelvic lymph node dissection, fails to appreciate that 30 per cent of pre-operative grades will differ from the final grade from the formalin-fixed uterine specimen, and estimating myoinvasion either by eyeballing or by frozen section also correlates poorly with the final histological result. Up to 38 per cent of Grade 1 tumours, 69 per cent of Grade 2 tumours and 78 per cent of Grade 3 tumours have their depth of myoinvasion underestimated by intraoperative gross inspection. A significant number of women deemed to be low risk preoperatively will demonstrate high-risk factors postoperatively.[18]

The modern approach to management of patients with endometrial cancer is to offer all patients who are medically fit, and not morbidly obese, the advantages of a formal staging procedure. After removing the uterus, if there is any evidence of myoinvasion on either gross or frozen section, then the staging procedure is completed. This comprises an assessment of the pelvic lymph nodes. Paraaortic lymph nodes are not routinely dissected. An omental biopsy or infracolic omentectomy may also be performed, particularly if the pre-operative histology suggests serous carcinoma.[19]

The reason why para-aortic nodes are not routinely dissected is that para-aortic node metastasis does not occur unless there are grossly positive pelvic nodes present, there is gross extrauterine spread to the adnexa or there is deep outer third myometrial invasion.[17]

By accurately defining disease spread via surgical staging, adjuvant irradiation therapy can be recommended to patients at high risk of recurrence due to extrauterine spread, while it can be confidently withheld from those patients without extrauterine spread, irrespective of whether high-risk local uterine factors are present.[20]

Patients who have had an adequate surgical staging and who are found to have their cancer strictly confined to the corpus are not offered adjuvant pelvic irradiation, as treatment is likely not to alter survival. Pelvic irradiation will reduce the likelihood of pelvic recurrence however and thus should be restricted to those patients with high risk factors.[21] The GOG has defined this high intermediate risk (HIR) as those with high grade, advanced age, deep myometrial invasion or with LVSI. Vaginal radiation therapy (brachytherapy) may be offered to those patients with high-grade tumours, deep myoinvasion and cervical or lower uterine segment involvement by tumour.[20, 22] The rationale for the use of local vaginal therapy or brachytherapy is to reduce the incidence of vaginal vault recurrences. There is strong evidence that this can be achieved, but again without an effect on overall survival.[23]

If surgical staging has not been undertaken, a substantial risk for lymph node metastasis exists if the final pathological evaluation of the uterus identifies superficial or intermediate myometrial invasion by grade 2–3 cancers, deep myometrial invasion by cancer of any grade, vascular space involvement and extension of tumour to the lower uterine segment or cervix or adnexa. Pelvic irradiation therapy should be considered in these situations. However, the addition of pelvic irradiation while not affecting survival does result in decreased local–regional recurrence.[24]

Prognosis

The majority of recurrences occur within the first 2 years post-treatment, and the majority of these occur at the vault. Most are symptomatic with abnormal bleeding and only occasionally are recurrences detected on surveillance vaginal vault cytology. These local recurrences are almost always salvaged with radiation therapy. Recurrence in a previously irradiated pelvis is not common, but as expected when this occurs prognosis is poor and many of these patients will have a component of distant relapse, making an attempt at radical exenterative surgery often pointless.

Most patients with early stage disease are cured of their disease with surgery alone. Whether the addition of pelvic irradiation to these patients actually improves survival is unlikely. An increasing amount of literature confirms that pelvic irradiation will reduce pelvic recurrences without affecting survival. For those patients with advanced or recurrent disease, cure is unlikely. Even those patients with apparent early and local recurrence will have a component of distant relapse. Hormonal therapy as well as cytotoxic chemotherapy may produce some useful palliative benefit.

Vulva cancer

Introduction

This is an uncommon cancer comprising 3–5 per cent of gynaecological malignancies, and less than 1 per cent of all malignancies in women. The majority of lesions are squamous cell carcinomas (80 per cent). Less common types include malignant melanoma, adenocarcinoma, usually Bartholin's gland, basal cell carcinoma and sarcoma.

It is a disease of older women, with an average age 65 years. It appears to be increasing in incidence in young women and those patients who are immune-suppressed, such as allograft renal transplantation recipients. Chronic vulval pruritus is the most common symptom, and may precede the presence of a mass or lump. Localized vulvar complaints may include pain, burning and discomfort when voiding.

Associated factors include obesity, hypertension, diabetes, increased sexual partners and warts. Thirty per cent will have an associated dysplasia elsewhere in the lower genital tract. A delay in diagnosis is not uncommon. Patients may present to local physicians with vulvar complaints and creams prescribed without proper assessment.

Lesions may be single or multifocal, unilateral or bilateral. They are divided into central and lateral lesions in view of different lymph drainage patterns. Spread patterns include local or direct extension, hematogenous or lymphatic. Lymphatic drainage is initially lateral, to superficial and deep inguinal–femoral nodes then pelvic nodes (usually medial external iliac group). The overall incidence of positive nodes is 30 per cent. Lymphatic channels can become blocked resulting in aberrant or retrograde lymph drainage. Pelvic nodes are positive only with positive groin nodes. The risk of pelvic lymph node metastases is small in the absence of ipsilateral positive groin nodes, with an overall risk 5 per cent. If the groin nodes are positive then the risk of pelvic nodes being positive is 20 per cent.

Natural history of disease

Presentation is usually with a prolonged history of vulva itch. A chronic itch–scratch cycle is common particularly in association with the lichen sclerosis. A large percentage of vulva cancers are initiated by high-risk HPV genotypes, analogous to cervical cancer. Indeed patients with vulva cancer have a high risk of having dysplasia or malignancy elsewhere in the lower genital tract. Vulva cancers tend to enlarge locally and then spread to the regional or inguinal lymph nodes.

Prognostic factors

Lymph node spread is the single most important prognostic factor in patients with superficial vulva cancer. Risk factors for groin metastases include high-grade tumours, suspicious, fixed or ulcerated regional nodes, the presence of LVSI, increasing age and increasing tumour thickness.[25] Many believe that an infiltrative growth is more aggressive than the papillary or exophytic type. The presence of positive groin nodes in general will result in a 50 per cent reduction in survival. In addition the presence of multiple positive groin nodes, particularly if both groins are involved, extension beyond the groin or extranodal spread and bulky disease are all associated with poor prognosis.

Prognostic factors increasing the risk of recurrence includes the presence of positive groin nodes, particularly if greater than three nodes are involved, tumour size greater than 4 cm, increasing tumour thickness, poor histologic grade (the proportion of undifferentiated tumour pattern), LVSI, clitoral or perineal location and clinically suspicious nodes. According to a linear logistic model of clinico–pathologic data in 272 patients, no lymph node metastases occurred in approximately one quarter of patients with a combination of low risk factors: i.e. no clinically suspicious nodes, negative capillary like space and non-midline vulvar cancers that were either Grade 1, and 1 to 5 mm thick or Grade 2, and 1–2 mm thick. In contrast all 10 patients with clinically suspicious nodes and Grade 4 tumours had positive groin nodes. It is implied that the risk of lymph node metastases is best determined by simultaneous evaluation of all risk factors rather than a single factor such as tumour thickness.[26]

Apparent local and early vulva cancer may recur in up to 30 per cent cases. Two-thirds of such recurrences occur locally on the vulva and are usually amenable to further surgical treatment. For those lesions that recur in the groin, while further treatment is provided, prognosis is poor. Patients with negative nodes have a 5-year survival of about 90 per cent; but this falls to about 50 per cent for patients with positive nodes.[27]

Therapies affecting prognosis

In patients with early stage vulva cancer, inadequate surgical excision can result in an increased risk of local recurrence. Lesions should be excised with at least a 1-cm tumour-free margin and the deep margin should be the inferior fascia of the urogenital diaphragm, which is coplanar with the fascia lata and the fascia over the symphysis pubis.[28] For T2/3 vulvar cancers, triple incision radical vulvectomy and inguinal lymphadenectomy provides similar survival to en bloc resection and is now the standard of care. Lymph node dissection is required for all cases with invasion greater than 1 mm.[29] Ipsilateral groin dissection is acceptable if the cancer is lateralized and there are no suspicious contralateral nodes.[30] All other cases need bilateral groin dissections performed. In performing a groin dissection, removal of the fascia lata is not necessary with the deep nodes located in the opening of the fossa ovalis, medial to the femoral vein.[31] Contralateral node metastases are extremely rare in lateral T1 and T2 tumours. Irradiation of the intact groin is inferior to groin dissection.[32]

Pelvic nodal metastases occur infrequently, unless the patient has (1) clinically suspicious (N2) groin nodes or (2) three or more positive unilateral groin nodes. Pelvic LND seems reasonable in patients with macroscopically positive groin nodes to (1) define the extent of disease so irradiation fields can be extended if necessary and (2) remove enlarged hypoxic, resistant tumour masses. Sentinel node assessment is receiving increasing attention, but remains an experimental procedure.[33]

Preoperative radiation therapy may be utilized in advanced primary lesions to decrease tumour bulk and in lesions close to the urethra and anus to lessen the risk of local recurrence. It is usually given with concurrent cisplatin and 5-fluorouracil.

Postoperatively patients with negative nodes and margin-free resections do not require further therapy. In some instances various features such as poorly differentiated cancers, large bulky tumours, those with diffusely infiltrative growth patterns, those with lymph-vascular space invasion or those with very small surgical margins (< 1 cm) may be selected for postoperative therapy based on concern for local relapse. Radiation therapy options would include whole pelvic irradiation centred low to include the vulva and soft tissues of the medial groins or vulva irradiation alone. If a unilateral dissection has been carried out, the contralateral groin may be dissected, radiated or observed. If nodal positivity is confirmed intraoperatively, one may consider pelvic node dissection or pelvic retroperitoneal exploration to remove any enlarged or suspicious nodes.[34] The prime indication for adjuvant postoperative radiotherapy is one or more positive groin nodes. When there is concern over the adequacy of excision (close margins) or the presence of LVSI after radical local excision, vulvar irradiation may be considered, or in the unusual situation where patients are unsuitable for surgery.

Prognosis

Overall 5-year survival for operable cases is about 70 per cent and the corrected 5-year survival rates are 90, 80, 50 and 15 per cent for stages I to IV. Extracapsular growth of lymph node metastases, two or more positive lymph nodes and greater than 50 per cent replacement of lymph nodes by tumour were predictors of poor survival. Patients with negative nodes have a 5-year survival of about 90 per cent; but this falls to about 50 per cent for patients with positive nodes.

The terminal phase of patients with advanced and recurrent vulva cancer may involve a local fungating lesion with bleeding, infection and pain together with manifestations of distant disease to the lungs, liver or bone.

References

1. Omura G, Brady M, Homesley H, Yordan E, Major F, Buchsbaum H. *et al.* Long term followup and prognostic factor analysis in advanced ovarian carcinoma: the Gynecologic Oncology Group experience. *J Clin Oncol* 1991; 9:1138–50.
2. Bristow R, Tomacruz R, Armstrong D, Trimble E, Montz F. Survival effect of maximal cytoreductive surgery for advanced ovarian carcinoma during the platinum era: a meta-analysis. *J Clin Oncol* 2002; 20:1248–59.

3. Junor E, Hole D, McNulty L, Mason M, Young J. Specialist gynaecologists and survival outcome in ovarian cancer: a Scottish national study of 1866 patients. *Br J Obstet Gynaecol* 1999; 106:1130–6.

4. Krebs H, Goplerud D. Surgical management of bowel obstruction in advanced ovarian cancer. *Obstet Gynecol* 1983; 61(3):327–30.

5. Delgado G, Bundy B, Zaino R, Sevin B, Creasman W, Major F. Prospective surgical-pathologic study of disease free interval in patients with stage Ib squamous cell carcinoma of the cervix: a Gynecologic Oncology Group Study. *Gynecol Oncol* 1990; 38:352–7.

6. Delgado G, Bundy B, Fowler W, Stehman F, Sevin B, Creasman W. *et al.* A prospective surgical pathological study of stage I squamous carcinoma of the cervix: a Gynecologic Oncology Group study. *Gynecol Oncol* 1989; 35:314–20.

7. Stehman F, Bundy B, DiSaia P, Keys H, Larson D, Fowler W. Carcinoma of the cervix treated with radiation therapy. *Cancer* 1991; 67:2776–85.

8. Ostor A. Natural history of cervical intraepithelial neoplasia: a critical review. *Int J Gynecol Pathol* 1993; 12(2):186–92.

9. Elliott P, Coppleson M, Russsell P, Liouros P, Carter J, MacLeod C. *et al.* Early invasive (FIGO stage Ia) carcinoma of the cervix: a clinico-pathologic study of 476 cases. *Int J Gynecol Oncol* 2000; 10:42–52.

10. Landoni F, Maneo A, Cormio G, Perego P, Milani R, Caruso O. *et al.* Class II versus class III radical hysterectomy in stage Ib-IIa cervical cancer: a prospective randomized study. *Gynecol Oncol* 2001; 80:3–12.

11. Weiser E, Bundy B, Hoskins W. Extraperitoneal versus transperitoneal selective paraaortic lymphadenectomy in the pretreatment surgical staging of advanced cervical carcinoma (a Gynecologic Oncology Group study). *Gynecol Oncol* 1989; 33:283–9.

12. Arrastia C, Fruchter R, Clark M, Maiman M, Remy J, Macasaet M. *et al.* Uterine carcinomasarcomas: incidence and trends in managment and survival. *Gynecol Oncol* 1997; 65:158–63.

13. Cosin J, Fowler J, Chen M, Paley P, Carson L, Twiggs L. Pretreatment surgical staging of patients with cervical carcinoma. The case for lymph node debulking. *Cancer* 1998; 82:2241–8.

14. Keys H, Bundy B, Stehman F, Okagaki T, Gallup D, Burnett A. *et al.* Radiation therapy with and without extrafascial hysterectomy for bulky stage IB cervical carcinoma: a randomized trial of the GOG. *Gynecol Oncol* 2003; 89(3):343–53.

15. Creasman W, Morrow C, Bundy B, Homesley H, Graham J, Heller P. Surgical pathologic spread patterns of endometrial cancer, a Gynecologic Oncology Group study. *Cancer* 1987; 60:2035–41.

16. Boronow R, Morrow C, Creasman W. Surgical staging in endometrial cancer: clinicopathologic findings of a prospective study. *Obstet Gynecol* 1984; 63:825–32.

17. Morrow C, Bundy B, Kurman R, Creasman W, Heller P, Homesley H. *et al.* Relationship between surgical-pathologic risk factors and outcome in clinical stage I and II carcinoma of the endometrium: a Gynecologic Oncology Group study. *Gynecol Oncol* 1991; 40(1)55–65.

18. Petersen R, Quinlivan J, Casper G, Nicklin J. Endometrial adenocarcinoma-presenting pathology is a poor guide to surgical management. *Aust NZ J Obstet Gynaecol* 2000; 40(2):191–4.

19. Fanning J, Nanavati P, Hilgers R. Surgical staging and high dose rate brachytherapy for endometrial cancer: limiting external radiotherapy to node positive tumors. *Obstet Gynecol* 1996; 87(6):1041–4.

20. Orr J, Holimon J, Orr P. Stage I corpus cancer: is teletherapy necessary? *Am J Obstet Gynecol* 1997; 176:777–89.

21. Keys H, JA R, Brunetto V, Zaino R, Spirtos N, Bloss J. *et al.* A phase III trial of surgery with or without adjunctive external pelvic radiation therapy in intermediate risk endometrial adenocarcinoma: a GOG study. *Gynecol Oncol* 2004; 92:744–51.

22. Orr J, Orr P, Taylor P. Surgical staging of endometrial cancer. *Obstet Gynecol* 1996; 39:656–68.

23. Creutzberg C, van Putten W, Koper P, Lybeert M, Jobsen J, Warlam-Rodenhuis C. *et al.* Surgery and postoperative radiotherapy versus surgery alone for patients with stage I endometrial carcinoma: multicentre randomised trial. *Lancet* 2000; 355:1404–11.

24. Creutzberg C, van Putten W, Koper P, Lybeert M, Jobsen J, Warlam-Rodenhuis C. *et al.* Survival after relapse in patients with endometrial cancer: results from a randomized trial. *Gynecol Oncol* 2003; 89(2):201–9.

25. Homesley H, Bundy B, Sedlis A, Yordan E, Berek J, Jahshan A. *et al.* Prognostic factors for groin node metastasis in squamous cell carcinoma of the vulva. A Gynecologic Oncology Group study. *Gynecol Oncol* 1993; 49:279–83.

26. Sedlis A, Homesley H, Bundy B, Marshall R, Yordan E, Hacker N. *et al.* Positive groin lymph nodes in superficial squamous vulvar cancer. A Gynecologic Oncology Group study. *Am J Obstet Gynecol* 1987; 156:1159–64.

27. Stehman F, Bundy B, Ball H, Clarke-Pearson D. Sites of failure and times to failure in carcinoma of the vulva treated conservatively: a Gynecologic Oncology Group study. *Am J Obstet Gynecol* 1996; 174:1128–33.

28. Heaps J, Fu Y, Montz F, Hacker N, Berek J. Surgical-pathologic variables predictive of local recurrence in squamous cell carcinoma of the vulva. *Gynecol Oncol* 1990; 38:309.

29. Burke T, Levenback C, Coleman R, Morris M, Silva E, Gershenson D. Surgical therapy of T1 and T2 vulvar carcinoma: further experience with radical wide excision and selective inguinal lymphadenectomy. *Gynecol Oncol* 1995; 57:215–20.

30. Andrews S, Williams B, DePriest P, Gallion H, Hunter J, Buckley S. *et al.* Therapeutic implications of lymph nodal spread in lateral T1 and T2 squamous cell carcinoma of the vulva. *Gynecol Oncol* 1994; 55:41–6.

31. Borgno G, Micheletti L, Barbero M, Cavanna L, Preti M, Valentino M. *et al.* Topographic distribution of groin lymph nodes. A study of 50 female cadavers. *J Reprod Med* 1990; 35(12):1127–9.

32. Stehman F, Bundy B, Thomas G, Varia M, Okagaki T, Roberts J. *et al.* Groin dissection versus groin radiation in carcinoma of the vulva: a Gynecologic Oncology Group study. *Int J Radiat Oncol Biol Phys* 1992; 24:389–96.

33. de Hullu J, Hollema H, Piers D, Verheijen R, van Diest P, Mourits M. *et al.* Sentinel lymph node procedure is highly accurate in squamous cell carcinoma of the vulva. *J Clin Oncol* 2000; 18:2811–16.

34. Homesley H, Bundy B, Sedlis A, Adcock L. Radiation therapy versus pelvic node resection for carcinoma of the vulva with positive groin nodes. *Obstet Gynecol* 1986; 68(6):733–40.

18

Brain cancer

Hiroko Ohgaki

Introduction

Tumours of the nervous system amount to less than 2 per cent of the total human cancer burden, their overall annual incidence being in the range of 7–9 new cases per 100,000 population. More than 40 histological types of nervous system tumours have been classified by the World Health Organization (WHO),[1] and this makes difficult the identification of factors with unequivocal prognostic value. The most frequent histological types of malignant brain tumour are diffusely infiltrating gliomas in adults and medulloblastomas in children. Among gliomas, glioblastoma is the most frequent, with an incidence rate of about 3 cases per 100,000 population and year.[2–4] Medulloblastoma is a malignant, invasive embryonal tumour of the cerebellum, which manifests preferentially in children[1] with an incidence rate of 0.2–0.3 cases per 100,000 population and year.[3] It accounts for approximately 20 per cent of paediatric central nervous system (CNS) neoplasms.[5] During recent decades, numerous studies have described genetic alterations in addition to conventional clinical and histopathological criteria. In this chapter, known prognostic factors are summarized for astrocytic and oligodendroglial gliomas and medulloblastomas.

Diffusely infiltrating astrocytomas

Diffusely infiltrating astrocytomas consist of three major entities: low-grade astrocytoma (WHO grade II), anaplastic astrocytoma (WHO grade III), and glioblastoma (WHO grade IV). These gliomas are the most frequent intracranial tumours, which account for more than 60 per cent of all primary brain tumours. Diffusely infiltrating astrocytomas typically manifest in adults and may arise at any site in the CNS, but preferentially in the cerebral hemispheres. They have a wide range of histopathological features and biological behaviour, but they diffusely infiltrate adjacent brain structures and have an inherent tendency for malignant progression, with glioblastoma being the most malignant phenotypic end point.[1] These diffusely infiltrating astrocytomas must be strictly distinguished from the pilocytic astrocytoma (WHO grade I) of children and adolescents which is more confined, preferentially affects the cerebellum and CNS midline structures, lacks a tendency for malignant progression and has a more favourable clinical outcome.

Low-grade astrocytoma, also termed diffuse astrocytoma or low-grade diffuse astrocytoma, typically affects young adults and is characterized by a high degree of cellular differentiation. Anaplastic astrocytoma is characterized by focal or dispersed anaplasia and marked proliferative potential.[1] Low-grade and anaplastic astrocytomas show a consistent tendency to progress to glioblastoma.[1]

Glioblastoma is the most malignant astrocytic tumour and is composed of poorly differentiated neoplastic astrocytes. Histopathological features include cellular polymorphism, nuclear atypia, brisk mitotic activity, microvascular proliferation, and necrosis. It may develop from low-grade or anaplastic astrocytomas (secondary glioblastoma), but much more frequently manifests after a short clinical history *de novo*, with no evidence of a less malignant precursor lesion (primary glioblastoma).[1, 4]

Factors affecting prognosis

Disease-related factors

Histological grading The histological grade of diffusely infiltrating astrocytomas is predictive of survival. Figure 18.1 shows population-based data on survival for low-grade astrocytoma, anaplastic astrocytoma, and glioblastoma.[4, 6]

Histological features Low-grade astrocytomas with a significant fraction of gemisto-cytes (gemistocytic astrocytomas) tend to undergo malignant progression more rapidly than the ordinary fibrillary astrocytoma,[6–8] despite the fact that the majority of neoplastic gemistocytes are in a non-proliferative state. Several studies suggest that the presence and extent of necrosis in glioblastomas correlates with poor clinical outcome.[9] An oligoden-droglial component is predictive of better survival of patients with anaplastic astrocytoma[10] and glioblastoma.[11]

Tumour size The size of tumour appeared to be an important predictive factor in a study of 379 low-grade glioma patients (astrocytomas, oligodendrogliomas, and mixed oligoastrocytomas) in two multicentric randomized trials conducted by the European Organization for Research and Treatment of Cancer (EORTC).[16] In glioblastomas, larger tumour size (> 5 cm) is predictive for a poor prognosis.[13, 17]

Proliferation There is a close correlation between the tumour growth fraction and histological grade, with mean values of MIB1 labeling index of 3.8 per cent for low-grade diffuse astrocytomas,

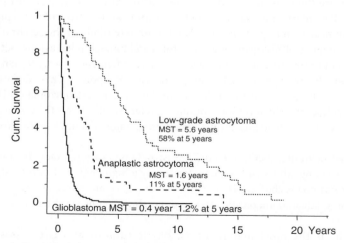

Figure 18.1 Population-based data on survival of patients with low-grade astrocytoma (WHO grade II), anaplastic astrocytoma (WHO grade III), and glioblastoma (WHO grade IV).[4, 6]

18.4 per cent for anaplastic astrocytomas, and 31.6 per cent for glioblastomas.[29] Analysis of a wide range of astrocytic tumours showed a gross correlation of proliferation with clinical outcome.[30, 31]

Genetic alterations The presence of *TP53* mutations in low-grade astrocytomas is not a predictor of patients' clinical outcome,[6, 8] although some studies have found a shorter time interval before progression in patients with low-grade astrocytomas carrying a *TP53* mutation.[32] In one study, non-gemistocytic low-grade astrocytomas with a codon 175 *TP53* mutation had a significantly worse prognosis compared with tumours carrying mutations at any other site.[8]

For glioblastomas, while some hospital-based studies showed no association between *TP53* status and outcome,[33, 34] one study with 97 glioblastoma cases showed that the presence of *TP53* mutations was a favourable prognostic factor.[35] In a recent population-based study, univariate analysis indicated that the presence of *TP53* mutations was predictive of longer survival, but age-adjusted multivariate analysis revealed no difference in survival between patients with or without *TP53* mutations.[4] In several studies, LOH 10q has been associated with poorer survival of glioblastoma patients.[4, 35] In contrast, mutations in the *PTEN* gene at 10q23 were not associated with prognosis of glioblastoma patients.[4, 33, 35] The predictive value of *EGFR* amplification in glioblastomas remains unclear. A meta-analysis of seven studies with 395 glioblastomas did not reveal a significant predictive value of *EGFR* amplification,[36] but several studies have suggested that *EGFR* amplification is predictive in certain age groups of glioblastoma patients.[33, 34] A recent population-based study indicated that the presence of *EGFR* amplification does not affect survival of glioblastoma patients in any age group.[4] Findings regarding the predictive value of *p16*^{INK4a} homozygous deletion in glioblastomas are also inconsistent. In a recent population-based study, both univariate and multivariate analysis failed to show any predictive value of homozygous *p16*^{INK4a} deletion.[4] The combination of LOH 1p/19q defined glioblastoma patients with significantly better survival.[35]

Patient-related factors

Age For patients with low-grade astrocytoma[6, 12] or glioblastoma,[4, 13, 14] young age at diagnosis has been consistently predictive of a more favourable clinical course. In one study, long-term glioblastoma survivors had a mean age of 45 years, significantly younger than all glioblastoma patients combined.[15] In a recent population-based study,[4] younger patients (< 50 years) showed significantly longer survival (median 8.8 months) than older patients (> 50 years, 4.1 months), and even among patients older than 50 years, age continues to be a significant predictive factor of poor survival of glioblastoma patients (Figure 18.2).

Pre-operative status Low-grade astrocytoma with epilepsy as the single symptom appears to have a better prognosis than if accompanied by other symptoms.[18] Conversely, presentation with a neurological deficit is associated with a worse prognosis than presentation with seizures or pressure symptoms alone.[19] A higher score (≥70) for pre-operative Karnofsky Performance Status (KPS) has consistently been shown to be significantly associated with longer survival in glioblastoma patients.[14, 20] Median survival of patients with malignant glioma (grade III or IV) with KPS 70, 80, 90 and 100 were 14.5, 17.0, 19.2, and 22.2 months, respectively.[14]

Impact of treatment on prognosis

Surgery

Total resection is a significant predictive factor of longer survival in low-grade astrocytoma patients.[7, 18] Survival rates at 1, 2, 3, and 4 years following surgery were 100, 96, 96 and 96 per cent

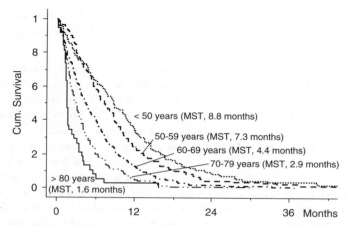

Figure 18.2 Older age is a significant predictive factor of survival of glioblastoma patients at the population level.[4]

for patients who underwent gross total resection and 86, 77, 77 and 64 per cent for patients with subtotal resection.[7] Other authors maintain that at least for a subset of patients, diagnostic biopsy may be equally effective if followed by external radiation[21] or brachytherapy.[22] For glioblastomas, evaluation of the extent of resection as a prognostic factor has given conflicting results, but there is some evidence that complete resection favours longer survival.[17, 23]

Adjuvant therapy

For low-grade astrocytomas, the potential effect on patient survival of adjuvant radio- or chemotherapy has been discussed for many years and is still uncertain.[24, 25] Many oncology centres, particularly in North America, routinely apply adjuvant therapy,[26] while others, particularly in Europe, prefer a wait and see approach, recommending radiotherapy only after evidence of progression to anaplastic astrocytoma. The latter view is supported by a study showing no significant difference in survival between patients who did and those who did not receive radiotherapy for supratentorial fibrillary astrocytomas.[27] Survival among 13 patients with supratentorial low-grade astrocytomas treated immediately after diagnosis and 17 patients initially followed up and treated only after clinical or radiological progression was identical (63 per cent survival rate after 5 years).[18]

Postoperative radiotherapy increases the mean survival of glioblastoma patients by 3–4 months.[28] Additional chemotherapy may improve survival. In a meta-analysis of 12 randomized clinical trials, the overall survival rate of high-grade glioma patients (glioblastomas and anaplastic astrocytomas) was 40 per cent at 1 year and slightly higher (46 per cent) after combined radio- and chemotherapy.[20]

Oligodendrogliomas

Oligodendroglioma (WHO grade II) is a well differentiated, slowly growing diffusely infiltrating tumour of adults, typically located in the cerebral hemispheres and composed predominantly of cells morphologically resembling oligodendroglia. Anaplastic oligodendroglioma (WHO grade III) is an oligodendroglioma with focal or diffuse histological features of malignancy and a less favourable prognosis.[1]

Factors affecting prognosis

Tumour-related factors

Histological grading The WHO grading system recognizes only two grades of oligodendroglial tumours: WHO grade II for well differentiated and WHO grade III for anaplastic oligodendrogliomas. Grading according to WHO has been shown to be significantly predictive of survival[37, 38] (Figure 18.3).

Tumour size and location The size of oligodendroglioma does not appear to be correlated with either survival or histological grade.[42] Location in the frontal lobe has been found to confer a more favourable prognosis.[40, 42, 43] Multivariate analyses showed that 5-year survival of patients with oligodendroglioma in the frontal and non-frontal localizations were 40 and 10 per cent, respectively.[40]

Proliferation Many studies have focused on the prognostic significance of the growth fraction (Ki-67/MIB-1 labelling index) in patients with oligodendroglial tumours.[37, 38, 40] In a study of 89 oligodendroglioma patients, the 5-year survival rate was 83 per cent among patients whose oligodendrogliomas had an MIB-1 labelling index of < 5 per cent but only 24 per cent among those with tumours with an index above 5 per cent.[37]

Genetic alterations For anaplastic oligodendrogliomas, it is well established that the presence of LOH 1p/19q is a significant predictor of susceptibility to chemotherapy and better survival of patients.[46-48] However, for WHO grade II oligodendrogliomas, the data are less clear. In a study of 36 oligodendroglioma cases, Smith et al.[49] reported that patients with combined loss of

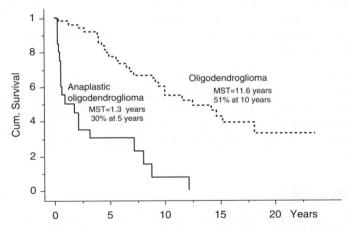

Figure 18.3 Population-based data on survival of patients with oligodendroglioma and anaplastic oligodendroglioma. Data are from a population-based study in the Canton of Zurich, Switzerland (Ohgaki H. *et al:* unpublished results).

1p and 19q had better overall survival. Similarly, Felsberg *et al.*[48] showed that LOH 1p and 19q was associated with longer survival in patients with low-grade oligodendroglial tumours. Sasaki *et al.*[50] evaluated 1p status in 44 WHO grade II oligodendrogliomas and found that 14 cases had been treated with chemotherapy at the time of clinical or radiological tumour progression, with 13 being evaluable for response to therapy. Of these, 10 of 11 cases with LOH 1p had responded to PCV, whereas neither case without LOH 1p had responded. Buckner *et al.*[51] carried out phase II trials of PCV as initial therapy for 31 patients with low-grade oligodendroglioma or oligoastrocytoma and observed that LOH 1p/19q was not associated with response to PCV. In a recent population-based study, in which patients were not treated with chemotherapy but 25 per cent of patients received radiotherapy, LOH 1p/19q was not predictive of patient survival in either univariate or multivariate analyses.[6]

Homozygous deletions of the *p16^{INK4a}* gene were primarily detected in those anaplastic oligodendrogliomas that lacked 1p and 19q losses.[46] Patients whose tumours had *p16^{INK4a}* deletions generally had shorter survival.[46] Decreased p16^{INK4a} expression was associated with poor survival of oligodendroglioma patients.[52]

Patient-related factors

Age Younger age at surgery (< 40 or 50 years) is associated with longer survival in oligodendroglioma patients.[39, 40] The median survival for patients younger than 20 years was 17.5 years and that for the group older than 60 years was 13 months.[41]

Performance score Higher postoperative Karnofsky scores (> 90) were associated with longer survival; oligodendroglioma patients without neurological deficits had a 5-year survival of 43 per cent, compared with 5 per cent among those with deficits.[43]

Impact of treatment on prognosis

Surgery: extent of resection

In most studies, an association was found between the extent of resection and longer survival, for both oligodendroglioma and oligoastrocytoma.[37, 43] The 19 patients who underwent gross total resection of their tumour had a median survival time and 5- and 10-year survival rates of 12.6 years, 74 and 59 per cent, compared to 4.9 years, 46 and 23 per cent, respectively, for the 63 who had subtotal resection.[44]

Chemotherapy

Both oligodendroglioma grade II and anaplastic oligodendroglioma are chemosensitive, with a 60–70 per cent rate of response to treatment with PCV (procarbazine, CCNU and vincristine).[45] Anaplastic oligodendrogliomas with allelic loss on chromosome 1 or with combined allelic losses on 1p and 19q are typically sensitive to PCV chemotherapy and show longer survival.[46–48]

Medulloblastoma

Medulloblastoma is a malignant invasive embryonal tumour of the cerebellum with preferential manifestation in children, and a peak of occurrence at 7 years of age.[1] It has an inherent tendency to metastasize via CSF pathways. Medulloblastomas correspond histologically to WHO grade IV.

Factors affecting prognosis

Tumour-related factors

Tumour size and location Patients with lateral tumours had a better prognosis than patients with midline tumours with brainstem infiltration.[53] Brainstem involvement did not appear predictive of disease-free survival independently, the 94 children with brainstem involvement having a similar probability of recurrence to the 174 children without brainstem disease in the SIOP I study.[63] Extent of disease at diagnosis of medulloblastomas (favouring localized disease) was an important prognostic factor in adults (age > 15 years).[64]

Histological features Desmoplastic medulloblastomas were associated with a somewhat better outcome in some series,[53, 54] but with poorer prognosis in others.[55] This discrepancy may be explained by the fact that in some of these studies tumours were classified as desmoplastic on the basis of an increased amount of collagen and reticulin fibres but without the typical nodular pattern of this variant. One study confirmed the favourable prognosis for the rare cases of extensive nodularity, while lesser degrees of nodularity or desmoplasticity were not associated with a statistically significant survival advantage.[56]

The large-cell variant of medulloblastoma appears to be biologically aggressive[57] and survival of children bearing this variant is significantly shorter.[56, 58] In a study with 330 cases from the Pediatric Oncology Group, significant anaplasia was identified in 24 per cent of cases and was strongly associated with shorter survival time.[56]

Proliferation Medulloblastomas with a BrdU labeling index (LI) of >20 per cent have been reported to have a worse prognosis.[66] In a multivariate analysis of postoperative survival of adult medulloblastoma patients, PCNA and Ki-67 LI had no prognostic value.[55] Mitotic percentage index was an independent prognostic factor for childhood medulloblastoma.[67]

Genetic alterations c-*MYC* mRNA expression is frequent (approx. 40 per cent) in medulloblastomas,[68] while c-*MYC* amplification is infrequent (5–8 per cent).[68, 69] In a study of 77 medulloblastomas from the Children's Oncology Group, all four paediatric medulloblastoma patients with c-*MYC* amplification died of clinically aggressive neoplasms within 7 months of diagnosis.[69] Medulloblastomas with *MYC* amplification were resistant to therapy and had a fatal outcome.[70] There is a significant association between anaplastic/large-cell tumours and *MYC* amplification, which is associated with aggressiveness in medulloblastomas.[71, 72] High c-MYC mRNA expression was also significantly associated with tumour anaplasia[73] and was a significant prognostic factor for poor clinical outcome in primitive neuroectodermal tumour (PNET) and medulloblastomas.[73, 74] In contrast, one study of 86 cases of medulloblastoma showed that c-MYC and N-MYC expression were not associated with prognosis.[75]

Children with medulloblastomas expressing no or little TrkC mRNA had a 4.8-fold greater risk of death than children with high TrkC expression.[76] One study of 87 PNET and medulloblastomas showed that high TrkC mRNA expression was associated with a higher 5-year cumulative survival rate than was low TrkC mRNA expression (89 vs 46 per cent).[77] When compared with established clinical prognostic factors and laboratory variables of potential prognostic significance, TrkC mRNA expression was the single most powerful predictor of outcome (hazard ratio, 4.81, p < 0.0001), exceeding all clinical prognostic factors.[77] The combination of low MYC mRNA expression and high TrkC mRNA expression identified a good-outcome group of PNET/medulloblastoma patients with 100 per cent progression-free survival after a median follow-up of 55 months.[74]

Correlations have been reported between LOH 17p and poor response to therapy,[78] and shortened survival time of medulloblastoma patients.[79] In one study, LOH 17p was associated with metastatic disease.[70] Several studies have shown that *c-erbB-2* overexpression is associated with poor prognosis of medulloblastoma patients.[71, 80]

Patient-related factors

Age and sex There was no difference between the survival rates of infants (age < 2 years) and of children (> 2 years),[59] but patients older than 10 years had a better prognosis than those aged 10 or less.[53] In analyses of 156 medulloblastomas in patients older than 18 years of age, the 5- and 10-year event-free survival rates were 61 and 48 per cent, respectively, and these were similar to those observed in children.[54] Other studies have shown better survival in adults than in children.[60, 61]

Girls with medulloblastoma have a much better outcome than boys.[62, 63] Disease-free survival was better in girls than in boys, the 10-year survival rates being 57 and 40 per cent, respectively, in the Multicentre Control Trial of the International Society of Pediatric Oncology (SIOP I).[63] Similarly, in adults (> 15 years) with medulloblastoma, the 5-year survival rate was 92 per cent for females vs 40 per cent for males.[64]

Impact of treatment on prognosis

Extent of surgical resection was predictive of better prognosis in paediatric patients with medulloblastoma.[59, 62] In the SIOP I study, patients undergoing total or subtotal excision tended to have better outcome than those in whom only a partial excision could be performed.[63] Taylor *et al.*[65]) carried out a large multicentre randomized clinical trial in medulloblastoma patients (3–16 years) to assess event-free survival (EFS) after chemotherapy following radiotherapy (RT) compared with RT alone. EFS was significantly better for chemotherapy and RT, with EFS of 78.5 per cent at 3 years and 74.2 per cent at 5 years, compared with 64.8 per cent and 59.8 per cent, respectively, for RT alone.[65]

References

1. Louis DN, Ohgaki H, Wiestler OD, Cavenee WK, Burger PC, Jouvet A, Scheithauer BW, Kleihues P. *WHO Classification of Tumors of the Central Nervous System*. IARC. Lyon, 2007.

2. Ohgaki H, Kleihues P. Epidemiology and etiology of gliomas. *Acta Neuropathol* 2005; 109:93–108.

3. Central Brain Tumor Registry of the United States. *Central brain tumor registry of the United States* (CBTRUS). Available at http://www.cbtrus.org, published 2002.

4. Ohgaki H, Dessen P, Jourde B, Horstmann S, Nishikawa T, Di Patre PL, Burkhard C, Schuler D, Probst-Hensch NM, Maiorka PC, Baeza N, Pisani P, Yonekawa Y, Yasargil MG, Lutolf UM, Kleihues P. Genetic pathways to glioblastoma: a population-based study. *Cancer Res* 2004; 64:6892–9.

5. Lantos PL, Louis DN, Rosenblum MK, Kleihues P. Tumours of the nervous system. In DI Graham and PL Lantos (eds) *Greenfield's neuropathology*, 7th edn, pp. 767–1052. London: Arnold, 2002.

6. Okamoto Y, Di Patre PL, Burkhard C, Horstmann S, Jourde B, Fahey M, Schuler D, Probst-Hensch NM, Yasargil MG, Yonekawa Y, Lutolf U, Kleihues P, Ohgaki H. Population-based study on incidence, survival rates, genetic alterations of low-grade astrocytomas and oligodendrogliomas. *Acta Neuropathol* 2004; 108:49–56.

7. Peraud A, Ansari H, Bise K, Reulen HJ. Clinical outcome of supratentorial astrocytoma WHO grade II. *Acta Neurochir (Wien)* 1998; 140:1213–22.

8. Peraud A, Kreth FW, Wiestler OD, Kleihues P, Reulen HJ. Prognostic impact of TP53 mutations and P53 protein overexpression in supratentorial WHO grade II astrocytomas and oligoastrocytomas. *Clin Cancer Res* 2002; 8:1117–24.

9. Barker FG, Davis RL, Chang SM, Prados MD. Necrosis as a prognostic factor in glioblastoma multiforme. *Cancer* 1996; 77:1161–6.

10. Donahue B, Scott CB, Nelson JS, Rotman M, Murray KJ, Nelson DF, Banker FL, Earle JD, Fischbach JA, Asbell SO, Gaspar LE, Markoe AM, Curran W. Influence of an oligodendroglial component on the survival of patients with anaplastic astrocytomas: a report of Radiation Therapy Oncology Group 83–02. *Int J Radiat Oncol Biol Phys* 1997; 38:911–14.

11. Hilton DA, Penney M, Pobereskin L, Sanders H, Love S. Histological indicators of prognosis in glioblastomas: retinoblastoma protein expression and oligodendroglial differentiation indicate improved survival. *Histopathology* 2004; 44:555–60.

12. Shafqat S, Hedley Whyte ET, Henson JW. Age-dependent rate of anaplastic transformation in low-grade astrocytoma. *Neurology* 1999; 52:867–9.

13. Fazeny-Dorner B, Wenzel C, Veitl M, Piribauer M, Rossler K, Dieckmann K, Ungersbock K, Marosi C. Survival and prognostic factors of patients with unresectable glioblastoma multiforme. *Anticancer Drugs* 2003; 14:305–12.

14. Weller M, Muller B, Koch R, Bamberg M, Krauseneck P. Neuro-Oncology Working Group 01 trial of nimustine plus teniposide versus nimustine plus cytarabine chemotherapy in addition to involved-field radiotherapy in the first-line treatment of malignant glioma. *J Clin Oncol* 2003; 21:3276–84.

15. Scott JN, Rewcastle NB, Brasher PM, Fulton D, Hagen NA, MacKinnon JA, Sutherland G, Cairncross JG, Forsyth P. Long-term glioblastoma multiforme survivors: a population-based study. *Can J Neurol Sci* 1998; 25:197–201.

16. Karim AB, Maat.B, Hatlevoll R, Menten J, Rutten EH, Thomas DG, Mascarenhas F, Horiot JC, Parvinen LM, van Reijn M, Jager JJ, Fabrini MG, van Alphen AM, Hamers HP, Gaspar L, Noordman E, Pierart M, van Glabbeke M. A randomized trial on dose–response in radiation therapy of low-grade cerebral glioma: European Organization for Research and Treatment of Cancer (EORTC) Study 22844. *Int J Radiat Oncol Biol Phys* 1996; 36:549–56.

17. Hulshof MC, Koot RW, Schimmel EC, Dekker F, Bosch DA, Gonzalez GD. Prognostic factors in glioblastoma multiforme. Ten years experience of a single institution. *Strahlenther Onkol* 2001; 177:283–90.

18. van Veelen ML, Avezaat CJ, Kros JM, van Putten W, Vecht C. Supratentorial low grade astrocytoma: prognostic factors, dedifferentiation, the issue of early versus late surgery. *J Neurol Neurosurg Psychiatry* 1998; 64:581–7.

19. Danks RA, Chopra G, Gonzales MF, Orian JM, Kaye AH. Aberrant p53 expression does not correlate with the prognosis in anaplastic astrocytoma. *Neurosurgery* 1995; 37:246–54.

20. Stewart LA. Chemotherapy in adult high-grade glioma: a systematic review and meta-analysis of individual patient data from 12 randomised trials. *Lancet* 2002; 359:1011–18.

21. Lunsford LD, Somaza S, Kondziolka D, Flickinger JC. Brain astrocytomas: biopsy, then irradiation. *Clin Neurosurg* 1995; 42:464–79.

22. Kreth FW, Faist M, Rossner R, Volk B, Ostertag CB. Supratentorial World Health Organization grade 2 astrocytomas and oligoastrocytomas. A new pattern of prognostic factors. *Cancer* 1997; 79:370–9.

23. Bouvier-Labit C, Chinot O, Ochi C, Gambarelli D, Dufour H, Figarella-Branger D. Prognostic significance of Ki67, p53 and epidermal growth factor receptor immunostaining in human glioblastomas. *Neuropathol Appl Neurobiol* 1998; 24:381–8.

24. Trautmann TG and Shaw EG. Supratentorial low-grade glioma: is there a role for radiation therapy? *Ann Acad Med Singapore* 1996; 25:392–6.

25. Loiseau H, Dartigues JF, Cohadon F. Low-grade astrocytomas: prognosis factors and elements of management. *Surg Neurol* 1995; 44:224–7.

26. Shaw EG. The low-grade glioma debate: evidence defending the position of early radiation therapy. *Clin Neurosurg* 1995; 42:488–94.

27. Hilton DA, Love S, Barber R, Ellison D, Sandeman DR. Accumulation of p53 and Ki-67 expression do not predict survival in patients with fibrillary astrocytomas or the response of these tumors to radiotherapy. *Neurosurgery* 1998; 42:724–9.

28. Rainov NG, Dobberstein KU, Bahn H, Holzhausen HJ, Lautenschlager C, Heidecke V, Burkert W. Prognostic factors in malignant glioma: influence of the overexpression of oncogene and tumor-suppressor gene products on survival. *J Neurooncol* 1997; 35:13–28.

29. Wakimoto H, Aoyagi M, Nakayama T, Nagashima G, Yamamoto S, Tamaki M, Hirakawa K. Prognostic significance of Ki-67 labeling indices obtained using MIB-1 monoclonal antibody in patients with supratentorial astrocytomas. *Cancer* 1996; 77:373–80.

30. Hoshino T, Ahn D, Prados MD, Lamborn K, Wilson CB. Prognostic significance of the proliferative potential of intracranial gliomas measured by bromodeoxyuridine labeling. *Int J Cancer* 1993; 53:550–5.

31. Prados MD, Krouwer HG, Edwards MS, Cogen PH, Davis RL, Hoshino T. Proliferative potential and outcome in pediatric astrocytic tumors. *J Neurooncol* 1992; 13:277–82.

32. Watanabe K, Sato K, Biernat W, Tachibana O, von Ammon K, Ogata N, Yonekawa Y, Kleihues P, Ohgaki H. Incidence and timing of *p53* mutations during astrocytoma progression in patients with multiple biopsies. *Clin Cancer Res* 1997; 3:523–30.

33. Smith JS, Tachibana I, Passe SM, Huntley BK, Borell TJ, Iturria N, O'Fallon JR, Schaefer PL, Scheithauer BW, James CD, Buckner JC, Jenkins RB. PTEN mutation, EGFR amplification, outcome in patients with anaplastic astrocytoma and glioblastoma multiforme. *J Natl Cancer Inst* 2001; 93:1246–56.

34. Simmons ML, Lamborn KR, Takahashi M, Chen P, Israel MA, Berger MS, Godfrey T, Nigro J, Prados M, Chang S, Barker FG, Aldape K. Analysis of complex relationships between age, p53, epidermal growth factor receptor, survival in glioblastoma patients. *Cancer Res* 2001; 61:1122–28.

35. Schmidt MC, Antweiler S, Urban N, Mueller W, Kuklik A, Meyer-Puttlitz B, Wiestler OD, Louis DN, Fimmers R, von Deimling A. Impact of genotype and morphology on the prognosis of glioblastoma. *J Neuropathol Exp Neurol* 2002; 61:321–8.

36. Huncharek M, Kupelnick B. Epidermal growth factor receptor gene amplification as a prognostic marker in glioblastoma multiforme: results of a meta-analysis. *Oncol Res* 2000; 12:107–12.

37. Dehghani F, Schachenmayr W, Laun A, Korf HW. Prognostic implication of histopathological, immuno-histochemical and clinical features of oligodendrogliomas: a study of 89 cases. *Acta Neuropathol* 1998; 95:493–504.

38. Wharton SB, Hamilton FA, Chan WK, Chan KK, Anderson JR. Proliferation and cell death in oligodendrogliomas. *Neuropathol Appl Neurobiol* 1998; 24:21–8.

39. Shimizu KT, Tran LM, Mark RJ, Selch MT. Management of oligodendrogliomas. *Radiology* 1993; 186:569–72.

40. Kros JM, Hop WC, Godschalk JJ, Krishnadath KK. Prognostic value of the proliferation-related antigen Ki-67 in oligodendrogliomas. *Cancer* 1996; 78:1107–13.

41. Westergaard L, Gjerris F, Klinken L. Prognostic factors in oligodendrogliomas. *Acta Neurochir (Wien)* 1997; 139:600–5.

42. Kros JM, Pieterman H, Van Eden CG, Avezaat CJ. Oligodendroglioma: the Rotterdam-Dijkzigt experience. *Neurosurgery* 1994; 34:959–66.

43. Schiffer D, Dutto A, Cavalla P, Bosone I, Chio A, Villani R, Bellotti C. Prognostic factors in oligodendroglioma. *Can J Neurol Sci* 1997; 24:313–19.

44. Shaw EG, Scheithauer BW, O'Fallon JR, Tazelaar HD, Davis DH. Oligodendrogliomas: the Mayo Clinic experience. *J Neurosurg* 1992; 76:428–34.

45. van den Bent MJ, Kros JM, Heimans JJ, Pronk LC, Van Groeningen CJ, Krouwer HG, Taphoorn MJ, Zonnenberg BA, Tijssen CC, Twijnstra A, Punt CJ, Boogerd W. Response rate and prognostic factors of recurrent oligodendroglioma treated with procarbazine, CCNU, vincristine chemotherapy. *Neurology* 1998; 51:1140–5.

46. Cairncross JG, Ueki K, Zlatescu MC, Lisle DK, Finkelstein DM, Hammond RR, Silver JS, Stark PC, Macdonald DR, Ino Y, Ramsay DA, Louis DN. Specific genetic predictors of chemotherapeutic response and survival in patients with anaplastic oligodendrogliomas. *J Natl Cancer Inst* 1998; 90:1473–9.

47. Bauman GS, Ino Y, Ueki K, Zlatescu MC, Fisher BJ, Macdonald DR, Stitt L, Louis DN, Cairncross JG. Allelic loss of chromosome 1p and radiotherapy plus chemotherapy in patients with oligoden-drogliomas. *Int J Radiat Oncol Biol Phys* 2000; 48:825–30.

48. Felsberg J, Erkwoh A, Sabel MC, Kirsch L, Fimmers R, Blaschke B, Schlegel U, Schramm J, Wiestler OD, Reifenberger G. Oligodendroglial tumors: refinement of candidate regions on chromosome arm 1p and correlation of 1p/19q status with survival. *Brain Pathol* 2004; 14:121–30.

49. Smith JS, Perry A, Borell TJ, Lee HK, O'Fallon J, Hosek SM, Kimmel D, Yates A, Burger PC, Scheithauer BW, Jenkins RB. Alterations of chromosome arms 1p and 19q as predictors of survival in oligoden-drogliomas, astrocytomas, mixed oligoastrocytomas. *J Clin Oncol* 2000; 18:636–45.

50. Sasaki H, Zlatescu MC, Betensky RA, Johnk LB, Cutone AN, Cairncross JG, Louis DN. Histopathological-molecular genetic correlations in referral pathologist-diagnosed low-grade 'oligodendroglioma'. *J Neuropathol Exp Neurol* 2002; 61:58–63.

51. Buckner JC, Gesme D Jr, O'Fallon JR, Hammack JE, Stafford S, Brown PD, Hawkins R, Scheithauer BW, Erickson BJ, Levitt R, Shaw EG, Jenkins R. Phase II trial of procarbazine, lomustine, vincristine as initial therapy for patients with low-grade oligodendroglioma or oligoastrocytoma: efficacy and associations with chromosomal abnormalities. *J Clin Oncol* 2003; 21:251–5.

52. Miettinen H, Kononen J, Sallinen P, Alho H, Helen P, Helin H, Kalimo H, Paljarvi L, Isola J, Haapasalo H. CDKN2/p16 predicts survival in oligodendrogliomas: comparison with astrocytomas. *J Neurooncol* 1999; 41:205–11.

53. Sure U, Berghorn WJ, Bertalanffy H, Wakabayashi T, Yoshida J, Sugita K, Seeger W. Staging, scoring and grading of medulloblastoma. A postoperative prognosis predicting system based on the cases of a single institute. *Acta Neurochir (Wien)* 1995; 132:59–65.

54. Carrie C, Lasset C, Alapetite C, Haie Meder C, Hoffstetter S, Demaille MC, Kerr C, Wagner JP, Lagrange JL, Maire JP. *et al.* Multivariate analysis of prognostic factors in adult patients with medulloblastoma. Retrospective study of 156 patients. *Cancer* 1994; 74:2352–60.

55. Giordana MT, Cavalla P, Chio A, Marino S, Soffietti R, Vigliani MC, Schiffer D. Prognostic factors in adult medulloblastoma. A clinico-pathologic study. *Tumori* 1995; 81:338–46.

56. Perry A. Medulloblastomas with favourable versus unfavourable histology: how many small blue cell tumor types are there in the brain? *Adv Anat Pathol* 2002; 9:345–50.

57. Giangaspero F, Rigobello L, Badiali M, Loda M, Reini L, Basso G, Zorzi F, Montaldi A. Large-cell medulloblastomas. A distinct variant with highly aggressive behavior. *Am J Surg Pathol* 1992; 16:687–93.

58. Ozer E, Sarialioglu F, Cetingoz R, Yuceer N, Cakmakci H, Ozkal S, Olgun N, Uysal K, Corapcioglu F, Canda S. Prognostic significance of anaplasia and angiogenesis in childhood medulloblastoma: a pediatric oncology group study. *Pathol Res Pract* 2004; 200:501–9.

59. Cervoni L, Cantore G. Medulloblastoma in pediatric age: a single-institution review of prognostic factors. *Childs Nerv Syst* 1995; 11:80–4.

60. Brandes AA, Palmisano V, Monfardini S. Medulloblastoma in adults: clinical characteristics and treatment. *Cancer Treat Rev* 1999; 25:3–12.

61. Abacioglu U, Uzel O, Sengoz M, Turkan S, Ober A. Medulloblastoma in adults: treatment results and prognostic factors. *Int J Radiat Oncol Biol Phys* 2002; 54:855–60.

62. Weil MD, Lamborn K, Edwards MS, Wara WM. Influence of a child's sex on medulloblastoma outcome. *JAMA* 1998; 279:1474–6.

63. Tait DM, Thornton Jones H, Bloom HJ, Lemerle J, Morris Jones P. Adjuvant chemotherapy for medulloblastoma: the first multi-centre control trial of the International Society of Paediatric Oncology (SIOP I). *Eur J Cancer* 1990; 26:464–9.

64. Le QT, Weil MD, Wara WM, Lamborn KR, Prados MD, Edwards MS, Gutin PH. Adult medulloblastoma: an analysis of survival and prognostic factors. *Cancer J Sci Am* 1997; 3:238–45.

65. Taylor RE, Bailey CC, Robinson K, Weston CL, Ellison D, Ironside J, Lucraft H, Gilbertson R, Tait DM, Walker DA, Pizer BL, Imeson J, Lashford LS. Results of a randomized study of preradiation chemotherapy versus radiotherapy alone for nonmetastatic medulloblastoma: The International Society of Paediatric Oncology/United Kingdom Children's Cancer Study Group PNET-3 Study. *J Clin Oncol* 2003; 21:1581–91.

66. Ito S, Hoshino T, Prados MD, Edwards MS. Cell kinetics of medulloblastomas. *Cancer* 1992; 70:671–8.

67. Gilbertson RJ, Jaros E, Perry RH, Kelly PJ, Lunec J, Pearson AD. Mitotic percentage index: a new prognostic factor for childhood medulloblastoma. *Eur J Cancer* 1997; 33:609–15.

68. Herms J, Neidt I, Luscher B, Sommer A, Schurmann P, Schroder T, Bergmann M, Wilken B, Probst-Cousin S, Hernaiz-Driever P, Behnke J, Hanefeld F, Pietsch T, Kretzschmar HA. C-MYC expression in medulloblastoma and its prognostic value. *Int J Cancer* 2000; 89:395–402.

69. Aldosari N, Bigner SH, Burger PC, Becker L, Kepner JL, Friedman HS, McLendon RE. MYCC and MYCN oncogene amplification in medulloblastoma. A fluorescence in situ hybridization study on paraffin sections from the Children's Oncology Group. *Arch Pathol Lab Med* 2002; 126:540–4.

70. Scheurlen WG, Schwabe GC, Joos S, Mollenhauer J, Sorensen N, Kuhl J. Molecular analysis of childhood primitive neuroectodermal tumors defines markers associated with poor outcome. *J Clin Oncol* 1998; 16:2478–85.

71. Ellison D. Classifying the medulloblastoma: insights from morphology and molecular genetics. *Neuropathol Appl Neurobiol* 2002; 28:257–82.

72. Leonard JR, Cai DX, Rivet DJ, Kaufman BA, Park TS, Levy BK, Perry A. Large cell/anaplastic medulloblastomas and medullomyoblastomas: clinicopathological and genetic features. *J Neurosurg* 2001; 95:82–8.

73. Soria JC, Jang SJ, Khuri FR, Hassan K, Liu D, Hong WK, Mao L. Overexpression of cyclin B1 in early-stage non-small cell lung cancer and its clinical implication. *Cancer Res* 2000; 60:4000–4.

74. Grotzer MA, Hogarty MD, Janss AJ, Liu X, Zhao H, Eggert A, Sutton LN, Rorke LB, Brodeur GM, Phillips PC. MYC messenger RNA expression predicts survival outcome in childhood primitive neuroectodermal tumor/medulloblastoma. *Clin Cancer Res* 2001; 7:2425–33.

75. Gajjar A, Hernan R, Kocak M, Fuller C, Lee Y, McKinnon PJ, Wallace D, Lau C, Chintagumpala M, Ashley DM, Kellie SJ, Kun L, Gilbertson RJ. Clinical, histopathologic, molecular markers of prognosis: toward a new disease risk stratification system for medulloblastoma. *J Clin Oncol* 2004; 22:984–93.

76. Grotzer MA, Janss AJ, Phillips PC, Trojanowski JQ. Neurotrophin receptor TrkC predicts good clinical outcome in medulloblastoma and other primitive neuroectodermal brain tumors. *Klin Padiatr* 2000; 212:196–9.

77. Grotzer MA, Janss AJ, Fung K, Biegel JA, Sutton LN, Rorke LB, Zhao H, Cnaan A, Phillips PC, Lee VM, Trojanowski JQ. TrkC expression predicts good clinical outcome in primitive neuroectodermal brain tumors. *J Clin Oncol* 2000; 18:1027.

78. Cogen PH and McDonald JD. Tumor suppressor genes and medulloblastoma. *J Neurooncol* 1996; 29:103–12.

79. Steichen-Gersdorf E, Baumgartner M, Kreczy A, Maier H, Fink FM. Deletion mapping on chromosome 17p in medulloblastoma. *Br J Cancer* 1997; 76:1284–7.

80. Gilbertson R, Wickramasinghe C, Hernan R, Balaji V, Hunt D, Jones-Wallace D, Crolla J, Perry R, Lunec J, Pearson A, Ellison D. Clinical and molecular stratification of disease risk in medulloblastoma. *Br J Cancer* 2001; 85:705–12.

19

Non-Hodgkin's lymphoma

Charles Dumontet and Catherine Thieblemont

Introduction

Non-Hodgkin's lymphomas (NHL) constitute a diverse set of syndromes characterized by their morphology as well as their immunological, cytogenetic and molecular characteristics. The chances of cure are good in certain subtypes such as diffuse large cell lymphoma (DLCL) with an overall 5-year survival of approximately 60 per cent. Most of the prognostic work in lymphoma, as reflected in this chapter, relates to identifying the predictors of response to therapy. Despite this, lymphoma is still a common cause of cancer death, but little research has been done on prognostic factors in patients likely to be referred to palliative care (those with recurrent disease). In this situation the survival has historically been 3–4 months, although new salvage therapies are enabling up to 50 per cent of relapsing patients to survive 5 years. (Evans, Lancet 12/7/03, 362(9378):139–146). Whereas the previous Working Formulation (WF) tended to be used to distinguish lymphomas with diverse prognoses on the basis of the percentage of large cells and the presence or absence of follicularity, the recent WHO classification has not been conceived as being a prognostic tool.

A variety of clinical and biological prognostic factors have been reported in lymphoproliferative syndromes in general and in NHL in particular. Validation of selected parameters on large series, confirmation of the independent prognostic power and the feasibility of evaluating the marker in routine clinical practice have all influenced the choice of the parameters most generally used today. Conversely novel markers, identified by molecular biology methods such as transcriptome analyses, have recently been identified and could lead to novel paradigms in defining patient subgroups in terms of prognosis.

The International Prognostic Index

The International Prognostic Index (IPI) has been the result of a large international collaboration aiming to identify a simple and robust index, based on clinical and biological data available at diagnosis, strongly correlated with patient outcome, that is the likelihood of cure.[1] This index is built on five parameters which include age, stage, number of extranodal sites, serum lactic dehydrogenase (LDH) values and performance status. The age-adjusted index is designed for younger patients with NHL. LDH, performance status and disease stage have been used to stratify patients in prospective clinical trials. Initially designed for patients with untreated diffuse large B-cell lymphoma, the IPI has been applied to a variety of other situations, including other types of lymphoma as well as pretreated patients. The IPI also carries strong predictive power for patients with peripheral T cell lymphoma,[2] but Aviles et al. found no evidence that the IPI was relevant in a series of 108 patients with angiocentric T cell/ NK cell lymphoma.[3] According to the IPI, disease recurrence is unlikely for scores of 0–1, moderately low for 2, moderately high for 3, and high if 4–5.

Analysis of IPI factors

Tumour dissemination is classified into 'localized disease', corresponding to stage I or stage II, and 'disseminated disease', corresponding to stage III or stage IV disease. A number of extranodal sites of two or more is one of the adverse factors of the IPI. Stage IV disease is defined by extranodal disease. Lymphoma involvement can concern any type of tissue: bone marrow involvement is the most frequent. Central nervous system localizations are of poor prognosis. Weak diffusion of chemotherapeutic agents within the CNS is at least partially responsible for the poor prognosis of CNS localizations.

The age limit used in the IPI is 60 years. A recurrent issue is whether advanced age is of poor prognosis because elderly patients receive inadequate therapy or whether it is in itself an adverse factor. Reports analysing dose intensity of chemotherapy in elderly agents suggest that elderly patients receiving appropriate therapy have a prognosis similar to that of younger patients receiving similar therapy.[4]

Serum lactic dehydrogenase values are generally believed to reflect tumour mass, possibly because of spontaneous tumour lysis. LDH values increase rapidly when tumour lysis is caused by therapy. Threshhold values used in the IPI are those defining increased values in a given laboratory. The fold increase in LDH values is not taken into account, although it is has been shown that patient outcome is strongly correlated with the level of serum LDH. LDH values have been incorporated in most scoring systems for patients with NHL.[5]

Patient performance status (PS), evaluated using the Eastern Cooperative Oncology Group (ECOG) scale, is defined as a poor prognosis factor when equal or greater than 2. This easily evaluated parameter is a powerful indicator both of the consequences which the tumour has on the host and of the host's ability to tolerate therapy.

It is of interest to consider those parameters which have not been incorporated in the IPI. Classical parameters such as 'tumour burden' for example, which have been shown to be correlated with patient outcome for decades in diseases such as Burkitt's lymphoma, are not identified as such in the IPI.[6] The localization of extranodal diseases is not taken into account either, although certain localizations are known to carry a worse prognosis. The existence of a predisposing state, in particular a disorder of the immune system, is not taken into account to define prognosis. More importantly in terms of therapeutic tolerance, the possible existence of significant comorbidities such as heart, renal or hepatic failure are not taken into account to define prognosis, although the administration of curative therapy is directly dependent on the integrity of these systems.

Limitations of the IPI

Among the limitations of the IPI are the fact that all of its components are dichotomic. For example LDH levels will be considered as an adverse factor even if they are slightly elevated, although it is well documented that strongly increased LDH values are more pejorative than lower values. Another significant limitation is that there is no loading for the parameters. Performance status is likely to be the most powerful and significant parameter but carries no extra weight in comparison to other factors. Furthermore, other relatively simple to obtain and powerful parameters such as $\beta2$-microglobulin have not been included in the IPI.

For patients with low-grade lymphoma entities, such as marginal zone lymphoma or small lymphocytic lymphoma, no specific prognostic parameters have been described and physicians have used the IPI to define a therapeutic strategy. However, in our experience with splenic marginal zone lymphoma (MZL), none of these criteria (age, PS, stage, number of extranodal sites, and

LDH level) was associated with outcome.[7] Other prognostic factors such as level of leukocytes (> 30 or > 20.10^9/L, lymphocytes < 4 or > 20 10^9/L, β2 microglobulin level, presence of serum monoclonal component) were described as adverse prognostic factors.[8, 9]

Applications of the IPI in situations other than untreated patients with DLCL

In spite of these caveats, the IPI has proven to be useful in a wide array of situations. Initially designed to stratify patients with diffuse large cell lymphoma at diagnosis, the IPI has demonstrated its prognostic value in this same patient population at relapse, and in Hodgkin's disease.[10]

Conversely the IPI is poorly adapted to follicular lymphoma, the most common indolent subtype. Median survival rates in this disease are in the 10 year range, although outcomes vary widely. The critical step in optimizing therapy for this heterogeneous disease is the definition of patient groups associated with favourable or unfavourable prognosis. The IPI has been demonstrated to be of poor discriminatory power, with only few patients falling into the high-risk IPI group.[11] The Follicular International Prognostic Index (FLIPI) was thus defined as the result of an important international effort, analysing more than 4000 patients.[12] Five parameters have been identified:

1. involvement of more than four nodal areas
2. elevated LDH
3. age greater than 60 years
4. stage III or IV, and
5. haemoglobin levels less than 120g/L.

Other prognostic factors

The IPI provides a robust and simple score to guide clinicians for the treatment of patients with NHL. However a variety of other parameters have been identified, including biological factors.

Serum β2 microglobulin is increased in a number of lymphoproliferative diseases, including NHL, chronic lymphocytic leukaemia, and myeloma. In patients with multiple myeloma serum β2 microglobulin is one of the most powerful prognostic factors, both at diagnosis and before high-dose therapy.[13] In patients with NHL β2 microglobulin is also a powerful predictive factor, in particular in patients with follicular lymphoma. In splenic MZL, serum β2 microglobulin has been reported to be one of the prognostic parameters of overall survival. Serum β2 levels have been reported to be predictive of prognosis and relapse in patients with diffuse large B-cell lymphoma.[14, 15]

Serum LDH values are routinely considered irrespectively of their isoform content. In a series of patients with NHL, we showed that isoforms 2 and 3 are preferentially altered in patients with NHL. Isoforms 4 and 5, on the other hand, were increased in patients in whom myeloid regeneration was observed. Alterations in isoforms 2 and 3 were found to be correlated with freedom from progression and overall survival. The isoform 3 content was also found to retain its predictive value in patients with high total serum LDH values.

Among cytokines, interleukin 6 has also been the focus of research as it appears to be regularly increased in the serum of patients with NHL.[16] A polymorphism in the promoter region of the IL-6 gene (-176) was shown to be correlated both with incidence and outcome in patients with NHL.[17] Studying 122 patients with Hodgkin's disease, Vassilakopoulos et al. have shown that serum IL-10 was increased in 45 per cent of patients at diagnosis and was an independent prognostic factor of survival.[18] The tumour necrosis factor (TNF)-ligand system has also been shown to be correlated with patient outcome in NHL.[19] Juszczinsky *et al.* have reported that polymorphisms of HLA class II DRB1*02 allele and TNF were correlated with patient outcome. In particular TNF polymorphism (-308A) was the only genotype associated with high values of TNF and the TNF receptors p55 and p75.[20] The presence of TNF -308A was associated with a low complete response rate as well as with a shorter freedom from progression and overall survival.

Other biological parameters have also been reported in patients with NHL. Adida *et al.* analysed survivin expression in a series of 222 patients with diffuse large B-cell lymphoma.[21] Patients whose tumours expressed survivin displayed significantly worse 5-year overall survival rate. Survivin remained an independent prognostic factor even when the IPI was taken into account. BAL (B Agressive Lymphoma), a protein involved in B-cell migration, has been identified by differential display in patients with poor outcome.[35] Peripheral blood lymphopenia has been shown to be correlated with stage in patients with Hodgkin's disease but not with prognosis.[22] CA 125 is not only a reliable marker for staging and assessing tumour activity in NHL, but is also predictive of decreased event-free and overall survival.[23] BLyS and its receptors have been reported to be correlated with patient outcome in patients with NHL.[24] BLyS levels were found to increase as tumours progressed towards a more aggressive phenotype. Patients with high BLyS levels were found to have poorer response to therapy and shorter overall survival. BLyS receptors (BCMA, TACI, BAFF-R) were found to be expressed in all NHL samples.

Microarray analyses in NHL

The majority of prognostic factors analysed in patients with NHL are either descriptive of disease extension or of biological and clinical consequences that the tumour induces in the host. Current treatment decisions do not take into account the biological profile of the patient's individual tumour. Conversely refinement in the definition of separate entities on the basis of cytogenetic, immunological and molecular characteristics involves breaking down 'lymphomas' into a growing number of distinct syndromes for which appropriate therapies can be designed.

It is anyone's guess to what extent and in how much time data gathered from pangenomic microarray analyses will impact on the way patients are routinely treated for lymphoma. The considerable progress of 'targeted therapies', currently represented by anti-CD20 monoclonal antibodies in patients with B-cell lymphoma, is clearly the first step in a series of novel treatments which will take into account the biological properties of the tumour. This however is still far from being a 'personalized therapy' in the sense that each patient's disease is considered as having a different biological profile leading to a different type of therapy. In this respect we can expect that novel potent prognostic factors will be identified by microarray approaches and that some alterations identified by this method will lead to original therapies. As an example, important advances have been achieved within the diffuse large B-cell lymphoma subtype with the recent description of the cell of origin subtypes – related to the germinal centre B-cell signature or to the activated B-cell signature – associated with significantly different prognoses.[25] Application of this gene profiling categorization in routine practice.is already available with immunohistochemical tools using three antibodies (CD10, bc16 and MUM1).[26] Other lymphoma subtypes, such as follicular lymphoma, mantle cell lymphoma and splenic marginal zone lymphoma, have been analysed with gene expression profiling to determine prognostic factors with interesting findings but not direct application yet in routine practice.[27–29] Defining therapy truly customized to each patient would first require a considerable diversity of active compounds, which we do not have today. It is likely that customized therapy will first rely on personalized dosing and scheduling, on the basis of individual genotypic profiling, rather than on tumour phenotype.

Significance of prognostic factors

Prognostic factors are generally interpreted as reflecting tumour aggressivity, tumour mass or consequences of tumour on the host. Conversely in a disease which is potentially curable such as DLCL, it is possible that some prognostic factors correspond to factors of resistance to therapy.

Since the description of combination chemotherapy, diffuse large B-cell lymphoma is considered to be a curable disease.[30] This is not the case for all lymphoma subtypes, and the possibility that some patients are cured of such diseases as follicular NHL or mantle cell lymphoma remains controversial and, in any event, rare. The outcome of patients with diffuse large cell lymphoma is well described by an increasing number of clinical and biological parameters, the most recent of which have been provided by the analysis of the transcriptome of tumour cells. This raises the interesting issue of whether prognostic factors can also be considered as factors predictive of chemoresistance.

Parameters related to tumour mass or localization can fairly simply be related to chemoresistance. Indeed bulky tumours associated with high serum LDH values are likely to be poorly vascularized and partly anoxic, resulting in poor diffusion and efficacy of antimitotic compounds against tumour cells. Extranodal sites such as the CNS may also be associated with reduced drug diffusion. Conversely localizations such as bone marrow appear to be accessible to drug diffusion and other mechanisms are likely to be involved in the relative resistance of lymphoma cells localized in the marrow. An interesting hypothesis is that of a potential protective role of the marrow microenvironment.

Factors predictive of sensitivity to therapy

A given factor is predictive of chemoresistance when it distinguishes tumour response after exposure to a given compound or family of compounds. Predictive factors can be distinguished from prognostic factors in that they are specific for a limited number of compounds and that they are predictive of response. Prognostic factors are related to adverse prognosis, independently of the type of treatment administered, and are associated with poor survival or progression-free survival.

There are few validated factors predictive of chemoresistance in patients with NHL. Expression of the Pgp efflux pump, a member of the ABC transporter family, is responsible for the classical multidrug resistance phenotype which concerns commonly used compounds such as anthracyclines, vinca alkaloids and etoposide. Expression of the *mdr1* gene, which codes for Pgp protein, is frequent in NHL.[31] LRP, another transport pump, has been reported to be expressed in approximately a quarter of NHL samples.[32] Conversely there are no validated parameters predictive of resistance to methotrexate, cyclophosphamide or platinum compounds in patients with NHL. Data obtained in patients with acute lymphoblastic leukaemia or solid tumours treated with platinum compounds suggest that other parameters could also be of use to predict resistance to non-MDR substrates in patients with NHL.

With the advent of therapeutic monoclonal antibodies, a novel issue concerns the identification of parameters predictive of response or resistance to these biomolecules. Monoclonal antibodies are likely to be cytotoxic through a variety of mechanisms including membrane target signalling, antibody-dependent complement-mediated cytotoxicity and accessory cell-mediated cytotoxicity. It has recently been reported that polymorphisms in the Fc receptor were predictive of response to rituximab in patients with follicular NHL.[33] Ongoing studies are likely to identify other parameters predictive of response to monoclonal antibody therapy in the future.

Factors predictive of toxicity

Chemotherapy-induced toxicity constitutes one of the major limitations of therapy in patients with DLCL. Toxicity can schematically be distinguished as 'early', occurring during or in the immediate aftermath of chemotherapy, or 'late'. Early toxicities are evaluated using international toxicity scales covering both reversible and irreversible toxicities. Late toxicities are well identified though less well classified and include myelodysplastic syndromes and secondary malignancies, cardiac toxicity and neurological toxicity. A legitimate question is whether most visceral toxicities described as 'late' are actually sequelae of early visceral toxicities which were not observed early in the course of treatment.

Predictors of early death

Early death, defined by death from whatever cause during the first 3 months of treatment, remains a critical problem, in particular in fragile patients with aggressive disease. We reported that age, ECOG performance status, serum LDH values, serum albumin, as well as leukocyte and haemoglobin values were independent factors of early death.[34] An early death index was designed, enabling the evaluation of the individual risk of early death in young (range 2–31 per cent risk of early death) and elderly (range 5–53 per cent) patients. This index allows the identification of patients with very low and very high risks of early death, thereby allowing specific precautions in subgroups of patients.

Conclusion

Clinicians caring for patients with NHL are faced with the considerable heterogeneity of patient outcome. Once the subtype of NHL has been established, some patients will be considered as potentially curable while for others prolonged remission will be the main goal. In all cases therapeutic decisions will take into account the patient's age, performance status and existing comorbidities. Current prognostic factors will assist the clinician in choosing the intensity of therapy. However, there are currently no factors which allow us to tailor therapy in terms of sensitivity to specific compounds. Additional research, analysing both patient gene polymorphisms and the biological properties of the tumour, is required to allow individual therapy of patients with NHL.

Acknowledgements

The authors acknowledge the support of the Comité de la Drôme of the Ligue Contre le Cancer and the Fondation de France for their support.

References

1. Project TIN-H s LPF. A predictive model for aggressive non-Hodgkin's lymphoma. *N Engl J Med* 1993; 329:987–94.
2. Ansell SM, Habermann TM, Kurtin PJ, Witzig TE, Chen MG, Li CY, Inwards DJ, Colgan JP. Predictive capacity of the International Prognostic Factor Index in patients with peripheral T-cell lymphoma. *J Clin Oncol* 1997; 15:2296–301.
3. Aviles A, Diaz NR, Neri N Cleto S, Talavera A. Angiocentric nasal T/natural killer cell lymphoma: a single centre study of prognostic factors in 108 patients. *Clin Lab Haematol* 2000; 22:215–20.
4. Kovner F, Merimsky O, Inbar M, Soyfer V, Cahan Y, Rachmani R, Chaitchik S. Prognostic importance of advanced age in aggressive non-Hodgkin's malignant lymphoma. *Oncology* 1996; 53:435–40.

5. Lopez-Guillermo A, Montserrat E, Reverter JC, Cervantes F, Escoda L, Tassies D, Blade J, Marin P, Sierra J, Ordi J. *et al.* Large-cell lymphoma: a study of prognostic factors and assessment of five recently proposed predictive systems. *Leuk Lymphoma* 1993; 10:101–9.

6. Magrath I, Lee YJ, Anderson T, Henle W, Ziegler J, Simon R, Schein P. Prognostic factors in Burkitt's lymphoma: importance of total tumor burden. *Cancer* 1980; 45:1507–15.

7. Thieblemont C, Felman P, Berger F, Dumontet C, Arnaud P, Hequet O, Arcache J, Callet-Bauchu E, Salles G, Coiffier B. Treatment of splenic marginal zone B-cell lymphoma: an analysis of 81 patients. *Clin Lymphoma* 2002; 3:41–7.

8. Troussard X, Valensi F, Duchayne E, Garand R, Felman P, Tulliez M, Henry-Amar M, Bryon P, Flandrin G. Splenic lymphoma with villous lymphocytes: clinical presentation, biology and prognostic factors in a series of 100 patients. Groupe Francais d'Hematologie Cellulaire (GFHC). *Br J Haematol* 1996; 93: 731–6.

9. Chacon J, Mollejo M, Munoz E, Algara P, Mateo M, Lopez L, Andrade J, Carbonero I, Martinez B, Piris M, Cruz M. Splenic marginal zone lymphoma: clinical characteristics and prognostic factors in a series of 60 patients. *Blood* 2002; 100;1648–54.

10. Vassilakopoulos TP, Nadali G, Angelopoulou MK, Siakantaris MP, Dimopoulou MN, Kontopidou FN, Karkantaris C, Kokoris SI, Kyrtsonis, MC, Tsaftaridis P, Pizzolo G, Pangalis GA. The prognostic significance of beta(2)-microglobulin in patients with Hodgkin's lymphoma. *Haematologica* 2002; 87;701–8; discussion 708.

11. Decaudin D, Lepage E, Brousse N, Brice P, Harousseau J, Belhadj K, Tilly H, Michaux L, Cheze S, Coiffier B, Solal-Celigny P. Low-grade stage III-IV follicular lymphoma: multivariate analysis of prognostic factors in 484 patients – a study of the groupe d'Etude des lymphomes de l'Adulte. *J Clin Oncol* 1999; 17;2499–505.

12. Solal-Celigny P, Roy P, Colombat P, White J, Armitage JO, Arranz-Saez R, Au WY, Bellei M, Brice P, Caballero D, Coiffier B, Conde-Garcia E, Doyen C, Federico M, Fisher RI, Garcia-Conde JF, Guglielmi C, Hagenbeek A, Haioun C, LeBlanc M, Lister AT, Lopez-Guillermo A, McLaughlin P, Milpied N, Morel P, Mounier N, Proctor SJ, Rohatiner A, Smith P, Soubeyran P, Tilly H, Vitolo U, Zinzani PL, Zucca E, Montserrat E. Follicular lymphoma international prognostic index. *Blood* 104;1258–65.

13. Facon T, Avet-Loiseau H, Guillerm G, Moreau P, Genevieve F, Zandecki M, Lai JL, Leleu X, Jouet JP, Bauters F, Harousseau JL, Bataille R, Mary JY. Chromosome 13 abnormalities identified by FISH analysis and serum β2-microglobulin produce a powerful myeloma staging system for patients receiving high-dose therapy. *Blood* 2001; 97;1566–71.

14. Aviles A, Zepeda G, Diaz-Maqueo JC, Rodriguez L, Guzman R, Garcia EL, Talavera A. Beta 2 microglobulin level as an indicator of prognosis in diffuse large cell lymphoma, *Leuk Lymphoma* 1992; 7;135–8.

15. Aviles A, Narvaez BR, Diaz-Maqueo JC, Guzman R, Talavera A, Garcia EL. Value of serum beta 2 microglobulin as an indicator of early relapse in diffuse large cell lymphoma, *Leuk Lymphoma* 1993; 9;377–80.

16. Kato H, Kinoshita T, Suzuki S, Nagasaka T, Hatano S, Murate T, Saito H, Hotta T. Production and effects of interleukin-6 and other cytokines in patients with non-Hodgkin's lymphoma. *Leuk Lymphoma* 1998; 29;71–9.

17. Cordano, P, Lake, A, Shield, L, Taylor, G. M, Alexander, F. E, Taylor, P. R, White, J, and Jarrett, R. F. Effect of IL-6 promoter polymorphism on incidence and outcome in Hodgkin's lymphoma, Br J Haematol. 128;493–5, 2005.

18. Sarris, A. H, Kliche, K. O, Pethambaram, P, Preti, A, Tucker, S, Jackow, C, Messina, O, Pugh, W, Hagemeister, F. B, McLaughlin, P, Rodriguez, M. A, Romaguera, J, Fritsche, H, Witzig, T, Duvic, M, Andreeff, M, and Cabanillas, F. Interleukin-10 levels are often elevated in serum of adults with Hodgkin's disease and are associated with inferior failure-free survival, Ann Oncol. 10;433–40, 1999.

19. Warzocha, K, Salles, G, Bienvenu, J, Barbier, Y, Bastion, Y, Doche, C, Rieux, C, and Coiffier, B. Prognostic significance of TNF alpha and its p55 soluble receptor in malignant lymphomas, Leukemia. 11 Suppl 3;441–3, 1997.

20. Juszczynski, P, Kalinka, E, Bienvenu, J, Woszczek, G, Borowiec, M, Robak, T, Kowalski, M, Lech-Maranda, E, Baseggio, L, Coiffier, B, Salles, G, and Warzocha, K. Human leukocyte antigens class II and tumor necrosis factor genetic polymorphisms are independent predictors of non-Hodgkin lymphoma outcome, Blood. 100;3037–40, 2002.

21. Adida, C, Haioun, C, Gaulard, P, Lepage, E, Morel, P, Briere, J, Dombret, H, Reyes, F, Diebold, J, Gisselbrecht, C, Salles, G, Altieri, D. C, and Molina, T. J. Prognostic significance of survivin expression in diffuse large B-cell lymphomas, Blood. 96;1921–5, 2000.

22. Ayoub, J. P, Palmer, J. L, Huh, Y, Cabanillas, F, and Younes, A. Therapeutic and prognostic implications of peripheral blood lymphopenia in patients with Hodgkin's disease, Leuk Lymphoma. 34;519–27, 1999.

23. Bairey, O, Zimra, Y, Kaganovsky, E, Shaklai, M, Okon, E, and Rabizadeh, E. Microvessel density in chemosensitive and chemoresistant diffuse large B-cell lymphomas, Med Oncol. 17;314–8, 2000.

24. Novak, A. J, Grote, D. M, Stenson, M, Ziesmer, S. C, Witzig, T. E, Habermann, T. M, Harder, B, Ristow, K. M, Bram, R. J, Jelinek, D. F, Gross, J. A, and Ansell, S. M. Expression of BLyS and its receptors in B-cell non-Hodgkin lymphoma: correlation with disease activity and patient outcome, Blood. 104;2247–53. Epub 2004 Jul 13, 2004.

25. Alizadeh, A, Eisen, M, Davis, R, Ma, C, Lossos, I, Rosenwald, A, Boldrick, J, Sabet, H, Tran, T, Yu, X, Powell, J, Yang, L, Marti, G, Moore, T, Hudson, J. J, Lu, L, Lewis, D, Tibshirani, R, Sherlock, G, Chan, W, Greiner, T, Weisenburger, D, Armitage, J, Warnke, R, and Staudt, L, et al. Distinct types of diffuse large B-cell lymphoma identified by gene expression profiling, Nature. 403;491–2, 2000.

26. Hans, C, Weisenburger, D, Greiner, T, Gascoyne, R, Delabie, J, Ott, G, Muller-Hermelink, H, Campo, E, Braziel, R, Jaffe, E, Pan, Z, Farinha, P, Smith, L, Falini, B, Banham, A, Rosenwald, A, Staudt, L, Connors, J, Armitage, J, and Chan, W. Confirmation of the molecular classification of diffuse large B-cell lymphoma by immunohistochemistry using a tissue microarray, Blood. 103;275–82, 2004.

27. Rosenwald, A, Wright, G, Wiestner, A, Chan, W, Connors, J, Campo, E, Gascoyne, R, Grogan, T, Muller-Hermelink, H, Smeland, E, Chiorazzi, M, Giltnane, J, Hurt, E, Zhao, H, Averett, L, Henrickson, S, Yang, L, Powell, J, Wilson, W, Jaffe, E, Simon, R, Klausner, R, Montserrat, E, Bosch, F, Greiner, T, Weisenburger, D, Sanger, W, Dave, B, Lynch, J, Vose, J, Armitage, J, Fisher, R, Miller, T, LeBlanc, M, Ott, G, Kvaloy, S, Holte, H, Delabie, J, and Staudt, L. The proliferation gene expression signature is a quantitative integrator of oncogenic events that predicts survival in mantle cell lymphoma, Cancer Cell. 3;185–97, 2003.

28. Dave S, Wright G, Tan B, Rosenwald A, Gascoyne R, Chan W, Fisher R, Braziel R, Rimsza L, Grogan T, Miller T, LeBlanc M, Greiner T, Weisenburger D, Lynch J, Vose J, Armitage J, Smeland E, Kvaloy S, Holte H, Delabie J, Connors J, Lansdorp P, Ouyang Q, Lister T, Davies A, Norton A, Muller-Hermelink H, Ott G, Campo E, Montserrat E, Wilson W, Jaffe E, Simon R, Yang L, Powell J, Zhao H, Goldschmidt N, Chiorazzi M, Staudt L. Prediction of survival in follicular lymphoma based on molecular features of tumor-infiltrating immune cells. N Engl J Med 2004; 351;2159–69.

29. Thieblemont C, Ballester B, Nasser V, Gazzo S, Doucet G, Felman P, Callet-Bauchu E, Berger F, Loi L, Salles G, Birnbaum D, Coiffier B, Houlgatte R. Gene expression profiling analysis in splenic marginal zone lymphoma allows to predict survival and histological transformation. In ASH Annual Meeting, Abstract 1125, San Diego, 2004,.

30. DeVita VT Jr, Canellos GP, Chabner B, Schein P, Hubbard SP, Young RC. Advanced diffuse histiocytic lymphoma, a potentially curable disease. Lancet 1975; 1;248–50.

31. Liu Q, Ohshima K, Kikuchi M. High expression of MDR-1 gene and P-glycoprotein in initial and re-biopsy specimens of relapsed B-cell lymphoma. Histopathology 2001; 38;209–16.

32. Filipits M, Jaeger U, Simonitsch I, Chizzali-Bonfadin C, Heinzl H, Pirker R. Clinical relevance of the lung resistance protein in diffuse large B-cell lymphomas. Clin Cancer Res 2000; 6;3417–23.

33. Cartron G, Dacheux L, Salles G, Solal-Celigny P, Bardos P, Colombat P, Watier H. Therapeutic activity of humanized anti-CD20 monoclonal antibody and polymorphism in IgG Fc receptor FcgammaRIIIa gene. *Blood* 2002; 99;754–8.

34. Dumontet C, Mounier N, Munck JN, Bosly A, Morschauser F, Simon D, Marit G, Casasnovas O, Reman O, Molina T, Reyes F, Coiffier B. Factors predictive of early death in patients receiving high-dose CHOP (ACVB regimen) for aggressive non-Hodgkin's lymphoma: a GELA study. *Br J Haematol* 2002; 118;210–7.

35. Aguia RC, Yakushijin Y, Kharbanda S, Salgia R, Fletcher JA, Shipp MA. BAL is a novel risk-related gene in diffuse large B-cell lymphomas that enhance cellular migration. *Blood* 2000; 96; 4328–34.

20

Leukaemia and myeloma

Paul Glare

Acute leukaemia

Introduction

Acute leukaemia occurs in two main forms: either acute lymphoblastic leukaemia (ALL) or acute myeloid leukaemia (AML), within which there are several subtypes. In the past, eight subtypes of AML were recognized (FAB criteria), referred to as M0 to M7, the lower the code number the more undifferentiated. M1 (undifferentiated myeloblastic without maturation) and M2 (differentiated myeloblastic) are the commonest. The FAB classification system is being replaced by WHO criteria based on cytogenic and molecular aspects of the disease.[1]

ALL is more common than AML and particularly common in children under the age of 5, although it may also be seen in young adults. Both forms of acute leukaemia represent neoplastic proliferation of immature cells within the bone marrow, either the lymphoblastic series (ALL) or a myeloid bone marrow stem cell (AML). The proliferating clone of malignant cells replaces normal bone marrow, resulting in bone marrow failure. This produces symptoms of anaemia, infection due to low white blood cell (WBC) count, and bleeding from thrombocytopenia. Leukaemic infiltration of other tissues may also occur, in particular the liver and spleen may be involved, peripheral lymphadenopathy is common and ALL has a high incidence of central nervous system (CNS) involvement. Chronic myeloid leukemia (CML), which represents a neoplastic proliferation of differentiated granulocytes, often transforms into an acute blastic phase. In around 70 per cent this will be AML, 25 per cent ALL and 5 per cent mixed. Patients with myeloproliferative disorders/myelodysplastic syndromes can also develop AML.

Prognostication in acute leukaemia is very difficult, because one needs to consider both the type of acute leukaemia and the specific therapy given. Modern management with combination chemotherapy and supportive care (antibiotics and blood products) means complete remissions will be achieved in the majority of patients and approximately half can be expected to be alive and free of leukaemia 5 years later. In a minority of cases, treatment barely changes the natural history of the disease. Without treatment, patients with acute leukaemia die within days to a few months.

Natural history

The proliferating clone of malignant cells resulting in acute leukaemia replaces normal bone marrow, resulting in progressive bone marrow failure and leukaemic infiltration of other tissues. B symptoms and diffuse bone pain are also common in AML.

Prognostic factors

The traditional prognostic factors for acute leukaemia were age and white cell count at presentation. It is now known that the white cell count is mainly determined by the genetic changes in the leukaemic cells. At the present time, three main prognostic factors are identified: age, cytogenetics and response to treatment.

Age

Older patients (> 55 years) have a worse prognosis. This is due partly to the disease being more resistant to chemotherapy in older people and also to their being less fit to withstand treatment.

Cytogenetics

Chromosomal changes can be a good or bad prognostic factor. Three types of changes have been shown to be good prognostic factors: patients with translocations 14;17 and 8;21, and inversion 16 have a good prognosis.[2, 3] Translocations of MLL and deletions of chromosome 5 and 7 are associated with poor outcomes.[4] Patients with normal cytogenetics have an intermediate risk.

New and promising cytogenetic prognostic markers include gene expression profile, over-expression of immunogenic antigens such as WT1, PRAME and BAALC, and cellular localization of mutant nucleophosmin (NPM).[5]

Treatment

Indicators of a good prognosis are the remission duration and response to therapy. People whose bone marrow goes back to normal after the first course of chemotherapy do better than those who still have some leukaemia left. Factors which can affect whether the remission is likely to be permanent, or whether there is a risk of relapse, include:

* the genetic changes in the leukaemic cell
* the time taken/number of treatments needed to achieve a complete remission
* the white blood cell count at the time of diagnosis
* age
* leukaemic cell surface markers.

Other prognostic factors

Indicators of a poor prognosis include:

* A high white cell count at presentation (> 100×10^9/l), which is a manifestation of certain adverse cytogenetic abnormalities (mutations of FLT3, *Kit* and *Ras* genes)
* Elevated LDH at presentation
* Patients developing extramedullary disease
* Disseminated intravascular coagulation (DIC) associated with promyelocytic leukaemia (French American British subtype (FAB) M3)
* Secondary leukaemia following the myelodysplastic syndrome or previous anti-cancer therapy
* The presence of drug resistance proteins
* Comorbidities.

Treatment affecting prognosis

Chemotherapy

Treatment of AML consists of induction chemotherapy in the form of daunorubicin, cytarabine and thioguanine/etoposide (DAT). This results in a complete remission in up to 85 per cent of cases.[6] This is followed by consolidation treatment with further courses of DAT or high-dose cytarabine.

Cure (in remission at 5 years) can be expected in 15–30 per cent cases. These overall figures mask a wide variety in outcomes, influenced by the prognostic factors, so that the chance of complete remission (CR) can range from 35–90 per cent and of cure from 5–80 per cent. A model for predicting chance of achieving a first remission based on these factors has recently been described.[7] The outcome of AML is modified by the precise therapy that is given for the specific genetic change. For example, patients with t(14;17), have the best prognosis when they are treated with all transretinoic acid, while t(8;21) and inv[16] are best treated with high dose ara C.[3, 4]

Bone marrow transplantation

The role of transplantation has changed in recent years. It used to be considered in selected patients after primary treatment, particularly those who achieve a second remission with standard chemotherapy. It is now known that allogeneic stem cell transplant can improve the outcome in intermediate and high-risk patients but is of little added value in the good risk patient.

Treatment of relapse

Although the outcome of patients with AML has improved because of cytarabine and anthracycline-based chemotherapy in combination with advanced supportive care and introduction of hemopoietic stem-cell transplantation, relapse continues to represent the leading cause of death in the majority of patients.[8]

Treatment of AML in first relapse is associated with relatively low response rates (CR 1–30 per cent, and cure < 5 per cent) unless a stem cell transplant is an option. Whenever second CR is attained, the median duration of the second relapse-free interval (RFI) is generally considerably shorter than the first RFI. Because only a minority of patiens who experience relapse will derive durable benefit from current re-induction therapy, it would be practically useful to estimate prognosis at the time of relapse, to facilitate therapeutic decision-making at this stage of the disease and guide individualized and investigational treatment strategies.

No standard care has yet been established for patients who relapse following a second CR. They have an overall median survival of 1–2 months with < 10 per cent alive at 1 year. Options include second line salvage therapy with repetitions of ara-C based combinations, Phase 1–II therapies, or palliative care. Response rates to second salvage therapy are of the order of 10–15 per cent with a duration of response of approximately 6 months, but up to 25 per cent die during re-induction.[9]

Short- and long-term prognosis

Without treatment, patients with acute leukaemia die within days to a few months. With treatment, the prognosis for acute leukaemia is better in childhood than for adults. ALL has a better prognosis than AML, with around 70 per cent of children cured compared to only 40 per cent with AML. In adults, long-term survival rates have been approximately half those in children, although with combination chemotherapy and/or transplantation cure rates of around 50 per cent are now to be expected for adults with AML achieving a remission.

Prognosis in advanced ALL

The prognosis in adults with ALL can be predicted from clinical and laboratory findings, especially the patient's age. Remission duration is an important determinant of long-term survival. Prognostic factors indicating a short duration of remission include:

1. Late achievement of complete remission (more than 4–5 weeks of therapy)
2. High WBC count at presentation
   - critical value for worse prognosis currently is 25,000–35,000 per μL
   - counts > 100,000 per μL are associated with poor prognosis

3. Age > 50 years

4. Cell markers

   ◆ possibly ALL with myeloid antigens (mixed lineage or hybrid)

   ◆ possibly pre-T-ALL

5. Chromosomal abnormalities (Ph-ALL: t [9;22], t [4;11]).

Additional factors reportedly affecting prognosis include organ involvement at presentation (extensive lymphadenopathy, hepatomegaly, splenomeglay, central nervous system involvement, mediastinal involvement), male gender, elevated lactate dehydrogenase (LDH), elevated gamma glutamyl transferase (GGT) levels, low platelet count, degree of bone marrow involvement, number of immature forms in the peripheral blood, weight loss and race.

The impact of some negative prognostic factors in the past has changed for the better with advances in treatment regimens.

Prognosis in advanced AML

Patients with a first relapse of AML have a 30 per cent chance overall of surviving 12 months and a 10 per cent chance of surviving 5 years, with a 25 per cent a chance of achieving a second remission if they are given re-induction therapy. A European co-operative group has developed a clinically useful prognostic scoring system for AML in first relapse, based on the multivariate analysis of 667 AML patients in first relapse among 1,540 newly diagnosed non-M3 AML patients (age 15 to 60 years) entered onto four successive chemotherapy studies.[8] The four clinically relevant parameters included in this index are:

◆ length of relapse-free interval after first complete remission

◆ cytogenetics at diagnosis

◆ age at relapse

◆ whether previous stem-cell transplantation was performed.

The effect of these factors on prognosis is shown in Table 20.1.

Table 20.1 Simplified prognostic score (0–14 points) for acute myeloid leukaemia at first relapse

Prognostic factor	Categories	Points
Duration of relapse-free interval from first complete remission	>18 months	0
	7–18 months	3
	<6 months	5
Cytogenetics at diagnosis	t(16;16) or inv(16)	0
	t(8;21)	3
	Other	5
Age at first relapse	<35 years	0
	36–45 years	1
	>45 years	2
Prior stem-cell transplantation before first relapse	Yes	0
	No	2

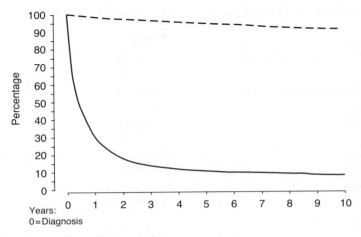

Figure 20.1 *Prognsotigram* curve for 6843 patients with AML.

A group from the M.D. Anderson Cancer Center in Houston have evaluated the outcome of patients with acute myelogenous leukaemia who underwent second salvage therapy.[9] The risk factors for poor short-term survival are:

1. Duration of first complete remission < 12 months

2. Duration of second complete remission < 6 months

3. Serum total bilirubin concentration > 1 mg/dL

4. Serum albumin concentration < 3.0 g/dL

5. Patient age > 60 years

6. > 50 per cent blasts in the bone marrow

7. Second salvage therapy given before 1991.

The greater the number of risk factors, the worse the prognosis (see Table 20.2).

For patients in first relapse, the European stratification system mentioned above defined three risk groups for long-term survival:

◆ A favourable prognostic group (score 0–6), representing < 10 per cent of cases: overall survival (OS) of 70 per cent at 1 year and 46 per cent at 5 years

◆ An intermediate-risk group (score 7–9), representing approximately one-quarter of cases with OS of 49 per cent at 1 year and 18 per cent at 5 years

◆ A poor-risk group (score 10–14), representing two-thirds of cases, with OS of 16 per cent at 1 year and 4 per cent at 5 years.

According to the MD Anderson study,[9] for patients undergoing second salvage therapy, the probability of surviving 1 year, according to risk group is:

◆ low risk (0–2 risk factors, 8 per cent cases) 22 per cent

◆ intermediate risk (3 risk factors, 20 per cent cases) 6 per cent

◆ high risk (4–7 risk factors, 72 per cent cases) 0 per cent.

Table 20.2 Prognosis in second relapsed AML, (adapted from Giles et al.[9])

Parameter	Finding	Points
Duration of first complete remission	>12 months	0
	<12 months	1
Duration of second complete remission	>6 months	0
	<6 months	1
Serum total bilirubin	<1 mg/dL	0
	>1 mg/dL	1
Serum albumin	>3.0 g/dL	0
	<3.0 g/dL	1
Age of the patient	<60 years of age	0
	>60 years of age	1
Percentage blasts in bone marrow	<50	0
	>50	1
Year of second salvage therapy	1991 or later	0
	Before 1991	1

For patients with MDS, the International Prognostic Scoring System (IPSS) can grade the severity of MDS.[10] IPSS 'scores' a patient's survival and the chances that his or her disease will transform to AML. The score is the sum of three factors:

1. the percentage of blasts in the bone marrow;
2. the results of cytogenetic tests
3. the type and amount of specific blood cells.

The score, when totalled, indicates three risk groups. For the high-risk group (score over 2.0), approximately 50 per cent patients will survive 4.5 months, 75 per cent developing AML within a year.

Myeloma

Introduction

Multiple myeloma (MM) is the malignant end of a spectrum of disease that results from the clonal proliferation of malignant B cells (plasma cells) at various stages of differentiation in the bone marrow.[11, 12] Up to 20 per cent of the bone marrow may be taken up by myeloma cells. MM is almost always accompanied by the presence in serum and/or urine of monoclonal immunoglobulins (IgG, IgM, IgA, IgD, IgE, or kappa/lambda light chains) or immunoglobulin fragments synthesized by the malignant plasma cell clone. Most patients also have lytic bone lesions.

In the US approximately 14,000 new cases are diagnosed annually, making up about 1 per cent of all cancers. The incidence may be increasing. Even though it is commonly considered a disease of the elderly, and is rare under the age of 40, the mean age at diagnosis is approximately 60. The highest incidence is in African American males.

Multiple myeloma is still essentially an incurable disease with generally a poor prognosis. The median survival is typically quoted as three years, but MM is in fact a heterogeneous disease,

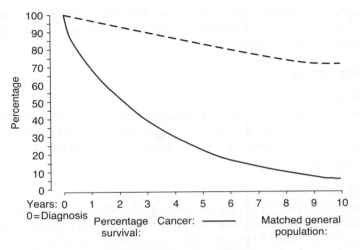

Figure 20.2 Prognostigram curve for 12000 patients with myeloma.

with survival ranging from less than 1 year to more than 10 years. Thus, an evaluation of the life expectancy of each patient with MM is important for at least two main reasons: (1) to predict the outcome, (2) to define the therapeutic strategy, and (3) to enrol homogeneous series of patients in clinical trials.

Natural history

The benign forms of plasma cell transformation – benign paraproteinemia or monoclonal gammopathy of uncertain significance – may be a forerunner of subsequent MM, as may plasmacytoma, the localized form of myeloma in which a single site of plasma cell proliferation occurs, forming a tumour mass. Up to 70 per cent patients with plasmacytoma go on to develop MM. There is also a subgroup of patients with indolent disease ('smouldering myeloma') who may have low-grade symptom-free disease for several years before entering a more aggressive phase.

The main clinical problems encountered by patients with MM are:

1. Hypercalcemia, occurring in up to 2/3 patients at some point

2. Lytic bone lesions, and pain

3. Bone marrow failure, resulting in:

   ◆ anaemia, with symptoms of fatigue and breathlessness,

   ◆ leukopenia, with a high risk of infections

   ◆ thrombocytopenia, with purpura and bleeding disorders.

Renal complications and neurological sequelae (spinal cord compression, sensory and motor neuropathies, high levels of paraprotein can cause hyperviscosity) occur less commonly. A rare complication of MM is amyloid formation, which can cause cardiac, nuerological and gastrointestinal dysfunction.

Evaluation for prognosis

For more than 30 years, tumour burden and proliferation rate have been the two key indicators for prognosis in MM, inferred from markers such as level of paraproteinin, number of lytic lesions, degree of anaemia, and serum calcium level were the main prognostic factors to be evaluated.[11] More recently β_2–microglobulin (B2M) and albumin have emerged as the most important factors to be measured.[13]

Prognostic factors

Clinical parameters

The favourable influence of a good performance status and young age (< 65 years) is well established. Patients younger than 40 years of age, though rare, with normal renal function and low B2M levels have a particularly good prognosis. By contrast neither gender nor race has prognostic significance.[14]

Laboratory markers

Paraprotein levels in serum and/or urine, haemoglobin, albumin, calcaemia, percent of bone marrow plasma cells, and number and size of lytic bone lesions all reflect tumour burden. These clinical parameters formed the basis for classifying patients into defined risk groups for more than 40 years.[15] Myeloma patients with a high LDH level follow a rapidly progressive course, a shortened time to relapse, and a decreased survival time.[16]

More recently, the role of β_2-microglobulin (B2M) as an important prognostic factor has been identified. B2M is the light chain of the class I histocompatibility antigens located on the membrane of all nucleated cells. It is also present in unbound form in the serum, is known to be increased in all lymphoproliferative diseases, and is probably produced by neoplastic cells. B2M is an expression of tumour burden and correlates with the traditional staging systems for assigning prognosis,[11] while multivariate analysis has shown B2M to carry the highest prognostic significance among all the parameters related to tumour burden. B2M serum values > = 6 mg/L are associated with shorter survival.[17] B2M and albumin form the basis of a new International Staging System for myeloma.[13]

Other prognostic markers

These include:

- Plasma cell morphology: immature or plasmablastic morphology and plasma cell aneuploidy implying a worse prognosis
- Plasma cell surface markers (immunophenotyping), although the data are conflicting
- Genetic changes: chromosome 13 deletion or 11q abnormalities have been associated with poor outcomes in a uniformly treated patient series
- Oncogenes: The K-ras proto-oncogene, the p53 suppressor gene, and over-expression of c-myc indicate molecular lesions in patients and confer a poor prognosis.
- Multidrug resistance
- Immune surveillance cells: low numbers of mature NK cells and CD4 T cells have been reported in advanced disease, while expanded T-cell clones that can recognize autologous idiotypic Ig structures are associated with an improved prognosis.
- Proliferative activity: the plasma cell proliferation rate reflects plasma cell DNA synthesis and is a marker of the intrinsic malignancy, rather than the tumour burden. It is usually evaluated by the labelling index (LI), and is also valuable in assigning prognosis. A high LI correlates with shorter survival. B2M and LI are independent variables:[18]
    (i) patients with both low B2M and low LI and treated with standard therapy: median survival of 71 months (classified as low risk),

(ii) patients at intermediate risk (only one variable high): median survival of 40 months,

(iii) patients with both variables high (high-risk MM): median survival of only 16 months.

- Interleukin-6 (IL-6) is a major growth factor for myeloma plasma cells that also stimulates hepatocytes to synthesize acute phase reactants like C-reactive protein (CRP), making CRP a simple, valid alternative to measuring LI. When combined with B2M, CRP can also be used to identify three risk groups:[19]

  (i)   low CRP and low B2M: median survival 54 months

  (ii) high CRP or B2M: median survival of 27 months,

  (iii) high CRP and B2M: survival of only 6 months.

Recently, molecular markers have been used to identify patients with multiple myeloma with high-risk disease who may require more aggressive management.[20] These include

- deletion of chromosome 13
- hypodiploidy
- t(4; 14) on flourescent in situ hybridization (FISH)
- t(14; 16) on FISH
- 17p(-) on FISH
- Plasma cell labelling index $> = 3$ per cent

Some 25–30 per cent of patients have one or more of these high-risk markers. The mean survival of a high-risk patient is 2–3 years, less than half the mean survival seen in low-risk patients.

Treatments affecting prognosis

Chemotherapy

For decades, treatment with the oral alkylating agent melphalan in combination with prednisone (MP) was the standard of care.[11, 12] On average, this regimen extends survival in myeloma patients from 7–9 months. However, nine identical trials of standard chemotherapy carried out in patients with comparable clinical stages, survival ranged from 19 to 42 months,[21] suggesting that clinically comparable patients with MM exhibit a wide variety of biologic characteristics. Thus, prognostic evaluation is important not only to predict patient outcome but also to guide the choice of therapy. MP is well tolerated even in elderly patients, but there are a number of problems with treating myeloma, including drug resistance and myelotoxicity.

Several attempts have been made to improve MP. Strategies usually involve adding or substituting different drugs, such as the vinca alkaloids (VCR, VBL) CPX, bleo and BCNU, or doxorubicin. Combination chemotherapy with several of these agents results in a higher response of tumour shrinkage and in selected populations, prolonged survival.

New agents

Major advances in understanding malignant plasma cell biology along with a recognition of the importance of the bone marrow microenvironment in supporting the growth of malignant cells has translated into a plethora of clinical trials examining targeted therapy with novel agents.[22] The key new agents are thalidomide, its derivative lenalidomide and the first-in-class proteasome inhibitor, bortezomib. For elderly patients or those unsuitable to undergo high-dose therapy, melphalan and prednisolone (MP) have until very recently been considered the gold standard therapy. The addition of thalidomide to this regimen (MPT) has improved complete response (CR) rates and PFS but at the cost of greater toxicity. A recent randomized controlled trial of 255 patients aged 60–85 years showed a response rate of 76 per cent with MPT compared with 47 per cent with MP.[23] Two-year event-free survival was also significantly improved (54 vs 27 per cent) with a non-significant trend to better overall survival. Venous thrombosis is the main toxicity, but can be reduced considerably (incidence 20 per cent down to 3 per cent) with low-molecular weight heparin (LMWH) prophylaxis.

Current approaches to management

Now the challenge for physicians managing patients with MM is not solely to understand the mechanisms, efficacy and toxicity of these various agents, but to negotiate the overlapping side-effects and determine the optimal sequence and combinations of these drugs for the individual patient.[22] To date, most of the clinical research has focused on patients with relapsed and refractory disease; however, ongoing trials are examining the role of these agents in previously untreated patients.

There is no simple 'one size fits all' treatment paradigm for myeloma, and indeed the treatment of patients with MM is evolving as a variety of drugs with differing mechanisms of action are becoming progressively available.[22] In general, the first decision is whether the patient is a suitable autologous peripheral blood progenitor cell (PBPC) transplant candidate. The low mortality of this procedure (< 1 per cent) means that patients up to the age of 70 years, depending on comorbidities, are considered for this treatment. For such patients, the first step is to induce a disease response with a dexamethasone-based regimen. The established regimen of infusional Vincristine Doxorubicin (Adriamycin) Dexamethasone (VAD) is losing favour (to avoid the need for i.v. access devices and the neuropathy that can occur with vincristine) and being replaced with oral regimens or even dexamethasone alone. The combination of thalidomide–dexamethasone for front-line therapy has no proven advantage over chemotherapy-based regimens.[22] Following stem cell collection and PBPC transplantation, patients will ultimately relapse usually within 2–4 years. Currently, the only choice apart from conventional chemotherapy regimens is thalidomide (alone or in combination); however, lenalidomide is likely to replace it as the primary second-line therapy when it becomes routinely available outside of clinical trials in the next few years. Bortezomib offers patients a third-line option.

For the non-transplant patients, oral MP was until the very recent past the gold standard of therapy. Thalidomide can be considered in patients who fail to obtain an optimal response. However, neurotoxicity can be a problem and may be severe, adversely influencing quality of life and also complicating future treatment options with agents that also exhibit this troublesome toxicity.

Short- and long-term prognosis

MM remains an incurable disease with median survival in the vicinity of 3–5 years, but with very heterogeneous survivals ranging from a few months to more than a decade. Prognostic staging systems for myeloma have been available for more than 40 years. The simplest ones use haemoglobin, performance status and blood urea nitrogen.[24]

The method of Durie and Salmon, devised more than 30 years ago, estimates tumour burden based on myeloma protein synthesis rates and a calculation of the total body tumour cell mass, based on haemoglobin, calcium, skeletal survey and monoclonal protein levels.[15] Criteria put patients into three groups, with median survivals of 64, 32, 6 months respectively (see Table 20.3).

The staging system for myeloma developed by Alexanian et al. is related to that of Durie and Salmon.[25] Baur et al. modified the Durie and Salmon staging system for multiple myeloma

Table 20.3 Durie and Salmon's classification system for myeloma (1975)

Stage	Criteria
I	All of the following ◆ haemoglobin >10 g/dL ◆ serum calcium < = 12 mg/dL ◆ X-ray: 0–1 bony lesions ◆ monoclonal protein: IgG <5 g/dL; IgA <3 g/dL; urine light chain excretion <4 g/24 hrs
II	Fits neither stage I or III
III	Any of the following ◆ haemoglobin <8.5 g/dL ◆ serum calcium >12 mg/dL ◆ extensive lytic bone lesions; widespread with fractures ◆ monoclonal protein: IgG >7 g/dL; IgA >5 g/dL; urine light chain excretion >12 g/24 hrs

by adding the magnetic resonance imaging (MRI) findings (number of lesions in spine and/or diffuse infiltration).[26] This provides a useful prognostic tool for patients with multiple myeloma and can help identify patients who may require more aggressive therapy. In one evaluation of this staging system, stage I patients had no deaths in 6 years, stage II had a median survival of 5 years and stage III a median of 15 months.

In the early 1990s, an Italian group developed a myeloma staging system based on clinical and histological findings.[27] The stages differed in total survival time, median survival and response to chemotherapy. Parameters, identified on multivariate analysis, were:

1. Bone marrow plasma cells: percentage, absolute number, absolute number of plasmablasts

2. Haemoglobin

3. Lytic bone lesions on X-rays

4. serum β-2-microglobulin

5. Bence–Jones proteinuria.

Scores are calculated to put patients into six groups with median survival ranging from 1–7 years.

Recently, the International Myeloma Working Group have also developed a staging system for multiple myeloma based on two easily measurable laboratory markers, serum levels of β2-microglobulin and albumin (see Table 20.4).[13]

Table 20.4 Prognosis from the International Staging System for myeloma

β2-microglobulin	Albumin	Stage	Median survival
<3.5 mg/dL	> = 3.5 g/dL	I	62 months
<3.5 mg/dL	<3.5 g/dL	II	44 months
3.5–5.5 mg/dL	NA	II	44 months
>5.5 mg/dL	NA	III	29 months

References

1. Harris NL, Jaffe ES, Diebold J. *et al.* The World Health Organization classification of hematological malignancies report of the Clinical Advisory Committee Meeting, Airlie House, Virginia, November 1997. *Mod Pathol* 2000; 13(2):193–207.

2. Tallman MS, Andersen JW, Schiffer CA. *et al.* All-trans retinoic acid in acute promyelocytic leukemia: long-term outcome and prognostic factor analysis from the North American Intergroup protocol. *Blood* 2002; 100(13):4298–302.

3. Byrd JC, Mrozek K, Dodge RK. *et al.* Pretreatment cytogenetic abnormalities are predictive of induction success, cumulative incidence of relapse, and overall survival in adult patients with de novo acute myeloid leukemia: results from Cancer and Leukemia Group B (CALGB 8461). *Blood* 2002; 100(13):4325–36.

4. Frohling S, Scholl C, Gilliland DG, Levine RL. Genetics of myeloid malignancies: pathogenetic and clinical implications. *J Clin Oncol* 2005; 23(26):6285–95.

5. Disperati P, Suarez-Saiz F, Khoury H, Minden MD. Leukemias. In MK Gospodarowicz, B O'Sullivan, LH Sobin, (eds) *Prognostic factors in cancer*, 3rd edn. Hoboken, NJ: Wiley-Liss; 2006; 291–300.

6. Jabbour EJ, Estey E, Kantarjian HM. Adult acute myeloid leukemia. *Mayo Clin Proc* 2006; 81(2):247–60.

7. Kantarjian H, O'Brien S, Cortes J. *et al.* Results of intensive chemotherapy in 998 patients age 65 years or older with acute myeloid leukemia or high-risk myelodysplastic syndrome: predictive prognostic models for outcome. *Cancer* 2006; 106(5):1090–8.

8. Breems DA, Van Putten WL, Huijgens PC. *et al.* Prognostic index for adult patients with acute myeloid leukemia in first relapse. *J Clin Oncol* 2005; 23(9):1969–78.

9. Giles F, O'Brien S, Cortes J. *et al.* Outcome of patients with acute myelogenous leukemia after second salvage therapy. *Cancer* 2005; 104(3):547–54.

10. Greenberg P, Cox C, LeBeau MM. *et al.* International scoring system for evaluating prognosis in myelodysplastic syndromes. *Blood* 1997; 89(6):2079–88.

11. Boccadoro M, Pileri A. Diagnosis, prognosis, and standard treatment of multiple myeloma. *Hematol Oncol Clin North Am* 1997; 11(1):111–31.

12. Bataille R, Harousseau JL. Multiple myeloma. *N Engl J Med* 1997; 336(23):1657–64.

13. Greipp PR, San Miguel J, Durie BG. *et al.* International staging system for multiple myeloma. *J Clin Oncol* 2005; 23(15):3412–20.

14. San Miguel JF, Gutierrez NC. Multiple myeloma. In MK Gospodarowicz, B O'Sullivan, LH Sobin, (eds) *Prognostic factors in cancer*, pp. Hoboken, NJ: Wiley-Liss, 2006; 301–06.

15. Durie BG, Salmon SE. A clinical staging system for multiple myeloma. Correlation of measured myeloma cell mass with presenting clinical features, response to treatment, and survival. *Cancer* 1975; 36(3):842–54.

16. Dimopoulos MA, Barlogie B, Smith TL, Alexanian R. High serum lactate dehydrogenase level as a marker for drug resistance and short survival in multiple myeloma. *Ann Intern Med* 1991; 115(12):931–5.

17. Bataille R, Durie BG, Grenier J. Serum beta2 microglobulin and survival duration in multiple myeloma: a simple reliable marker for staging. *Br J Haematol* 1983; 55(3):439–47.

18. Greipp PR, Lust JA, O'Fallon WM, Katzmann JA, Witzig TE, Kyle RA. Plasma cell labeling index and beta 2-microglobulin predict survival independent of thymidine kinase and C-reactive protein in multiple myeloma. *Blood* 1993; 81(12):3382–7.

19. Bataille R, Boccadoro M, Klein B, Durie B, Pileri A. C-reactive protein and beta-2 microglobulin produce a simple and powerful myeloma staging system. *Blood* 1992; 80(3):733–7.

20. Debes-Marun CS, Dewald GW, Bryant S. *et al.* Chromosome abnormalities clustering and its implications for pathogenesis and prognosis in myeloma. *Leukemia* 2003; 17(2):427–36.

21. Bergsagel DE. Is aggressive chemotherapy more effective in the treatment of plasma cell myeloma? *Eur J Cancer Clin Oncol* 1989; 25(2):159–61.

22. Kenealy M, Prince HM. Current status of new drugs for the treatment of patients with multiple myeloma. *Intern Med J* 2006; 36(12):781–9.

23. Palumbo A, Bringhen S, Caravita T. *et al.* Oral melphalan and prednisone chemotherapy plus thalidomide compared with melphalan and prednisone alone in elderly patients with multiple myeloma: randomised controlled trial. *Lancet* 2006; 367(9513):825–31.

24. Carbone PP, Kellerhouse LE, Gehan EA. Plasmacytic myeloma. A study of the relationship of survival to various clinical manifestations and anomalous protein type in 112 patients. *Am J Med* 1967; 42(6):937–48.

25. Alexanian R, Balcerzak S, Bonnet JD. *et al.* Prognostic factors in multiple myeloma. *Cancer* 1975; 36(4):1192–201.

26. Baur A, Stabler A, Nagel D. *et al.* Magnetic resonance imaging as a supplement for the clinical staging system of Durie and Salmon? *Cancer* 2002; 95(6):1334–45.

27. Pasqualetti P, Casale R, Collacciani A, Colantonio D. Prognostic factors in multiple myeloma: a new staging system based on clinical and morphological features. *Eur J Cancer* 1991; 27(9):1123–6.

21

Sarcoma

Katherine T. Morris and Murray F. Brennan

Introduction

Soft tissue sarcoma is a rare disease with approximately 10–12,000 cases per year in the US. The majority of patients with extremity sarcomas are cured by a single operation with or without the addition of adjuvant radiation therapy. However, depending on certain risk factors, some will go on to advanced disease and subsequent demise.

For the purposes of this chapter, we define a patient to have advanced sarcoma if they have systemic or nodal metastasis, large (> 10 cm), deep, and high-grade primary extremity tumours, or visceral or retroperitoneal sarcomas as these are known to have a less favourable prognosis.[1] Using this definition, 42 per cent of patients admitted to the Memorial Sloan Kettering Cancer Center (MSKCC) from 1 July 1982 to 30 June 2004 had advanced or high-risk sarcoma.

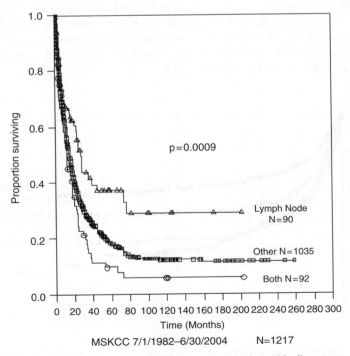

Figure 21.1 Comparison of actuarial survival based on presentation with distant metastasis, isolated lymph node metastasis, or combination of sites.

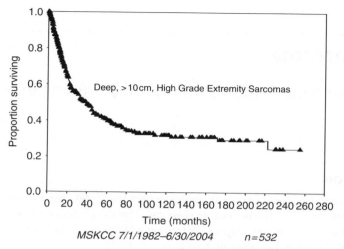

Figure 21.2 Actuarial survival of patients with high-grade, deep sarcomas over 10 cm in size.

Natural history

Patients presenting with systemic and/or nodal metastasis carry a poor prognosis (Figure 21.1), yet it is favourable compared to metastatic disease from other primary malignancies such as pancreatic cancer. The importance of risk factors are large size, depth, and high grade for extremity lesions, as shown in Figure 21.2. The high mortality for patients who have high-grade deep tumours > 10 cm is apparent. In 2000, we published our experience with survival for patients with retroperitoneal or visceral liposarcomas; documenting that site was an independent factor.[1] An updated survival curve for all patients with visceral, retroperitoneal, or intra-abdominal sarcomas treated at MSKCC is shown in Figure 21.3.

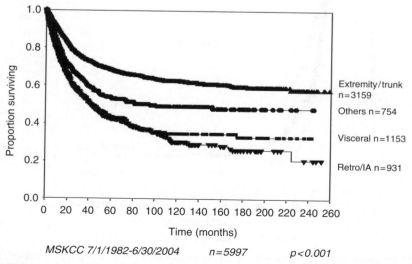

Figure 21.3 Comparison of actuarial survival based on location of sarcoma.

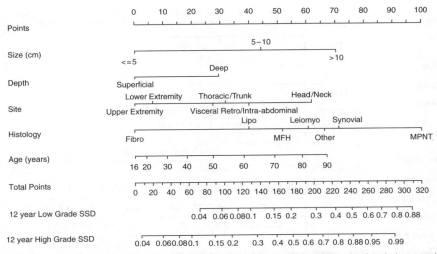

Instructons for physician. Locate the patient's tumor size on the size axis. Draw a line straight upwards to the **Points** axis to determine how many points towards sarcoma-specific death the patient receive for his tumor size. Repeat this process for the other axes, each time drawing straight upward to the **Points** axis. Sum the points achieved for each predictor and locate this sum on the **Total Points** axis. Draw a line straight down to either the Low grade or High grade axis to find the patient's probability of dying from sarcoma within 12 years assuming he or she does not die of another cause first. Instruction to patient: If we had 100 patients exactly like you, we would expect between <predicted percentage from nomogram – 8%>and <predicted percentage +8%> to die of sarcoma within 12 years if they did not die of another cause first, and death from sarcoma after 12 years is still possible.

Fibro, fibrosarcoma; Lipo, liposarcoma; Leiomyo, leiomyosarcoma; MFH, malignant fibrous histiocytoma; MPNT, malignant Peripheral-nerve tumor; Gr, grade; SSD, sarcoma-specific death.

Figure 21.4 Nomogram for estimating post-resection 12-year sarcoma-specific death. From Kattan W, Leung Dh, Brennan MF. Postoperative nomogram for 12-year sarcoma-specific death. *Journal of Clinical Oncology* 2002; 20(3):719–96. Reproduced with permission from the American Society of Clinical Oncology.

To assist clinicians in estimating a disease-specific survival for individual sarcoma patients with primary or recurrent tumours we have developed internally validated nomograms for soft tissue sarcoma. Figure 21.4 illustrates the nomogram for 12-year sarcoma-specific death for all patients with primary tumour presentation.[2] Instructions for use are contained in the legend. Figure 21.5 is the nomogram for probability of death for patients who have local recurrence.[3] A simple web-based program for using these nomograms is available free of charge at http://www.mskcc.org, search under "nomogram".

Factors affecting prognosis

Metastatic disease

A few well-defined factors affect prognosis for patients with sarcoma metastatic to either lymph nodes or distant sites, with a highly selected group of patients able to undergo R0 resection having up to 38 per cent 5-year actuarial survival.[4] The most common site for metastasis in sarcoma is the lungs, with 19 per cent of all extremity sarcoma patients having isolated pulmonary metastasis as their first site of distant recurrence.[5] Multivariate analysis of patient and tumour-related factors affecting prognosis for patients with pulmonary sarcoma metastasis shows age over 50, and the presence of a malignant peripheral nerve tumour or liposarcoma primary to be independent predictors of worse outcome. Disease-free interval of over 12 months and a low-grade primary tumour were independent predictors of improved outcome (see Table 21.1).[6]

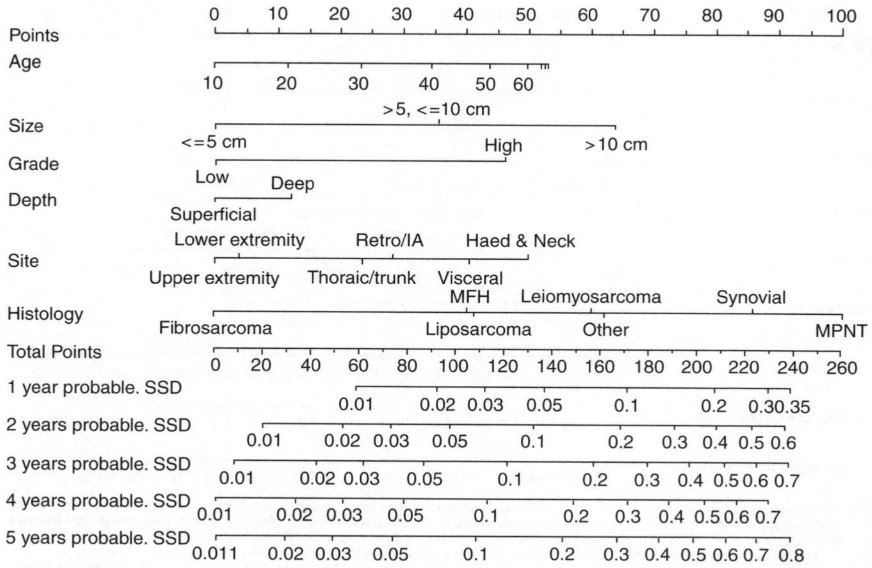

Figure 21.5 Nomogram for estimating post-resection survival following a local recurrence. From Kattan MW, Heller G, Brennan MF. A competing-risks nomogram for sarcoma-specific death following local recurrence. *Statistics in Medicine* 2003; 22:3515–25. Copyright John Wiley and Sons Limited. Reproduced with permission.

Table 21.1 Factors influencing survival after development of pulmonary metastases

Variable	Cox model p-value	Relative risk (95% CI)	Prognostic significance
Age > 50 years	0.008	1.30 (1.05–1.54)	Unfavourable
Malignant peripheral nerve tumour primary	0.03	1.50 (1.04–2.29)	Unfavourable
Liposarcoma primary	0.0003	1.71 (1.25–2.16)	Unfavourable
Disease free interval > 12 months	0.0006	0.71 (0.59–0.86)	Favourable
Low grade primary tumour	0.02	0.66 (0.46–0.95)	Favourable

From Billingsley KG, Burt MF, Jara E. *et al.* Pulmonary metastases from soft tissue sarcoma: analysis of patterns of disease and postmetastasis survival. *Annals of Surgery* 1999; 229(5):602–10. Reproduced with permission from Lippincott, Williams and Wilkins.

Table 21.2 Factors influencing prognosis in extremity sarcomas

Variable	5-year DSS rate (%)	Cox model p-value	RR (95% CI)
Size (cm)	85	0.0001	2.1 (1.5–3.0)
< 5	82		
5–10	61		
> 10			
Site			
Upper extremity – proximal	86	0.016	1.6 (1.3–2.0)
Upper extremity – distal	82		
Lower extremity – proximal	69		
Lower extremity – distal	78		
Depth			
Superficial	92	0.0002	2.8 (1.6–4.8)
Deep	69		
Grade			
Low	95	0.0001	4.0 (2.5–6.6)
High	66		
Histology			
Leiomyosarcoma	71	0.012	1.9 (1.1–3.0)
Malignant peripheral nerve tumour	51	0.0077	1.9 (1.2–3.2)

From Pisters PWT, Leung DH, Woodruff J, Shi W, Brennan MF. Analysis of prognostic factors in 1,041 patients with local-ized soft tissue sarcomas of the extremities. *Journal of Clinical Oncology* 1996; 15(2):646–52. Reproduced with permission from the American Society of Clinical Oncology.

High risk extremity disease

The overall prognostic factors important for outcome in patients with extremity sarcomas are defined. The multivariate analysis of a review of prognostic factors for distant recurrence for 1,041 patients with extremity sarcomas treated consecutively at MSKCC is summarized in Table 21.2.[7] This analysis also found that presentation with local recurrence was a weak adverse prognostic factor with a recurrence rate of 1.5 (95 per cent CI 1.0–2.2). Local recurrence of an extremity soft tissue sarcoma is known to be a poor prognostic factor[8] and patients suffering local recurrence after treatment for a high-grade or deep primary sarcoma were found to have a higher risk of later development of metastasis. These patients are good candidates for enrolment in trials of investigational adjuvant therapy. However "while local recurrence is a predictor of metastasis and death, a causal relationship cannot be presumed".[8] Multivariate analysis of prognostic factors for overall post-metastasis survival in patients with high-risk extremity disease revealed primary tumour size over 10 cm to be the only independent predictor of survival after development of metastasis.[7]

Visceral or retroperitoneal sarcomas

Visceral or retroperitoneal sarcomas present a different set of problems, with the most common cause of demise for patients being failure of locoregional control.[1] Stratification of risk factors for patients with retroperitoneal sarcomas using the AJCC TNM system, validated for extremity sarcomas only, has proven limited. Retroperitoneal or visceral sarcomas are deep by definition, rarely under 5 cm by time of diagnosis, and have lymph node metastasis less than 2 per cent of the time.[9] A recent publication suggests a different manner to risk stratify patients with retroperitoneal sarcomas based on an analysis of 124 patients treated at multiple centres and 107 treated at a single tertiary care centre. Patients were grouped into a clinicopathologic scale as follows: Class I – low-grade tumour, completely resected (R0 or R1 resection), without metastasis, Class II – high-grade tumour, completely resected, without metastasis, Class III – low- or high-grade, incomplete resection, no metastasis, and Class IV – low- or high-grade, complete or incomplete resection, presence of metastasis. Survival based on these four classes is shown in Figure 21.6.[10]

The initial prognostic significance of high-grade in retroperitoneal sarcomas was confirmed in an analysis of 500 patients treated at MSKCC.[11] Over 60 per cent of the patients in this group had high-grade tumours, with 60 per cent also being over 10 cm at diagnosis. While liposarcoma was the most common histologic subtype (41 per cent), there were a considerable number of other histologies represented. High grade and histologic subtype of liposarcoma were the only tumour-related factors showing significant association with local recurrence or distant metastasis-free survival on multivariate analysis of patients with resectable disease.

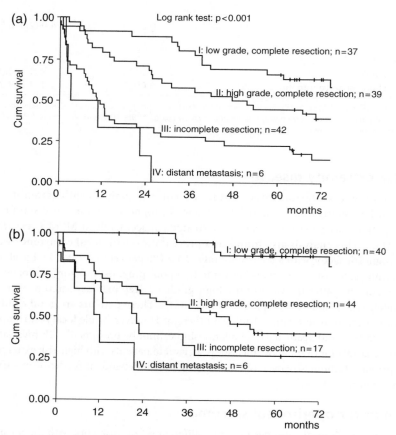

Figure 21.6 Overall actuarial survival of retroperitoneal sarcoma patients by clinicopathologic class in multiple and single institution study. From van Dalen T, Hennipman A, van Coevorden F. et al. Evaluation of a clinically applicable post-surgical classification system for primary retroperitoneal soft tissue sarcoma: analysis of 500 patients treated and followed at a single institution. *Annals of Surgery* 2004; 228(3):355–65. Reproduced with permission from Lippincott, Williams and Wilkins.

Even retroperitoneal sarcoma patients with disease-free survivals of 5 years will have an ongoing risk of recurrence, with 40 per cent recurring within the next 5 years.[9] For patients with disease-free survivals of 5 years, the only predictor of long-term freedom from tumour-related mortality was complete resection, although age less than 50 years at initial surgery and the presence of a high-grade tumour were significantly associated with increased risk of distant metastasis on multivariate analysis.

Therapies affecting prognosis

Metastatic disease

Patients with metastatic sarcoma benefit most if surgical extirpation of metastasis is an option. Review of the treatment of pulmonary metastasis from sarcoma at Memorial Sloan Kettering reveals a median survival of 33 months with complete resection, significantly different from 16 months for patients undergoing incomplete resection and 11 months for patients without resection ($p < 0.001$).[6] The number of metastasis or need for bilateral resections did not influence survival once operation was embarked on providing R0 resection obtained, and repeat complete resection of pulmonary metastasis can also offer actuarial median survivals of up to 65 months in highly selected patients.[12]

A multivariate analysis of prognostic factors for patients undergoing repeat resection of pulmonary metastasis reveals that ability to completely resect all lesions is the most favourable prognostic factor. There are three preoperatively available pieces of information to assist in risk stratification (low grade, 1–2 metastasis, and largest metastasis under 2 cm – see Table 21.3). Patients with zero or one of these adverse factors had a median disease specific survival (DSS) of 65 months in this analysis, while those with all three poor prognostic factors had only a median DSS of 10 months, suggesting this population would be an excellent one to consider for experimental adjuvant therapy.[12]

High-risk extremity disease

As the primary treatment for extremity sarcomas, surgery has the main role. The significance of positive microscopic margins for extremity sarcomas is emphasized in a report analysing 2,084 patients with localized primary soft tissue sarcoma, 73 per cent of which originated in the extremity or superficial trunk. With a median follow up of 50 months and a negative resection margin in 78 per cent of patients, a positive microscopic margin was associated with a near doubling in the prevalence of local recurrence (15 per cent with negative margin and 28 per cent with positive margin, $p < 0.001$) and an increase in the risk of distant recurrence and disease-related

Table 21.3 Factors influencing prognosis after repeat resection of pulmonary metastases from sarcoma

Variable	Cox model p-value	Relative risk (95% CI)	Prognostic significance
Complete re-resection	< 0.0001	0.21 (0.10–0.44)	Favourable
Low grade primary	0.045	0.29 (0.09–0.97)	Favourable
1–2 metastasis	0.012	0.38 (0.20–0.73)	Favourable
Largest metastasis < 2 cm	0.004	0.42 (0.22–0.83)	Favourable

From Weiser MR, Downey RJ, Leung DH, Brennan MF. Repeat resection of pulmonary metastases in patients with soft tissue sarcoma. *Journal of the American College of Surgeons* 2000; 191(2):184–90. Reproduced with permission from the American College of Cardiology Foundation.

death (18 vs 29 per cent p < 0.001). A significant decrease in local recurrence-free survival for patients with positive margins was observed for all histologic subtypes except fibrosarcoma and for all locations except the retroperitoneum, confirming the importance of margins as a prognostic factor in extremity sarcomas. Interestingly, 72 per cent of patients with positive resection margins had no local recurrence. Independent predictors of a positive margin in this study were no prior excision, size over 10 cm, deep tumours, and fibrosarcoma histopathology (likely due to a 40 per cent positive margin rate for desmoids, included in the fibrosarcoma group).[13]

As patients with extremity sarcomas and positive resection margins are at higher risk for local recurrence, many recommend adjuvant therapy for these patients, especially where repeat resection would not be an option. Unfortunately, while confirmed to reduce local recurrence in other prospective, randomized studies of the addition of radiation therapy to patients with positive margin resection,[14–15] a survival benefit has not been shown,[16] leading some authors to advocate strongly for selective use of adjuvant radiotherapy for cases where a local recurrence would lead to a de-functionalizing surgery as opposed to merely a repeat resection.

Visceral or retroperitoneal sarcoma

The ability to achieve a gross complete resection of these tumours is the best prognostic factor. With the exception of retroperitoneal liposarcomas, complete gross resection is the only appropriate surgical goal. Radiation therapy remains limited by damage to adjacent structures, and traditional chemotherapy has yet to prove effective. For the most common histologic subtype of retroperitoneal sarcoma, liposarcoma, however, severe symptoms and death from local spread are significant problems. While incomplete gross resection is not recommended for other sarcomas, for this tumour, it can serve a purpose. A retrospective review comparing patients with incomplete resection to those with no resection found partial resection to be an independent factor for increased survival (median survival 26 vs 4 months). In addition, pre-operative symptoms were successfully palliated in 75 per cent of patients undergoing incomplete resection, demonstrating the appropriateness of selective operation for this population.[17]

Short- and long-term prognosis

As indicated in Figure 21.1, patients with distant metastases from sarcomas have a median survival of approximately 1 year, with approximately one-third alive at 2 years, and a 10–15 per cent chance of survival to 5 years. Some long-term survivors are seen.

References

1. Linehan DC, Lewis JJ, Leung DH, and Brennan MF. Influence of biologic factors and anatomic site in completely resected liposarcoma. *Journal of Clinical Oncology* 2000; 18(8):1637–43.

2. Kattan MW, Leung DH, Brennan MF. Postoperative nomogram for 12-year sarcoma-specific death. *Journal of Clinical Oncology* 2002; 20(3):791–6.

3. Kattan MW, Heller G, Brennan MF. A competing-risks nomogram for sarcoma-specific death following local recurrence. *Statistics in Medicine* 2003; 22:3515–25.

4. van Geel AN, Pastorino U, Jauch JW. *et al.* Surgical treatment of lung metastases: The European Organization for Research and Treatment of Cancer-Soft Tissue and Bone Sarcoma Group Study of 255 Patients. *Cancer* 1996; 77(4):675–82.

5. Gadd MA, Casper ES, Woodruff JM, McCormack PM, Brennan MF. Development and treatment of pulmonary metastases in adult patients with extremity soft tissue sarcoma. *Annals of Surgery* 1993; 218(6):705–12.

6. Billingsley KG, Burt ME, Jara E *et al.* Pulmonary metastases from soft tissue sarcoma: analysis of patterns of disease and postmetastasis survival. *Annals of Surgery* 1999; 229(5):602–10.

7. Pisters PWT, Leung DH, Woodruff J, Shi W, Brennan MF. Analysis of prognostic factors in 1,041 patients with localized soft tissue sarcomas of the extremities. *Journal of Clinical Oncology* 1996; 14(5):1679–89.

8. Lewis JJ, Leung D, Heslin M, Woodruff JM and Brennan MF. Association of local recurrence with subsequent survival in extremity soft tissue sarcoma. *Journal of Clinical Oncology* 1997; 15(2):646–52.

9. Heslin MJ, Lewis JJ, Nadler E, *et al.* Prognostic factors associated with long-term survival for retroperitoneal sarcoma: implications for management. *Journal of Clinical Oncology* 1997; 15(8):2832–9.

10. van Dalen T, Hennipman A, van Coevorden F, *et al.* Evaluation of a clinically applicable post-surgical classification system for primary retroperitoneal soft-tissue sarcoma. *Annals of Surgical Oncology* 2004; 11(5):483–90.

11. Lewis JJ, Leung D, Woodruff JM, Brennan MF. Retroperitoneal soft-tissue sarcoma: analysis of 500 patients treated and followed at a single institution. *Annals of Surgery 1998;* 228(3):355–65.

12. Weiser MR, Downey RJ, Leung DH, Brennan MF. Repeat resection of pulmonary metastases in patients with soft-tissue sarcoma. *Journal of the American College of Surgeons* 2000; 191(2):184–90.

13. Stojadinovic A, Leung D, Hoos A, Jaques DP, Lewis JJ, Brennan MF. Analysis of the prognostic significance of microscopic margins in 2,084 localized primary adult soft tissue sarcomas. *Annals of Surgery* 2002; 235(3):424–34.

14. Pisters PW, Harrison LM, Leung DH, Woodruff JM, Casper ES, Brennan MF. Long-term results of a prospective randomized trial of adjuvant brachytherapy in soft tissue sarcoma. *Journal of Clinical Oncology* 1996; 14(3):859–68.

15. Yang JC, Chang AE, Baker AR, *et al.* Randomized prospective study of the benefit of adjuvant radiation therapy in the treatment of soft tissue sarcomas of the extremity. *Journal of Clinical Oncology* 1998; 16(1):197–203.

16. Alektiar KM, Velasco J, Zelefsky MJ, Woodruff JM, Lewis JJ, Brennan MF (2000). Adjuvant radiotherapy for margin-positive high-grade soft tissue sarcoma of the extremity. *International Journal of Radiation Oncology, Biology, Physics* 2000; 48(4):1051–8.

17. Shibata D, Lewis JJ, Leung DH, Brennan MF. Is there a role for incomplete resection in the management of retroperitoneal liposarcomas? *Journal of the American College of Surgeons* 2001; 193(4):373–9.

22

Unknown primary

Jonathan E. Dowell

Introduction

In the majority of cancer patients, the organ in which the malignancy developed is evident at presentation. However, some patients present with cancer that has metastasized, and the primary tumour site cannot be identified. Cancer from an unknown primary site (CUP) represents 2–3 per cent of all cancer diagnoses. While certain subgroups of patients with this diagnosis benefit from specific therapeutic approaches, unfortunately, these subgroups constitute only a small minority (10–15 per cent) of the patients with CUP.[1] Treatment options for the remainder of patients are limited and the prognosis for this group is poor.

Natural history

While CUP represents a heterogeneous group of clinical presentations, certain features are characteristic. CUP is typified by a unique biology that results in the development of metastatic disease prior to signs or symptoms referable to an obvious primary site and prior to radiographic evidence of a primary. Therefore, patients frequently present with a brief history of non-specific complaints that fail to elucidate the origin of the tumour. In most patients with CUP, the primary is never identified during the patient's lifetime, and even after autopsy, it remains obscure in up to 20 per cent of patients.

Additional distinguishing features of CUP are the presence of widespread metastatic disease as well as unusual sites of metastases. More than 30 per cent of CUP patients present with three or more sites of metastasis, while fewer than 15 per cent of patients with metastatic disease from a known primary present with three or more organs involved. In addition, autopsy series have shown that patients with CUP more frequently have unexpected sites of metastases (e.g. skin, heart, kidney) when compared with their counterparts with known primary sites.[2, 3]

Factors affecting prognosis

The most critical prognostic feature in CUP is histology. Though CUP is commonly thought to include only carcinomas, a small number of patients (5 per cent) will be given a diagnosis of 'poorly differentiated neoplasm' on their initial biopsy. In this group of patients, additional pathological evaluation to exclude a more treatable histology such as lymphoma is essential. Given the wide variety of immunohistochemical antibodies now available, distinguishing between carcinoma and lymphoma is rarely difficult, but in select cases, repeat biopsy may be required to secure a precise diagnosis. Not surprisingly, those patients ultimately found to have lymphoma enjoy a distinctly superior prognosis.

The vast majority of patients with CUP have carcinoma. Within this group, approximately 10–15 per cent present with clinical features that place them in a better prognostic subset.

Women with peritoneal carcinomatosis

In women that present with malignant ascites and peritoneal carcinomatosis, the origin of the tumour is typically the ovaries. However, in some, no ovarian or other primary tumour is evident. This syndrome has gone by several names, including papillary carcinoma of the peritoneum, multifocal extraovarian papillary carcinoma, and primary peritoneal carcinoma. The histology is that of a serous or papillary carcinoma and is often indistinguishable from ovarian cancer.

Women with this clinical presentation should be treated as though they have ovarian cancer. Numerous small series have demonstrated that an approach that includes aggressive surgical debulking followed by systemic platinum-based chemotherapy results in outcomes similar to that seen with ovarian cancer of an equivalent stage. In these series, median survivals range from 11–24 months and 5-year survival rates of 15–20 per cent are reported.[1, 2, 4]

An occasional man or woman will present with a similar clinical picture but with a histology more consistent with a gastrointestinal primary, such as a mucin–producing or signet-ring adenocarcinoma. These tumours are typically less responsive to chemotherapy, and the outcome for these patients is considerably worse.

Women with axillary lymph node metastases

Women who present with unilateral axillary lymph nodes as the only site metastatic carcinoma and no evident primary site should be assumed to have stage II breast cancer. With aggressive local therapy to the ipsilateral breast (surgery and/or radiation) and standard adjuvant chemotherapy for breast cancer, the outcome is identical to that of patients with node-positive breast cancer. As with breast cancer, prognosis is heavily determined by the extent of nodal involvement, but with appropriate treatment, greater than 50 per cent of these patients can be cured.[1, 2, 4, 5]

Women with multifocal metastases that include axillary lymph nodes may have metastatic breast cancer. While curative treatment for these patients is not available, they appear to benefit from hormonal therapy or chemotherapy directed against breast cancer, and their prognosis is probably superior to that of the majority of patients with CUP.

Patients with squamous cell carcinoma in cervical lymph nodes

An occasional patient will present with squamous cell carcinoma in high or mid-cervical lymph nodes and no apparent primary site after careful panendoscopic evaluation. These patients are typically managed with a strategy similar to that used in head and neck cancer. For those patients with no evidence of metastatic disease outside of the neck, treatment generally consists of radical neck dissection followed by radiation, either to the ipsilateral neck only or a more extensive field that includes all of the area from the nasopharynx to the clavicles bilaterally. In modern series that have evaluated this approach, long-term local tumour control rates of 50–70 per cent and 5–year survival rates of 40–60 per cent are reported.[1, 4, 5]

In patients with lower cervical or supraclavicular lymph node metastases from squamous cell carcinoma, the prognosis is worse, presumably because of the increased likelihood that the primary tumour is in the lung. However, if this is the only site of metastatic disease, approximately 10–15 per cent of patients achieve long-term survival with an aggressive approach that includes surgery followed by radiation or radiation alone.[5]

Patients with squamous cell carcinoma in inguinal lymph nodes

In rare instances, a patient will present with poorly differentiated or squamous cell carcinoma in inguinal lymph nodes and no clear primary site after careful examination of the most likely sites of origin including the lower extremity, anorectal and genital regions. In this setting, if the tumour has not spread beyond the inguinal area, retrospective series suggest that surgery alone or followed by radiation can produce long-term survival in approximately 25 per cent of patients.[1]

Men with possible prostate cancer

In men with CUP and predominantly blastic bone metastases, a diagnosis of prostate cancer should be considered. Evaluation should include serum Prostate Specific Antigen (PSA) and staining of the biopsy material for PSA and other prostate specific markers. Even if serum or tumour markers of prostate cancer are absent, a trial of hormonal therapy is warranted as there are reports of durable tumour response with this approach.

In addition, in men with CUP and atypical clinical presentations for prostate cancer, the presence of serum or tumour PSA may predict for response to hormonal treatment. Retrospective series suggest that some of these patients benefit from hormonal manipulation and probably have a survival that is superior to that of the average patient with CUP.[1, 4]

Patients with a single site of metastatic disease

In patients who present with what appears to be a solitary site of metastatic carcinoma from an unknown primary site, consideration should be given to aggressive local therapy. Depending on the organ involved, this typically includes surgery and/or radiation. While the majority of these patients will eventually relapse, there are reports of long-term durable survival with this approach.[4]

Patients with neuroendocrine carcinoma

Neuroendocrine carcinoma from an unknown primary site appears to include three distinct groups of patients.[4] The first are those that present with predominantly liver and/or bone disease and histological features consistent with a low-grade well-differentiated carcinoid or pancreatic islet cell tumour. These tumours are typically indolent and progress slowly over many years. As with carcinoid or islet cell tumours with known primaries, chemotherapy has limited efficacy (response rates < 10 per cent in most series) and does not alter survival. Patients with symptomatic hormone production may benefit from treatment with octreotide.

The second group includes those patients with a histologic diagnosis of small cell carcinoma and no apparent primary in the lung or elsewhere. Even in the absence of a lung primary, the majority of these patients will respond to treatment for small cell lung cancer with platinum analogues and etoposide, with response rates as high as 80 per cent and case reports of long-term survival described.[4, 6]

The final subset of patients are those with poorly differentiated carcinoma with neuroendocrine features identified only by immunohistochemistry or electron microscopy. In the only published series of these patients, tumour response rates in excess of 60 per cent were reported with platinum-based chemotherapy and long-term disease-free survival was seen in 10 per cent.[6] Whether this subgroup of neuroendocrine carcinoma truly represents a subset of CUP with better prognosis ideally requires confirmation in larger prospective studies.

The extragonadal germ cell tumour syndrome

In rare instances, a patient with a poorly differentiated carcinoma presents with clinical features consistent with a metastatic extragonadal germ cell tumour but has atypical histology that makes a definitive diagnosis impossible. This 'syndrome' was first described in 1981 and includes the following features:

- occurs in men under the age of 50

- tumour with a midline distribution (mediastinum, retroperitoneum) and/or with multiple pulmonary nodules

- the duration of symptoms is short (< 3 months) and/or there is a history of rapid tumour growth

- serum levels of alphafetoprotein and/or beta human chorionic gonadotropin are elevated

- a good response to prior chemotherapy or radiotherapy has been demonstrated.

Few patients display all of these features, but in those felt to possibly have the syndrome, treatment with platinum-based chemotherapy regimens that are used for germ cell tumours is warranted. With this approach, objective tumour responses are seen in the majority of patients (100 per cent in the initial series) and long-term survival can be achieved.[1, 4, 7]

Patients with poorly differentiated carcinoma or poorly differentiated adenocarcinoma

Approximately 30 per cent of patients with CUP will be given a histologic diagnosis of poorly differentiated carcinoma (PDC) or poorly differentiated adenocarcinoma (PDA). Patients with this diagnosis constitute a heterogeneous group of clinical presentations and outcomes. Whether they are a subset of CUP with an especially good prognosis is controversial.

Hainsworth and colleagues published a series of 220 patients with PDC or PDA from an unknown primary site and concluded that this group should be considered to have a superior outcome to those patients with CUP that have well-differentiated tumours. In this series, patients received platinum-based chemotherapy, and an objective tumour response rate of 63 per cent and an actuarial 10-year survival of 16 per cent were observed. A multivariate analysis of all 220 patients identified predominant tumour location in the retroperitoneum or peripheral lymph nodes, only one or two metastatic sites, negative smoking history, and younger age as being independent predictors of an excellent outcome.[8]

Of note, this series was initially designed to include only patients with presentations characteristic of the extragonadal germ cell tumour syndrome and was subsequently modified to include all CUP patients with PDC or PDA. As a result, approximately 25 per cent of patients in the series had features consistent with an extragonadal germ cell tumour. An additional confounding feature is that the study began enrolling patients in 1978, prior to the routine use of immunohistochemistry (IHC). A subsequent analysis of the early patients' diagnostic material with IHC discovered that several of the long-term survivors actually had histologies that are particularly sensitive to chemotherapy, such as lymphoma and germ cell tumour.[4]

Lenzi and colleagues at the M.D. Anderson Cancer Center performed a more recent and larger retrospective review of all 1400 CUP patients seen between 1987 and 1994.[9] All patients had extensive pathologic review, including IHC. They found no survival advantage or particular sensitivity to chemotherapy for the group of patients with PDC or PDA.

A comparison of the patients' clinical features from both series reveals some important differences. In the Hainsworth series, the median age of the population was 39, 83 per cent of patients were male, and 39 per cent of patients had the mediastinum or retroperitoneum as the *dominant* site of disease. Conversely, in the Lenzi series, the median age was 60, only 54 per cent of the patients were male, and only 27 per cent had *any* mediastinal or retroperitoneal involvement. The Hainsworth series therefore included a group of younger, predominantly male patients many of whom likely had extragonadal germ cell tumours. Several other small series have also suggested that CUP patients with PDC or PDA may be especially sensitive to platinum chemotherapy. However, with advent of IHC to correctly identify histology in patients previously labelled PDC or PDA, and with the ability to recognize those patients with features of the extragonadal germ cell tumour syndrome, it is unlikely that the remainder of patients with PDC or PDA represent a subset of CUP with a better prognosis.

A number of prognostic factors have been identified in those CUP patients that do not fall into one of the treatable subsets mentioned above. Abbruzzese and colleagues retrospectively evaluated 657 consecutive CUP patients seen at their institution and, in a multivariate analysis, found that male gender, an increasing number of metastatic sites, liver metastases, supraclavicular lymph node metastases, and adenocarcinoma histology were independent predictors of an adverse prognosis.[10] This same group has also published the results of a classification and regression tree analysis of 1000 CUP patients. This method uses recursive partitioning to determine the effect of specific clinical and histological variables on survival. The 'default tree' for this analysis is shown in Figure 22.1. As an example, the longest surviving subgroup (group 1 in Figure 22.1) in their analysis had a median survival of 40 months and included those patients with nonadenocarcinoma histology, < 2 metastatic sites, and no liver, bone, adrenal, or pleural metastases. Conversely, those patients with liver involvement, histology other than neuroendocrine carcinoma, and age > 61.5 years had a median survival of 5 months (group 10).[11] While this model is a potentially effective tool for ascertaining prognosis in CUP patients, its complexity prevents easy applicability in daily practice, and it has not been validated in an independent set of patients.

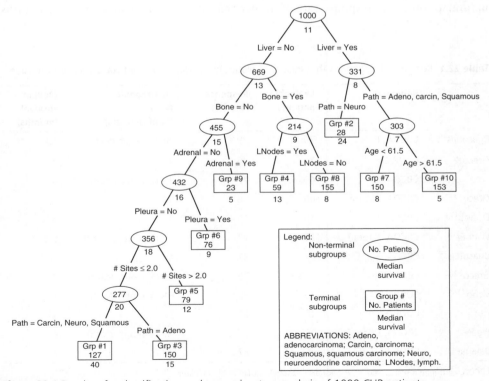

Figure 22.1 Results of a classification and regression tree analysis of 1000 CUP patients.

   Culine and colleagues have also devised a prognostic model for CUP. In a multivariate analysis of 150 unselected patients, they identified only an elevated serum lactate dehydrogenase (LDH) and a performance status greater than 1 as independent predictors of poor outcome. In this model, patients with a normal LDH and a performance status of 0 or 1 had a median survival of 11.7 months and a 1-year survival of 45 per cent. Those patients with a performance status > 1 or an elevated LDH had a median survival of 3.9 months and a 1-year survival of 11 per cent. The model was then validated on an independent set of 116 CUP patients and very similar results were obtained.[12] Although generated from a relatively small number of patients, this classification schema remains the only one in CUP to be validated in an independent patient set and does provide a simple method for identifying two groups of patients with distinctly different prognoses.

Therapies affecting prognosis

For those CUP patients that do not fall into one of the treatment responsive subsets outlined above, the utility of chemotherapy is unproven. No large phase III randomized trials to identify a survival or palliative benefit from treatment have been undertaken. Innumerable small phase II trials have evaluated virtually every conceivable chemotherapy drug and combination in CUP. Objective tumour response rates typically range from 0–40 per cent with resultant median survivals of 3–10 months. These modest results often come with significant toxicity.

   More recent studies have incorporated newer agents, such as the taxanes, into treatment regimens for these patients. One such regimen includes a combination of carboplatin (Paraplatin™), paclitaxel (Taxol™) and oral etoposide (Vepesid™). In CUP patients treated with this combination, an objective response rate of 48 per cent and a median survival of 11 months

Table 22.1 Recent CUP regimens that include a platinum analogue with a taxane and/or etoposide

	Regimen	Evaluable patients	Response rate (%)	Neutropenic fever (% of patients)	Median survival (months)
Briasoulis[15]	CBCDA, P	70	39	NR (2 septic deaths)	13
Greco[16]	CDDP, D	23	26	12	8
	CBCDA, D	40	22	13 (2 septic deaths)	8
Greco[13]	CBCDA, P, E (oral)	66	48	17	11
Dowell[17]	CBCDA, E	16	19	29	6.5
Warner[18]	CBCDA, E (oral)	33	23	12 (2 septic deaths)	5.6
Briasoulis[19]	CBCDA, Epi, E	62	37	NR	10.0
Greco[20]	CBCDA, P, G	113	25	10 (1 septic death)	9
Voog[21]	CDDP, E	25	32	NR (1 septic death)	8
Liu[22]	CDDP, E	20	25	30	4
Piga[23]	CBCDA, Doxo, E	102	27	NR (1 septic death)	9
Balana[24]	CDDP, E, G	30	37	20	7.2

CBCDA, carboplatin (Paraplatin™); P, paclitaxel (Taxol™); CDDP, cisplatin (Platinol™); D, docetaxel (Taxotere™); E, etoposide (Vepesid™); G, gemcitabine (Gemzar™); Doxo, doxorubicin (Adriamycin™); NR, not reported.

were reported.[13] Unfortunately, additional trials that have also evaluated combinations of a platinum analogue with etoposide or a taxane demonstrated much less impressive results and, at times, serious toxicity (Table 22.1).

While on the surface some of the results with newer regimens appear superior to those seen with best supportive care or with older chemotherapy combinations, this remains unproven. Given the inherent selection bias in clinical trials of chemotherapy, it is impossible to accurately estimate the impact of treatment on survival from small phase II trials. The hope is that selected patients with a good performance status may derive some advantage from chemotherapy, but supportive care without chemotherapy remains a reasonable option in this group.

Short- and long-term prognosis

If one excludes the special subsets of CUP patients outlined above, the prognosis for the remainder of patients is grim. In a review of 1000 CUP patients treated at a single institution from 1987–1994, the median survival of the population was 11 months and 11 per cent of patients survived 5 years. [11] While instructive, this data is probably somewhat biased by the fact that it comes from a referral centre that sees a large number of patients who are well enough to travel long distances to receive their care. Population-based registries from Europe and the US typically report median survivals of 4–5 months, 1-year survivals of 15–30 per cent and 5-year survivals of 5 per cent in unselected patients with CUP.[2, 14] Even if one includes the more treatable subsets of patients with CUP, it is unlikely that more than 10 per cent of the entire CUP population achieves long-term disease free survival.

References

1. Dowell JE. Cancer from an unknown primary site. *Am J Med Sci* 2003; 326:35–46.
2. Pavlidis N. Cancer of unknown primary: biological and clinical characteristics. *Ann Oncol* 2003; 14(Suppl 3):11–18.
3. van de Wouw AJ, Jansen RL, Speel EJ, Hillen HF. The unknown biology of the unknown primary tumour: a literature review. *Ann Oncol* 2003; 14:191–6.
4. Greco FA, Hainsworth JD. Cancer of unknown primary site. In VJ Devita, S Hellman, S Rosenberg S (eds) *Cancer: principles and practice of oncology*, pp. 2537–60. Philadelphia, PA: Lippincott, Williams, & Wilkins, 2001.
5. Brigden ML, Murray N. Improving survival in metastatic carcinoma of unknown origin. *Postgrad Med* 1999; 105(63–4):67–74.
6. Hainsworth JD, Johnson DH, Greco FA. Poorly differentiated neuroendocrine carcinoma of unknown primary site. A newly recognized clinicopathologic entity. *Ann Intern Med* 1988; 109:364–71.
7. Richardson RL, Schoumacher RA, Fer MF, Hande KR, Forbes JT, Oldham RK, Greco F. A. The unrecognized extragonadal germ cell cancer syndrome. *Ann Intern Med* 1981; 94:181–6.
8. Hainsworth JD, Johnson DH, Greco FA. Cisplatin-based combination chemotherapy in the treatment of poorly differentiated carcinoma and poorly differentiated adenocarcinoma of unknown primary site: results of a 12-year experience. *J Clin Oncol* 1992; 10:912–22.
9. Lenzi R, Hess KR, Abbruzzese MC, Raber MN, Ordonez NG, Abbruzzese JL. Poorly differentiated carcinoma and poorly differentiated adenocarcinoma of unknown origin: favorable subsets of patients with unknown-primary carcinoma? *J Clin Oncol* 1997; 15:2056–66.
10. Abbruzzese JL, Abbruzzese MC, Hess KR, Raber MN, Lenzi R, Frost P. Unknown primary carcinoma: natural history and prognostic factors in 657 consecutive patients. *J Clin Oncol* 1994; 12:1272–80.

11. Hess KR, Abbruzzese MC, Lenzi R, Raber MN, Abbruzzese JL. Classification and regression tree analysis of 1000 consecutive patients with unknown primary carcinoma. *Clin Cancer Res* 1999; 5:3403–10.

12. Culine S, Kramar A, Saghatchian M, Bugat R, Lesimple T, Lortholary A, Merrouche Y, Laplanche A, Fizazi K. Development and validation of a prognostic model to predict the length of survival in patients with carcinomas of an unknown primary site. *J Clin Oncol* 2005; 20:4679–83.

13. Greco FA, Burris HA 3rd, Erland JB, Gray JR, Kalman LA, Schreeder MT, Hainsworth J. D. Carcinoma of unknown primary site. *Cancer* 2000; 89:2655–60.

14. van de Wouw, A. J, Janssen-Heijnen, M. L, Coebergh, J. W, Hillen, H. F. Epidemiology of unknown primary tumours; incidence and population-based survival of 1285 patients in Southeast Netherlands, 1984–1992. *Eur J Cancer* 2002; 38:409–13.

15. Briasoulis, E, Kalofonos, H, Bafaloukos, D, Samantas, E, Fountzilas, G, Xiros, N, Skarlos, D, Christodoulou, C, Kosmidis, P, Pavlidis, N. Carboplatin plus paclitaxel in unknown primary carcinoma: a phase II Hellenic Cooperative Oncology Group Study. *J Clin Oncol* 2000; 18:3101–7.

16. Greco FA, Erland JB, Morrissey LH, Burris HA 3rd, Hermann RC, Steis R, Thompson D, Gray J, Hainsworth JD. Carcinoma of unknown primary site: phase II trials with docetaxel plus cisplatin or carboplatin. *Ann Oncol* 2000; 11:211–15.

17. Dowell JE, Garrett AM, Shyr Y, Johnson DH, Hande KR. A randomized Phase II trial in patients with carcinoma of an unknown primary site. *Cancer* 2001; 91: 592–7.

18. Warner E, Goel R, Chang J, Chow W, Verma S, Dancey J, Franssen E, Dulude H, Girouard M, Correia J, Gallant G. A multicentre phase II study of carboplatin and prolonged oral etoposide in the treatment of cancer of unknown primary site (CUPS). *Br J Cancer* 1998; 77:2376–80.

19. Briasoulis E, Tsavaris N, Fountzilas G, Athanasiadis A, Kosmidis P, Bafaloukos D, Skarlos D, Samantas E, Pavlidis N. Combination regimen with carboplatin, epirubicin and etoposide in metastatic carcinomas of unknown primary site: A Hellenic Co-Operative Oncology Group Phase II Study. *Oncology* 1998; 55:426–30.

20. Greco FA, Burris HA 3rd, Litchy S, Barton JH, Bradof JE, Richards P, Scullin DC Jr, Erland JB, Morrissey LH, Hainsworth JD. Gemcitabine, carboplatin, and paclitaxel for patients with carcinoma of unknown primary site: a Minnie Pearl Cancer Research Network study. *J Clin Oncol* 2002; 20:1651–6.

21. Voog E, Merrouche Y, Trillet-Lenoir V, Lasset C, Peaud PY, Rebattu P, Negrier S. (2000). Multicentric phase II study of cisplatin and etoposide in patients with metastatic carcinoma of unknown primary. *Am J Clin Oncol* 2000; 23:614–16.

22. Liu JM, Chen YM, Chao Y, Liu SM, Tiu CM, Wu HW, Chiou TC, Hsieh RK, Chen LT, Whang-Peng J. Continuous infusion cisplatin and etoposide chemotherapy for cancer of unknown primary site (CUPS) in Taiwan, a region with a high prevalence of endemic viral infections. *Jpn J Clin Oncol* 1998; 28:431–5.

23. Piga A, Nortilli R, Cetto GL, Cardarelli N, Fedeli SL, Fiorentini G, D'Aprile M, Giorgi F, Parziale AP, Contu A, Montironi R, Gesuita R, Carle F, Cellerino R. Carboplatin, doxorubicin and etoposide in the treatment of tumours of unknown primary site. *Br J Cancer* 2004; 90:1898–904.

24. Balana C, Manzano JL, Moreno I, Cirauqui B, Abad A, Font A, Mate JL, Rosell R. A phase II study of cisplatin, etoposide and gemcitabine in an unfavourable group of patients with carcinoma of unknown primary site. *Ann Oncol* 2003; 14:1425–9.

23

Melanoma

Anne Hamilton and Katherine Clark

Introduction

Melanoma is one of the most common cancers. In the US, it accounts for 4.3 per cent of cancer incidence and 1.5 per cent of cancer mortality.[1] The worldwide highest incidences of melanoma occur in Australia and New Zealand.

In New South Wales (Australia), melanoma ranks second in incidence only to breast cancer in women, and prostate cancer in men. It accounts for 10 per cent of all new cancer cases, representing a lifetime risk of 1 in 29. The incidence in New South Wales is increasing in both men and women, although mortality is holding stable, accounting for 3 per cent of cancer deaths. The stable mortality rate is likely to be due to aggressive public awareness of the importance of reporting changing skin lesions and early detection programmes of the harmful effects of sun exposure.[2]

While early detection of melanoma provides an excellent chance for long-term survival, once it has become disseminated the prognosis is universally poor.

Natural history

General considerations

It seems melanoma occurs as a result of childhood sun exposure, with episodes of childhood sunburn especially implicated. Other risk factors include Caucasian race, blue eyes and fair skin, male gender, a family history of melanoma, a personal prior history of melanoma, large numbers of naevi and other skin cancers, and immunosuppression.

Initially, the majority of individuals present with a pre-existing skin lesion that has changed in appearance or character, usually occuring over a period of months. Observed changes include darkening of the colours, increases in height and width, or new onset of itching or bleeding. In 5 per cent of cases, the primary lesion is never found and patients present with metastatic disease.

The natural course of melanoma is directed by a variety of features, which are dependant upon characteristics of the primary tumour and characteristics of the affected individual.

Patterns of spread

Three clinical patterns of spread are recognized for melanoma:

- In-transit or satellite metastases (direct spread)
- Spread to locoregional lymph nodes (lymphatic spread)
- Distant metastases (haematogenous spread).

Satellite metastases are defined as metastatic nodules that develop within two centimetres (cm) of the original cutaneous lesion. These may be within the dermis, subcutaneous tissue or the adjacent blood vessels. The presence of satellite lesions is associated with an increased incidence of lymph node involvement and local recurrence. Satellite lesions form the first site of relapse in about 10 per cent of cases.

When satellite lesions are located greater than 2 cm from the primary, they become re-classified as in-transit metastases. In-transit metastases develop prior to locoregional lymph node invasion, and occur as the site of first relapse in about 50 per cent. Once lymph node involvement is documented, haematogenous spread will occur in 20 per cent of patients.

About a third of patients do not follow this pattern of local relapse, but will present with distant metastases as their first sign of relapse.

Location of primary and subsequent sites of metastases

The location of the primary melanoma predicts metastatic sites. Primary melanomas of the lower limbs and head and neck region are more likely to be associated with satellite or in-transit spread. However, patients with primary lesions of the upper extremities or of the trunk are more likely to develop distant metastases as their first site of recurrence.

Metastases from melanoma have been documented in nearly every organ in the body. The most common sites of disease are soft tissue and lymph node, bone, lung, liver, adrenal, and the central nervous system (CNS) (parenchyma as well as the leptomeninges). Melanoma is noteworthy, however, for its frequent involvement of unusual metastatic sites, including the small bowel and colon, pancreas, heart, kidney, thyroid, and eye.[3]

Time to metastases

The time to metastases from the development of the original tumour is variable. Patients who develop locoregional metastases (satellite lesions, local lymph node invasion) are more likely to develop metastases in less than 2 years from diagnosis of the original lesion. However, the third of patients who develop distant metastases as their first site of relapse are more likely to develop problems over more than 2 years.[4]

Factors affecting prognosis

Early stage disease

In NSW (Australia), primary melanoma is now associated with long-term survival of more than 90 per cent.[2] As previously noted, this is most likely due to public awareness campaigns of the importance of changes in skin lesions.

In both early and late stages of the disease, there is increasing recognition that the accurate prognostication of affected individuals depends on individual characteristics and features of the melanotic lesion.

At diagnosis, important prognostic features of the lesion that should be included in the initial pathology report include the lesion's histology and growth phase, thickness of the primary lesion (Breslow's thickness), ulceration, depth of invasion (Clark's level), mitotic rate, presence of activated lymphocytes, features of regression, phase of growth and the absence or presence of lymph node spread, vascular or lymphatic spread and the presence of satellites. Other important prognostic features of the affected individual that must be taken into account are age, gender and anatomical site of the primary tumour.[4]

Prognostic factors in metastatic disease

Once melanoma has become disseminated the prognosis is universally poor, with the median survival expected to measure approximately 8 months, with only 2–3 per cent of patients with advanced disease alive at 5 years. In the patients with metastatic disease, there have been attempts to identify subgroups with better or worse prognosis, though the data is still limited.

Patient related prognostic factors

Gender

Male gender has been identified as being associated with a poorer prognosis in both early and advanced disease. This is a trend that has long been noted, with the different survival rates attributed to both earlier diagnosis in women, an increased rate of thin disease at diagnosis and an as yet unidentified biological factor. In advanced disease, male gender is associated with reduced survival of 1–2 months compared to similar aged women, regardless of other prognostic factors.[6]

Age and comorbidities

Age seems to be an independent prognostic indicator with elderly patients (> 60 years). Older patients are more likely to be diagnosed with ulcerated and thicker primaries. In later stage disease, poorer prognosis may reflect decreased options, with patients less likely to be considered for surgery and other tumour-modifying therapies.[7]

Performance status

Performance status is widely used as a prognostic marker in cancer medicine. It is not surprising in advanced melanoma that patients with poor performance status have been statistically identified as a group with poor prognosis, although this information is largely extrapolated from survival data from treatment studies. The difference in survival for patients with a good performance status compared to those with poor functional status is measured in months.[8, 12, 18]

Psychological factors

Psychological factors have been reported as influencing prognosis in metastatic disease.[29] In this group, prospectively collected data suggests patients who display the following characteristics are more likely to have longer survival than patients at equal disease stage:

- patients who reported that the goal of their treatment was cure
- patients who minimized the effect of cancer on their lives
- patients who harboured anger towards their diagnosis
- married patients
- patients who reported their cancer was not difficult to live with
- patients who reported better quality of life.

Although the subjects included in this work were at similar stages in terms of their disease burden, the authors acknowledge that sicker patients were not included and there is no detail as to the participant's functional status. Other important prognostic indicators that were not included in this work include the time to relapse and the serum lactate dehydrogenase (LDH) levels. The differences seen in the two groups of patients may well have reflected the differing behaviours of their diseases.

Other work examining the psychology of patients with melanoma in the last year of life suggests that as patients become sicker they become more fatigued, experience greater difficulties coping with activities of living and may experience greater mood changes as a result.[30]

Tumour-related prognostic factors

AJCC (TNM) stage

◆ Sites of metastases

◆ LDH.

The M classification identifies patients with distant metastases. However, even in this group, there are variables, which suggest better or worse prognosis. Therefore, the staging system has divided the M or metastatic category into three subcategories:

◆ M1, which stages non-visceral metastases and includes distant skin, subcutaneous or lymph node metastases

◆ M2, which includes patients with lung metastases

◆ M3, which includes all other visceral and distant metastases.

The sites of metastases have been examined prospectively, retrospectively and in meta-analysis. Overall, visceral metastases appear to have a much poorer prognosis than metastases to skin and the subdermis. As a group, the prognosis of patients with metastases to gastrointestinal tract, the liver, bone and brain rarely exceeds 8 months, with the poorest prognosis associated with the subgroups of central nervous system and liver disease. The range of observed survival rates for patients with liver disease is 2–8 months, with central nervous system involvement survival measured between 4–8 months. The presence of lung and pleural metastases is less clear. Survival has been over a range that is measured between 6 months to 2 years. The best long-term survival for patients with metastatic disease is best when metastases are isolated to the skin or lymph nodes, with these patients's survival reported between 7 months to 2 years.

In addition to the sites of metastases, the number of visceral metastases carries prognostic information. Not surprisingly, the number of sites appears to be a highly significant predictor of poor outcomes for patients. Isolated disease involving the skin or lungs may be associated with a 10–12 month survival, compared with an 8-month survival with single visceral metastases. However, involvement of two or more sites suggests survival duration will fall to 6 months and this is worse of more than two sites are involved.

LDH is a highly predictive serological marker in metastatic melanoma. The presence of an elevated LDH greater than 10 per cent of normal upgrades any M to the next highest M.

LDH reflects tumour activity and tumour turnover. Elevated levels are associated with greater tumour burdens and much worse outlooks. An elevated LDH to the upper limit of normal at the time of diagnosis of metastatic disease is associated with poor prognosis. Rapidly escalating levels of LDH may be seen in patients who are deteriorating rapidly.[7, 10–13]

Disease-free interval

Tumour behaviour is also reflected in a measure of time from the original diagnosis to the time of first relapse. A short space between to first relapse or from a change from local disease to distant metastases is associated with poorer outlooks. Patients who develop recurrent disease in less than 36 months have an expected 5-year survival of only 17 per cent compared to 30 per cent if the time to relapse is greater than 36 months. Additionally, patients who progress within 36 months from regional to distant metastases have an expected median survival of 18 months, compared to 24 months for those who progress from negative node status to distant disease.

Therapies affecting prognosis

It is unclear whether systemic therapy has any impact on prognosis in metastatic melanoma. A Cochrane review of systemic treatments for metastatic cutaneous melanoma, last updated in 2003, identified no studies that compared systemic therapy to either placebo or best supportive care in the metastatic setting,[18] and no such studies have been published since. Dacarbazine has been used as the reference agent in most recent studies of new agents or drug combinations in the metastatic setting, and is associated with response rates in the order of 10–20 per cent, and overall survival of 6–9 months. Alternative agents, such as platinum, temozolamide and fotemustine have not appreciably improved on these figures. Studies of biochemotherapy have demonstrated no survival advantage over single-agent cytotoxics, although higher response rates and some prolongation of time to disease progression have been noted in some studies.[19–22]

Despite this, several studies indicate that those patients who exhibit an objective response to therapy for metastatic disease have a better prognosis than those with stable or progressive disease on treatment.[23, 24] The lack of prognostic impact of systemic therapies in this disease is therefore likely to be largely statistical in nature, and can be explained by a combination of factors. First, the percentage of responding patients is small with all interventions, so that any survival effect in responders is diluted in the larger population. Second, unless a significant proportion of responding patients are in the group that dies earlier than the population median, the median will not move. Finally, as the tail of survival curves in metastatic melanoma studies can be long (up to 10 per cent of patients are alive at 2-year follow-up, and up to 5 per cent survive 5 years),[25–27] and as follow-up is usually abandoned after 12–24 months in studies done in the metastatic setting, any prognostic effect from response to therapy in the patients with indolent disease is unlikely to be detected.

Thus, new strategies for assessing drug effect in melanoma are needed. First, prognostic factors for very long survival need to be identified, as these patients probably don't need therapy, and should be excluded from studies of new therapies in the first instance. Second, biological markers for response to the therapy being studied need to be identified in melanoma. Such predictive markers might then be used to enrich study populations with patients at high probability of responding to therapy, so that higher response rates might be achieved. Finally, randomized discontinuation study designs that filter out non-responders should be considered.[28] In an example of such a trial design, all eligible patients would receive an initial 6–9 weeks of a new drug. Patients with progressive disease come off study, while those with stable or responding disease are randomized to either continue therapy, or switch to placebo. Efficacy would be assessed only in those patients who have reached the randomization milestone. Alternatives to this design include treatment with a combination of DTIC and a new drug initially, followed by randomization between continued combination therapy, or cessation of the new drug with continuation of DTIC alone in non-progressing patients, or treatment with a combination of DTIC and a new drug initially, followed by randomization between the two single agents after the first response assessment.

Short- and long-term prognosis

The currently most important evidence-based prognostic factors for patients at diagnosis have been classified into the generally accepted American Joint Committee on Cancer (AJCC) Melanoma Staging System. The current version of the AJCC system was released in 2002 after an international panel of experts reviewed the best available scientific evidence and correlated it with large databases.[8] The review was undertaken in response to concerns that the previous 1997 AJCC Melanoma Staging System was failing to take into account more recently confirmed important prognostic factors. The result is the now universally accepted staging classification. Widespread acceptance and use of this system is imperative ensure universal standards of practice and to enable communication between clinicians, both clinically and when performing and reporting research. This system improves identification of patients at risk for recurrent disease or poor outcomes, strengthens recommendations for treatment and allows provision of the best available prognostic information for patients and their families.

The current AJCC classification is based on the tumour, lymph node and presence of metastases staging system (TNNM).

The main features of this system are:

- The thickness of the primary lesion (measured in millimeters), expressed as Brelsow's thickness
- Whether or not the lesion is ulcerated
- The level of invasion, but only in tumours < 1 mm thick (expressed as Clark's level)
- The number of positive lymph nodes (both macroscopic and microscopically involved)
- The presence of satellite lesions and in transit metastases
- The LDH levels in metastatic disease
- The location of metastatic deposits.

The T category is calculated from the thickness of the lesion, the absence or presence of ulceration, and the level of invasion.

The thickness of the lesion is described in millimeters (mm) or Breslow's thickness and has repeatedly been proven to be a strong and reliable predictor of prognosis, with the most recent staging system dividing the statistically important depth of tumours into < 1.0 mm, 1.01–2.0 mm, 2.01–4.0 mm and > 4.0 mm. So strong is the association between tumour thickness and survival that when the 10-year mortality rates of melanomas are considered compared to thickness of the primary tumour, an almost linear graph results. Why tumour thickness is such a reliable indicator of prognosis is unclear. Suggestions include the theories that thicker tumours may have more rapid growth patterns or thicker tumours are representative of a delayed diagnosis (lead time bias).

The other major consideration of the T stage is the absence or presence of ulceration. Ulceration is defined as the absence of an intact epidermis overlying the primary melanoma. The presence of ulceration carries a high risk of metastases and is a sufficiently poor prognostic factor to upgrade the T staging to the next highest T category, as detailed in the Table 23.1.

Ulceration occurs in about 25 per cent of primary melanomas. It is a highly significant predictor of poorer outcomes, especially in men. The most likely reason for this is that the presence of ulceration leads to underestimation of the thickness of the lesion.

The level of invasion of the cutaneous and subcutaneous tissue is refered to as the Clark's level. It was previously regarded as an important prognostic factor, whatever the thickness of the primary tumour was. However, more recently, it has been suggested that only in "thin" (< 1.0 mm) tumours does the level of invasion carry prognostic significance. The level of invasion or Clark's level of invasion is therefore still reported, but because of the wide range of variability in recording it, it is only factored into the T staging when the tumour is thin. In this situation, a thin melanoma, with a Clark's thickness of greater than or equal to IV are upgraded to the next T category (Table 23.2).

The N classification is one of the most important predictors of survival and has been identified as the area that is associated with the most degree of variability. Within the N category, there are three subgroups based on the presence of nodal involvement (either microscopic or macroscopic), the presence of satellite metastases, and the characteristics of the primary lesion (the absence or presence of ulceration and tumour thickness).

Table 23.1 AJCC Staging of melanoma (2002)

Stage	Nodes	Satellite or in-transit metastasis	Without ulceration	With ulceration	Distant metastasis
0	Negative	Absent	*In situ*	–	Absent
IA	Negative	Absent	< 1.0mm AND Clark II or III	–	Absent
IB	Negative	Absent	< 1.0mm AND Clark IV or V	< 1.0mm	Absent
	Negative	Absent	1.01–2.0mm	–	Absent
IIA	Negative	Absent	2.01–4.0mm	1.01–2.0mm	Absent
IIB	Negative	Absent	> 4.0mm	2.01–4.0mm	Absent
IIC	Negative	Absent	–	> 4.0mm	Absent
IIIA	1–3 positive (microscopic)	Absent	Any	–	Absent
IIIB	1–3 positive (microscopic)	Absent	–	Any	Absent
	1–3 nodes (macroscopic)	Absent	Any	–	Absent
	negative	Present	Any	Any	Absent
IIIC	1–3 positive (macroscopic)	Absent	–	Any	Absent
	≥4 positive	Absent	Any	Any	Absent
	Positive	Present	Any	Any	Absent
IV	Any	Any	Any	Any	Present

The 2002 AJCC staging re-categorized the absence or presence of nodal involvement (histologically and clinically) and the number of nodes rather than the size of the involved lymph nodes as important, highlighting the importance of sentinel lymph node mapping.

Sentinel lymph node mapping allows clinicians to identify the first lymph node that receives lymphatic drainage from a region and undertake a biopsy of this node. A microscopic diagnosis of nodal invasion can be made. This is considered the most sensitive indicator of lymphatic

Table 23.2 Table of Clark's thickness

Level I	**Intraepidermal growth with intact basement membrane**
Level II	Invasion of the papillary dermis
Level III	Tumour involvement filling the papillary dermis and invasion of the junction between the papillary and reticular dermis
Level IV	Invasion of the tumour into the reticular dermis
Level V	Invasion of tumour into the subcutaneous fat

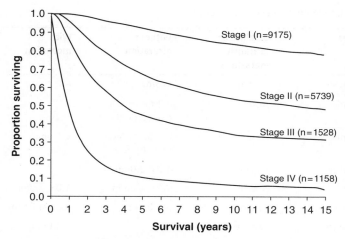

Figure 23.1 Fifteen-year survival curves for the Melanoma Staging System comparing localized melanoma (stages I and II), regional mestastases (stage III), and distant metastases (stage IV). The numbers in parentheses are the numbers of patinets from the AJCC melanoma staging database used to calculate the survival rates. The differences between the curves are highly significant ($p < 0.0001$).

metastases and this process has considerably improved the ability of clinicians to provide prognostic information. Histologically negative nodes have a 5-year survival rate of 93 per cent compared to 67 per cent if sentinel node sampling is positive.

The number of affected nodes carries prognostic significance. If only one node is involved, 5- year survival is estimated at about 40 per cent. In comparison, if more than five nodes are involved 5-year survival falls to around 15 per cent.

The M category relies upon the estimation of the serum LDH and the sites of metastases. These are discussed in more detail under prognostic factors associated with advanced disease.

The TNM groups are classified into I, II, III or IV stage disease. The estimated 5-year survival of these groups is 93, 68, 45 and 11 per cent respectively,[4, 9, 10] see Figure 23.1.

References

1. SEER Cancer Statistics Review 1975–2002.

2. Cancer in NSW; Incidence and mortality 2003.

3. Leiter U et al. *Journal of Surgical Oncology* 2004; 86:172–8.

4. de Braud F, Khayat D, Kroon B. *et al*. Malignant melanoma. *Critical Reviews in Oncology/Haematology* 2003;47:35–63.

5. Scolyer RA, Thompson JF, Stretch JR. *et al*. Pathology of melanocytic lesions; new, controversial and clinically important issues. *Journal of Surgical Oncology* 2004; 86:200–11.

6. Ahmed I. Malignant melanoma; prognostic indicators. *Mayo Clinic Proceedings* 1997; 72:356–61.

7. Swetter SM, Geller AC, Kirkwood JM. Melanoma in the older person. *Oncology (Huntington)* 2004; 18:1196–7.

8. Schuchter L, Schultz D, Delray J. *et al*. A prognostic model for predicting 10-year survival in patients with primary melanoma. *Archives of Internal Medicine* 1996; 125:369–75.

9. Thompson JF, Shaw HM, Hersey P, Scolyer RA. The history and future of melanoma staging. *Journal of Surgical Oncology* 2004; 86:224–35.

10. Balch CM, Soong SJ, Atkins MB. *et al.* An evidence-based staging system for cutaneous melanoma. *CA Cancer J Clinicians* 2004; 54:131–49.

11. Thompson JF, Scolyer RA, Kefford. Cutaneous melanoma. *Lancet* 2005; 365:686–701.

12. Lomuto M, Calabrese P, Giulani A. prognostic signs in melanoma; state of the art. *European Journal of Dermatology and Venereology* 2004; 18:291–300.

13. Calonjie E. Best Practice No 162. The histological reporting of melanoma. *Journal of Clinical Pathology* 2005; 53:587–90.

14. Fearfield LA, Rowe A, Francis N. *et al.* Clinico–pathological features of relapsing very thin melanoma. *Clinical and Experimental Dermatology* 2001; 26:686–95.

15. Azzola MF, Shaw HM, Thompson JF, Soong SJ. *et al.* Tumor mitotic rate is a more powerful prognostic indicator than ulceration in patients with primary cutaneous melanoma. *Cancer* 2003; 97:1488–98.

16. Hussein MR. Tumour-infiltrating lymphocytes and melanoma tumorigenesis; an insight. *British Journal of Dermatology* 2005; 153:18–21.

17. Nguyen TH. Mechanisms of metastasis. *Clinics in Dermatology* 2004; 22:209–16.

18. Crosby T, Fish R, Coles B. *et al. Systemic treatments for metastatic cutaneous melanoma.* The Cochrane Database of Systemic Reviews 2004; 4.

19. Middleton MR, Grob JJ, Aaronson N. *et al.* Randomized phase III study of temozolomide versus dacarbazine in the treatment of patients with advanced metastatic malignant melanoma. *J Clin Oncol* 2000; 18(1):158–66.

20. Avril MF, Aamdal S, Grob JJ. *et al.* Fotemustine compared with dacarbazine in patients with disseminated malignant melanoma; a phase III study. *J Clin Oncol* 2004; 22(6):1118–25.

21. Kirkwood JM, Bedikian AY, Millward MJ. *et al.* Long-term survival results of a randomized multinational phase 3 trial of dacarbazine with or without BCL-2 antisense (oblimersen sodium) in patients with advanced malignant melanoma. Proc ASCO 2005. *J Clin Oncol* 2005; 23(16S):711s (abstract 7506).

22. Eigentler TK, Caroli UM, Radny P. *et al.* Palliative therapy of disseminated malignant melanoma; a systematic review of 41 randomised clinical trials. *Lancet Oncol* 200; 4:748–59.

23. Falkson CI, Falkson HC. Prognostic factors in metastatic malignant melanoma. *Oncology* 1998; 55:59–64.

24. Ryan L, Kramar A, Borden E. Prognostic factors in metastatic melanoma. *Cancer* 1993; 71:2995–3005.

25. Brand CU, Ellwanger U, Stroebel W. *et al.* Prolonged survival of 2 years or longer for patients with disseminated melanoma. *Cancer* 1997; 79:2345–53.

26. Manola J, Atkins M, Ibrahim J. *et al.* Prognostic factors in metastatic melanoma; a pooled analysis of Eastern Cooperative Oncology Group trials. *J Clin Oncol* 2000; 18:3782–93.

27. Lee ML, Tomsu K, Von Eschen KB. Duration of survival for disseminated malignant melanoma; results of a meta-analysis. *Melanoma Research* 2000; 10:81–92.

28. Rosner GL, Stadler W, Ratain MJ. Randomized discontinuation design; application to cytostatic antineoplastic agents. *J Clin Oncol* 2002; 20(22):4478–84.

29. Butow PN, Coates AS, Dunn SM. Psychological predictors of survival in metastatic melanoma. *Journal of Clinical Oncology* 1999; 17:2256–63.

30. Brown JE, Brown RF, Miller RM. *et al.* Coping with metastatic melanoma; the last year of life. *Psycho-Oncology* 2000; 9:283–92.

Part III

Prognosis in palliative care

24

Bone secondaries

Edward Chow and Albert Yee

Introduction

Bone metastases are a frequent complication of cancer. They are clinically apparent in about 50 per cent of all cancer patients and have been reported in 70–85 per cent of cancer patients at autopsy. Pain arising from bone metastases is the most common symptom requiring treatment in cancer patients. Fifty to seventy-five per cent of patients with bone metastases suffer from severe pain. As reflected in a consensus statement from a National Cancer Institute Workshop, the under-treatment of cancer pain is a serious and neglected public health problem. Treatment involves multiple care providers including medical and radiation oncologists, pain specialists, surgeons, and other healthcare professionals. Unfortunately a multidisciplinary co-ordinated approach across these specialties is currently lacking in the management of bone metastases. Moreover, the collaboration and exchange of research information between the basic and clinical scientists have been inadequate.

With advances in effective systemic treatment and supportive care, survival of patients with bone metastases has improved substantially. Certain subsets of patients with bone metastases (e.g. breast and prostate cancer with predominately bone or bone-only metastases) have life expectancies that range from 2–5 years. Successful management of bone metastases during these years is essential for reducing the skeletal complications and for maximizing patient quality of life.

Natural history of the condition

The symptoms of bone metastases are often severe, and develop earlier in the clinical course of patients with cancer than symptoms due to either liver or lung metastases. Complications of skeletal metastases are common and can seriously impair patient quality of life and function. Pain and impaired mobility occur in 65–75 per cent of patients with bone metastases;[1] fractures of weight-bearing long bones occur in 10–20 per cent;[1] hypercalcaemia occurs in 10–15 per cent;[1,2] and spinal cord or nerve root compression occurs in 5 per cent.[3]

There is a propensity for certain primary malignancies that possess a predilection for bony metastases. The classic 'benzene-ring' description by anatomical location of thyroid cancer, breast/lung cancer, renal/colon cancer, and prostate cancer features those malignancies that tend to spread to bone. Bone is the first site of relapse in more than 80 per cent of prostate and around 50 per cent of breast cancer patients.

Certain malignancies, such as thyroid cancer and renal cell carcinoma, tend to be vascular tumours that are important when considering a potential surgical procedure in the treatment of impending or pathologic fracture. There is also variation in the longevity of patients who present with skeletal metastases. As such, these are important variables that need to be considered prior to making a decision regarding patient care. The goal is to improve patient quality of life and palliation.

Factors affecting prognosis

In the past, patients with bone metastases, particularly those with pathological fractures, had short lifespans. An aggressive treatment approach was therefore not warranted.

In 1981, Harrington reported that the average survival for patients with bone metastases referred for orthopaedic fixation increased from 7 months to 19 months between 1960 and 1980.[4] Median survival for patients with bone metastases range widely, depending on the primary cancer: prostate, 29.3 months; breast, 22.6 months; renal-cell, 11.8 months; lung, 3.6 months.[4]

Certain subsets of patients with bone metastases have even longer life expectancies.

About 20 per cent of breast cancer patients predominantly experience either bone or bone-only metastases, and the 5-year survival rate can be as high as 45 per cent. Patients with bone-only metastases have a median survival of 52 months.[5–7]

Bony metastases from prostate cancer can be controlled by hormone manipulation for an average of 36 months. Hormone-resistant prostate cancer patients survive for 6–9 months on average.[8]

Clinical experience has shown that not only patients with breast and prostate cancers generally survive longer when compared with patients with lung cancer, but also patients with bone-only metastases live longer than those with visceral metastases.

However, once bone-related complications occur, such as pathological fractures, spinal cord compression or hypercalcaemia of malignancy, the median survival will be shortened to 12, 4 and 3 months respectively in women with breast cancer.[9] This is generally true for other primaries too.

Performance status has been shown to correlate with duration of survival. Symptoms comprising part of the 'terminal cancer syndrome' including anorexia and shortness of breath were strong predictors of poor survival.

The time interval between first diagnosis of cancer and diagnosis of metastatic disease may reflect the aggressiveness of the disease. The age of the patient may influence not only recommendations for treatment, but also prediction of their remaining lifespan.

Therapies affecting prognosis

Pain medication

The initial management includes the use of simple analgesics and non-steroidal anti-inflammatory agents, titrating to stronger opioids guided by patients' pain response and the analgesic ladder. Dexamethasone may also be helpful. Adjuvant analgesics such as amitriptyline and gabapentin should be considered if there is a neuropathic component. Adequate analgesics can often provide pain relief and better quality of life provided side-effects of analgesics are attended and managed. Unfortunately, a substantial portion of patients with bone metastases is undermedicated with analgesics when referred to palliative radiotherapy clinics.[10, 11] Input from pain specialists is crucial in the management of painful bone metastases.

Bisphosphonates

Bisphosphonates are potent inhibitors of bone resorption. The results of randomized controlled trials comparing a bisphosphonate with either placebo or no treatment in secondary prophylaxis (i.e. in patients with established bone metastases) have shown that once bone metastases are present, the use of bisphosphonates in addition to first-line chemotherapy or hormonal therapy can significantly reduce skeletal related events.[12–18]

A recent meta-analysis of 33 studies that included patients with bone metastases from many different tumour types found bisphosphonate treatment significantly reduced the odds ratios for fracture (0.65; 95 per cent C.I. 0.55–0.78), need for radiotherapy (0.67; 0.57–0.79), and incidence of hypercalcaemia (0.54; 0.36–0.71).[19]

The American Society of Clinical Oncology guidelines recommend breast cancer patients with plain radiographic evidence of bone destruction for intravenous pamidronate 90 mg delivered over 2 hours or zoledronic acid 4 mg over 15 minutes every 3 to 4 weeks.[20] Cancer Care Ontario guidelines also endorse this except in patients with a short expected survival (i.e., less than six months) who have well-controlled bone pain.[21]

In a placebo-controlled randomized clinical trial, long-term treatment with 4 mg of zoledronic acid has been shown to be safe and provide sustained benefits for men with metastatic hormone-refractory prostate cancer.[22] Details of the efficacy of bisphosphonates have been described in the previous chapters.

Radiation therapy

External beam local radiotherapy

Radiation therapy has long been employed in the management of bone metastases including relief of bone pain, prevention of impending fractures and promotion of healing in pathological fractures. Stabilization of bony destruction occurs in 80 per cent and reossification takes place in 50 per cent of patients after radiotherapy.

Palliation of bone metastases comprises a significant workload in the specialty of radiation oncology. External beam radiation therapy is effective and cost-efficient in relieving symptomatic bone metastases. The most commonly employed schemes to treat bone metastases include a single 8 Gy, 20 Gy in 5 daily fractions, 30 Gy in 10 daily fractions and 40 Gy in 20 daily fractions. Numerous randomized trials have been conducted on dose-fractionation schedules of palliative radiotherapy. Despite that, there is still no uniform consensus on the optimal dose fractionation scheme.

Retrospective series have documented prompt improvement in pain in 80–90 per cent of patients with various dose fractionations without causing significant haematological or gastrointestinal side-effects. One of the first randomized studies on bone metastases was conducted by Radiation Therapy Oncology Group (RTOG). The initial analysis of this trial (RTOG 74–02) concluded that a low dose short-course schedule was as effective in pain relief as more aggressive high-dose protracted schedules.[23] However, this study was criticized for using physician-based pain assessment. A re-analysis of the same set of data, grouping solitary and multiple bone metastases, using the end point of pain relief and taking into account of analgesic intake and retreatment, concluded that the number of radiation fractions was significantly associated with complete pain relief.[24] This conclusion was directly contrary to the initial report, making the choice of end points very important in defining the outcome of clinical trials.[25]

Several prospective randomized trials that compared the efficacy of different dose-fractionation schedules have subsequently been performed. They included the recent large-scale multi-centre trials comparing the efficacy of a single 8 Gy treatment against multiple treatments. The UK Bone Pain Working Party found no difference in the degree and duration of pain relief in this study of 765 patients randomized to receive either a single treatment or five fractionated treatments.[26] The Dutch Bone Metastases Study included 1171 patients and found no difference in pain relief or the quality of life following a single 8 Gy or 24 Gy in six daily radiation treatments.[27]

One critical review on the subject of radiation dose fractionation suggested that protracted fractionated radiotherapy, given over 2–4 weeks, results in more complete and durable pain relief.[28] This was performed because of concerns regarding the influence of length of survival on the durability of pain relief. It was unclear whether higher radiation doses were necessary for durable pain relief in patients who survived longer.

The recent meta-analyses showed no significant difference in complete and overall pain relief between single and multi-fraction palliative radiotherapy for bone metastases.[29, 30] No dose–response relationship could be detected by including data from trials that evaluated several different radiation schedules. The meta-analysis reported that the complete response rates (absence of pain after radiotherapy) were 33.4 and 32.3 per cent after single and multi-fraction radiation treatment respectively, while the overall response rates were 62.1 and 58.7 per cent, respectively. The latter became 72.7 and 72.5 per cent respectively when the analysis was restricted to evaluated patients alone. Most patients will experience pain relief in the first 2–4 weeks after radiotherapy, be it single or multiple fractionations.[29] However, the retreatment and pathological fracture rates were higher in single fraction treatments.[30]

How, then, are radiation oncologists to prescribe treatment? The answer most likely resides within the clinical circumstances and individual wishes of each patient. There is no doubt that in patients with short life expectancy, protracted schedules are a burden. However, in patients with a longer expected survival, such as breast and prostate cancer patients with bone metastases only, other parameters need to be taken into account. Since re-treatment rates are known to be higher following a single versus multiple fractions, about 25 versus 10 per cent respectively, patients with good performance status may wish to share the decision-making process. A recent survey of patients with bone metastases has suggested that patients are not prepared to trade off long-term outcomes in favour of a shorter treatment course.[31] Durability of pain relief was more important than short-term 'convenience' factors. Patients prefer multiple treatments up front in hopes of avoiding re-treatment. However, they need to be aware of the potential physician bias of more readiness to retreat after single fraction accounting for the difference in retreatment rates in the trials.

Wide-field/half-body external beam radiation

Patients with bone metastases can have multiple sites of disease and present with diffuse symptoms affecting several sites. Wide-field/half-body external beam radiation (HBI) has been used to treat patients with multiple painful bone metastases. Single fraction HBI has been shown to provide pain relief in 70–80 per cent of patients. Pain relief is apparent within 24–48 hours. Toxicities include minor bone marrow suppression and gastrointestinal side-effects such as nausea and vomiting in upper-abdominal radiation that may be controlled with ondansetron or dexamethasone. Pulmonary toxicity is minimal provided the lung dose is limited to 6 Gy (corrected dose). Fractionated HBI was investigated in a phase II study that compared a single fraction (n = 14) with fractionated HBI (25–30 Gy in a 9–10 fractions) (n = 15). Pain relief was achieved in over 94 per cent of patients. At 1 year, 70 per cent in the fractionated and 15 per cent in the single fraction group had pain control; retreatment was required in 71 and 13 per cent for the single and fractionated group, respectively. A randomized trial of 499 patients compared local radiation alone versus local radiation plus a single fraction of HBI. The study documented a lower incidence of new bone metastases (50 vs 68 per cent) and fewer patients requiring further local radiotherapy at 1 year after HBI (60 vs 76 per cent).[32]

Systemic radiation – radioisotopes

An alternative approach to the palliation of multiple bone metastases is the administration of a bone-seeking radioactive isotope that is taken up at sites of bone metastases with osteoblastic activity. The isotopes deliver the radiation dose through the release of beta particles; their range of radiation is only a few millimetres, thereby concentrating their dose within the bone metastases and delivering little dose to the adjacent normal bone marrow. The radiation half-life is about 50 days in the metastasis and only 14 days in the normal bone marrow.

Systemic radiation using radioisotopes such as strontium, samarium and rhenium has been used increasingly to palliate bone pain and improve the quality of life in these patients. These agents are particularly useful among patients with multiple symptomatic metastases. Because the radiation is localized to the metastases, radioisotopes can be used for re-irradiation when there are concerns about normal tissue tolerance to further external beam radiation. Also, improved outcomes and cost-effectiveness have been demonstrated when radioisotopes have been combined with external beam radiation. The Trans-Canada Study comparing external beam radiation alone or in combination with Strontium-89 for bone metastases demonstrated better pain relief and reduced need for external beam radiation to other sites in the latter group.[33] Convenience to the patient is the other key advantage because radioisotope therapy is administered as a single injection. With normal bone marrow parameters, re-treatment with radioisotope therapy is also possible because the adjacent normal tissues do not receive any radiation dose.

A flare of pain, like that seen with hormonal therapy in breast cancer, may precede the relief of symptoms. It may take up to 1–2 months before there is relief of symptoms. Because of this, patients should have a life expectancy that allows the benefit of the relief of symptoms. Contraindications to bone-seeking radioisotopes include compromised bone marrow tolerance defined as a platelet count < 60,000/mL, white count < 2.5×10^3/mL, disseminated intravascular coagulation, or myelosuppressive chemotherapy within the previous month. Because bone-seeking radioisotopes do not penetrate to soft tissues, they are also contraindicated for treatment of soft tissue metastases or epidural extension with spinal cord compression. As with external beam radiation, an impending pathological fracture should be evaluated for surgical stabilization. Impending or established pathological fractures and cord compressions are acute emergencies to be managed by surgical or radiation oncology teams. Once the fracture or compression is stabilized, radioisotopes may be appropriate therapy for ongoing palliation of pain.

Complications of bone metastases – localized external beam radiotherapy for pathological and impending fractures

Pathological fractures are handled with orthopaedic stabilization whenever possible. Surgery rapidly controls pain and returns that patient to mobility. Elective orthopaedic stabilization has reportedly resulted in good pain relief and sustained mobility in up to 90 per cent of patients. Early identification of patients with a high risk of fracture is especially important. A fracture of the weight-bearing long bones can be a devastating event, even in a healthy person. Prophylactic orthopaedic fixation is often advised to avoid the trauma of a pathological fracture. The operative procedure has fewer complications and less impact on functional outcome.

The criteria often used to determine fracture risk in long bones include:

◆ Persistent or increasing local pain despite radiotherapy, particularly when aggravated by functional loading

◆ A solitary, well-defined lytic lesion greater than 2.5 cm

◆ A solitary, well-defined lesion circumferentially involving more than 50 per cent of the cortical bone

◆ Metastatic involvement of the proximal femur associated with a fracture of the lesser trochanter.

Although radiotherapy provides pain relief and tumour control, it does not restore bone stability. Postoperative radiotherapy is usually recommended after surgical stabilization of a pathologic fracture. Patients who are without visceral metastases and who have a relatively long survival (e.g. > 3 months) are more likely to benefit from postoperative radiotherapy. Because the entire bone is at risk for microscopic involvement and the procedure involved in rod placement may seed the bone at other sites, the length of the entire rod used for bone stabilization should be included in the radiation field. When the radiation fields are more limited, instability of the rod, resulting in pain and need for re-operation, can result from recurrent osteolytic metastases outside the radiation portal.

Orthopaedic surgery

The main indications for consideration of surgical treatment of bony metastases are painful lesions that are refractory to non-surgical therapies, significant pre-critical lesions that pose risk for pathologic fracture (i.e. impending pathologic fracture), and pathological fractures. There are several principles that are important in the surgical treatment of pathologic fracture. Internal fixation (plates, screws, intramedullary rods, etc.) of pathological fractures is temporary. The device will fail from repetitive cyclical implant loading unless the bone heals. Bony healing is slower than for fractures through normal bone. Surgical strategies are often required to optimize initial implant stability (e.g. bone cement/polymethyl-methacrylate, bone grafting). Additional neo-adjuvant or adjuvants are required to tip the balance in favor of bony repair (e.g. radiation therapy, chemotherapy).

Management of specific fractures

In the upper extremity, symptomatic lesions without fracture can often be managed by splinting, radiation therapy, and physiotherapy to maintain active range of motion. Following fracture, glenohumeral lesions require a form of shoulder arthroplasty (e.g. hemiarthroplasty) with adjuvant radiation therapy. Humeral shaft fractures are often treated by plate and screw fixation or an intramedullary rod and bone cement augmentation is often employed. Again, adjuvant radiation therapy can readily be applied postoperatively, in particular, if an intramedullary rod is inserted as minimal surgical incisions are required around the shoulder and elbow. Shoulder and elbow contractures are common and early range of joint motion should be encouraged. Pathological lesions distal to the elbow are uncommon as are lesions in the lower extremity distal to the knee.

In the lower extremity, over 50 per cent of pathological fractures occur in the proximal femur. Lesions in the femoral neck, intertrochanteric and subtrochanteric area should almost always be prophylactically stabilized because of the high stresses placed across this anatomic location. Pathologic fractures of weight-bearing long bones typically require surgical treatment as a part of the treatment solution because of the profound impact of stability on ambulatory capacity and function. Primarily pelvic or periacetabular lesions can often be managed by radiation therapy. These are difficult areas to access surgically. When present in the weight-bearing dome of the acetabulum, surgical reconstruction often involves more complex total hip replacement/arthroplasty. Preparation for special 'revision-type' implants (acetabular roof ring, bone cement, calcar replacing femoral components) to compensate bone loss issues makes functional results following total hip replacement not as favourable compared to total hip replacement performed for osteoarthritis of the hip. Pathological fractures of the femoral and tibial shaft are best treated by surgical stabilization. As with the conventional trauma population, intramedullary rod fixation has become the standard of care in the management of such fractures. The distinct advantages of intramedullary rod fixation include the minimal surgical exposures. The technique maintains the vascularity of the bone without periosteal stripping. The implant is a 'load-sharing' device which has advantages for healing, and also often permits patients to be immediately ambulatory on the surgically treated limb following the procedure. A general principle in bone metastases is acknowledging the goal of palliation and that lesions elsewhere in the same bone may develop over time. As such, a common principle is to span the entire long bone, which in considering the femur would include cephalomedullary nail fixation which provides additional fixation into the femoral neck and head. Fat and tumour emboli to lung can occur during intramedullary reaming for insertion of the intramedullary rod. As such, perioperative respiratory management is important when dealing with fractures through weight-bearing long bones.

In the vertebral column, a more distinct consideration in addition to issues of stability is the potential for neurologic compromise. High-risk precritical vertebral lesions posing risk for pathological burst fracture, epidural compression with resultant spinal cord compression and paralysis should be aggressively treated. Conventional spinal surgery may involve a surgical decompression (anterior, posterior, or combined), however, the primary goal is to achieve stability. Spinal stability is afforded by surgical arthrodesis and spinal instrumentation. Conventional spinal surgery for the treatment of vertebral metastases is often a complex surgical procedure. The surgical outcomes can be significant in patient pain relief and quality of life, however the results are better at restoring spinal stability and assisting with pain control versus the ability of a decompression to reverse neurological damage that has occurred.[34, 35] However, radiation therapy does not adequately address significant bony compression and its use is limited in relatively radioresistant tumours (eg. renal carcinoma). The timing of surgery, radiation therapy (neo-adjuvant versus adjuvant) is often debated. Prognostically, conventional spinal surgery in the face of tissues previously irradiated has a three- to fourfold increase in wound complications when compared to those individuals who have not had prior irradiation.[34, 36]

Newer minimal invasive surgical (MIS) approaches that include vertebroplasty and kyphoplasty have provided a means of augmenting spinal stability without the morbidity and aforementioned complexities associated with conventional spinal surgery.[37] The ability of percutaneous injection of polymethylmethacrylate (bone cement) to mechanically stabilize pathological fractures of the vertebral column is a therapy that can provide excellent early pain relief and does not unduly delay adjuvant radiation therapy. The complications of vertebroplasty, however, appear to be greater than its use in osteoporosis.[38–41] The procedure can also be an effective salvage in those patients where radiation therapy was unable to adequately control symptoms.[42] There are newer strategies in minimal access surgery, and current research holds future promise in techniques such as laser ablation, photodynamic therapy, and other strategies to lower the risks associated with vertebroplasty. Indeed, the vertebroplasty approach has been adapted to other anatomic locations such as pelvis lesions that are difficult to access surgically in the 'cementoplasty' approach.[43, 44]

The multidisciplinary approach and mutual collaborative discussions between medical oncologist, radiation oncologist, and surgeon is required to derive a treatment plan best suited for the individual, considering the patient and fracture. At our tertiary cancer centre, we have established a multidisciplinary bone metastases clinic – the ultimate one-stop shop for our cancer patients with bone metastases.[45]

Chemotherapy and hormonal therapy

Chemotherapy should be considered in patients with chemosensitive tumours such as multiple myeloma, small cell lung cancer, lymphoma and germ cell tumours. In pre- and postmenopausal breast cancer women with bone metastases who relapse on tamoxifen, chemotherapy offers a potential chance of further response. The increasing role of chemotherapy has been documented in recent randomized trials not only to improve pain and quality of life, but also in prolonging survival such as in advanced hormone-refractory prostate cancer. When given with prednisone, treatment with docetaxel every 3 weeks led to superior survival and improved rates of response in terms of pain, serum prostatic specific antigen (PSA) level, and quality of life, as compared with mitoxantrone plus prednisone.[46] Hormonal therapy is also of benefit in the management of symptomatic bone metastases from prostate cancer, breast cancer and endometrial cancer. Details can be found in their respective chapters.

Short-term prognosis

Bisphosphonates and palliative radiotherapy are commonly employed to palliate bone metastases in breast cancer. It has been observed that responders to bisphosphonates and palliative radiotherapy present with different baseline biochemical markers of bone turnover when compared with those of non-responders. The change in these biochemical markers during the treatment course is also different for responders and non-responders. There is a suggestion that biochemical markers could be a predictor for response to treatment interventions.

Markers of bone remodelling have been shown to be suppressed by anti-resorptive therapy, and the response of these bone markers has been applied to monitoring therapy for bone metastases.

A myriad of new markers of bone metabolism assayed from either serum or urine specimens of patients with bone metastases are currently available for clinical investigation. Among the novel markers used to assess bone resorption are products of bone collagen breakdown that include: (1) the pyridinium cross-links: pyridinoline (PYD) and deoxypyridinoline (DPD), (2) N-telopeptide (NTX), and (3) C-telopeptide (CTX). These bone resorption markers have largely replaced urinary hydroxyproline as the preferred biochemical markers of bone turnover in the clinical laboratory.

Vinholes *et al.* in a double blind, placebo-controlled study evaluated the efficacy of pamidronate on pain relief from bone metastases. Patients with a persistent elevation of urinary NTX level had poor pain relief.[47]

Lipton *et al.* studied 21 patients placed on pamidronate therapy. Over the course of 4–6 months, NTX concentrations in 12 of the patients decreased to levels within the normal reference range of pre-menopausal women, whereas in the remaining nine patients the marker did not reach normality. Those with normalization of NTX levels had a lower bone fracture rate (5/12 – 42 per cent) than the other cohort with elevated bone markers (8/9 – 89 per cent). Furthermore, in the patients in whom the marker normalized, there was progression of disease in bone in only 25 per cent (3/12) of the patients compared with 78 per cent (7/9) of patients in whom the NTX remained elevated.[48]

Vinholes *et al.* in another study evaluated 37 patients with newly diagnosed bone metastases from breast cancer randomized to oral pamidronate or placebo in addition to anti-cancer therapy for assessment of response and identification of progression. An increase of NTX of 30 per cent predicted progression of disease. In a similar prospective study of 97 patients, of whom 53 were breast cancer patients, with metastatic bone disease, Costa *et al.* again observed that a 50 per cent increase in NTX correlated significantly with radiograph diagnosis of bone metastases progression. Serial measurements of the newer markers of bone resorption hold promise in helping the clinician to more rapidly assess which patients are responding to systemic therapy than do traditional radiograph techniques.[49, 50]

In the recent UK Bone Pain Radiotherapy Trial, 22 patients were entered into a supplementary study to establish the effects of local radiotherapy for metastatic bone pain on markers of osteoclast activity, particularly the pyridinium crosslinks pyridinoline and deoxypyridinoline, the latter being specific for bone turnover. Urine samples were collected before and one month after radiotherapy. Patients were treated with either a single 8 Gy or 20 Gy in five daily fractions. Pain response was scored with validated pain charts completed by patients.[51]

Urinary pyridinium concentrations were compared with pain response. In the non-responding patients, baseline concentrations of both pyridinoline and deoxypyridinoline were higher than responders, and rose further after treatment, whereas in responders, the mean values remained unchanged. This resulted in significant differences between responders and non-responders for both indices after treatment (p = 0.027). The authors conclude that radiotherapy-mediated inhibition of bone resorption, and thus osteoclastic activity could be a predictor for pain response.

Further research is required to eventually allow physicians to employ the biochemical markers to predict the response and monitor the progress to systemic interventions and radiation therapy.

Long-term prognosis

We analysed prospectively 16 factors in 395 patients seen in a dedicated palliative radiotherapy clinic in a large tertiary cancer centre using Cox's proportional hazards regression model.[52] Bone metastases were diagnosed in 70 per cent of these patients.

Six prognostic factors had a statistically significant impact on survival: primary cancer site, site of metastases, Karnofsky Performance Score (KPS), and fatigue, appetite and shortness of breath scores from the modified Edmonton Symptom Assessment Scale. Risk group stratification was performed: (1) by assigning weights to the prognostic factors based on their levels of significance; and (2) by the number of risk factors present. The weighting method provided a Survival Prediction Score (SPS), ranging from 0 to 32. The survival probability at 3, 6 and 12 months was 83, 70, and 51 per cent respectively for patients with SPS < 13 (n = 133); 67, 41, and 20 per cent for patients with SPS 14–19 (n = 129); and 36, 18, and 4 per cent for patients with SPS ≥ 20 (n = 133) (p < 0.0001) (Table 24.1, Figure 24.1).

Corresponding survival probabilities based on number of risk factors were: 85, 72, and 52 per cent (< 3 risk factors) (n = 98); 68, 47, and 24 per cent (4 risk factors) (n = 117); and 46, 24, and 11 per cent (≥5 factors) (n = 180) (p < 0.0001) (Table 24.2, Figure 24.2).

Based on the final model, we generated three risk groups with different probabilities of survival using two different methods: (1) partial score method (Table 24.3) and (2) number of risk factors method (Table 24.4). The first method took into account the different prognostic weightings whereas the second assumed equal weighting among the six prognostic factors. Examples of using the SPS for specific patients are as follows:

> The SPS for a patient with breast cancer, bone metastases only, KPS = 70, fatigue score of 5, appetite score of 4 and shortness of breath score of 3 was: 0 + 0 + 0 + 4 + 0 +2 = 6 (Group A). The number of risk factors for her was 2 (Group 1).
>
> The SPS for a patient with prostate cancer, bone metastases only, KPS = 40, fatigue score of 9, appetite score of 6 and shortness of breath score of 2 was: 5 + 0 + 6 + 5 + 0 +2 = 18 (Group B). The number of risk factors for him was 4 (Group II).

Table 24.1 Risk groups based on the survival prediction scores (SPS)

Risk groups (SPS)	N	Survival at 3 months (%) (95% CI)	Survival at 6 months (%) (95 % CI)	Survival at 12 months (%) (95 % CI)	Median survival in weeks (95% CI)	P-value
A (0–13)	133	83 (77–90)	70 (62–78)	51 (42–60)	53 (38–70)	< 0.0001
B (14–19)	129	67 (59–76)	41 (33–50)	20 (13–27)	19 (17–26)	
C (20–32)	133	36 (28–44)	18 (11–24)	4 (1–7)	8 (6–10)	

N, number of patients.

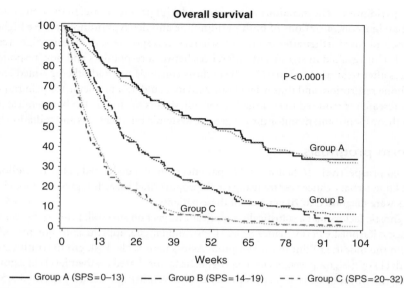

Figure 24.1 Risk group stratification by partial score method. Survival experiences of the three groups of patients identified by the SPS. Average estimated survival probabilities from Cox's model (dotted lines) and the actual outcome estimated by the Kaplan–Meier method (bold lines). SPS, survival perdiction scores.

Another patient with lung cancer, both bone and visceral metastases, KPS = 30, fatigue score of 10, appetite score of 9 and shortness of breath score of 9, had a SPS of 6 + 6 + 6 + 5 + 4 + 4 = 31 (Group C). He had 6 risk factors (Group III).

Their corresponding predicted survival can be obtained from Tables 24.3 and 24.4.

Our model based on simple clinical covariates proved to be effective in predicting survival and statistically significant in a multivariate analysis. The external validation is ongoing.

In summary, the advance in the care of patients with bone metastases not only requires a multidisciplinary approach of all the healthcare professionals involved, but also a reliable predictive model.

Table 24.2 Risk groups based on the total number of risk factors method

Risk groups (total number of risk factors)	N	Survival at 3 months (%) (95% CI)	Survival at 6 months (%) (95% CI)	Survival at 12 months (%) (95% CI)	Median survival in weeks (95% CI)	P-value
I (0–3)	98	85 (78–92)	72 (63–81)	52 (42–63)	62 (41–70)	< 0.0001
II (4)	117	68 (60–77)	47 (38–57)	24 (16–32)	24 (18–29)	
III (5–6)	180	46 (38–53)	24 (18–31)	11 (6–16)	11 (9–14)	

N, number of patients.

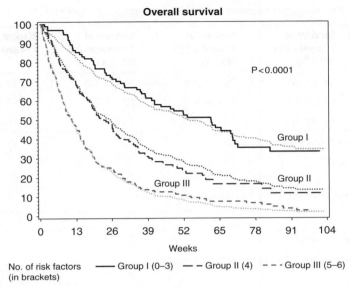

Figure 24.2 Risk group stratification by number of risk factors. Survival experiences of the three groups of patients identified the number of risk factors. Average estimated survival probabilities from Cox's model (dotted lines) and the actual outcome estimated by the Kaplan–Meier method (bold lines).

Table 24.3 Pocket reference table for survival prediction score (SPS)

	Partial score
1. Primary cancer site	
Breast	0
Prostate	5
Lung	6
Others	7
2. Site of metastases	
Bone only	0
Others	6
3. KPS	
> 50	0
≤ 50	6
4. Fatigue score	
0–3	0
4–7	4
8–10	5
5. Appetite score	
0–7	0
8–10	4
6. Shortness of breath score	
0	0
1–3	2
4–10	4

Table 24.3 (continued) Pocket reference table for survival prediction score (SPS)

Risk groups (SPS)	Survival at 3 months (%) (95% CI)	Survival at 6 months (%) (95% CI)	Survival at 12 months (%) (95 % CI)	Median survival (weeks) (95% CI)
A (0–13)	83 (77–90)	70 (62–78)	51 (42–60)	53 (38–70)
B (14–19)	67 (59–76)	41 (33–50)	20 (13–27)	19 (17–26)
C (20–32)	36 (28–44)	18 (11–24)	4 (1–7)	8 (6–10)

SPS, Sum of partial scores of the above six groups.

Table 24.4 Pocket reference table for number of risk factors

Six risk factors

1. Non breast cancer patients

2. Sites of metastases other than bone only

3. KPS ≤ 50

4. Fatigue score 4–10

5. Appetite score 8–10

6. Shortness of breath score 1–10

Risk groups (total number of risk factors)	Survival at 3 months (%) (95% CI)	Survival at 6 months (%) (95% CI)	Survival at 12 months (%) (95% CI)	Median survival in weeks (95% CI)
I (0–3)	85 (78–92)	72 (63–81)	52 (42–63)	62 (41–70)
II (4)	68 (60–77)	47 (38–57)	24 (16–32)	24 (18–29)
III (5–6)	46 (38–53)	24 (18–31)	11 (6–16)	11 (9–14)

References

1. Body JJ. Metastatic bone disease: clinical and therapeutic aspects. *Bone* 1992; 13(Suppl 1):S57–62.

2. Bilezikian JP. Management of acute hypercalcemia. *N Engl J Med* 1992; 326:1196–203.

3. Orr FW, Kostenick P, Sanchez-Sweatman OH, Singh G. Mechanisms involved in the metastasis of cancer to bone. *Breast Cancer Res Treat* 1993; 25:151–63.

4. Harrington KD. Prophylactic management of impending fractures. In KD Harrington KD (ed.) *Orthopedic Management of Metastatic Bone Disease*, pp. 283–307. St. Louis: CV Mosby; 1988.

5. Perez JE, Machiavelli M, Leone BA, Romero A, Rabinovich MG, Vallejo CT, Bianco A, Rodriguez R, Cuevas MA, Alvarez LA. Bone-only versus visceral-only metastatic pattern in breast cancer: analysis of 150 patients. *Am J Clin Oncl* 1990; 13:294–8.

6. Yamishita K, Ueda T, Komatsubara Y, Koyama H, Inaji H, Yonenobu K, Ono K. Breast cancer with bone-only metastases: visceral metastases-free rate in relation to anatomic distribution of bone metastases. *Cancer* 1991; 68:634–7.

7. Yamashita K, Ueda T, Komatsubara Y, Koyama H, Inaji H, Ono K, Yonenobu K (1992). A classification of bone metastases from breast cancer. In A Uchida, K Ono (eds) *Recent advances in musculoskeletal oncology*, pp. 254 Berlin: Springer-Verlag, 1992.

8. Yamishita K, Denno K, Ueda T, Komatsubara Y, Kotake T, Usami M, Maeda O, Nakano S, Hasegawa Y. Prognostic significance of bone metastases in patients with metastatic prostate cancer. *Cancer* 1993; 71:1297–302.

9. Coleman R, Rubens R. The clinical course of bone metastases from breast cancer. *British Journal of Cancer* 1987; 55:61–6.

10. Chow E, Connolly R, Franssen E, Fung KW, Vachon M, Andersson L, Schueller T, Stefaniuk K, Szumacher E, Hayter C, Pope J, Finkelstein J, Danjoux C. Prevalence of underdosage of cancer bone pain in patients referred for palliative radiotherapy and its potential implications in radiotherapy trials. *Annals The Royal College of Physicians and Surgeons of Canada* 2001; 34:217–22, 34: 290.

11. Yau V, Chow E, Davis L, Holden L, Schueller T, Danjoux C. Pain management in cancer patients with bone metastases remains a challenge. *Journal of Pain and Symptom Management* 2004; 27(1):1–3.

12. Conte P, Latreille L, Mauriac L. *et al.* Delay in progression of bone metastases in breast cancer patients treated with intravenous pamidronate: results from a multinational randomized controlled trial. *Journal of Clinical Oncology* 1996; 14:2552–9.

13. Diel I, Solomayer E, Costa S, Gollan C, Goerner R, Wallwiener D. *et al.* Reduction in new metastases in breast cancer with adjuvant clodronate treatment. *New England Journal of Medicine* 1998; 339:357–63.

14. Hortobagyi G, Theriault R, Porter L, Blayney D, Lipton A, Sinoff C. *et al.*. Efficacy of pamidronate in reducing skeletal complications in patients with breast cancer and lytic bone metastases. *New England Journal of Medicine* 1996; 335:1785–791.

15. Hortobagyi G, Theriault R, Lipton A, Porter L, Blayney D, Sinoff C. *et al.* Long-term prevention of skeletal complications of metastatic breast cancer with pamidronate. *Journal of Clinical Oncology* 1998; 16:2038–44.

16. Lipton A, Theriault RL, Hortobagyi GN, Simeone J, Knight RD, Mellars K, Reitsma DJ, Heffernan M, Seaman JJ. Pamidronate prevents skeletal complications and is effective palliative treatment in women with breast carcinoma and osteolytic bone metastases: long term follow-up of two randomized, placebo-controlled trials. *Cancer* 2000; 88(5):1082–90.

17. Paterson A, Powles T, Kanis J, McCloskey E, Hanson J, Ashley S. Double-blind controlled trial of oral clodronate in patients with bone metastases from breast cancer. *Journal of Clincal Oncology* 1993; 11:59–65.

18. Theriault RL, Lipton A, Hortobagyi GN, Leff R, Glück S, Stewart JF, Costello S, Kennedy I, Simeone J, Seaman JJ, Knight RD, Mellars K, Heffernan M, Reitsma DJ, for the Protocol 18 Aredia Breast Cancer Study Group. Pamidronate reduces skeletal morbidity in women with advanced breast cancer and lytic bone lesions: a randomized, placebo-controlled trial. *Journal of Clinical Oncology* 1999; 17(3):846–54.

19. Ross JR, Saunders Y, Edmonds PM. *et al.* Systematic review of role of bisphosphonates on skeletal morbidity in metastatic cancer. *BMJ* 2003; 327:469–72.

20. Bruce E, Hillner, James N, Ingle, Rowan T, Chlebowski, Julie Gralow, Gary C, Yee NA, Janjan JA, Cauley BA, Blumenstein KS, Albain A, Lipton SB. American Society of Clinical Oncology 2003 Update on the role of bisphosphonates and bone health issues in women with breast cancer *J of Clin Oncol* 2003; 21(21):4042–57.

21. Breast Cancer Disease Site Group. Use of bisphosphonates in patients with bone metastases from breast cancer. CCO Practice Guideline Initiative. 2004, Available at http://www.hiru.mcmaster.ca/ccopgi/guidelines/bre/cpg1_11.html.

22. Saad F, Gleason DM, Murray R, Tchekmedyian S, Venner P, Lacombe L, Chin JL, Vinholes JJ, Goas JA, Zheng M; Zoledronic Acid Prostate Cancer Study Group. Long-term efficacy of zoledronic acid for the prevention of skeletal complications in patients with metastatic hormone-refractory prostate cancer. *Natl Cancer Inst* 2004; 96(11):879–82.

23. Tong D, Gillick L, Hendrickson F. The palliation of symptomatic osseous metastases: final results of the study by the Radiation Therapy Oncology Group. *Cancer* 1982; 50:893–9.

24. Blitzer P. Reanalysis of the RTOG study of the palliation of symptomatic osseous metastases. *Cancer* 1985; 55:1468–72.

25. Chow E, Wu JS, Hoskin P, Coia LR, Bentzen SM, Blitzer PH. International consensus on palliative radiotherapy endpoints for future clinical trials in bone metastases. *Radiother Oncol* 2002; 64(3): 275–80.

26. Bone Pain Trial Working Party. 8 Gy single fraction radiotherapy for the treatment of metastatic skeletal pain: randomized comparison with multi-fraction schedule over 12 months of patient follow-up. *Radiother Oncol* 1999; 52:111–21.

27. Steenland E, Leer J, van Houwelingen H. *et al.* The effect of a single fraction compared to multiple fractions on painful bone metastases: a global analysis of the Dutch Bone Metastasis Study. *Radiother Oncol* 1999; 52:101–9.

28. Ratanatharathorn V, Powers W, Moss W. *et al.* Bone metastasis: review and critical analysis of random allocation trials of local field treatment. *Int J Radiat Oncol Biol Phys* 1999; 44:1–18.

29. Wu J, Wong R, Johnston M, Bezjak A, Whelan T. Meta-analysis of dose-fractionation radiotherapy trials for the palliation of painful bone metastases. *Int J Radiat Oncol Biol Phys* 2002; 55(3): 594–605.

30. Sze WM, Shelley MD, Held I. *et al.* Palliation of metastatic bone pain: single fraction versus multifraction radiotherapy-a systematic review of randomized trials. *Clin Oncol (R Coll Radiol)* 2003; 15:345–52.

31. Barton MB, Dawson R, Jacob S, Currow D, Stevens G, Morgan G. Palliative radiotherapy of bone metastases: an evaluation of outcome measures. *J Eval Clin Pract* 2001; 7(1): 47–64.

32. Poulter C, Cosmatos D, Rubin P. *et al.* A report of RTOG 8206: A phase III study of whether the addition of single dose hemibody irradiation to standard fractionated local field irradiation is more effective than local field irradiation alone in the treatment of symptomatic osseous metastases. *Int J Radiat Oncol Biol Phys* 1992; 23:207–14.

33. Porter A, McEwan A, Powe J. Results of a randomized phase III trial to evaluate the efficacy of Strontium-89 adjuvant to local field external beam irradiation in the management of endocrine-resistant metastatic prostate cancer. *Int J Radiat Oncol Biol Phys* 1993; 25:805–13.

34. Wai EK, Finkelstein JA, Tangente RP, Holden L, Chow E, Ford M. *et al.* Quality of life in surgical treatment of metastatic spine disease. *Spine* 2003; 28(5):508–12.

35. Wise JJ, Fischgrund JS, Herkowitz HN, Montgomery D, Kurz LT. Complication, survival rates, and risk factors of surgery for metastatic disease of the spine. *Spine* 1999; 24(18):1943–51.

36. Ghogawala Z, Mansfield FL, Borges LF. Spinal radiation before surgical decompression adversely affects outcomes of surgery for symptomatic metastatic spinal cord compression. *Spine* 2001; 26(7):818–24.

37. Fourney DR, Schomer DF, Nader R, Chlan-Fourney J, Suki D, Ahrar K. *et al.* Percutaneous vertebroplasty and kyphoplasty for painful vertebral body fractures in cancer patients. *J Neurosurg Spine* 2003; 98(1):21–30.

38. Amar AP, Larsen DW, Esnaashari N, Albuquerque FC, Lavine SD, Teitelbaum GP. Percutaneous transpedicular polymethylmethacrylate vertebroplasty for the treatment of spinal compression fractures. *Neurosurgery* 2001; 49(5):1105–14; discussion 1114–15.

39. Mathis JM, Barr JD, Belkoff SM, Barr MS, Jensen ME, Deramond H. Percutaneous vertebroplasty: a developing standard of care for vertebral compression fractures. *Am J Neuroradiol* 2001; 22(2):373–81.

40. Rodriguez-Catarino M. Percutaneous vertebroplasty – a new method for alleviation of back pain. *Lakartidningen* 2002; 99(9):882–90.

41. Ratliff J, Nguyen T, Heiss J. Root and spinal cord compression from methylmethacrylate vertebroplasty. *Spine* 2001; 26(13):E300–2.

42. Chow E, Holden L, Danjoux C, Yee A, Vidmar M, Connolly R. *et al.* Successful salvage using percutaneous vertebroplasty in cancer patients with painful spinal metastases or osteoporotic compression fractures. *Radiother Oncol* 2004; 70(3):265–7.

43. Harty JA, Brennan D, Eustace S, O'Byrne J. Percutaneous cementoplasty of acetabular bony metastasis. *Surgeon* 2003; 1(1):48–50.

44. Hodge JC. Cementoplasty and the oncologic population. *Singapore Med J* 2000; 41(8):407–9.

45. Chow E, Finkelstein J, Connolly R, Andersson L, Pope J, Axelrod T, Stephen D, Szumacher E, Wong R, Hayter C, Danjoux C. New combined bone metastases clinic: the ultimate one-stop for cancer patients with bone metastases. *Current Oncology* 2000; 7: 205–8.

46. Tannock IF, de Wit R, Berry WR, Horti J, Pluzanska A, Chi KN, Oudard S, Theodore C, James ND, Turesson I, Rosenthal MA, Eisenberger MA, TAX 327 Investigators. Docetaxel plus prednisone or mitoxantrone plus prednisone for advanced prostate cancer. *N Engl J Med* 2004; 351(15):1488–90.

47. Vinholes J, Guo CY, Purohit OP, Eastell R, Coleman RE. Metabolic effects of pamidronate in patients with metastatic bone disease. *Br J Cancer* 1996; 73(9):1089–95.

48. Lipton A, Demers L, Curley E, Chinchilli V, Gaydos L, Hortobagyi G, Theriault R, Clemens D, Costa L, Seaman J, Knight R. Markers of bone resorption in patients treated with pamidronate. *Eur J Cancer* 1998; 34(13):2021–6.

49. Vinholes JJ, Purohit OP, Abbey ME, Eastell R, Coleman RE. Relationships between biochemical and symptomatic response in a double-blind randomised trial of pamidronate for metastatic bone disease. *Ann Oncol* 1997; 8(12):1243–50.

50. Vinholes J, Guo CY, Purohit OP, Eastell R, Coleman RE. Evaluation of new bone resorption markers in a randomized comparison of pamidronate or clodronate for hypercalcemia of malignancy. *J Clin Oncol* 1997; 15(1):131–8.

51. Hoskin PJ, Stratford MRL, Folkes LK. *et al.* Effect of local radiotherapy for bone pain on urinary markers of osteoclast activity. *Lancet* 2000; 355:1428–9.

52. Chow E, Fung KW, Panzarella T, Bezjak A, Danjoux C, Tannock I. A predictive model for survival in metastatic cancer patients attending an out-patient palliative radiotherapy clinic. *International Journal of Radiation Oncology, Biology and Physics* 2002; 53(5):1291–302.

25

Brain secondaries

Andrew Broadbent and George Hruby

Introduction

In adults, brain metastases are about 10 times more frequent than primary brain tumours[1] and when appropriately managed are the direct cause of death in only 30–50 per cent of those affected.[2] They are detected either through the staging process, or more commonly following investigation of symptoms such as headache or focal weakness.

Numerically, lung, breast, renal cell and colon cancers account for the majority of brain metastases. Autopsy series comparing patterns of metastatic spread have shown that melanoma has a higher rate of spread to brain compared with other cancers.[3] These reported rates of brain metastasis range from 10–50 per cent for most malignancies,[4] and up to 75 per cent in those patients with disseminated melanoma.[1, 5]

Previously at least 50 per cent of those afflicted were thought to have multiple lesions.[6] Newer studies with better imaging techniques suggest that this may in fact be closer to 80 per cent.[7] Melanoma, lung cancer and breast cancer commonly present with multiple lesions, whilst renal cell cancer may present as a single lesion.[8] Almost 80 per cent of brain metastases are located in the supratentorial area; other sites of spread include the cerebellum (10–15 per cent) and brain stem (1–5 per cent). With the exception of small cell lung cancer, brain metastases tend to occur in patients who already have systemic metastases.[9]

The prognosis of a patient with brain metastases having conservative (supportive) treatment that does not involve corticosteroids or radiotherapy is thought to be approximately 4 weeks. This figure is based on one historical series.[10] Management options range from observation to craniotomy (in appropriate candidates) and include steroids, whole brain radiotherapy (WBRT), stereotactic radiosurgery (SRS) and/or chemotherapy and other systemic agents. Whole brain radiotherapy is the mainstay of treatment for brain metastases. Despite many clinical trials aimed at improving treatment outcomes, the median survival remains 3–6 months. More recently, other modalities of treatment such as radiosurgery and chemotherapy have been added, and are still being evaluated.

The natural history of brain metastases

Haematogenous spread is the commonest mechanism of spread, with deposition of metastases tending to occur at the interface of grey and white matter and also the watershed areas. These are the areas where the blood vessels are at their narrowest. Direct extension is the other method, whereby the tumour breaches the dura. This is reported in tumours arising from the base of skull or vertebrae, and in head and neck cancers.

A model on how brain metastases are established and grow is still being developed. Currently the 'seed and soil' hypothesis appears to be the best model. This has three principles in its definition.

1. Cancers are heterogeneous and have subpopulations of cells that have different properties that assist metastases

2. The process of dissemination self-selects those cells that will survive in a 'new' environment.

3. Successful implantation and growth of the metastasis depends on multiple factors such as angiogenesis and homeostatic mechanisms controlled by the tumour.

This has been supported by studies in animal models which show that the tumour cells must reach the vasculature of the brain, attach to the endothelial cells of the microvasculature, then extravasate to the parenchyma, proliferate due to growth factors and induce new blood vessel formation.[11]

The blood–brain barrier (BBB) may be the rate-limiting step in this model. This barrier not only limits the penetration of chemotherapy agents, but there is animal model evidence that it provides resistance to cell migration which may be due to the presence of laminin, fibronectin and type IV collagen as well as the basement membrane.[12] Damage to the BBB from ischemia, oedema or surgery may increase the ability of metastases to migrate across.[13, 14]

As cerebral scanning is not routinely performed unless symptomatic, most patients have symptoms at diagnosis. The symptoms are variable depending on area of deposition. Symptoms may include headache, cognitive changes, focal weakness, speech difficulties and reduced coordination.

Features of end stage disease from cerebral metastases include symptoms of raised intracranial pressure (nausea, vomiting, headaches that are worse in the mornings etc.), increasing focal symptoms from tumour mass, (weakness, sensory changes, speech, cranial nerve dysfunction and ataxia), epilepsy and cognitive dysfunction.

Late signs from raised intracranial pressure include coning of the cerebral peduncles with resultant change to a deep coma and a Cheyne–Stokes respiratory pattern, suggesting a prognosis of a few hours.

Without treatment, cerebral metastases are the cause of death in most patients, however treatment with radiotherapy may reduce this to less than 50 per cent.[15] Use of corticosteroids may temporarily delay the progression of symptoms by reducing oedema, usually with significant response by 24 hours of commencing, and peak effect within 5 days. Up to 70 per cent of patients will benefit from the use of corticosteroids, particularly those with oedema causing raised intracranial pressure, rather than focal signs.[16] There is no proven link between response to steroids and response to radiotherapy.

Quality of life decisions need to be considered regarding treatment. Steroid side-effects of cushingnoid features, PUD, proximal myopathy, osteoporosis, poor wound healing, mood changes and hypertension are the main ones to consider. Short-term side-effects secondary to WBRT such as alopecia, fatigue, nausea, scalp erythema, radiation parotitis and skin dryness may occur. Long-term side-effects such as cognitive impairment and ataxia are generally not an issue due to poor survival.

As only approximately 25 per cent of patients with cerebral metastases will develop seizures,[15] anti-epileptics are not usually commenced as prophylaxis. There is no evidence that they prevent first time seizures when caused by metastases.

Factors affecting prognosis

Prognostic factors have been identified in the management of brain metastases in several studies. Those most consistently reported include performance status, number of brain metastases, resection, the presence of extracranial disease and age.[2, 17] Factors such as site of primary[18, 19] and

Table 25.1 Univariate prognostic factors in brain metastases[2]

Covariate	Comparison	p-value
Brain metastases	Alone versus with other metastases	< 0.0001
Karnofsky Performance Status	> = 70 versus < 70	< 0.0001
Age	< 65 versus > = 65	< 0.0001
Primary site	Breast versus lung and others	0.001
Primary lesion	Controlled versus uncontrolled	< 0.0001
Histology	Squamous and small cell versus others	< 0.0001
Neurologic function	No dysfunction versus some dysfunction	< 0.0001
Total radiation dose	> = 52 Gy versus < 52 Gy	< 0.0001
Time interval from diagnosis of primary to brain metastases	< 2 years versus > 2 years	0.004

From Gaspar L, Scott C, Rotman M, Asbell S, Phillips T, Wasserman T. *et al*. Recursive partitioning analysis (RPA) of prognostic factors in three Radiation Therapy Oncology Group (RTOG) brain metastases trials. *Radiation, Oncology, Biology and Physics* 1997; 37(4):745–51. Reproduced with permission of Elsevier Inc. (c) 1997.

histology[20] are more variably reported. Both Lagerwaard[18] and Priestman[19] found that breast cancer patients survived longer than those with lung cancer, although other studies have not confirmed this.

Gaspar[2] retrospectively examined a multicentre database comprising 1200 patients pooled from three consecutive randomized RTOG trials performed between 1979 and 1993. All trials involved various dose/fractionation regimes of WBRT, some patients also received radiosensitizers.[21–23] On univariate analysis (see Table 25.1), prognostic factors indicate a survival difference according to KPS, age, number of brain metastases, status and site of origin of primary lesion, and the time interval between presentation of primary and brain metastases.

After multivariate analysis three classes of patients were derived based on the four following prognostic factors: Karnofsky performance status (KPS), primary tumour status, presence of extracranial metastases and patient age. These three categories (or classes) were subsequently validated,[24] and corroborated by Neider.[25] In Neider's study (of 528 patients treated at a single German institution with either WBRT or surgery and WBRT), only 3 per cent of patients fell into the most favourable category (class 1).

The categories are defined as follows:

- Class 1 is age < 65, KPS ≥ 70, controlled primary and no extracranial metastases.
- Class 2 is defined as those patients, who were neither class 1 nor 3.
- Class 3 is KPS < 70, irrespective of age, primary status or metastases.

The median survival for classes 1, 2 and 3 was 7.1, 4.2, and 2.3 months respectively. It must be noted that although classes 1 and 3 are clearly delineated, class 2 covers a wider range of survivals. Neider noted that class 2 patients with controlled primary tumours had median survivals approaching those of class 1 patients.

Despite the limitations noted above, these categories would appear to be the best guide in terms of prognostication for those being considered for WBRT. It may also be helpful in selecting patients for more or less aggressive treatments.

Therapy affecting prognosis

Survival with cerebral metastases is generally poor, with very few long-term survivors. The survival data for some representative studies is summarized in Table 25.2, and further discussed in the following sections.

Table 25.2 Selected survival studies by treatment allocation

Study	Treatment	Number of patients	Median survival (months)
Radiotherapy			
Borgelt et al. 1981[34]	WBRT 1200 cGy/1 fr	26	3.5
	WBRT 2000 cGy/5 fr	129	2.8 p > 0.05
WBRT alone versus Surgery			
Patchell et al. 1990[37]	WBRT alone	23	3.5
	WBRT + surgery	25	10 p = <0.01
Vecht et al. 1994[49]	WBRT alone	31	6.5
	WBRT + surgery	32	10.5 p = 0.04
Mintz et al.[30]	WBRT alone	41	6
	WBRT + surgery	41	5.5 p = 0.24
Surgery alone versus Surgery and WBRT			
Patchell et al. 1998[41]	Surgery alone	46	10.5
	Surgery + WBRT	49	12 p = 0.39
Stereotactic radiosurgery			
Kondziolka et al. 1999[28]	WBRT	14	7.5
	WBRT and SRS	13	11 p = 0.22
Andrews et al 2004(40) (single brain metastasis)	WBRT	94	4.9
	WBRT and SRS	92	6.5 p = 0.0393
Chemotherapy			
Antonadou et al. 2002[45]	WBRT (for metastatic cancer to the brain)	21	7
	WBRT and temozolamide	24	8.6 p = 0.447
Robinet et al. 2001[44]	Early WBRT (for metastatic non-small cell cancer to the brain)	85	5.25
	Delayed WBRT with chemotherapy chemotherapy	86	6 p = 0.83
Radiosensitizers			
Mehta et al. 2002[47]	3000 cGy/10 fr	208	4.9
	3000 cGy/10 fr and motexafin gadolinium	193	5.2 p = 0.48
Suh et al. 2005[48]	WBRT	250	4.4
	WBRT and efaproxiral	265	5.4 p = 0.16

Corticosteroids

There are no randomizsed controlled trials (RCT) of steroids versus best supportive care, and there is only one randomized trial of steroids with or without WBRT.[26] This trial of steroids with or without WBRT included only 48 patients, it lacked statistical analysis, and the trial predated computed tomoraphy (CT) scanning. Median survival in this trial was 10 versus 14 weeks for the steroid alone and combined treatment arms respectively (no p value stated).

WBRT

In a systematic review on the effectiveness of WBRT, Pease[27] has suggested that with no treatment there is a survival of approximately of 1 month in patients managed with best supportive care only. The use of corticosteroids may increase survival time for up to 2 months, although there is no randomized evidence to support this.

The treatment of brain metastases from solid tumours with whole brain radiotherapy (WBRT) and corticosteroids is a recognized standard treatment. Despite reported response rates of 50–75 per cent, survival is poor, with a median survival of 3–6 months after radiotherapy for those with multiple metastases.[28, 29, 30, 31] Response to radiotherapy may take up to 1 month and during this time, up to 30 per cent of patients will die from their extracranial disease.[32]

Effects of dose

Radiotherapy regimens used for the treatment of brain secondaries vary, however altered dose/fractionation schedules do not consistently influence survival in randomized trials.[33, 34, 35, 36] In a systematic review and meta-analysis, Tsao reviewed nine RCTs studying various dose-fractionation schedules for WBRT. There was no difference in survival outcomes. Furthermore, in the Lagerwaard study (the largest retrospective cohort), where 76 per cent of patients received either 30 Gy in 10 fractions or 20 Gy in 5 fractions, dose was also not found to be significant.

Craniotomy

Three randomized trials have examined the role of metastatectomy in single brain metastases in addition to WBRT. In 1990, Patchell[37] demonstrated, in a study of 48 patients with KPS > 70, a survival of approximately 10 months for those having resection versus 3.5 months in those without resection (p < 0.01). Noordijk[38] confirmed this finding in a study of 63 evaluable patients (with good performance status) with median survivals of 10 months with resection compared to 6 months without (p = 0.04). In the largest series, Mintz[30] randomized 84 patients but did not find any significant difference in survival. Median survival for both arms was only 5–6 months. However, this study included patients with fair to good (KPS 50 or more) performance status (suggesting that extracranial disease may have been a significant contributor to mortality), which may have limited the potential benefit of more aggressive CNS treatment. In contrast to the other two trials, the Patchell trial was the only one that mandated MRI to confirm the CT finding of a single lesion.

In appropriately selected patients, the above results appear to be generalizable. In 2 retrospective WBRT series, the survival for patients with a single brain metastasis treated with surgery and WBRT was 8–9 months versus 3–4 months for WBRT alone.[18, 20] In our experience, patients undergoing resection for more than one metastasis (n = 22) had a median survival of 5 months compared to 8 months for those who had resection of a single brain metastasis (p = 0.01).

There are other reasons for removing or debulking metastases, for example, obstructive hydrocephalus can be improved. Reduction of steroid requirements and improving some neurological symptoms are other possible benefits. In the case of a solitary brain metastasis without a known primary site, there is a case for resection to establish histological confirmation. However, it should be noted that not all metastases can be resected due to their anatomical position.

Stereotactic radiosurgery

A retrospective series and one RCT suggest improved outcomes with the use of stereotactic radiosurgery.[28, 39] Again benefit appears confined to those with solitary metastasis and excellent performance status. The RTOG 95–08 RCT[40] examined those with 1–3 metastases (in those with metastases deemed unresectable or where trial patients were not medically fit for surgery) randomized to either WBRT alone (167 patients) or WBRT + SRS boost (164 patients). In this trial, the addition of SRS improved survival in patients with a single lesion, from 4.9 (WBRT alone) to 6.5 months (WBRT + SRS). Those further selected patients who had both a single lesion on MRI and were Gaspar class 1, had a median survival of 9.6 months (46 patients with WBRT alone) versus 11.6 months (45 patients with WBRT and SRS).

Addition of WBRT to craniotomy

Patchell's[41] subsequent 1998 trial of 95 patients showed improved intracranial control with surgical resection (reduction in brain tumour recurrence) and WBRT when compared to resection alone, although there was no significant difference in length of functional independence with the addition of WBRT. Median survival was not significantly different between the two treatment arms, 12 months for postoperative radiotherapy, and 10.5 months without.

Chemotherapy

Traditional chemotherapy agents have not been a standard treatment for brain metastases for several reasons, including the role of the blood–brain barrier, resistance to chemotherapy, and systemic side-effects reducing quality of life. Several studies have shown an increased tumour response rate, but no increase in survival.[42–44]

A newer agent, temozolamide, which easily crosses the blood–brain barrier and has fewer toxic side-effects, has recently been studied. One study of 45 patients comparing temozolamide plus WBRT with WBRT alone showed an increased response rate, but no increase in survival.[45] Thalidomide has also been studied in a dose-finding trial, but without any survival benefit.[46]

Radiosensitizers

Tsao[8] examined the combinations of WBRT and radiosensitizers (five randomized controlled trials). Consistent with the absence of a dose response with WBRT alone, the combination treatment did not enhance survival; neither did addition of chemotherapy with WBRT (5 RCT). One of these studies involved over 400 patients in a randomized trial of motexafin gadolinium and whole-brain radiation therapy,[47] where survival increased from 4.9 months to 5.2 months, although without statistical significance.

Most recently, the use of efaproxiral,[48] a non-cytotoxic radiosensitizer and a modifier of the hypoxic state in a study of over 500 patients, did not improve survival statistically significantly when added to WBRT.

Short- and long-term prognosis

Briefly, those treated with best supportive care including corticosteroids survive 1–2 months with little hope of long-term survival (LTS). Patients selected for WBRT will generally survive

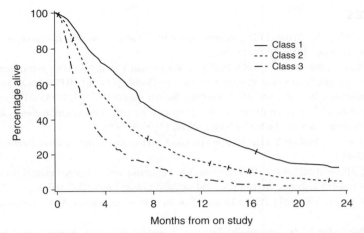

Figure 25.1 Survival curve for RPA classes from Gaspar's analysis. From Gaspar L, Scott C, Rotman M, Asbell S, Phillips T, Wasserman T. *et al*. Recursive partitioning analysis (RPA) of prognostic factors in three Radiation Therapy Oncology Group (RTOG) brain metastases trials. *Radiation, Oncology, Biology and Physics* 1997; 37(4):745–51. Reproduced with permission of Elsevier Inc. (c) 1997.

2–7 months with rare LTS. Finally those highly selected patients who undergo craniotomy and/or SRS may survive up to 1 year with a few LTS.

For patients treated with WBRT, Lagerwaard[18] quoted a median survival of 3.4 months with 1 and 2 year survivals of 12 and 4 per cent respectively. Outcomes in the Priestman[19] trial were somewhat poorer with a median survival of 79 days, and a 6-month survival of either 17 or 25 per cent depending upon radiotherapy schedule. As one of the treatment arms consisted of 12 Gy in two fractions, the patients referred to this study may have been less favourable. In previous RTOG studies, the median survival ranged from 18–20 weeks.[33, 36]

Gaspar's[2] analysis of survival for the three prognostic classes were 7.1 months, 4.2 months and 2.3 months respectively. Figure 25.1 shows the survival curves for the three classes from Gaspar's analysis, where even the best prognostic group has a 2-year survival of less than 20 per cent.

The small numbers in the three trials of WBRT[30, 37, 49] with or without surgical resection, which consisted of highly selected patients, make it difficult to generalize the results. Reported 2 year survivals are less than 20 per cent.[37, 49]

Patchell's 1998[41] trial of postoperative WBRT for single brain metastases did not document long term or 2-year survival. Length of time until tumour recurrence, and time to death due to neurological causes were improved in the adjuvant radiotherapy arm.

Long-term survival for patients with WBRT and a radiosurgery boost was examined in a RTOG trial.[40] Patients with either one metastasis, class 1 prognostic factors or those whose largest metastases was less than 2 cm in diameter and who had SRS and WBRT had the best survival. The 2-year survival for the above patients was less than 20 per cent.

Future studies will need to look at the impact on quality of life and functional status. It is not so easy to differentiate the beneficial effects of dexamethasone versus WBRT in the short term.[50] Further work, particularly in the palliative situation, might be to better define the patients for whom radiotherapy is inappropriate.

References

1. Walker AE, Robins M, Weinfeld FD. Epidemiology of brain tumors: the national survey of intracranial neoplasms. *Neurology* 1985; 35(2):219–26.

2. Gaspar L, Scott C, Rotman M, Asbell S, Phillips T, Wasserman T. *et al.* Recursive partitioning analysis (RPA) of prognostic factors in three Radiation Therapy Oncology Group (RTOG) brain metastases trials. *International Journal of Radiation Oncology, Biology, Physics* 1997; 37(4):745–51.

3. Patel JK, Didolkar MS, Pickren JW, Moore RH. Metastatic pattern of malignant melanoma. A study of 216 autopsy cases. *American Journal of Surgery* 1978; 135(6):807–10.

4. Pickren J, Lopez G, Tsukada Y, Lane W. Brain metastases: an autopsy study. *Cancer Treatment Symposia* 1983; 2:295–313.

5. Amer MH, Al-Sarraf M, Baker LH, Vaitkevicius VK. Malignant melanoma and central nervous system metastases: incidence, diagnosis, treatment and survival. *Cancer* 1978; 42(2):660–8.

6. Delattre JY, Krol G, Thaler HT, Posner JB. Distribution of brain metastases. *Archives of Neurology* 1988; 45(7):741–4.

7. Schaefer PW, Budzik RF Jr, Gonzalez RG. Imaging of cerebral metastases. *Neurosurgery Clinics of North America* 1996; 7(3):393–423.

8. Tsao MN, Lloyd NS, Wong RK, Rakovitch E, Chow E, Laperriere N. *et al.* Radiotherapeutic management of brain metastases: a systematic review and meta-analysis. *Cancer Treatment Reviews* 2005; 31(4):256–73.

9. Puduvalli VA, TS. Mangement of patients with brain metastases. In SBE Booth (ed.) *Primary and metastatic brain tumours*, pp. 31–57. Oxford: Oxford University Press; 2004.

10. DiStefano A, Yong Yap Y, Hortobagyi GN, Blumenschein GR. The natural history of breast cancer patients with brain metastases. *Cancer* 1979; 44(5):1913–8.

11. Schackert G, Fidler IJ. Site-specific metastasis of mouse melanomas and a fibrosarcoma in the brain or meninges of syngeneic animals. *Cancer Research* 1988; 48(12):3478–84.

12. Bernstein JJ, Woodard CA. Glioblastoma cells do not intravasate into blood vessels. *Neurosurgery* 1995; 36(1):124–32; discussion 132.

13. Zhang ZG, Zhang L, Jiang Q, Zhang R, Davies K, Powers C. *et al.* VEGF enhances angiogenesis and promotes blood–brain barrier leakage in the ischemic brain. *Journal of Clinical Investigation* 2000; 106(7):829–38.

14. Dietrich WD. The importance of brain temperature in cerebral injury. *Journal of Neurotrauma* 1992; 9(Suppl 2):S475–85.

15. Posner JB. Pathogenesis of central nervous system paraneoplastic syndromes. *Revue Neurologique* 1992; 148(6–7):502–12.

16. Gutin PH. Corticosteroid therapy in patients with cerebral tumors: benefits, mechanisms, problems, practicalities. *Seminars in Oncology* 1975; 2(1):49–56.

17. Auchter RM, Lamond JP, Alexander E, Buatti JM, Chappell R, Friedman WA. *et al.* A multiinstitutional outcome and prognostic factor analysis of radiosurgery for resectable single brain metastasis. *International Journal of Radiation Oncology, Biology, Physics* 1996; 35(1):27–35.

18. Lagerwaard FJ, Levendag PC, Nowak PJ, Eijkenboom WM, Hanssens PE, Schmitz PI. Identification of prognostic factors in patients with brain metastases: a review of 1292 patients. *International Journal of Radiation Oncology, Biology, Physics* 1999; 43(4):795–803.

19. Priestman TJ, Dunn J, Brada M, Rampling R, Baker PG. Final results of the Royal College of Radiologists' trial comparing two different radiotherapy schedules in the treatment of cerebral metastases. *Clinical Oncology (Royal College of Radiologists)* 1996; 8(5):308–15.

20. Broadbent AM, Hruby G, Tin MM, Jackson M, Firth I. Survival following whole brain radiation treatment for cerebral metastases: an audit of 474 patients. *Radiotherapy & Oncology* 2004; 71(3):259–65.

21. Sause WT, Crowley JJ, Morantz R, Rotman M, Mowry PA, Bouzaglou A. *et al.* Solitary brain metastasis: results of an RTOG/SWOG protocol evaluation surgery + RT versus RT alone. *American Journal of Clinical Oncology* 1990; 13(5):427–32.

22. Komarnicky LT, Phillips TL, Martz K, Asbell S, Isaacson S, Urtasun R. A randomized phase III protocol for the evaluation of misonidazole combined with radiation in the treatment of patients with brain metastases (RTOG-7916). *International Journal of Radiation Oncology, Biology, Physics* 1991; 20(1):53–8.

23. Phillips TL, Scott CB, Leibel SA, Rotman M, Weigensberg IJ. Results of a randomized comparison of radiotherapy and bromodeoxyuridine with radiotherapy alone for brain metastases: report of RTOG trial 89–05. *International Journal of Radiation Oncology, Biology, Physics* 1995; 33(2):339–48.

24. Gaspar LE, Scott C, Murray K, Curran W. Validation of the RTOG recursive partitioning analysis (RPA) classification for brain metastases. *International Journal of Radiation Oncology, Biology, Physics* 2000; 47(4):1001–6.

25. Nieder C, Nestle U, Motaref B, Walter K, Niewald M, Schnabel K. Prognostic factors in brain metastases: should patients be selected for aggressive treatment according to recursive partitioning analysis (RPA) classes? *International Journal of Radiation Oncology, Biology, Physics* 2000; 46(2):297–302.

26. Horton J, Baxter DH, Olson KB. The management of metastases to the brain by irradiation and corticosteroids. *American Journal of Roentgenology, Radium Therapy & Nuclear Medicine* 1971; 111(2):334–6.

27. Pease NJ, Edwards A, Moss LJ. Effectiveness of whole brain radiotherapy in the treatment of brain metastases: a systematic review. *Palliative Medicine* 2005; 19(4):288–99.

28. Kondziolka D, Patel A, Lunsford LD, Kassam A, Flickinger JC. Stereotactic radiosurgery plus whole brain radiotherapy versus radiotherapy alone for patients with multiple brain metastases. *International Journal of Radiation Oncology, Biology, Physics* 1999; 45(2):427–34.

29. Kurtz JM, Gelber R, Brady LW, Carella RJ, Cooper JS. The palliation of brain metastases in a favorable patient population: a randomized clinical trial by the Radiation Therapy Oncology Group. *International Journal of Radiation Oncology, Biology, Physics* 1981; 7(7):891–5.

30. Mintz AH, Kestle J, Rathbone MP, Gaspar L, Hugenholtz H, Fisher B. *et al.* A randomized trial to assess the efficacy of surgery in addition to radiotherapy in patients with a single cerebral metastasis. *Cancer* 1996; 78(7):1470–6.

31. Hall WA, Djalilian HR, Nussbaum ES, Cho KH. Long-term survival with metastatic cancer to the brain. *Medical Oncology|Medical Oncology (Totowa)* 2000; 17(4):279–86.

32. Edwards A, Gerrard G. The management of cerebral metastases. *Eur J. Pall Care* 1998; 5(1):7–11.

33. Borgelt B, Gelber R, Kramer S, Brady LW, Chang CH, Davis LW. *et al.* The palliation of brain metastases: final results of the first two studies by the Radiation Therapy Oncology Group. *International Journal of Radiation Oncology, Biology, Physics* 1980; 6(1):1–9.

34. Borgelt B, Gelber R, Larson M, Hendrickson F, Griffin T, Roth R. Ultra-rapid high dose irradiation schedules for the palliation of brain metastases: final results of the first two studies by the Radiation Therapy Oncology Group. *International Journal of Radiation Oncology, Biology, Physics* 1981; 7(12):1633–8.

35. Haie-Meder C, Pellae-Cosset B, Laplanche A, Lagrange JL, Tuchais C, Nogues C. *et al.* Results of a randomized clinical trial comparing two radiation schedules in the palliative treatment of brain metastases. *Radiotherapy & Oncology* 1993; 26(2):111–16.

36. Gelber RD, Larson M, Borgelt BB, Kramer S. Equivalence of radiation schedules for the palliative treatment of brain metastases in patients with favorable prognosis. *Cancer* 1981; 48(8):1749–53.

37. Patchell RA, Tibbs PA, Walsh JW, Dempsey RJ, Maruyama Y, Kryscio RJ. *et al.* A randomized trial of surgery in the treatment of single metastases to the brain. *New England Journal of Medicine* 1990; 322(8):494–500.

38. Noordijk EM, Vecht CJ, Haaxma-Reiche H, Padberg GW, Voormolen JH, Hoekstra FH. *et al*. The choice of treatment of single brain metastasis should be based on extracranial tumor activity and age. *International Journal of Radiation Oncology, Biology, Physics* 1994; 29(4):711–17.

39. Jyothirmayi R, Saran FH, Jalali R, Perks J, Warrington AP, Traish D. *et al*. Stereotactic radiotherapy for solitary brain metastases. *Clinical Oncology (Royal College of Radiologists)* 2001; 13(3):228–34.

40. Andrews DW, Scott CB, Sperduto PW, Flanders AE, Gaspar LE, Schell MC. *et al*. Whole brain radiation therapy with or without stereotactic radiosurgery boost for patients with one to three brain metastases: phase III results of the RTOG 9508 randomised trial. *Lancet* 2004; 363(9422):1665–72.

41. Patchell RA, Tibbs PA, Regine WF, Dempsey RJ, Mohiuddin M, Kryscio RJ. *et al*. Postoperative radiotherapy in the treatment of single metastases to the brain: a randomized trial. *JAMA* 1998; 280(17):1485–9.

42. Postmus PE, Haaxma-Reiche H, Smit EF, Groen HJ, Karnicka H, Lewinski T. *et al*. Treatment of brain metastases of small cell lung cancer: comparing teniposide and teniposide with whole-brain radiotherapy – a phase III study of the European Organization for the Research and Treatment of Cancer Lung Cancer Cooperative Group. *Journal of Clinical Oncology* 2000; 18(19):3400–8.

43. Bernardo G, Cuzzoni Q, Strada MR, Bernardo A, Brunetti G, Jedrychowska I. *et al*. First-line chemotherapy with vinorelbine, gemcitabine, and carboplatin in the treatment of brain metastases from non-small cell lung cancer: a phase II study. *Cancer Investigation* 2002; 20(3):293–302.

44. Robinet G, Thomas P, Breton JL, Lena H, Gouva S, Dabouis G. *et al*. Results of a phase III study of early versus delayed whole brain radiotherapy with concurrent cisplatin and vinorelbine combination in inoperable brain metastasis of non-small cell lung cancer: Groupe Francais de Pneumo-Cancerologie (GFPC) Protocol 95–1. *Annals of Oncology* 2001; 12(1):59–67.

45. Antonadou D, Paraskevaidis M, Sarris G, Coliarakis N, Economou I, Karageorgis P. *et al*. Phase II randomized trial of temozolomide and concurrent radiotherapy in patients with brain metastases. *Journal of Clinical Oncology* 2002; 20(17):3644–50.

46. Hwu WJ, Krown SE, Panageas KS, Menell JH, Chapman PB, Livingston PO. *et al*. Temozolomide plus thalidomide in patients with advanced melanoma: results of a dose-finding trial. [see comment] [erratum appears in *J Clin Oncol* 2002; 20(15):3361]. *Journal of Clinical Oncology* 2002; 20(11):2610–5.

47. Mehta MP, Rodrigus P, Terhaard CH, Rao A, Suh J, Roa W. *et al*. Survival and neurologic outcomes in a randomized trial of motexafin gadolinium and whole-brain radiation therapy in brain metastases. *Journal of Clinical Oncology* 2003; 21(13):2529–36.

48. Suh JH, Stea B, Nabid A, Kresl JJ, Fortin A, Mercier JP. *et al*. Phase III study of efaproxiral as an adjunct to whole-brain radiation therapy for brain metastases. *Journal of Clinical Oncology* 2006; 24(1):106–14.

49. Vecht CJ, Haaxma-Reiche H, Noordijk EM, Padberg GW, Voormolen JH, Hoekstra FH. *et al*. Treatment of single brain metastasis: radiotherapy alone or combined with neurosurgery? *Annals of Neurology* 1993; 33(6):583–90.

50. Bezjak A, Adam J, Barton R, Panzarella T, Laperriere N, Wong CS. *et al*. Symptom response after palliative radiotherapy for patients with brain metastases. *European Journal of Cancer* 2002; 38(4):487–96.

26

Leptomeningeal disease

Vicki Jackson and Lida Nabati

Leptomeningeal metastases are an important, yet relatively infrequent, complication of malignancy. Leptomeningeal metastases are found in 5 per cent of all patients with cancer,[1] but are believed to be increasing in frequency, due to more successful treatment options for the underlying malignancy. Prolonged survival, coupled with improvements in neuroimaging, has increased the detection of leptomeningeal metastases. Overall, leptomeningeal metastasis suggests a very poor prognosis, with a median survival of 1 month for untreated patients.[1] The range of survival for patients with leptomeningeal metastases is quite broad (Table 26.1), with some patients surviving months to even years after diagnosis. The variability of survival appears to be related to the type and chemosensitivity of the primary tumour.

The leptomeninges consist of the pia and arachnoid membrane. Metastases to these structures are often a late complication of both solid and haematologic malignancies, as well as from primary central nervous system (CNS) tumours. Although leptomeningeal metastases can be the result of any malignancy, the tumours most commonly associated with leptomeningeal metastases include small cell and non-small cell lung cancer, breast cancer, melanoma and non-Hodgkin's lymphoma[2] (Table 26.2). The high frequency of leptomeningeal metastases in acute lymphoblastic leukemia has led to prophylactic treatment in children and adults.

Natural history

Patients with leptomeningeal metastases commonly present with headache, change in mental status or localizing neurologic signs and symptoms at more than one level of the neuroaxis. Cranial nerve abnormalities occur in over 50 per cent of patients at the time of diagnosis.[3] Pain affects 80 per cent of patients, with diffuse headache in 25 per cent and pain in a spinal, radicular, or meningeal pattern in 50 per cent.[2, 4]

Table 26.1 Range and median survival reported in selected treatment series

Study	Survival range	Median survival
Jayson et al.[7]	1–1261 days	77 days
Wasserstrom et al.[3]	1–29 months	5.8 months
Herrlinger et al.[6]	–	4.8 months
Fizazi et al.[8]	?–868 days	67 days
Grant et al.[19]	2–33 weeks	9 weeks
Grossman et al.[15]	14 days–110.5+ weeks†	15.9, 14.1 weeks*

† One patient still alive at last follow-up at 110.5+ weeks.

* Respective median survival for patients treated with methotrexate and thiotepa.

Table 26.2 Frequency of leptomeningeal metastasis by primary malignancies

Primary malignancy	Frequency (%)
Lung	15
Small cell lung cancer	1
Non-small cell lung cancer	
Breast	5
Skin melanoma	5
Head and neck	1
Prostate	Rare
Leukaemia	5–15
Lymphoma	6

Adapted from Kesari S. and Batchelor T. (2003) Leptomeningeal metastases. *Neurol Clin N Am* 21, 25–66; with permission.

In general, patients with leptomeningeal metastases die from complications of systemic disease. Another 5–10 per cent die from treatment-related complications.[1] While numerous treatment modalities exist, few have been shown in randomized trials to significantly impact neurologic status, quality of life or survival. Factors affecting prognosis, as well as therapies affecting survival and outcome, are discussed below.

Diagnosis and evaluation

Advances in radiologic imaging have improved our ability to diagnose leptomeningeal metastases. On gadolinium-enhanced magnetic resonance imaging (MRI), patients with leptomeningeal metastases demonstrate enhancement of the leptomeninges, ventricular surface, cranial nerves or spinal roots.

The diagnosis of leptomeningeal metastases is confirmed by the presence of malignant cells in cerebrospinal fluid (CSF). However, not all patients with leptomeningeal metastases will have malignant cells detectable in the CSF: 50 per cent of patients have an initial lumbar puncture (LP) that is negative for malignant cells, but about 90 per cent will have a positive cytologic exam after three LPs.[3] Hence, multiple LPs are often necessary to make a definitive diagnosis. Initial CSF studies frequently reveal increased protein, reduced glucose, a lymphocytic pleocytosis and an elevated opening pressure.[2]

Experts recommend that patients with leptomeningeal metastases have a CSF flow study to help determine the appropriateness of intrathecal treatment (IT).[5] Subarachnoid CSF block occurs in up to 70 per cent of patients and is a poor prognostic sign.[2] CSF block is an indicator of greater overall tumour burden and makes IT less effective because chemotherapeutic agents are not able to penetrate all affected CNS sites.[5]

Factors affecting prognosis

Tumour type

The presence of leptomeningeal metastases disease generally indicates a poor prognosis. However, survival depends on many factors, the most important of which is tumour type.

Median survival for patients with leptomeningeal metastases arising from non-small cell lung cancer is 6 months, from breast cancer is 7.5 months and from non-AIDS related lymphoma is 10 months[1] (Table 26.3).

Prognosis for breast cancer patients with leptomeningeal metastasis is better than for patients with other solid tumours who develop leptomeningeal metastases,[3, 6] probably due to greater chemosensitivity of breast cancer. Though lobular type tumours are the less common form of breast cancer, in patients with breast cancer and leptomeningeal metastases, they are represented to a greater extent.[7, 8]

Other factors affecting prognosis

Studies have identified multiple other factors that influence prognosis, however there is little consensus in the literature. Presented here are the factors that have been consistently shown to be of prognostic import (Table 26.4).

In a retrospective multivariate analysis of 58 breast cancer patients with leptomeningeal metastases, five markers of poor prognosis were identified. These were an age greater than 55, the presence of lung metastases, a reduced CSF glucose level, an elevated CSF protein level and cranial nerve involvement.[8] Another study found that the extent of pre-treatment CNS disease was the best predictor of response to combined modality therapy.[10] This is supported by research showing that a block of CSF flow, due to bulky CNS disease, suggests a poor prognosis.[11] Sherman et al. found that pre-treatment cognitive status, assessed by neuropsychological testing, was not only predictive of survival but also useful in tracking disease course over time.[12]

Performance status (PS) is also an important prognostic factor.[7] Data is conflicting about its independent correlation with survival.[12, 13] PS appears to be most important in determining appropriateness for treatment, which, in turn, may influence survival. Many studies exclude patients with a poor performance status for treatment, and current NCCN guidelines recommend stratifying patients into poor or acceptable treatment risk categories based on PS.[5]

Therapies affecting survival

Treatment is often unsuccessful due to the presence of diffuse CNS disease, as well as the difficulty associated with delivering treatment to all affected sites. Additionally, leptomeningeal metastases often occur late in the course of treatment for the primary tumour, when the tumour is more likely to be resistant to many standard chemotherapeutic option.

To date, no placebo-controlled randomized trials have been done, and there appears to be little consensus on optimal treatment regimens. In two studies of aggressively treated leptomeningeal metastases, 30 per cent of patients survived less than 6 weeks.[9, 13] Nevertheless, the literature generally supports improved survival for patients who are aggressively treated.[3, 6, 7, 9] For patients

Table 26.3 Median survival in months with leptomeningeal metastases by primary malignancy

Primary malignancy	Herrlinger et al.	Median survival Wasserstrom et al.	Chamberlain
All	4.8	5.8	–
Breast	11.3	7.2	7.5
Lung	1.8	4.0	6*
Melanoma	4.7	3.6	4

* Non-small cell lung cancer.

Table 26.4 Factors affecting prognosis

Poor prognosis	Favourable prognosis
Advanced age	Longer duration of CNS symptoms
Poor performance status	Absence of CNS disease on imaging
Progressive systemic disease	Absence of elevated CSF protein
Bulky CNS disease with CSF block	Concurrent systemic chemotherapy
Cranial nerve involvement	Longer duration of CNS symptoms[21]

with a favourable risk profile, treatment options include symptomatic treatment plus systemic, intrathecal or intraventricular chemotherapy.[5]

Intrathecal/intraventricular chemotherapy

Methotrexate, cytarabine and thio-TEPA are the most commonly used intrathecal and intraventricular therapies for leptomeningeal metastases. It remains controversial as to whether intrathecal or intraventicular administration of chemotherapy confers a survival advantage for patients with leptomeningeal metastases originating from solid tumours. Some studies have shown that this treatment does not add survival advantage.[14, 15] Other studies have shown that, for patients carefully selected to participate in randomized trials receiving intrathecal or intraventricular treatment, median survival was 2–4 months.[15, 16, 17]

Two factors appear to influence durable response to treatment. The first is a clinically significant response to systemic chemotherapy,[9, 14] and the second is the absence of bulky CNS disease. Unobstructed CSF flow appears to be important to allow chemotherapy to penetrate the entire CNS.

In a study of 25 patients with breast cancer and leptomeningeal metastases, median survival improved from 8 to 22 weeks, for patients treated aggressively with whole brain irradiation and aggressive intrathecal and intraventricular chemotherapy, compared with patients treated with whole brain irradiation, with or without intrathecal chemotherapy.[18]

Systemic chemotherapy alone

Systemic chemotherapy has been shown to have a positive impact on survival.[6, 8, 19] According to one study, this benefit was seen only in patients without evidence of subarachnoid lesions, by imaging, or evidence of extra-CNS deposits.[6] This may be due to the fact that leptomeningeal metastases break down the blood–brain barrier, allowing systemic chemotherapy to enter the CSF.

Novel therapies

Other novel therapies exist, including intrathecal administration of immunotherapy agents (e.g. monoclonal antibodies, cytokines) and targeted toxins. Therapies in development include viral-mediated gene therapy, monoclonal antibodies to tumour antigens, signal transduction inhibitors, as well as systemic chemotherapy combined with techniques to disrupt the blood–brain barrier.[2]

Burdens of treatment

It is important to note that treatment is not without its burdens. Patients undergoing aggressive intrathecal and intraventricular treatment may have prolonged survival, without an improvement in the underlying deficits, and may have a worsening of neurologic symptoms, due to the direct CNS toxicity from the treatment.[20] Treatment toxicities include aseptic and bacterial meningitis and chemotherapy-related leukoencephalopathy and myelopathy. Additionally, the burden of continued treatment, given a short life expectancy, may not be a reasonable trade-off for many patients. The literature gives little attention to end points other than survival. End points such as neurologic status, clinical response, and quality of life may be of greater importance.

Therapies affecting outcome

Goals of palliative treatment for leptomeningeal metastases include improvement of pain, and stabilization of neurologic status and cranial nerve palsies. It is felt that approximately half of all patients benefit from treatment, with a resultant stabilization or an improvement in clinical status.[3, 6] Cytologic remission does not always correlate with clinical or neurologic response.

Given the overall poor prognosis for survival and symptom burden, even with aggressive treatment, the importance of intensive supportive care cannot be over emphasized. Supportive care may include corticosteroids, analgesics, anticonvulsants, radiation therapy to symptomatic sites, ventriculoperitoneal shunting and referral to hospice.

It is important to consider outcomes not only for the patients but also for those caring for them. Unfortunately, significant neurologic impairment often persists despite treatment. Significant delirium can make caring for a patient at home extremely challenging for family members, necessitating that end of life care take place in an institutional setting.

Conclusions

Leptomeningeal metastases are becoming an increasingly common complication of malignancy. Unfortunately, clearly effective treatment regimens are not available. A multitude of factors have been investigated, as possible predictors of prognosis, with the aims of targeting treatments to those who are likely to benefit from them. Despite these efforts, survival remains poor, even for carefully selected treatment groups.

The most important prognostic indicators are underlying tumour type and chemosensitivity. Tumours such as breast cancer and lymphoma are the most likely to benefit from treatment, provided that CSF flow studies indicate that intrathecal or intraventricular therapy would be able to reach all affected sites.

Several limitations exist in the current literature. These include the small number of randomized prospective controlled trials, the fact that early studies were done prior to the widespread availability of MRI, that most studies group patients with varying tumour histology and, finally, that survival is often used as end point in clinical investigations when quality of life, neurologic status, clinical response or stabilization of disease would be more appropriate end points.

References

1. Chamberlain MC. Leptomeningeal metastases: A review of evaluation and treatment. *J Neurooncol* 1998; 37:271–84.
2. Kesari S, Batchelor T. Leptomeningeal metastases. *Neurol Clin N Am* 2003; 21:25–66.
3. Wasserstrom WR, Glass JP, Posner JB. Diagnosis and tretment of leptomeningeal metastases from solid tumors: experience with 90 patients. *Cancer* 1982; 49:759–72.
4. Kaplan JG, DeSouza TG, Farkash A. *et al*. Leptomeningeal metastases: comparison of clinical features and laboratory data of solid tumors, lymphomas and leukemias. *J Neurooncol* 1990; 9:225–9.

5. NCCN. Central nervous system cancer guidelines, *The complete library of NCCN oncology practice guidelines*, CD-ROM. Rockledge, PA. 2001. To view most recent version of the guideline, go online to http://www.nccn.org.

6. Herrlinger U, Förschler H, Küker W. *et al.* Leptomeningeal metastasis: survival and prognostic factors in 155 patients. *J Neurol Sci* 2004; 223:167–78.

7. Jayson GC, Howell A, Harris M, Morgenstern G, Chang J, Ryder WD. Carcinomatous meningitis in patients with breast cancer. An aggressive disease variant. *Cancer* 1994; 74:3135–41.

8. Fizazi K, Asselain B, Vincent-Salomon A. *et al.* Meningeal carcinamatosis in patients with breast carcinoma. *Cancer* 1996; 77:1315–23.

9. Boogerd W, Hart AAM, van der Sande JJ, Engelsman E. Meningeal carcinomatosis in breast cancer. Prognostic factors and influence of treatment. *Cancer* 1991; 67:1685–95.

10. Chamberlain MC, Kormanik P. Carcinomatous meningitis secondary to breast cancer: predictors of response to combined modality therapy. *J Neurooncol* 1997; 35:55–64.

11. Chamberlain MC, Kormanik PA. Prognostic signifigance of coexistent bulky metastatic central nervous system disease in patients with leptomeningeal metastases. *Arch Neurol* 1997; 54:1364–8.

12. Sherman, AM, Jaeckle K, Meyers CA. Pretreatment cognitive performance predicts survival in patients with leptomeningeal disease. *Cancer* 2002; 95:1311–16.

13. Sause WT, Crowley John, Harmon JE *et al.* Whole brain irradiation and intrathecal Methotrexate in the treatment of solid tumor leptomeningeal metastases – A Southwest Oncology Group Study. *J Neurooncol* 1988; 6:107–12.

14. Siegal T, Lossos A, Pfeffer R. Leptomeningel metastases: analysis of 31 patients with sustained off-therapy response following combined-modality therapy. *Neurology* 1994; 44:1463–9.

15. Grossman SA, Finkelstein DM, Ruckdeschel JC, Trump DL, Moynihan T, Ettinger DS. Randomized prospective comparison of intraventricular methotrexate and thiopeta in patients with previously untreated neoplastic meningitis. *J Clin Oncol* 1993; 11:561–9.

16. Glantz MJ, LaFallette S, Jaeckle KA *et al.* Randomized trial of a slow-release versus a standard formulation of cytarabine for the intrathecal treatment of lymphomatous meningitis. *J Clin Oncol* 1999; 17:3110–16.

17. Glantz MJ, Jaeckle KA, Chamberlain MC *et al.* A randomized controlled trial comparing intrathecal sustained-release cytarabine (DepoCyt) to intrathecal methotrexate in patients with neoplastic meningitis from solid tumors. *Clin Cancer Res* 1999; 5:3394–402.

18. Yap H-Y, Yap B-S, Tashima CK, DiStefano A, Blumenschein GR. Meningeal carcinomatosis in breast cancer. *Cancer* 1978; 42:283–6.

19. Grant R, Naylor B, Greenberg HS. Clinical outcome in aggressively treated meningeal carcinomatosis. *Arch Neurol* 1994; 51:457–61.

20. Siegal T. Leptomeningeal metastases: rationale for systemic chemotherapy or what is the role of intra-CSF-chemotherapy? *J Neurooncol* 1998; 38:151–7.

21. Balm M, Hammack J. Leptomeningeal carcinomatosis: presenting features and prognostic factors. *Arch Neurol* 1996; 53:626–32.

27

Liver metastases

Angela Byrne and Michael J. Lee

Metastasis is the most common neoplasm affecting the adult liver, and the liver itself is the second most common site for malignant spread of disease after the lymph nodes. The dual blood supply and microvasculature of the liver contribute to this spread, as the fenestrations in the sinusoidal epithelium allow a foothold for tumour cells arriving via the bloodstream.[1] The liver may be the site of metastasis from virtually any primary malignant neoplasm, but the most common primary sites are the colon, stomach, pancreas, breast, eye and lung. In children, the most common liver metastases are from neuroblastomas, Wilms tumours, or leukaemia (Table 27.1).

Natural history of liver metastases

The main factors that dictate the mode of invasion include the adhesiveness of different types of cells, the inability of some cells to survive in the bloodstream, the pressure on surrounding tissues and host tissue destruction by enzymes released by tumour cells. The destruction of liver tissue by cancer cells and their metastases is related to the release of a variety of proteinases from the cancer cells so that in the early stages of tumour implantation, the malignant cells lie in close proximity to the diffusible nutrients. The pathologic anatomy of metastases resembles that of the primary neoplasm and metastases often show the same degree of vascularity as that of the primary lesion.[2] In addition, blood flow is said to increase relative to the normal parenchyma in all metastases, even hypovascular tumours. Large metastases tend to displace the surrounding vessels, and they may compress or occlude portal venous branches. They may also outgrow their blood supply, causing hypoxia and necrosis at the centre of the lesion. Metastatic tumours may be expanding or infiltrative and may vary in size, shape, vascularity, and growth pattern. They vary because of differences in blood supply, haemorrhage, cellular differentiation, fibrosis, and necrosis. Up to 15 per cent of patients have tumour thrombi that occlude the portal or hepatic veins. In the presence of mucin secretion and necrosis, metastases can develop calcification that is detectable radiographically.[3]

Factors affecting prognosis

Several factors influence the incidence and pattern of liver metastases. These include the patient's age and sex, the primary site, the histologic type, and the length of existence of the primary tumour. Some malignant lesions such as colonic carcinoma, carcinoid, and hepatocellular carcinoma may present with lesions confined to the liver, however most tumours that metastasize to the liver, such as breast and lung cancers, have often spread to other sites at the same time. The true prevalence of liver metastases is unknown as most autopsy figures reflect the end stage of the disease. However at autopsy, depending on the primary tumour type, 30–70 per cent of patients with cancer at post mortem have liver metastases. The male to female ratio for colon

Table 27.1 Tumours that metastasise to liver

Lymphoma (especially AIDS related)
HCC
Pancreatic carcinoma
Lung (particularly adenocarcinoma)
Cervix
Melanoma
Nasopharyngeal carcinoma
Kaposi sarcoma
Myeloma deposits
Cystadenocarcinoma ovary
Cystadenocarcinoma pancreas
Leiomyosarcoma
Squamous cell carcinoma
Testicular carcinoma
Granulosa cell ovarian tumour
Mucinous adenocarcinoma of the colon
Pancreatic carcinoma
Gastric carcinoma
Neuroblastoma
Cholangiocarcinoma
Breast carcinoma
Renal cell carcinoma
Carcinoid
Choriocarcinoma
Pancreatic islet cell tumours
Wilms tumour
Myeloma deposit
Hepatic chloroma

cancer is 3:2 and for the majority of other metastasizing tumours is 1:1. Liver metastases usually affect patients aged between 50 and 70 with a mean of 69 years for rectal cancer, 30–70 years for breast cancer, 71 years for colon cancer and neuroblastoma 6–9 years.[4]

Factors that significantly predict a poor prognosis on univariate analysis included coexisting symptomatic liver disease, deranged liver function tests, the presence of ascites, histological grade 3 disease at primary presentation, advanced age, oestrogen receptor (ER) negative tumours, carcinoembryonic antigen of over 1000 ng ml and multiple versus single liver metastases.

In colorectal metastases, independent prognosticators of survival are Dukes' stage, number of metastases, and serum concentrations of carcinoembryonic antigen, alkaline phosphatase, and albumin. Significant differences have been found in cumulative overall survival between patients assigned to good, moderate, and poor prognoses depending on the above pararmeters, with Dukes A disease, a single liver metastasis and near normal blood results indicating a good prognosis. However, no patient with poor prognosis and only 19.7 per cent of patients with moderate prognosis are seen to survive 5 years, compared with 62.5 per cent of patients with good prognosis.[5]

Hepatic involvement by metastatic disease and the duration of survival appear to be inversely related. Many patients die of cancer as a result not only of metastases, but also recurrence of their primary neoplasm and treatment with cytotoxic drugs. In most patients with cancer, the cause of death is usually indirect and not due to an overwhelming metastatic burden. The most common causes of death in cancer patients are chest or urinary tract infections, usually as a result of Gram-negative organisms. The infections usually result from impairment in lymphatic drainage caused by metastases. In addition, paraneoplastic syndromes occur in up to 75 per cent of patients which can lead to electrolyte imbalance and deterioration of the patients' condition. For the most part, patients die with their metastases and not from them.

Diagnosis of metastases

The accurate detection of metastatic disease at the time of diagnosis or during treatment is critical to patient management. Early identification[4] provides the opportunity for resection, which at least in the case of colorectal carcinoma has been shown to prolong survival. In addition, image-guided therapies are evolving and can play both a curative and a palliative role.

Ultrasound has traditionally been widely used in diagnosis. In general, findings using this modality are non-specific, with focal or diffuse parenchymal changes, hepatomegaly or nodularity[6] (Figure 27.1). Computed tomography (CT), which is widely available and familiar, is the mainstay of hepatic imaging. Using a bolus injection of iodinated contrast material, three distinct phases of parenchymal enhancement are seen – arterial, portal and equilibrium. Effects of arterial enhancement are seen at 20–30 seconds after contrast material injection. Liver enhancement is minimal during this latter phase. During the portal venous phase, beginning 60–70 seconds after injection, liver parenchymal enhancement peaks because of portal venous inflow. Most liver metastases are identified during this phase as focal areas of low attenuation (Figure 27.2). Decreasing vascular and parenchymal enhancement and loss of lesion–liver contrast mark the equilibrium phase.[7]

Magnetic resonance imaging (MRI) has become increasingly attractive as a primary imaging technique as it offers high intrinsic lesion–liver contrast, technical versatility and multiplanar capability, although its use currently lags far behind that of CT as a technique for general liver imaging. Extracellular agents for imaging include a variety of paramagnetic chelates of gadolinium. Tissue-specific agents that have been approved for use include magafodipir, a hepatobililiary-positive agent and ferumoxides, a reticuloendothelial agent (Figure 27.3). The T_1 and T_2 signal intensities of metastases are variable but are usually prolonged, resulting in hypo- to isointensity on T_1-weighted[5] sequences and iso- to hyperintensity on T_2 weighted sequences.[8]

Recently positron emission tomography (PET) using [18F]-2-deoxy-2-fluoro-d-glucose (FDG) has emerged as a promising diagnostic modality, particularly in recurrent colorectal cancer (Figure 27.4a, b). Indeed it can change management in up to 30 per cent of patients with potentially resectable metastases, mainly by detecting previously unknown extrahepatic disease. Furthermore, it is useful in the follow-up of patients who undergo resection, as it is extremely sensitive in detecting residual or recurrent malignancy and appears predictive for response to therapy. PET is becoming more available and more widely used.[9]

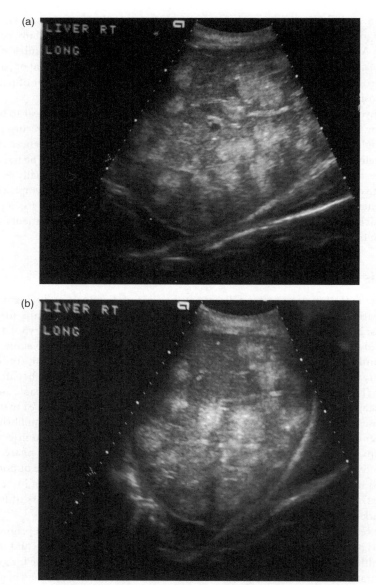

Figure 27.1 Ultrasound images showing multiple hyperechoic lesions involving all segments of the liver, in a patient with metastatic colorectal disease.

In general, diagnosing metastases is well performed with helical CT during the portal venous phase using a bolus injection. If there is suspicion of hypervascular lesions, the addition of unenhanced and arterial images is beneficial. Multiphase scanning also aids in characterization. Biopsy may be required in small or problematic lesions. MR is also useful with equivococal studies. In general, a dynamic-enhanced sequence using gadolinium should be included with T_1 and T_2 sequences.

(a)

(b)

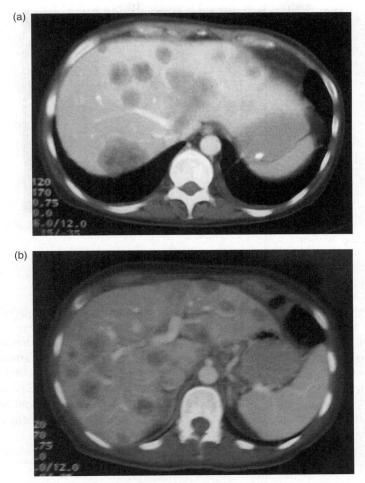

Figure 27.2 Computed tomography showing low attenuation areas within the liver corresponding to multiple liver metastases.

Therapies affecting prognosis

Therapy directed at the liver to control or eliminate the predominant site of disease should theoretically translate into improved survival. Unfortunately, because of a variety of adverse conditions, only 15 per cent of patients with metastases from colon cancer can undergo curative liver resection. Therefore, staging is an important prerequisite in selecting patients and accurate evaluation should be performed as to the local extent and distribution within the liver. Involvement of the porta hepatis and central portal vein indicate unresectability. Recurrence of liver metastases after resection occurs in up to 60 per cent of cases after a median of 9–12 months. This may occur if adequate margins have not been achieved, or occult metastases were undetected at the time of surgery. Only 33 per cent of these recurrent lesions are resectable resulting in an overall 3-year survival rate of 33 per cent. This demonstrates that re-resection

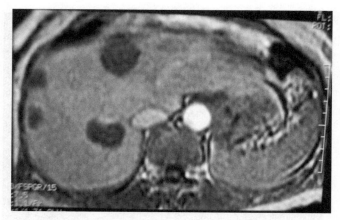

Figure 27.3 Magnetic resonance imaging pre-contrast shows areas of low signal within the liver, raising the possibility of metastases.

can provide improved long-term survival rates in a carefully selected group of patients. Selection criteria for re-resection are the same as for primary hepatectomy.[10]

Because of these high rates of recurrence, the use of adjuvant chemotherapy has been recommended. A randomized study comparing surgery versus adjuvant continuous hepatic arterial infusion with 5-fluorouracil (5-FU) and continuous systemic infusion of 5-FU demonstrated an improvement in 3-year disease-free survival in patients with colorectal metastases of 58 versus 34 per cent.[11] Recent early studies testing incorporation of irinotecan or oxaliplatin into hepatic arterial chemotherapy (HAC) either as additional systemic treatment or as integral

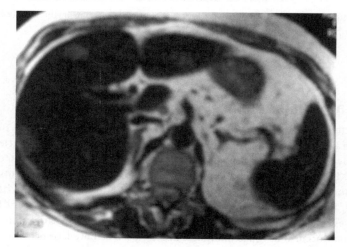

Figure 27.4 Magnetic resonance imaging post-iron oxide administration reveals areas of high signal within the liver consistent with metastases.

components of the HAC infusional regimen confirmed feasibility, safety and efficacy with response rates between 30 and 60 per cent being reported in some series. Other studies showed the combination with internal irradiation with lipiodol I-131 and biologic agents such as cytokines could be achieved with tolerable toxicity. Pre-operative chemotherapy, however with 5-FU, folinic acid and oxaliplatin, can lead to a 40 per cent 5-year survival rate. Thus, pre-operative multimodal therapy allows better survival rates.[12]

If a patient has multiple metastases or is not suitable for resection there are other therapy options available. Thermoablative methods are generally limited to those with five or fewer lesions. Ideal tumours are smaller than 2.5 cm, completely surrounded by normal liver parenchyma and at least 1 cm away from large hepatic vessels and the bile duct. Hepatic cryosurgery involves the delivery of subfreezing temperatures through penetrating or surface cryoprobes in which a cryogen is circulated. Cell death is induced by cooling the probe tip down to −190° Celsius. Ice-balls up to 8 cm in diameter can be created and freezing is usually carried out twice, generally by ultrasound guidance. Prognosis after cryotherapy is favourable when it is combined with other treatment modalities such as resection or chemotherapy, with 52 per cent survival at 2 years.[13] Radiofrequency ablation involves an alternating electric current which is operated in the radiofrequency range and can induce focal ablation. Temperatures in excess of 50° Celsius are produced which leads to coagulative necrosis and tissue ablation of up to 5 cm, and multiple ablations within a single setting can be achieved. These devices can be used percutaneously with the use of conscious sedation and ultrasound guidance. Results of various clinical series have been promising with a 52–67 per cent complete ablation rate at 1 year and survival rates of 96, 64 and 40 per cent at 1, 3 and 5 years. Precise placement of the probe is of crucial importance for induction of complete ablation and radiological guidance is used for optimum effect. Complication rates vary between 3 and 8 per cent in most studies. Death is very rare and usually occurred in patients with large volume of tumour whereby renal failure, sepsis and disseminated intravascular coagulation (DIC) took place. Minor complications of fever, leukocytosis and transient abnormalities in liver function tests occurred in the majority of patients.[14]

Overall, however, surgery remains the treatment of choice for potentially resectable tumours. Chemotherapy with 5-FU is part of standard care and minimally invasive techniques have promising results in patients with limited disease who are not surgical candidates and are an additional treatment option, particularly in patients with colorectal cancer as their primary tumour.

Short- and long-term prognosis for survival

Due to the high incidence of colon cancer, most of the available data relates to metastases arising from colorectal tumours. The results obtained with resection of these hepatic metastases provide compelling evidence that this is the treatment of choice. Of patients presenting with recurrent colorectal cancer, 80 per cent will have hepatic metastases and in 30 per cent, the liver is the most frequent and only site of relapse. Up to a quarter of patients present with synchronous metastases. Retrospective surveys have shown a variable natural history with a median survival of up to 24 months in patients with untreated liver metastases. Currently surgery offers the only possibility for cure with a mean 5-year survival rate of 30 per cent, ranging from 16–45 per cent. In one study, actuarial survival rates at 2 years were 83 per cent, at 3 years 55 per cent and at 5 years 29 per cent. In addition, with improved operative and postoperative care, leading to decreased morbidity, resection is a safe and efficient procedure. When combined with pre-operative chemotherapy, the survival rate may increase to 40 per cent. If thermoablative techniques such as cryotherapy are used, particularly with resection, the prognosis may be up to 52 per cent at 5 years.

Table 27.2 Prognosis of liver metastases, according to primary site of the tumour

Colorectal	29–52% at 5 years
Breast	2 years median
Gastric	7 months
Pancreaticobiliary	1 year
Melanoma	25% at 5 years
Ovarian	12 months
Carcinoid	67% at 5 years

Radiofrequency ablation techniques are still being investigated but currently survival rates of 96, 64 and 40 per cent have been seen at 1, 3 and 5 years.[15]

Breast cancer has a significant tendency to spread to the liver. Unfortunately, it is often inappropriate to surgically remove cancer that has spread from the breast to the liver due to other extrahepatic disease. The median survival of patients with this form of metastatic disease rarely exceeds 2 years. In liver metastases from breast cancer, factors that indicate possible positive effects of resection include the liver being the first and only site to which the cancer has spread, the absence of tumour in the lymph nodes around the liver and curative resection. Studies have shown that in selected patients with liver metastases from breast cancer, an aggressive surgical approach is associated with favourable long-term survival. The overall 2- and 5-year survival rates were 86 and 61 per cent, respectively, whereas the 2- and 5-year disease-free survival rates were 39 and 31 per cent.[16]

Thermoablative treatments have also been used. Magnetic resonance (MR) guided laser ablation for less than five liver lesions have shown high local tumour control and survival rates. These include median survival of 4.3 years, 1-year survival of 96 per cent, 2-year survival of 80 per cent, 3-year survival of 63 per cent and 5-year survival of 41 per cent. As part of a treatment plan for breast cancer that has spread to the liver, one should consider using chemotherapy before and/or after liver resection. As treatment, whole-body control with chemoendocrine therapy is fundamental. In chemotherapy, anthracyclines are the first choice and taxanes are the second, but the use of herceptin for herceptest-positive patients should be considered. Achieving a temporary partial response is possible, although cure is almost impossible. The prognosis of patients with unresectable multiple metastasis to the liver is poor; the 3- and 5-year survival rates are 22 and 11 per cent, respectively.[17]

Previous clinical experience indicates that resection of liver metastases of noncolorectal gastrointestinal (GI) tract adenocarcinomas is not effective in treating the disease. If cancer of the GI tract has spread to the liver, it is very common that the disease is also elsewhere in the liver, in the peritoneum or lungs. Fluoroucil-based combination therapy is often the only real treatment option for gastric metastases to the liver. Median survival of unilobar metastasis is 7.8 months and 4.3 months for bilobar involvement. Gastrectomy might prolong survival in patients with unilobar metastasis, but not in patients with bilobar disease. Chemotherapy could prolong the survival in patients without gastrectomy, but not the survival after gastrectomy. Poor prognostic factors have been found to be alkaline phosphatase greater than 100, concomitant peritoneal disease and a performance status of less than 2 on a quality of life (QoL) questionnaire. In one study, 1-year survival for good, moderate, and poor risk groups were 48.5, 25.7, and 11 per cent, respectively and pretreatment physical, role functioning, and global QoL predicted survival.[18]

Hepatic metastases from pancreatobiliary cancer have a dismal patient prognosis of approximately 1 year after diagnosis. For hepatic metastases from biliary cancer, hepatic resection has been performed in a small number of patients, resulting in a median survival time of less than 12 months. In most series previously reported, the treatment for hepatic metastases from pancreatobiliary malignancies was systemic and regional chemotherapy, especially hepatic arterial infusion chemotherapy. However, there is no evidence suggesting a beneficial effect of cancer chemotherapy on prognosis. Therefore new therapeutic modalities will be required to improve the outcome of the treatment of hepatic metastases of pancreatobiliary cancer.[19]

Malignant melanoma is a unique tumour that may be regulated and controlled by the body's own cancer-fighting system. For this reason, very aggressive approaches are taken to treat these types of tumours, which can be surgically removed. This approach may be further supported by the promising, newly emerging adjuvant therapies being studied for melanoma treatment. An example is cisplatin chemotherapy and polyvinyl[11] sponge particles which are injected intra-arterially to the liver. Recent scientific data on the resection of isolated liver metastases of melanoma indicate a 5-year survival benefit of between 25–35 percent when compared to historical stage IV melanoma controls. Distant metastases are unusual at presentation and during the course of ovarian carcinoma. Significant risk factors for the development of distant metastases are seen to be stage, grade, and lymph node involvement. Median survival from diagnosis of distant disease averages 12 months. The most important prognostic factor associated with survival has been documented as the interval time between diagnosis of ovarian cancer and documentation of distant metastases.[20]

Carcinoid tumours were first described more than a century ago, but the treatment of patients with advanced disease remains a challenge to physicians. The overall 5-year survival rate for all patients with carcinoid tumours regardless of the site has been reported to be 67.2 per cent. The prognosis of patients with early stage disease is good and surgical resection is the standard form of treatment. The resection of local or regional metastases can result in cure for some cases. However, patients with metastatic dissemination have poor outcomes as chemotherapy is generally ineffective. Surgical resection of isolated hepatic metastases, surgical hepatic artery ligation or hepatic chemo-embolization produce responses in selected patients.[21]

Approximately 70 per cent of all patients with neuroblastoma have metastatic disease at diagnosis. The prognosis for patients with neuroblastoma is related to their age at diagnosis, clinical stage of disease, and (in patients older than 1 year) regional lymph node involvement. Other conventional prognostic variables include the site[12] of the primary tumour and tumour histology. Children of any age with localized neuroblastoma and infants younger than 1 year with advanced disease and favourable disease characteristics have a high likelihood of long-term, disease-free survival. Older children with advanced-stage disease, however, have a significantly decreased chance for cure despite intensive therapy. As an example, aggressive multi-agent chemotherapy has resulted in a 2-year survival rate of approximately 20 per cent in older children with stage IV neuroblastoma.[22]

Overall, the only curative procedure for hepatic metastases is resection, but as few patients are suitable for this, other methods of treatment such as thermoablation and chemotherapy are used. Supportive palliative care should be available for those patients who are not cured so that the least amount of discomfort and morbidity are caused.

References

1. Leveson SH, Wiggins PA, Giles GR. Deranged liver blood flow patterns in the detection of liver metastases. *Br J Surg* 1985; 72(2):128–30.

2. Edmondson HA, Peters RL. Tumours of the liver: pathologic features. *Semin Roentgenol* 1983; 18(2):75–83.

3. Edmondson HA, Craig JR. Neoplasm of the liver. In L Schiff, ER Schiff (eds) *Diseases of the liver*, 8th edn, pp. 1109–58. Philadelphia, PA: JB Lippincott, 1987.

4. Weiss LA. A pathobiologic overiew of metastasis. *Semin Oncol* 1977; 4:5–17.

5. Schindl M, Wigmore SJ, Currie EJ, Laengle F, Garden OJ. Prognostic scoring in colorectal cancer liver metastases: development and validation. *Arch Surg* 2005; 140(2):183–9.

6. Kinkel K, Lu Y, Both M. Detection of hepatic metastases from cancers of the gastrointestinal tract by using noninvasive imaging methods (US, CT, MR imaging, PET): a meta-analysis. *Radiology* 2002; 224(3):748–56.

7. Baron RL. Understanding and optimizing use of contrast material for CT of the liver. *AJR* 1994; 163:323–31.

8. Sica GT, Hoon J, Ros P. CT and MR imaging of hepatic metastases. *AJR* 2000; 174:691–8.

9. Arulampalam T, Costa D, Visvikis D. The impact of FDG-PET on the management algorithm for recurrent colorectal cancer. *Eur J Nucl Med* 2001; 28(12):1758–65.

10. Schlag PM, Benhidjeb. Resection and local therapy for liver metastases, *Best Practice and Research Clinical Gastroenterology* 2002; 16(2):299–317.

11. Kemeny MM. Prospective randomized study of surgery alone versus continuous hepatic infusion of FUDR and continuous systemic infusion of 5-FU after hepatic resection for colorectal liver metastases. *Proceedings of the American Society for Clinical Oncology* 1999; 18:264a(1012).

12. Bismuth H, Adam R, Levi F. et al. Resection of nonresectable liver metastases from colorectal cancer after neoadjuvant chemotherapy. *Annals of Surgery* 1996; 351:509–22.

13. Adam R, Akpinar E, Jahann M. Place of cryosurgery in the treatment of malignant tumours. *Annals of Surgery* 1997; 225:39–50.

14. McGahan JP, Dodd GD. Radiofrequency ablation of the liver. *AJR* 2001; 176:3–16.

15. Schlag PM, Benhidjeb. Resection and local therapy for liver metastases. *Best Practice and Research Clinical Gastroenterology* 2002; 16(2):299–317.

16. Wyld L, Gutteridge E, Pinder SE, James JJ, Chan SY, Cheung KL, Robertson JF, Evans AJ Prognostic factors for patients with hepatic metastases from breast cancer. *Br J Cancer* 2003; 89(2):284–90.

17. Mack MG, Straub R, Eichler K, Sollner O, Lehnert T, Vogl TJ. Breast cancer metastases in liver: laser-induced interstitial thermotherapy–local tumor control rate and survival data. *Radiology* 2004; 233(2):400–9. Epub 2004 30 September.

18. Kwok CM, Wu CW, Lo SS, Shen KH, Hsieh MC, Lui WY. Survival of gastric cancer with concomitant liver metastases. *Hepatogastroenterology* 2004; 51(59):1527–30.

19. Ishii H, Furuse J, Nagase M, Yoshino M, Kawashima M, Satake M, Ogino T, Ikeda H. Hepatic arterial infusion of 5-fluorouracil and extrabeam radiotherapy for liver metastases from pancreatic carcinoma. *Hepatogastroenterology* 2004; 51(58):1175–8.

20. Cormio G, Rossi C, Cazzolla A, Resta L, Loverro G, Greco P, Selvaggi L. Distant metastases in ovarian carcinoma. *Int J Gynecol Cancer* 2003; 13(2):125–9.

21. Comaru-Schally AM, Schally AV. A clinical overview of carcinoid tumors: perspectives for improvement in treatment using peptide analogs. *Int J Oncol* 2005; 26(2):301–9.

22. Azizkhan RG, Haase GM. Current biologic and therapeutic implications in the surgery of neuroblastoma. *Semin Surg Oncol* 1993; 9(6):493–501.

28

Lung secondaries

David Currow and Christine Sanderson

Introduction

Metastases to the lung are a frequent complication of malignancy, occurring in 10–20 per cent of epithelial cancers, 50–70 per cent of sarcomas involving extremity, chest wall, or head and neck,[1] and in up to 90 per cent of those dying of osteosarcoma.[2] The natural history of metastatic lung disease varies enormously. The outcome for a particular individual depends on a combination of factors:

- the primary site of the malignancy, and its inherent aggressiveness
- the status of the underlying disease – if it is controlled at the primary site, and the presence of any metastases to other extrapulmonary sites
- the potential responsiveness of the underlying disease to local or systemic treatment
- history of any previous treatments for the cancer
- the location of the lung metastases, and their impact on respiratory function
- the patient's comorbidities and performance state, particularly any coexisting cardiorespiratory disease, and
- the potential resectability of the metastases.

As with all cancers, it can be difficult to separate the morbidity caused by local disease (in this case the respiratory tract) from the systemic manifestations of the cachexia/anorexia syndrome. Most people, even those with lung metastases, are most troubled by the whole-body manifestations of uncontrolled cancer, and progressive weakness from advanced malignancy itself also causes dyspnoea. Nonetheless, up to 50 per cent of lung metastases may be asymptomatic.[3] The presence of dyspnoea is an independent risk factor for shortened prognosis in advanced cancer.[4] The relationship between dyspnoea and the underlying neoplastic or intercurrent lung disease may not be in proportion to the damage to lung parenchyma.

There is little direct information within the literature regarding the prognostic impact of developing lung metastases. Most case series describing their natural history predate the availability of positron emission scanning (PET) to sensitively identify metastatic sites.[5] However, pathological studies of autopsy series from the pre-chemotherapy era provide some natural history data, suggesting that around 45 per cent of those people with lung metastases from any primary site will survive, untreated, for 1–6 months, and 20 per cent for 6–12 months. The 2-year survival, untreated, may be around 9 per cent.[3] The difference between ascertainment rates ante mortem and post mortem can be quite large, and we should differentiate between clinically significant and pathologically identified disease.

Natural history of cancer with lung metastases

Lung metastases are often regarded as an ominous prognostic development by both patients and clinicians, yet cancer that is metastatic to lung may itself have little apparent independent impact on prognosis, as in prostate cancer.[6] In a small number of cases surgical management may offer the prospect of cure or substantially prolonged survival.[7] In other cases disease modifying treatments – chemotherapy, radiotherapy or biological agents – may allow the disease to be controlled for a variable period, but only rarely cured.

Prognostic factors relating to the primary cancer

While many primary cancers have the potential to metastasize to lung, the implications vary enormously. Clinical outcomes differ according to the primary tissue type (e.g. epithelial, sarcomatous or germ cell). However, the most significant factor is the clinical aggressiveness of the primary tumour.

The time between initial diagnosis and the appearance of metastatic disease is an important prognostic factor in the outcome of lung metastases.[7] This reflects the biology of the underlying malignant process, in which early metastatic spread is a marker of aggressive disease behaviour. There are data that show genetic differences in cancers that mestastasize early, suggesting a very different biology. The presence of metastases at multiple sites or in lymph nodes also implies an aggressive disease process. Diseases with a long period between occurrence of the primary tumour and of any metastases are clinically more indolent, with a better prognosis. Pathological and biochemical features of the cancer's activity (e.g. grade and stage of the primary; markers associated with poor prognosis such as chromosomal abnormalities, or receptor status for breast cancer; and measures of catabolism such as raised LDH or CRP, or low albumin) all contribute evidence to build up a prognostic profile of the total impact of the disease.

Performance status

Performance status, weakness, and the cancer–cachexia syndrome are indicators of disease activity and its systemic impact. They are predictors of overall survival in this setting.[4] When a patient experiences deterioration in performance status, or other constitutional symptoms, more rapid disease progression is likely. They are also less able to tolerate either surgical or non-surgical management of their cancer, even if the intervention is palliative. Most people with rapidly progressive disease, unless the primary is highly likely to respond to systemic treatment, should be managed supportively, rather than attempting to modify the disease's course. If tumours are highly chemosensitive or radiosensitive, however, disease-modifying treatment may resolve constitutional symptoms and improve the patient's performance state. High grade lymphoma, germ cell tumours and small cell lung cancer – all of which can generate lung metastases – may fit this category.

Symptoms caused by lung disease

The consequence of the developing lung metastases depends also on the amount of respiratory compromise they cause directly. The effect on respiratory function of a solitary peripheral nodule can be contrasted with that of an extrinsic lesion obstructing a large airway that cannot be treated by stenting, or with that of lymphangitis carcinomatosis.[8] Pre-existing cardiorespiratory disease also magnifies the clinical impact of lung metastases. On the other hand, asymptomatic lung metastases may alter prognosis far less than metastases to other visceral sites, such as liver.[6, 9]

Infection

Obstructive processes predispose to recurrent infection that can be difficult to clear, and may result in the death of the patient if unable to be treated effectively. This is most likely in the setting of collapse/consolidation patterns caused by obstruction of a large airway by lung metastases.

Obstructive processes

Obstructing lesions caused by metastatic lung disease are predominantly extrinsic. Endobronchial lesions are rarer, but can occur with a range of primary sites including breast, kidney, and melanoma. Proximal lesions, and those impinging on the large airways, may have a dramatic course, presenting with stridor and severe respiratory distress. In selected patients, interventional techniques such as radiotherapy, laser ablation or stenting may improve quality of life considerably, although the impact on survival is not as clear-cut.[10] Distal lesions may be relatively asymptomatic, unless cardiorespiratory function is already impaired.

Pleural and pericardial effusions

Malignant effusions are commonly associated with lung or pleural metastatases, causing respiratory distress and chest wall symptoms. Recurrent pleural effusion has a poor prognosis, independent of tumour type, with a median survival of about 3 months, which worsens with deteriorating performance status.[11] Pericardial effusion may occur either alone or in association with pleural effusion. Malignant pericardial effusion may cause severe shortness of breath and occurs most commonly in lung cancer, breast cancer and haematological malignancies, with median survival following drainage of 3, 8, and 17 months respectively in one series.[12] There is evidence that systemic treatment, if appropriate, can improve the prognosis of patients with breast cancer and pericardial effusion.[13] Presentation with haemodynamic collapse or tamponade are very poor prognostic factors.[14] If the patient is well enough, a pericardial effusion should be drained for palliation of symptoms.

Lymphangitis carcinomatosis and respiratory failure

The majority of cases of lymphangitis carcinomatosis arise from a primary breast carcinoma. Stomach, lung and pancreatic cancers are other significant primary sites.[15, 16] Widespread infiltration by neoplastic cells into pulmonary lymphatics causes rapidly progressive shortness of breath and respiratory failure. Unless a cancer is exquisitely sensitive to systemic therapy (chemotherapy or biological agents including hormone therapy)[17] median prognosis is measured in weeks.

Prognostic factors relating to potential operability of lung metastases

In 1990 the International Registry of Lung Metastases (IRLM) was established to investigate outcomes of metastasectomy for pulmonary metastases.[18] The data relates to a small, carefully selected subgroup of patients who are fit enough for surgery. There are no prospective trials comparing surgery with other forms of treatment, or to no treatment, in similar groups of patients. Rarer tumours such as sarcomas, germ cell tumours and paediatric malignancies account for 40 per cent of the cases on the database. In the more common epithelial tumours, where the average age is older, and the pattern and behaviour of disease less favourable, few patients are selected for surgery.[7] Thus, despite their prevalence, colorectal cancers and breast cancers make up only about 20 per cent of the cases in the IRLM. It is therefore not possible to extrapolate from these data to the whole population of people with lung metastases.

Based on IRLM outcomes, the optimal candidate for lung metastasectomy would be someone in whom:

- disease is controlled at the primary site
- metastases are completely resectable, with adequate residual lung
- disease-free interval between the primary cancer and lung metastases is greater than 36 months.

In the relatively small group where complete resection was achieved, the overall survival for all pathologies at 5 years was 36 per cent: 22 per cent of these patients were long-term survivors at 15 years (median 35 months). When resection was incomplete, 5-year survival was only 13 per cent (median 15 months). Of the specific tumours treated, germ cell tumours had the best outcomes (68 per cent survival at 5 years), and melanomas the worst (21 per cent 5 year survival, median 19 months). Clinically indolent disease does best with metastasectomy, and this subset of people may also benefit from repeat metastasectomies if their disease continues to behave in a truly indolent manner.

In recent years the indications for metastesectomy have been broadened, and now may include resection of multiple – including bilateral – lung metastases, resection of lung metastases present at diagnosis of the primary disease, and repeated resections for recurrent lung metastases. Eligibility criteria for surgery continue to evolve, however they necessarily involve consideration of the patients' ability to tolerate the surgical procedure, and the technical operability of the metastases. Mortality and morbidity from the procedure also should be considered. Thirty-day mortality is still 1–2 per cent.

Number of lung metastases is a significant prognostic factor, although less important than resectability and disease-free interval. There was no difference in the survival of patients having ten or more lung metastases resected when compared with those who had four or more. Repeat resection is controversial, and the number of people who are likely to benefit is extremely small, comprising a very small percentage of an already highly selected subgroup. Although survival data for repeat resections looks astounding (44 per cent at 5 years, 29 per cent at 10 years), these are people with long disease-free intervals, control of all other known disease, and excellent functional status.

Some specific primary sites of cancer

Long-term survival following excision of lung metastases is possible in cancers of the oropharynx (squamous cell carcinoma), colon and kidney (adenocarcinomas), in sarcomas, and in germ cell tumours. In patients for whom surgery is not an option, the prognosis relates to the manage-ability of the underlying disease process.

Breast cancer

Visceral metastatic disease (liver, lung or brain) has a much poorer prognosis than the pattern of disease with bone metastases only. The tumour grade is prognostically important, although confounded by the fact that high-grade tumour pathology is more likely to spread to lung than any other site.[19] It also associated with less likelihood of the tumour being hormone-receptor positive, and with decreased disease-free interval. A further confounder is the pathological difficulty, of older case series distinguishing between new primary lung cancer and metastatic breast cancer.

Renal cell carcinoma

Lung is the most common metastatic site for renal cell carcinomas, accounting for more than 60 per cent of metastatic disease.[20] Metastatic renal cell carcinoma until recently had a very poor outlook, but with new agents systemic treatment may provide real benefits. Approximately one-third of people diagnosed with renal call carcinoma have metastatic disease at presentation, and another third will develop metastatic disease within 18 months of definitive treatment. Most findings of respiratory involvement are incidental. When the primary cancer is controlled and surgery is feasible, metastasectomy may improve survival.

Colon cancer

Between 10 and 20 per cent of people with metastatic colorectal cancer have lung involvement, which is not an independent prognostic indicator in this disease.[21] However, it is rarely the only site of metastatic disease. Newer chemotherapy options deliver modest survival advantages for those with good performance status. This improves prognosis, although improved level of function maintained over longer periods of time is also an important palliative outcome. Few of these patients, perhaps 2–4 per cent, are likely to be candidates for surgery.

Head and neck cancer

Most squamous cell carcinomas of the head and neck spread locoregionally, with lung metastases making up 80 per cent of all distant spread. Even in locally extensive disease the 5-year survival rates are above 30 per cent. Excision of solitary metastatic lung lesions also achieves 30–40 per cent 5-year survival rates.[22] Given the significant respiratory comorbidities of many people with head and neck cancer, this is an impressive result.

Prostate cancer

Pulmonary metastases are detected clinically in about 15 per cent, contrasting with a prevalence of about 60 per cent at autopsy.[6] Unlike breast cancer, the histological grade is generally lower with pulmonary metastases than with bone or lymph node pathology. Response to hormonal therapy in men with stage D2 disease and lung metastases was as good as, that of men with other sites of metastasis.

Melanoma

Survival of people with disseminated melanoma and lung metastases is very poor, with a higher relative risk of death even when adjusted for all other prognostic factors when compared to other cancers.[23]

Thyroid cancer

Occult pulmonary metastases of well-differentiated papillary or follicular thyroid cancers are curable with ^{131}I in 75 per cent; however nodules visible on chest X-ray have a much lower cure rate of about 10 per cent. Patients with solitary metastases from thyroid and other endocrine malignancies may be candidates for surgery.[24]

Pancreatic cancer

Pulmonary metastases are a late event in pancreatic cancer and survival is extremely poor. In one series there were no patients with resectable disease, which is consistent with the aggressive nature of this disease process.[24]

Germ cell tumour

In the surgical literature, germ cell tumours have the best outcomes from metastasectomy, with 63 per cent 10-year survival.[18] This reflects the fact that the majority of these tumours are potentially highly treatable, and presence of lung metastases without other poor prognostic factors does not result in a worse prognosis.[25]

Sarcoma

Soft tissue sarcomas are a heterogenous group of cancers. Median survival with metastatic disease is 11–15 months, but pulmonary metastasectomy may be curative in selected cases. If the patient is not a candidate for surgery, systemic treatment may offer a palliative and possibly a survival benefit.[26] Osteosarcomas tend to occur in a younger age group, with a peak in adolescence; 10–20 per cent will have macroscopic metastases at diagnosis[27] and about 50 per cent of those with lung metastases will be candidates for surgery with curative intent.[28]

References

1. Billingsley KG, Burt ME, Jara E *et al.* Pulmonary metastases from soft tissue sarcoma: analysis of patterns of diseases and post-metastasis survival. *Ann Surg* 1999; 229(5):602–10.

2. Jeffree GM, Price CH, Sissons H. The metastatic patterns of osteosarcoma. *Br J Cancer* 1975; 32(1):87–107.

3. Farrell JT. Pulmonary metastasis: a pathological, clinical, roentgenological study based on 78 cases seen at necropsy. *Radiology* 1935; 24:444–51.

4. Vigano A, Donaldson N, Higginson IJ, Bruera E, Mahmud S, Suarez-Almazor M. Quality of life and survival prediction in terminal cancer patients: a multicentre study. *Cancer* 2004; 101:1090–8.

5. Spira A, Ettinger DS. Multidisciplinary management of lung cancer. *NEJM* 2004; 350:379–92.

6. Nakamachi H, Suzuki H, Akakura K *et al.* Clinical significance of pulmonary metastases in stage D2 prostate cancer patients. *Prostate Cancer and Prostatic Diseases* 2002; 5:159–63.

7. Pastorino U, Buyse M, Friedel G *et al.* Long-term results of lung metastasectomy: prognostic analysis based on 5206 cases. *J Thorac Cardiovasc Surg* 1997; 113:37–49.

8. Emirgil C, Zsoldos S, Heineman HO. Effect of metastatic carcinoma to the lung on pulmonary function in man. *Am J Med* 1964; 36:382–94.

9. Sauter ER, Bolton JS, Willis GW, Farr GH, Sardi A. Improved survival after pulmonary resection of metastatic colorectal carcinoma. *J Surg Oncol* 1990; 43:135–8.

10. Seijo LM, Sterman DH. Interventional pulmonology. *NEJM* 2001; 344:740–8.

11. Burrows CM, Mathews WC, Colt HG. Predicting survival in patients with recurrent symptomatic malignant pleural effusions. *Chest* 2000; 117:1, 73–8.

12. Cullinane CA, Paz IB, Smith D, Carter N, Grannis FN. Prognostic factors in the surgical management of pericardial effusion in the patient with concurrent malignancy. *Chest* 2004; 125(4):1328–34.

13. Swanepoel E, Apffelstaedt JP. Malignant pericardial effusion in breast cancer: terminal event or treatable complication? *J Surg Oncol* 1997; 64:308–11.

14. Tsang TSM, Seward JB, Barnes ME, Bailey KR, Sinak LJ, Urban LH, Hayes SN. Outcomes of primary and secondary treatment of pericardial effusion in patients with malignancy. *Mayo Clin Proc* 2000; 75(3):248–53.

15. Harold JT. Lymphangitis carcinomatosa of the lungs. *QJM* 1952; 21(83):353–60.

16. Bruce DM, Heys SD, Eremin O. Lymphangitis carcinomatosa: a literature review. *J R Coll Surg* 1996; 41:7–13.

17. Fujita J, Yamagishi Y, Kubo A, Takigawa K, Yamaji Y, Takahara J. Respiratory failure due to pulmonary lymphangitis carcinomatosis. 1993; *Chest* 103:967–8.

18. Pastorino U. History of the surgical management of pulmonary metastases and development of the International Registry. *Seminars in Thoracic and Cardiovascular Surgery* 2002; 14(1):18–28.

19. Porter GJR, Evans AJ, Pinder SE, James JJ, Cornford EC, Burrell HC. *et al.* Patterns of metastatic breast carcinoma: influence of tumour histological grade. *Clin Radiol* 2004; 59:1094–8.

20. Ljungberg B, Alamdari F, Rasmuson T, Roos G. Follow-up guidelines for metastatic renal cell carcinoma based on the occurrence of metastases after radical nephrectomy. *Br J Urol* 1999; 84(4):405–11.

21. Penna C, Nordlinger B. Colorectal metastasis (liver and lung). *Surg Clin N Am* 2002; 82:1075–90.

22. Younes RN, Gross JL, Silva JF, Fernandez JAP, Kowalski LP. Surgical treatment of lung metastases of head and neck tumours. *Am J Surg* 1997; 174(4):499–502.

23. Leo F, Cagini L, Rocmans P, Cappello M, Van Geel AN, Maggi G. *et al.* Lung metastases from melanoma: when is surgical treatment warranted? *Br J Cancer* 2000; 83:5, 569–72.

24. Khan JH, McElhinney DB, Rahman SB, George TI, Clark OH, Merrick SH. Pulmonary metastases of endocrine origin: the role of surgery. *Chest* 1998; 114:526–34.

25. International Germ Cell Cancer Collaborative Group. International Germ Cell Consensus Classification: a prognostic factor-based staging system for metastatic germ cell cancers. *J Clin Oncol* 1997; 15(2):594–603.

26. Keohan ML, Taub RN Chemotherapy for advanced sarcoma: therapeutic decisions and modalities. *Semin Oncol* 1997; 24(5):572–9.

27. Ferguson WS, Goorin AM. Current treatment of osteosarcoma. *Cancer Invest* 2001; 19(3):292–315.

28. Pastorino U, Gasparini M, Tavecchio L, Azzarelli A, Mapelli S, Zucchi V. The contribution of salvage surgery to the management of childhood osteosarcoma. *J Clin Oncol* 1991; 9:1357–62.

29

Hypercalcaemia

Niklas Zojer and Martin Pecherstorfer

Introduction

Hypercalcaemia is defined as increase of serum calcium above the upper limit of normal range. In adults, the normal range of serum Ca is 2.1–2.7 mmol/L (or 8.4–10.6 mg/dl). Approximately 40 per cent of serum Ca is bound to albumin, 10 per cent is found in the form of inorganic complexes, while 50 per cent is circulating in the free, ionized form, which is the biologically active form. Abnormally high or low serum albumin levels can lead to the detection of false high or low total serum Ca levels (pseudohyper- or pseudohypocalcemia, respectively). In such cases, measurement of ionized Ca levels is useful (normal range 1.15–1.35 mmol/L or 4.6–5.4 mg/dl).

In healthy humans, the total serum calcium concentration is maintained within the narrow range of 2.1–2.7 mmol/L. Parathormone (PTH) is the central regulating hormone in this process. The secretion of PTH by the parathyroid responds inversely to changes in the serum level of ionized calcium. When serum calcium falls, the serum concentration of PTH increases, leading to increased bone resorption, increased renal calcium reabsorption and increased transformation of 25-hydroxy cholecalciferol (vitamin D) into the more active 1, 25 dihydroxy vitamin D (calcitriol) in the kidney.

In solid tumours, two types of hypercalcaemia of malignancy were differentiated previously:

1. The humoral hypercalcaemia, which was characterized by raised serum calcium levels in the absence of bone metastases, and

2. The local osteolytic variant, where neoplastic bone destruction was evident.

Recently, however, it has been shown that parathyroid hormone-related pro-tein (PTHrP) is the hormone responsible for increased bone resorption both in humoral and local osteolytic hypercalcaemia of malignancy.[1] The hypercalcaemia seen in hematologic cancers on the other hand is rarely related to the activity of PTHrP. Here, 1,25-dihydroxyvitamin D and cytokines such as interleukin (IL)-6 and tumor necrosis factor-β TNF-β may be the mediators of osseous breakdown. In myeloma, disruption of the RANKL/RANK and osteoprotegerin system has been implicated for development of osteolytic lesions and hypercalcaemia.[2] Also, secretion of osteoblast inhibiting factors (e.g. Dickkopf-1; DKK1) may play a role.[3]

Natural history of the condition

Tumour cells do not resorb bone directly but recruit the host's osteoclasts by humoral or paracrine mechanisms, e.g. secretion of PTHrP. PTHrP is a proteohormone which in its amino terminal region closely resembles PTH. This homology suffices to allow PTHrP to interact with the PTH receptor. PTHrP or other cytokines secreted by tumour cells act on osteoblasts (or bone marrow stromal cells), which react with an increased expression of RANKL on their surface and, probably, also with a decreased production of osteoprotegerin (OPG).[4] OPG is a soluble decoy 'receptor' of RANKL. After binding to OPG, RANKL cannot interact with RANK. Thus, the stimulating effects of RANKL on the osteoclast lineage are blocked by OPG.[5]

Besides increased bone resorption, an increased renal calcium reabsorption contributes to the development of hypercalcaemia in patients with tumours expressing PTHrP. PTHrP serum levels in normocalcaemic cancer patients lie within the normal range. In patients with solid tumours, the transition from normocalcaemia to hypercalcaemia is accompanied by a constant increase in the amount of PTHrP secreted and circulating in blood. In contrast, as mentioned above, in hypercalcaemic patients with hematologic tumours, PTHrP is elevated only in rare cases.[6]

Although PTHrP and PTH act through the same receptor in bone and kidney, there are clear differences between the syndromes of humoral hypercalcaemia of malignancy and primary hyperparathyroidism. In contrast to primary hyperparathyroidism, serum 1,25 dihydroxy vitamin D concentrations[7] and calcium absorption from the gut are decreased in patients with malignant hypercalcaemia, and there is a decrease in bone formation and decrease in serum chloride and metabolic alkalosis.[1] These differences may be due to modification of the effects of PTHrP by other factors produced by the tumour, such as IL-1, IL-6, transforming growth factor-α TGFα, and TNFα.

As the serum calcium concentration starts to rise subsequent to bone and renal effects of PTHrP and other factors, renal water reabsorption decreases progressively, resulting in polyuria. The loss of water leads to increased reuptake of sodium and calcium by the proximal tubuli of the kidney. Thus, the serum calcium concentration increases further, leading to a vicious cycle.

Symptoms of hypercalcaemia

The intensity and also the type of symptoms in hypercalcaemia depend on the height of the serum concentration of ionized calcium and also on the time interval in which the serum calcium reached its actual level.[8] Hypercalcaemic cancer patients usually present with symptoms if serum calcium exceeds 3.0 mmol/L. These symptoms can resemble symptoms of brain metastases. Most striking is the progressive impairment of the cerebral function: fatigue, dizziness, nausea, lethargy, somnolence, and coma. Other consequences of elevated serum calcium concern the gut (vomiting and constipation) and the kidney (polyuria and subsequent polydipsia).

Incidence

A main reason for the variability of estimates on the frequency of hypercalcaemia of malignancy is that most estimates are calculated as prevalence rates, rather than incidence rates. The frequency of hypercalcaemia determined in a hospital population over a period of time depends on the duration of the patients' illness (survival) and the frequency of testing for hypercalcaemia. Also, there may be a variation between hospitals due to patient selection (e.g. higher frequency of hypercalcaemia of malignancy in referral centres as compared to primary care centres). Hypercalcaemia of malignancy is estimated to occur in 10–40 per cent of cancer patients at some time during the course of their disease (prevalence). In contrast, the incidence of hypercalcaemia is much lower. Vassilopoulou-Sellin et al.[9] retrospectively studied 7667 patients registered for the first time at the M.D. Anderson Cancer Center. Hypercalcaemia was present in 1.15 per cent of patients. When analysed according to tumour type, hypercalcaemia was evident in 3.5 per cent of patients with renal cell/urinary tract cancer, 3.2 per cent of patients with myeloma, 1.6 per cent of patients with lung cancer and 0.9 per cent of breast cancer patients.

Impact of therapy on prognosis

Intravenous saline infusion, rehydration and volume expansion is the first important step of treatment and may yield reductions of the serum calcium level by 0.3–0.5 mmol/L within 48 hours. Henle loop-specific diuretics such as furosemid can be added and increase sodium-dependent renal calcium excretion but must be accompanied with adequate fluid repletion in order to counteract the negative effect of volume contraction on calciuresis. The intravenous application of a potent bisphosphonate, however, is today the mainstay of treatment of malignant hypercalcaemia.[10] Usually pamidronate (90 mg), ibandronate (4 mg), or zolendronate (4 mg) is given as a single infusion, which restores normocalcaemia within 5 days in 70–80 per cent of patients. Because of the potential nephrotoxicity, these bisphosphonates must be administered in sufficient volume over the recommended minimal infusion time.

The higher the initial serum calcium concentration, the lower the percentage of patients with normalized serum calcium following treatment with a defined dose of a bisphosphonate (BP).[11] By increasing the dose, the response rate to bisphosphonate treatment can be increased. Thus, in the majority of patients with tumour-associated hypercalcaemia, normocalcaemia can be restored by bisphosphonate treatment, although some studies have reported an association between high serum PTHrP levels and reduced response to BPs.[12–15] In contrast to the clear relationship between administered dose of an individual bisphosphonate and the proportion of patients becoming normocalcaemic following this treatment, a relationship between dose and time to relapse of hypercalcaemia was not demonstrated in randomized studies including more than 100 patients.[16–18]

Although effective treatment of hypercalcaemia of malignancy can alleviate the debilitating symptoms of this disorder, application of bisphosphonates or other anti-hypercalcemic agents was not shown to prolong survival in these patients (discussed in detail below). Only if effective, systemic anti-cancer treatment (e.g. chemotherapy) is applied, survival can be improved. However, it is strongly recommended that treatment with bisphophonates is not withheld from any patient with hypercalcaemia of malignancy. Improvement of performance status might allow later application of anti-cancer chemotherapy and symptom improvement in itself is an important treatment goal in palliative care.

Short- and long-term prognosis

Usually hypercalcaemia of malignancy indicates advanced disease and is therefore linked with a poor prognosis. However, in some of these patients a long-term survival has been observed. To identify these patients, it first is crucial to check for alternative causes of hypercalcaemia in patients with malignancy. Primary hyperparathyroidism was identified as underlying elevated serum Ca levels in some patients with cancer, and this was associated with a better outcome. In a series of 100 patients with breast cancer, measurement of serum calcium and serum PTH led to the diagnosis of hyperparathyroidism in 7 cases.[19] Coexistence of primary hyperparathyroidism and malignant disease has also been reported for other types of cancer, e.g., multiple myeloma and cutaneous T-cell lymphoma.[20–21] In a series of 47 hypercalcaemic cancer patients, median survival in those 7 patients with coexisting hyperparathyroidism was 817 days, compared to 33 days in the remaining 40 patients, in whom PTH was suppressed.[22]

Table 29.1 lists alternative causes of hypercalcaemia that should be ruled out before diagnosing hypercalcaemia of malignancy. Only true hypercalcaemia of malignancy, occurring either due to secreted factors as a paraneoplastic phenomenon or due to bone destruction directly, carries an adverse prognosis. However, even when hypercalcaemia of malignancy has been established,

Table 29.1 Alternative causes of hypercalcaemia

Primary hyperparathyroidism
Drugs (thiazide diuretics, calcium and vitamin D supplementation, vitamin A supplementation, lithium, tamoxifen-'flare phenomenon')
Hyperthyroidism
Immobilization
Sarcoidosis
Addison's disease
Acromegaly
Pseudo-hypercalcaemia (total Ca levels elevated, ionized Ca normal – when total protein is elevated)

there are certain factors by which patients can be stratified into risk groups with different survival. Critical factors are the nature of the underlying malignancy, presence or absence of visceral metastases and availability of specific anti-cancer treatment and performance status, among others (Table 29.2). Studies evaluating prognosis of patients with hypercalcaemia of malignancy are discussed below in detail.

Ralston et al.[23] studied 126 patients with cancer-associated hypercalcaemia, with tumour types including squamous cell carcinoma of the lung (34 per cent), breast cancer (17 per cent), myeloma (6 per cent), lymphoma (3 per cent), genitourinary cancer (12 per cent), lung cancer other than squamous (11 per cent), adenocarcinoma of unknown origin (8 per cent), head and neck cancer (4 per cent) and primary liver cancer (3 per cent) and pancreatic cancer (1 per cent). The median survival in patients with haematological tumours (myeloma and lymphoma) was 60 days compared with 38 days in patients with squamous cell carcinoma of the lung, 30 days in patients with breast cancer and 29 days in patients with other solid tumours. Other studies find a somewhat better survival for patients with hypercalcaemia in these disease groups. For example in the Mayo series,[24] myeloma patients with hypercalcaemia at presentation have a median survival of 23 months. This indicates that patient selection has a huge impact on median survival times when the patient number is small (e.g. in the study by Ralston et al. only eight patients with myeloma were included). For breast cancer the difference to other studies

Table 29.2 Prognosis in patients with hypercalcaemia of malignancy

	Favourable	Unfavourable
Underlying malignancy	Myeloma, B-cell lymphoma	Breast cancer, squamous cell cancer, renal cell carcinoma, T-cell lymphoma, others
Metastases	Bone	Visceral
Systemic anti-tumour treatment	Available	Not available
WHO performance score	0–1	2–4
Ca serum level	< 3 mmol/L	> 3 mmol/L
PTHrP	Normal	Elevated

is less pronounced, but here the series seems better balanced with a higher number of patients included (n = 22). In the study by Ralston et al., availability of anti-cancer treatment (26 patients) was associated with a better outcome with a median survival of 135 days, as compared to a median survival of 30 days for the whole group. Survival did not differ in patients treated with different anti-hypercalcaemic regimens. Although it may not prolong survival, effective antihypercalcaemic treatment did achieve symptomatic relief in the majority of patients (improvement of polyuria/polydipsia, central nervous system symptoms, constipation, nausea/vomiting, malaise and fatigue). After antihypercalcaemic treatment, the prevalence of symptoms related to hypercalcaemia (except pain) was significantly reduced. Of patients treated with corticosteroids alone only 26 per cent were discharged from hospital, while 70 per cent of those treated with pamidronate could be discharged.

In another study,[25] retrospective analysis identified 114 patients with tumour-induced hypercalcaemia. Forty per cent of the patients had breast cancer, 13 per cent lung cancer, 8 per cent renal cell cancer, 6 per cent myeloma, and the remaining 33 per cent of patients other tumour types including gynaecological and head and neck cancer. The median survival for the whole group was 55 days (range 3 days to more than 21 months). Eligibility for chemotherapy or hormone therapy was a prognostic factor, with median survival at 86 days for patients receiving such treatment and only 35 days for the group not receiving systemic anti-cancer treatment. Interestingly, median survival was also different for patients receiving or not receiving radiotherapy, and for patients achieving or not achieving normocalcemia. These findings might be due to the fact that a proportion of patients would have died before radiotherapy could have been instituted or normocalcaemia could have been achieved. It is unlikely that radiotherapy or normocalcaemia by itself would have exerted a positive effect on survival.

Serum-PTHrP levels were shown to have an impact on prognosis in hypercalcaemic cancer patients.[26] When stratified according to PTHrP levels, hypercalcaemic cancer patients with normal PTHrP levels had a median life expectancy of 66 days (n = 29), whereas median survival was 33 days in patients with elevated levels of PTHrP (n = 30). The first group included significantly more patients with breast cancer, whereas squamous cell cancer was the leading diagnosis in the group with elevated PTHrP levels. Visceral metastases were also more common in the group with elevated PTHrP levels. However, the duration of neoplastic disease was similar between the groups. It might be speculated that elevated PTHrP levels contribute to more aggressive tumour behaviour by either stimulating tumour growth or impairing the immunologic defence of the host. A higher resistance to chemotherapy also reflects the unfavourable biology of tumours producing PTHrP. Although a comparable number of patients in both groups received chemotherapy, objective tumour responses were only observed in the group with normal PTHrP levels.

Myeloma

In a retrospective analysis of 1027 myeloma patients diagnosed at the Mayo Clinic in Rochester, Minnesota,[24] 13 per cent of patients had a serum calcium level ≥ 11mg/dL at initial presentation. These patients had an adverse outcome, with a median survival of 23 months, compared with 35 months for myeloma patients with a serum calcium < 11 mg/dL at diagnosis. Besides its prognostic impact, evaluation of serum calcium levels is critical for allocating myeloma patients to stage I–III according to the Durie and Salmon classification system. Myeloma is classified as stage I disease when serum calcium is normal or < 10.5 mg/dL, while a serum calcium > 12 mg/dL defines patients as having stage III disease. In the initial staging of myeloma, the serum calcium level is an important risk factor, however long-term survival is possible in hypercalcaemic patients by applying effective anti-myeloma treatment. In myeloma patients with relapsed or chemotherapy-refractory disease, the presence of hypercalcaemia heralds a poor prognosis, but even in these patients salvage regimen (bortezomib, lenalidomide) can lead to remissions and prolonged survival. A quick control of hypercalcaemia is mandatory in myeloma patients, as these patients are at an increased risk for renal insufficiency. Hypercalcaemia and resulting nephrocalcinosis might be a triggering event for acute renal failure in this setting. Paraproteinemia, propensity to infections, analgesic drugs can also contribute to renal failure.

Breast cancer

Ten per cent of breast cancer patients developed hypercalcaemia in a large retrospective study.[27] All of these patients had metastatic disease, and 85 per cent had widespread skeletal involvement. It is well known that breast cancer patients with disease confined to the skeleton enjoy a favourable prognosis (median survival > 2 years) as compared to patients with visceral involvement. Prognosis is compromised in breast cancer patients when hypercalcaemia is present. In a single-centre study on 72 breast cancer patients diagnosed with hypercalcaemia between 1980 and 1992,[28] the median survival was only 4.5 months (range 0–61 months). In the subgroup with dominant visceral metastases the survival was even worse (median 2 months), while the subgroup of 34 patients with bone metastases only had a median survival of 10 months. Notably, more than 25 per cent of patients in this favourable subgroup were alive at 2 years. Other important prognostic factors in this setting seem to be the interval between first systemic relapse and hypercalcaemia (with a short interval indicating poor prognosis) and response to systemic anti-cancer therapy. In a similar study, Brada et al.,[29] analysed 93 breast cancer patients with hypercalcaemia seen between 1985 and 1997. Eighty-five of those patients (91 per cent) had metastatic disease. In contrast to the series reported by de Wit et al.[28] the majority of patients in this series had only mild hypercalcaemia (Ca < 3 mmol/L) – i.e. 65 per cent versus 24 per cent of patients. This might explain the more favourable outcome in the latter series (median survival 8.5 months). Brada et al. stratified patients according to three risk factors: serum calcium level, symptomatic status and presence of visceral metastases. Patients without symptoms, no evidence of visceral metastases and Ca < 3 mmol/L had the best prognosis with a median survival over 3.5 years. Those with one adverse prognostic feature had an intermediate prognosis with a median survival of 16 months, while patients presenting with two or more adverse features had a median survival of only 2.5 months.

Kristensen et al.[30] retrospectively analysed two cohorts of hypercalcaemic breast cancer patients, those diagnosed between 1986 and 1989 (period 1), before bisphosphonates were introduced into therapy of hypercalcaemia of malignancy, and a second cohort diagnosed between 1993 and 1996 (period 2). None of the patients from period 1 received bisphosphonates, while all but one patient from period 2 were treated with intravenous bisphosphonates with or without prednisolone or calcitonin. Normocalcaemia was achieved in a higher percentage of patients in a much shorter time in period 2 as compared to period 1 (days from diagnosis of hypercalcaemia to restoration of normocalcaemia 5 vs 19 in period 2 and period 1, respectively). However, survival of patients with severe hypercalcaemia (ionized serum Ca > 1.6 mmol/L) was not significantly different between the periods (2.2 months vs 1.4 months in period 2 and period 1, respectively), with virtually overlapping survival curves. The authors concluded that although normocalcaemia can be achieved quickly in a high percentage of hypercalcaemic breast cancer patients with bisphosphonates, this has no impact on overall prognosis. WHO performance status, extent of metastatic disease and availability of systemic anti-cancer treatment were prognostic factors in this cohort. Also, the authors presented evidence from period 1 that the severity of hypercalcaemia based on the ionized serum Ca level bears prognostic impact. Patients with a ionized Ca level less than 1.48 mmol/L (mild hypercalcaemia) had a survival of 17.7 months, patients with a ionized Ca level of 1.48–1.60 mmol/L (moderate hypercalcaemia) a survival of 2.5 months, and patients with a ionized Ca above 1.6 mmol/L (severe hypercalcaemia) a median survival of only 1.4 months. Median survival of all 193 patients from period 1 was 6.7 months. The findings underline the conclusions drawn by Ralston et al.,[23] that treatment of hypercalcaemia with bisphosphonates does not prolong survival, but must be recommended for symptom palliation.

Adult T-cell leukaemia/lymphoma

Hypercalcaemia is common in patients with adult T-cell leukaemia/lymphoma, occurring in 32 per cent of patients in a large retrospective study (n = 820).[31] This carries an adverse prognosis with a survival of less than 6 months. Survival of patients without hypercalcaemia is more than 1 year (median survival of the whole group 10 months).

B-cell non-Hodgkin's lymphoma

A retrospective study identified hypercalcaemia in 8 of 112 patients with B-cell non-Hodgkin's lymphoma (7.1 per cent).[32] Five patients with high-grade B-NHL had hypercalcaemia at presentation. All of these had advanced disease. Median survival of these patients was only 10 months, compared with 21 months for the patients with advanced high-grade B-NHL without hypercalcaemia (n = 47). None of the five patients with hypercalcaemia achieved a complete remission with standard chemotherapy or further intensive chemotherapy or radiotherapy.

Another patient with high-grade B-NHL had hypercalcaemia at relapse, as well as two patients with low-grade B-NHL. One of the latter patients relapsed with transformation to a high-grade histology (Richter's syndrome). All of these patients had only a poor response to therapy and a short survival.

Squamous cell carcinoma

Head and neck

The incidence of hypercalcaemia in patients with head and neck carcinoma was 2.9 per cent in a large retrospective study on 1438 patients.[33] Nearly all of these patients had squamous cell cancer, only one patient an undifferentiated carcinoma. None of the hypercalcaemic patients had adenocarcinoma. The incidence of hypercalcaemia was highest (8 per cent) in patients with cancer of the nasal cavity, followed by cancer of the tongue (4 per cent) and laryngeal cancer (3.7 per cent). Most of the patients had advanced disease with 90 per cent classified as stage IV. Prognosis of these patients seems poor, with a median survival of only 33 days. Patients with stage III who were treated locally by radiation therapy and/or surgical resection had a more favourable survival, as well as those patients responsive to chemotherapy.

Lung

Hypercalcaemia seems to indicate a poor prognosis, with a median survival of 38 days in the series of Ralston et al.[23]

Oesophagus

The incidence of hypercalcaemia in a retrospective series on 208 patients with squamous cell carcinoma of the oesophagus, for whom oesophageal resection was done, was 7.7 per cent (n = 16).[34] Bone metastases were evident in only 3 of these 16 patients. Survival at 1 year was 61.7 per cent and 18.2 per cent for patients without and with hypercalcaemia, respectively. Figures for 2 years are 37.8 per cent and 9.1 per cent, respectively.

Hepatocellular carcinoma

Hypercalcaemia was reported to occur in 5.3 per cent of patients with hepatocellular carcinoma.[35] Like other paraneoplastic syndromes, hypercalcaemia of malignancy is associated with an adverse outcome in this disease.

Renal cell carcinoma

In renal cell carcinoma there is an increasing tendency for hypercalcaemia as the stages progress. The incidence in stage I disease is 3 per cent, rising to 18.9 per cent in stage IV disease (overall incidence stage I–IV, 9.2 per cent).[36] In patients with resectable disease, hypercalcaemia resolves after surgery. With relapsing disease, reoccurrence of hypercalcaemia is common. Hypercalcaemia does not seem to have prognostic impact in stage I–III patients, as with effective surgery the tumour is removed completely. However, in stage IV disease median survival was shown to be 45 days in hypercalcemic patients (n = 7), compared to more than 9 months in patients with normal Ca levels (n = 30).

Other tumour entities

Other tumour entities which have infrequently been associated with hypercalcaemia of malignancy are gynaecological tumours, gastrointestinal tumours, bladder cancer and sarcoma, among others. Some of those tumour entities were included in studies looking at prognosis in an unselected cohort of patients with hypercalcaemia of malignancy (see above). Generally, hypercalcaemia of malignancy seems to herald a poor prognosis in practically all those tumour types, although survival figures were not stated individually.

Concluding remarks

Table 29.3 summarizes the results of studies discussed above. Except for newly diagnosed hypercalcemic myeloma patients, who have a median survival close to 2 years, survival of hypercalcaemic cancer patients can be measured in weeks to months. Treatment of hypercalcaemia of malignancy is associated with improvement or reversal of debilitating symptoms

Table 29.3 Survival of hypercalcaemic patients according to tumour type

Tumour entity	Number of patients studied	Survival (months)	Reference
Myeloma (at diagnosis)	133	23	24
Breast cancer	72	4.5	28
	93	8.5	29
	212	6.7	30
Adult T-cell L	262	< 6	31
High-grade B-NHL	5	10	32
Head and neck	42	1	33
Lung	43	1	23
Oesophagus	13	7	34
Renal cell carcinoma (stage IV)	7	1.5	35

of hypercalcaemia, however, the poor prognosis of patients is not affected. Hypercalcaemia indicates an aggressive biology of the underlying malignancy. PTHrP might play a role in conferring enhanced growth of cancer cells and resistance to therapy, but likely other cytokines are involved also.

References

1. Mundy GR, Guise TA. Hypercalcemia of malignancy. *Am J Med* 1997; 103:134–45

2. Croucher PI, Shipman CM, Lippitt J. et al. Osteoprotegerin inhibits the development of osteolytic bone disease in multiple myeloma. *Blood* 2001; 98:3534–40.

3. Tian E, Zhan F, Walker R. et al. The role of the Wnt-signaling antagonist DKK1 in the development of osteolytic lesions in multiple myeloma. *N Engl J Med* 2003; 349:2483–94.

4. Lacey DL, Timms E, Tan HL. et al. Osteoprotegerin ligand is a cytokine that regulates osteoclast differentiation and activation. *Cell* 1998; 93:165–76.

5. Simonet WS, Lacey DL, Dunstan CR. et al. Osteoprotegerin: a novel secreted protein involved in the regulation of bone density. *Cell* 1997; 89:309–19.

6. Kremer R, Shustik C, Tabak T, Papavasiliou V, Goltzman D. Parathyroid hormone-related peptide in hematologic malignancies. *Am J Med* 1996; 100:406–11.

7. Schilling T, Pecherstorfer M, Blind E, Leidig G, Ziegler R, Raue F. Parathyroid hormone-related protein (PTHrP) does not regulate 1,25 dihydroxyvitamin D levels in hypercalcemia of malignancy. *J Clin Endocrinol Metab* 1993; 76:801–3.

8. Shane E. Hypercalcemia: pathogenesis, clinical manifestations, differential diagnosis, and management. In *Primer on the metabolic bone disease and disorders of mineral metabolism*, 4th edn, pp. 183–7. An official publication of The American Society for Bone and Mineral Research. Philadelphia, PA: Lippincott, 1999.

9. Vassilopoulou-Sellin R, Newman BM, Taylor SH, Guinee VF (1993). Incidence of hypercalcemia in patients with malignancy referred to a comprehensive cancer center. *Cancer* 1993; 71:1309–12.

10. Pecherstorfer M, Brenner K, Zojer N. Current management strategies for hypercalcemia. *Treat Endocrinol* 2003; 2:273–92.

11. Thiebaud D, Jaeger P, Jacquet AF, Burckhardt P. Dose–response in the treatment of hypercalcemia of malignancy by a single infusion of the bisphosphonate AHPrBP. *J Clin Oncol* 1988; 6:762–8.

12. Gurney H, Grill V, Martin TJ. Parathyroid hormone-related protein and response to pamidronate in tumour-induced hypercalcemia. *Lancet* 1993; 341:1611–13.

13. Body JJ, Dumon JC, Thirion M, Cleeren A. Circulating PTHrP concentrations in tumour-induced hypercalcemia: influence on the response to bisphosphonate and changes after therapy. *J Bone Miner Res* 1993; 8:701–6.

14. Pecherstorfer M, Schilling T, Blind E. et al. Parathyroid hormone-related protein and life expectancy in hypercalcemic cancer patients. *J Clin Endocrinol and Metab* 1994; 78:1268–70.

15. Walls J, Ratcliffe WA, Howell A, Bundred NJ. Response to intravenous bisphosphonate therapy in hypercalcaemic patients with and without bone metastases: the role of parathyroid hormone-related protein. *Br J Cancer* 1994; 70:169–72.

16. Major P, Lortholary A, Hon J. et al. Zoledronic acid is superior to pamidronate in the treatment of hypercalcemia of maligancy: a pooled analysis of two randomized, controlled clinical trials. *J Clin Oncol* 2001; 19:558–67.

17. Pecherstorfer M, Herrmann Z, Body JJ. et al. Randomized phase II trial comparing different doses of the bisphosphonate ibandronate in the treatment of hypercalcemia of malignancy. *J Clin Oncol* 1996; 14:268–76.

18. Ralston SH, Thiebaud D, Herrmann Z. et al (1997). Dose–response study of ibandronate in the treatment of cancer-associated hypercalcemia. *Br J Cancer* 75, 295–300.

19. Fierabracci P, Pinchera A, Miccoli P. et al. Increased prevalence of primary hyperparathyroidism in treated breast cancer. *J Endocrinol Invest* 2002; 24:315–20.

20. Otsuka F, Hayakawa N, Ogura T. et al. A case of primary hyperparathyroidism accompanying multiple myeloma. *Endocr J* 1997; 44:105–9.

21. Albes B, Bazex J, Bayle-Lebey P, Benuet A, Lamant L. Primary hyperparathyroidism and cutaneous T-cell lymphoma: fortuitous association? *Dermatology* 2001; 203:162–4.

22. Hutchesson AC, Bundred NJ, Ratcliffe WA. Survival in hypercalcemic cancer patients with co-existing primary hyperparathyroidism. *Postgrad Med J* 1995; 71:28–31.

23. Ralston SH, Gallacher SJ, Patel U, Campbell J, Boyle IT. Cancer-associated hypercalcemia: morbidity and mortality. Clinical experience in 126 treated patients. *Ann Intern Med* 1990; 112:499–504.

24. Kyle RA, Gertz MA, Witzig TE. et al. Review of 1027 patients with newly diagnosed multiple myeloma. *Mayo Clin Proc* 2003; 78:21–33.

25. Ling PJ, A'Hern RP, Hardy JR. Analysis of survival following treatment of tumour-induced hypercalcaemia with intravenous pamidronate (APD). *Br J Cancer* 1995; 72:206–9.

26. Pecherstorfer M, Schilling T, Blind E. et al. Parathyroid hormone-related protein and life expectancy in hypercalcemic cancer patients. *J Clin Endocrinol Metab* 1994; 78:1268–70.

27. Coleman RE and Rubens RD. The clinical course of bone metastases from breast cancer. *Br J Cancer* 1987; 55:61–6.

28. De Wit S, Cleton FJ. Hypercalcemia in patients with breast cancer: a survival study. *J Cancer Res Clin Oncol* 1994; 120:610–14.

29. Brada M, Rowley M, Grant DJ, Ashley S, Powles TJ. Hypercalcaemia in patients with disseminated breast cancer. *Acta Oncol* 1990; 29:577–80.

30. Kristensen B, Ejlertsen B, Mouridsen HT, Loft H. Survival in breast cancer patients after the first episode of hypercalcaemia. *J Intern Med* 1998; 244:189–98.

31. No authors listed. Major prognostic factors of patients with adult T-cell leukemia-lymphoma: a cooperative study. Lymphoma Study Group (1984–1987). *Leuk Res* 1991; 15:81–90.

32. Majumdar G. Incidence and prognostic significance of hypercalcaemia in B-cell non-Hodgkin's lymphoma. *J Clin Pathol* 2002; 55:637–8.

33. Won C, Decker DA, Drelichman A, Al-Sarraf M, Reed ML. Hypercalcemia in head and neck carcinoma. Incidence and prognosis. *Cancer* 1983; 52:2261–3.

34. Kuwano H, Baba H, Matsuda H. et al. Hypercalcemia related to the poor prognosis of patients with squamous cell carcinoma of the esophagus. *J Surg Oncol* 1989; 42:229–33.

35. Oldenburg WA, Van Heerden JA, Sizemore GW, Abboud CF, Sheedy PF 2nd. Hypercalcemia and primary hepatic tumours. *Arch Surg* 1982; 117:1363–6.

36. Fahn HJ, Lee YH, Chen MT, Huang JK, Chen KK, Chang LS. The incidence and prognostic significance of humoral hypercalemia in renal cell carcinoma. *J Urol* 1991; 145:248–50.

30

Spinal cord compression

Nora Janjan, Anita Mahajan, Eric L. Chang,
Ian McCutcheon, Edward Lin, Prajnan Das,
Sunil Krishnan, and Edward Chow

Introduction

The issues related to the treatment of spinal cord compression from cancer present a paradigm for the treatment of all metastatic disease. The profound consequence of paralysis from spinal cord compression to the patient and their caregivers involves significant suffering and financial burden. Although by definition incurable, patients with metastatic disease benefit greatly from therapeutic strategies that prevent spinal cord compression, and that diagnose and treat spinal cord compression early to maintain functional status. Maintaining functional integrity in the cancer patient significantly reduces caregiver burden and societal costs.

The treatment of spinal cord compression must be differentiated from futile care that is defined as treatment that provides limited patient benefit, with the risk of toxicity often greater than the possibility of achieving the goal of therapeutic response. To be appropriate, treatment intent must be consistent with the clinical presentation, and have defined and achievable goals. Consistent with these precepts, the prevention, and early diagnosis and treatment of spinal cord compression, avoids emergency evaluations and hospitalizations, and has a defined achievable goal.[1]

Natural history of spinal cord compression

Pain is the initial symptom in approximately 90% of patients with spinal cord compression, and the development of spinal cord compression is associated with a poor overall prognosis. Paraparesis or paraplegia occurs in over 60%, sensory loss is noted in 70–80%, and 14–77% have bladder and/or bowel disturbances.[2–17] The extent of the epidural mass influences functional outcome because greater residual neurologic impairment results from a complete spinal cord block results than with a partial block.

The time from the original diagnosis to the development of metastatic spinal disease averages 32 months, and the average time is reported to be 27 months from diagnosis of skeletal metastases to spinal cord compression. The vertebral column is involved by metastatic tumour in 40% of patients who die of cancer. Approximately 70% of vertebral metastases involve the thoracic spine, 20% the lumbosacral region, and 10% the cervical spine. From a tumour registry of 121,435 patients, the cumulative probability of at least one episode of spinal cord compression occurring in the last 5 years of life was 2.5%.[4] The diagnosis of spinal cord compression was associated with a doubling of the time spent in hospital in the last year of life.

Pain can be present for months to days before neurological dysfunction evolves. Unlike degenerative joint disease which primarily occurs in the low cervical and low lumbar regions, pain due to epidural spinal cord compression can occur anywhere in the spinal axis, and is aggravated by recumbency. Weakness can signal the rapid progression of symptoms and 30% of patients with weakness become paraplegic within 1 week. Rapid development of weakness, defined as occurring in less than 2 months, most commonly occurs in lung cancer, while breast and prostate cancers can progress more slowly. Neurological deficits can develop within a few hours in up to 20% of patients with spinal cord compression.[2, 4, 7–18] The rate of development of motor symptoms correlates with therapeutic improvement. Motor function improved among 86% of patients who had >14-day time to development of symptoms. Only 29% improved when motor deficits developed over 1 to 7 days before the diagnosis of spinal cord compression. Improvements occurred in only 10% if motor deficits developed over 8 to 14 days.

Among 153 consecutive cases of spinal cord compression in one study, 37% of patients had breast cancer, 28% had prostate cancer, 18% had lung cancer, and 17% had other solid tumours.[2] The time between primary tumour diagnosis and development of spinal cord compression was dependent on tumour type, with the shortest time associated with lung cancer and the longest time for breast cancer. Lung cancer patients had the most severe functional deficits with more than 50% totally paralyzed. Breast cancer patients were ambulatory 59% of the time. More severe disturbances in gait occurred when the time between the interval from the diagnosis of the primary tumour and spinal cord compression was short. Total blockage of the spinal cord occurred in 54%, and 46% had partial blockage. Total paralysis was present in 43 patients, 31 could move their legs but could not walk, 19 were able to walk with assistance, and 60 could walk unassisted. Sensory exam of the legs was normal in 34, slight disturbances were present in 84, and total lack of pain perception occurred in 35 patients. After radiation, 40 were totally paralyzed, 20 could move their legs without being able to walk, 17 were able to walk with assistance, and 76 had unassisted gait. The median survival time was 3.4 months. Survival was dependent on time from primary tumour diagnosis, ambulatory function at diagnosis and after treatment.

Prognostic factors in spinal cord compression

Prognostic factors and survival were evaluated among 60 consecutive patients with metastatic spinal cord compression. Factors such as age, discharge destination, primary tumour site, other metastases, comorbidities, and haemoglobin and albumin levels had no significant influence on survival time. Median survival time was 4.1 months once the diagnosis of metastatic spinal cord compression was made, with the exception of gastrointestinal cancer patients with a median survival time of 0.6 months.[19] The type of primary tumour did have a direct influence, however, on the interval between the diagnosis of the primary tumour and the diagnosis of spinal cord compression due to metastatic disease.[2] Factors important to survival in another study, determined among 153 consecutive patients with metastatic spinal cord compression, included time from primary tumour diagnosis until spinal cord compression (although tumour type itself was not a factor), and ambulatory function at the time of diagnosis and after treatment.[2]

Unlike bone metastases involving other sites, the prognostic factors for spinal cord compression are specific to functional outcome. The Scottish Cord Compression Group surveyed outcomes one month after treatment for spinal cord compression among 128 patients.[20] Median survival of all patients was 59 days (range 43–75 days), and 13% of those treated for spinal cord compression had died within a month of treatment. For ambulatory patients, median survival was 151 days (range 80–222 days), median survival for those walking with assistance was 71 days (range 46–96 days), and was 35 days (range 26–44 days) those unable to walk at diagnosis of spinal cord compression (Figure 30.1). The median Karnofsky performance status was 50 (range 40–60) and was the poorest for patients with lung cancer. The pace of care was dependent on

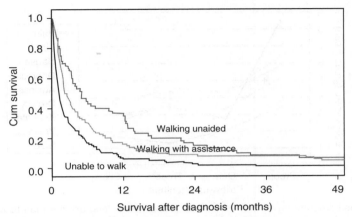

Figure 30.1 Survival in relation to mobility level at diagnosis of spinal cord compression. From Conway R, Graham J, Kidd J, Levack P, and other members of the Scottish Cord Compression Group. What happens to people after malignant cord compression? Survival, function, quality of life, emotional well-being and place of care 1 month after diagnosis. *Clinical Oncology* 2007; 19:56–62.

mobility at diagnosis. Ambulatory patients generally remained at home while those requiring assistance with walking and paralyzed patients generally required institutional care. Mobility and bladder function at diagnosis was predictive of function after radiation for spinal cord compression; only 7% of paralyzed patients regained full mobility and only 28% of catheterized patients regained full bladder function. Pain was unrelieved in 47% and 18% continued to have severe pain. Quality of life measures were strongly correlated with functional status, yet only 8% were anxious or depressed.

Prognosis has a significant influence regarding the decision for surgical intervention of spinal cord compression. The Tokuhasi and Tomita scores can accurately predict survival after surgery for metastatic spinal cord compression. There were six clinical parameters including Karnofsky index, number of extraspinal bone metastases, number of metastases in the vertebral body, metastases to the major internal organs, primary site of cancer, severity of spinal cord palsy. A Tokuhashi score of 4 or more, or a Tomita score of 6 or less predicted a 76% 3-month survival.[21–23] These findings were confirmed when postoperative outcomes were evaluated among 987 patients who underwent surgical treatment of spinal cord compression. Significant improvements in pain, and quality of life parameters were noted using the Edmonton Symptoms Assessment Scale (Figure 30.2). Primary cancers of the lung, melanoma, and upper gastrointestinal tumours with median survival rates of 87 days, 69.5 days and 56 days, respectively.[20] Intermediate survivorship of 223 days and 346 days were found for prostate cancer and breast cancer, respectively. The longest survival was in patients with lymphoma (706 days) and myeloma (591 days). Increasing age and primary lung cancer were risk factors for death within 30 days of surgery. Preoperative neurological deficits were found to be an independent determinant of a worse prognosis when confounding factors were taken into account. Patients with preoperative neurological deficits were 19% more likely to die. When surgery was performed for persistent neurological deficits after radiation, 71% of patients were more likely to get a postoperative infection.

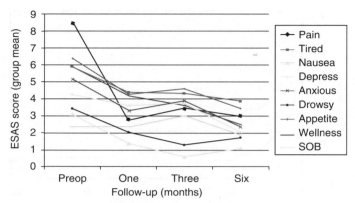

Figure 30.2 The Edmonton Symptom Assessment scores before, and up to 6 months in follow-up after surgical intervention for spinal cord compression. From Finkelstein JA, Ford MH. Diagnosis and management of pathological fractures of the spine. *Current Orthopedics* 2004; 18:396–405.

Assessment for prognosis

Any cancer patient with back pain, especially with known metastatic involvement of the vertebral bodies, should be suspected as having spinal cord compression. The risk of spinal cord compression exceeds 60% among patients with back pain and plain film evidence of vertebral collapse due to metastatic cancer. Epidural spinal cord disease is documented in 17% of asymptomatic patients who have an abnormal bone scan but normal plain films. When vertebral metastases are present on both on bone scan and plain film, 47% of asymptomatic patients will have epidural disease.[8] A magnetic resonance imaging (MRI) scan to rule out spinal cord compression should be performed in symptomatic patients with osteoblastic changes on plain film even if the vertebral contour and bone scan are normal (Figure 30.3).

Bone scans are a sensitive and specific method of detecting bone metastases, but MRI is the best available technique for evaluating the bone marrow, neoplastic invasion of the vertebrae, the central nervous system and peripheral nerves.[18] Positron emission tomography (PET)

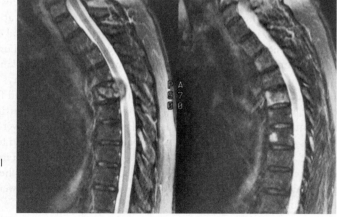

Figure 30.3 MRI of the spine demonstrating epidural extension from vertebral bone metastases on the left. The MRI on the right does not show spinal cord compression but osteoplastic disease is noted.

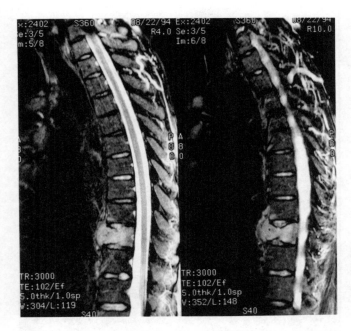

Figure 30.4 Osteoblastic involvement, demonstrated on MRI of the spine, associated with vertebral collapse with breast cancer.

[18]F-flurordeoxyglucose has also found unsuspected spinal cord compression, later confirmed on MRI, in a study among melanoma patients.[19] Bone or other metastases rarely fail to be detected when radiographic diagnosis is pursued. When radiographic confirmation of malignancy is equivocal, bone biopsy should be considered.

Radiographic determination of the involved spinal levels is critical to radiation treatment planning.[24] Clinical determination of the location of epidural spinal cord compression is incorrect in 33% of cases. Plain film radiographs will show involvement of more than one spinal level in about one-third of patients. If the results of MRI, tomographic studies, and surgical findings are included, over 85% of patients will have multiple sites of vertebral involvement. Bone scans fail to detect bone metastases 13% of the time because bone scans image the osteoblastic, not the osteolytic, components of bone metastases. When there was evidence of spinal metastases on bone scan, 49% had more extensive disease on MRI. While spinal cord compression is caused by soft tissue epidural metastases in 75% of cases, the remaining 25% of cases are caused by bone collapse.[13] Computed tomography (CT) usually finds metastases in the posterior portion of the vertebral body. With plain X-rays, the destruction of the pedicles is the most common finding that identifies spine metastases, but CT imaging has shown that destruction of the pedicles occurs only in combination with involvement of the vertebral body. Osteoblastic bony expansion, commonly seen in both prostate and breast cancers, can result in spinal cord compromise as well as osteolytic vertebral compression fractures (Figure 30.4). MRI findings correlated with stage of multiple myeloma, the β_2 microglobulin level, the type of chain, and the response to therapy.[25]

Therapies affecting prognosis

Treatment of spinal cord compression includes emergent corticosteriods, radiotherapy and/or neurosurgical intervention. Radiotherapy is the treatment of choice for most cases of spinal cord compression,[26] which is a radiotherapeutic emergency (Figure 30.5). More sophisticated treatment planning can allow sparing of adjacent normal structures (Figure 30.6).

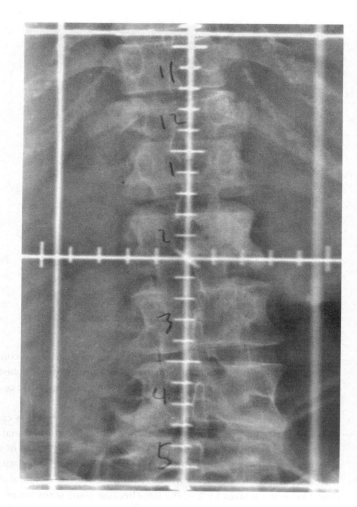

Figure 30.5 Typical radiation portal to treat disease involvement in the vertebral bodies and epidural region.

Radiation

Radiation for spinal cord compression is delivered by external beam therapy (linear accelerators, Cobalt[60] units) that administers with a prescribed number of daily fractions over several weeks. A variety of radiation energies and biological characteristics are now available to help localize treatment to the areas at risk and exclude uninvolved normal tissues.[27]

Using conventional radiation techniques, radiation for vertebral metastases commonly were prescribed to 5 cm below the skin surface using [60]Cobalt or 6MV photons. However, mean depths from MRI scans of 20 patients equalled 5.5 cm for the posterior spinal canal, 6.9 cm for the anterior spinal canal, and 9.6 cm for the anterior vertebral body. Based on the radiation dose distributions, a metastatic lesion in the anterior vertebral body could receive a radiation dose that is significantly lower than that prescribed unless radiation dose distributions are considered.

Generally photons are used to treat spinal cord compression. Occasionally electron beam therapy is used in paediatric cases, and proton beam radiation is now becoming available for the treatment of spinal cord tumours in some comprehensive cancer centres. Stereotactic radiosurgery provides a high dose of photon radiation to a small, well-defined area. Using radiosurgery,

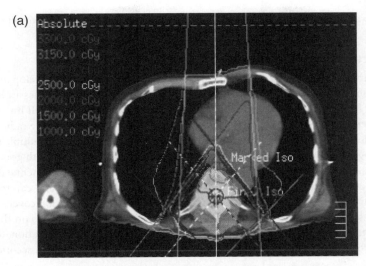

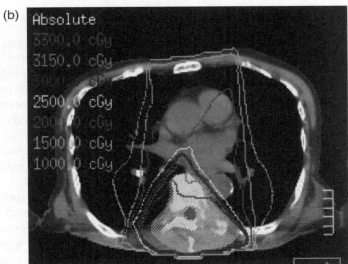

Figure 30.6 CT-based treatment planning using a wedge pair technique that reduces the radiation exit dose to the heart to less than 2500 cGy, and the oesophagus which is demarcated in the lower view.

the vertebral body can receive 20 Gy while less than 0.5 cm³ of the spinal cord is exposed to 8 Gy of radiation. Combined with kyphoplasty, radiosurgery is able to relieve pain in 92% of patients during a 7 to 20 month follow-up period.

Radiation beams diverge as they penetrate through the body such that the field that exits the body is larger than the field that enters the body. If spinal metastases occur above a previously radiated area of the spinal cord, the new radiation field must be matched to the prior radiation field, accounting for the divergence of the radiation beam. Extreme precision is required when administering radiation, especially when the radiation treatment must match a previously radiated segment of the spinal cord. Issues regarding reirradiation are especially important in palliative therapy.[3, 28]

Tolerance to radiation depends on the type of tissue treated. There are two types of normal tissues.

Acute-reacting tissues

These are rapidly proliferating tissues like mucosal surfaces, and usually develop an inflammatory radiation reaction during the course of treatment. Acute radiation toxicities are a function of the dose per fraction, total dose, and the area and volume of tissue irradiated. If mucosal surfaces like the upper aerodigestive tract, bowel and bladder can be excluded from the radiation portals, acute radiation side-effects can be significantly reduced whether a single or multiple fractions are prescribed. A more protracted course of radiation is still used for patients with good prognostic factors who require treatment over the spine and other critical sites.[29] Experimental data suggests that acute-responding tissues recover radiation injury in a few months and can tolerate additional radiation therapy later. However, there is considerable variability in recovery from radiation among late-reacting tissues like the spinal cord. This recovery depends on the technique used, the organ irradiated, the volume irradiated, the initial total dose of radiation, the radiation dose given with each fraction, and the time interval between the initial and second courses of radiation.

Late-reacting tissues

Late-reacting tissues like brain and spinal cord, liver, and muscle do not proliferate, and generally do not develop a significant inflammatory reaction during the radiation course. With regard to the radiation tolerance of the spinal cord, the potential for the development of radiation myelitis with total radiation doses represents the limiting factor in the treatment of large tumour burdens near or involving the spinal canal.[30] The total dose to the spinal cord is generally limited to 4000 cGy administered at 200 cGy per fraction to minimize any risk of irreversible radiation injury to the spinal cord, especially among patients who have received chemotherapy or need to have a significant length of spinal cord irradiated. A steep curve based on total radiation dose predicts the risk of developing radiation myelopathy; a small increase in total radiation dose can result in a large increased risk for radiation myelopathy. The length of spinal cord that needs to be irradiated significantly affects the late radiation tolerance of the spinal cord. Clinical and experimental experience has failed to demonstrate any difference in radiosensitivity in different segments of the spinal cord. The risk of radiation myelitis in the cervico–thoracic spine is less than 5% when 6000 cGy is administered at 172 cGy per fraction, or 5000 cGy is given with daily fractions of 200 cGy per fraction. The effects of tumour or mechanical trauma to the spinal cord, compromising blood flow and causing oedema, also reduce the late radiation tolerance of the spinal cord to radiation. Vasogenic oedema of the spinal cord and nerve roots can be caused by compression injury. Metastatic epidural compression results in vasogenic spinal cord oedema, venous haemorrhage, loss of myelin, and ischaemia, and increases synthesis of prostaglandin E_2, that can be inhibited by steroids or non-steroidal anti-inflammatory agents. Other consequences of pathologic compression include haemorrhage, loss of myelin and ischaemia. Retreatment of a previously irradiated segment of spinal cord results in high risk for radiation-induced myelopathy because other neurological pathways cannot compensate for an injury to a specific level of the spinal cord. Experimental data has shown that the time course and the extent of long-term recovery from radiation are dependent on the specific type and age of tissue.

Equivalent normal tissue effects can be achieved with a variety of radiation treatment schedules.[26] The following clinical radiation schedules are used to treat spine metastases: 2000 cGy is delivered in 5 fractions, 3000 cGy is administered in 10 fractions, 3500 cGy in 14 fractions or 4000 cGy in 20 fractions. The late radiation effects on the spinal cord are would be equal to giving 2800 cGy, 3600 cGy, and 3900 cGy, respectively at 200 cGy per fraction. This shows that as the radiation dose per fraction increases, the late radiation toxicities also increase rapidly.

Complete pain relief after radiation is achieved in 73% of spine metastases, compared with 88% of metastases in long bones and 67% of pelvic bone metastases,[32, 33] while the functional outcome is dependent on the level of symptoms at the time radiation is administered. The mean time to pain relief was 35 days in 108 breast cancer patients. Accounting for the limited prognosis, metastatic spinal cord compression has been treated either with a single 8 Gy fraction or 5 4 Gy fractions. The median time to recurrence was 6 months among 62 patients with a range of 2 to 40 months.[3] Retreatment consisted of another single 8 Gy fraction, or 5 more fractions of either 3 Gy or 4 Gy. Motor function improved in 40%, and it was stable in an additional 45%; 38% of the nonambulatory patients regained the ability to walk. This more efficient radiation treatment schedule provides sufficient tumour regression for neurological improvement.

Recurrent symptoms at a different spinal level occurred in more than three-quarters of patients treated with radiation and within 6 months of the initial treatment.[15] Persistent pain after radiotherapy for vertebral metastases should be investigated to exclude the possibility of progressive disease in or outside the radiation portal, or mechanical spinal instability because of a vertebral compression fracture. Changes seen in the bone marrow on MRI after palliative radiotherapy initially includes decreased cellularity, oedema and haemorrhage followed by fatty replacement and fibrosis.[31] These well-defined changes on MRI after radiotherapy can be distinguished from those seen with progressive disease.

The projected length of survival is the critical issue for radiation dose and schedule for palliative radiation for bone metastases. In one study, only 12 of 245 patients were alive at the time of analysis with approximately 50% alive at 6 months, 25% at 1 year, 8% at 2 years and 3% at 3 years after palliative radiation. For breast cancer patients the survival rates at these time points after palliative radiation were 60%, 44%, 20%, and 7%, respectively. For prostate cancer, the survival rates were 60% at 6 months, 24% at 1 year and there were no patients who survived 2 years. In the RTOG trial the median survival for solitary bone metastases was 36 weeks and was 24 weeks for multiple bone metastases.[34] The RTOG study also demonstrated that the level of pain correlated with prognosis among patients with multiple bone metastases. This survival difference may be an important observation because unrelieved pain and the resultant sequelae of immobility may contribute to mortality as well as morbidity.

Surgery

A statistically significant improvement in functional outcome occurs with laminectomy and radiotherapy in treatment of epidural spinal cord compression over either modality alone for selected clinical presentations. Laminectomy has been recommended to promptly reduce tumour volume in an attempt to relieve compression and injury of the spinal cord and provide stabilization to the spinal axis. The rate of tumour regression following radiotherapy is too slow in these cases to effect recovery of lost neurologic function, and radiation therapy cannot relieve compression of the spinal column due to vertebral collapse. After radiation alone to treat a partial spinal cord block, 64% of patients regain ambulation, 33% have normalization of sphincter tone, 72% are pain free, and median survival is 9 months. With a complete spinal cord block only 27% will have improvement in motor function and 42% will continue to have pain after radiation alone. In paraparetic patients who undergo laminectomy and radiation, 82% regain the ability to walk, 68% have improved sphincter function, and 88% have relief of pain.

Laminectomy is indicated with rapid neurologic deterioration, tumour progression in a previously irradiated area, stabilization of the spine, paraplegic patients with limited disease and good probability of survival, and to establish a diagnosis. Adjuvant radiotherapy is often given to treat microscopic residual disease after neurosurgical intervention.[35–37] Surgical restoration of the vertebral alignment may be required due neurologic compromise and pain caused by progressive vertebral collapse. Vertebral collapse may occur due to cancer or mechanical vertebral instability after tumour regression (Figure 30.7). Appropriate diagnostic studies and intervention should be pursued with persistent pain because the neurologic compromise and pain from vertebral instability can be as devastating as that with epidural spinal cord metastases.

Surgery often is the only available option for therapy because previously administered radiation may preclude further radiotherapy in the region of the malignant spinal cord compression.

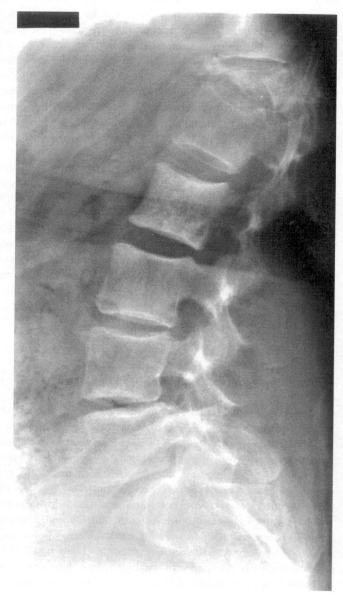

Figure 30.7 Compression fraction of the twelfth thoracic vertebral body following an initial pain-free interval after palliative radiation. Recurrent back pain was caused by spinal instability due to vertebral weakness with rapid tumour regression resulting in the compression fracture.

This is often the case in lung cancer because metastases are located in the thoracic spine in over 70% cases, and many of these patients have received mediastinal irradiation. Early involvement by the radiotherapist in the management of the patients with suspected spinal cord involvement is important to allow time to obtain prior radiotherapy records, determine if further radiation is possible and expedite the clinical decision-making process. Using stereotactic conformal radiotherapy and intensity-modulated radiation therapy to total doses of 39 Gy, reirradiation results in 95% local control at 12 months follow-up.[38,39] Half of the patients had neurologic improvement, and 13 of 16 patients had relief of pain. No significant late toxicity was reported.

Percutaneous vertebroplasty

Percutaneous vertebroplasty is another alternative that injects bone cement into structurally weakened vertebrae to provide biomechanical stability.[40] The effect of vertebroplasty on vertebral bulge, a measure of posterior vertebral body wall motion, was reduced by up to 62%. Tumour location affected both the vertebral bulge and the axial vertebral displacement. Posterior movement of the tumour and tumour shape caused the greatest increased the vertebral bulge.

Short- and long-term prognosis

Median survival among patients with spinal cord compression ranges between 3 and 7 months with a 36% probability for a 1-year survival. For specific types of cancer, the mean survival time is 14 months for breast cancer, 12 months in prostate cancer, 6 months in malignant melanoma, and 3 months in lung cancer once epidural spinal cord compression is diagnosed.[8, 11, 15–18]

The severity of weakness at presentation is the most significant factor for recovery of function.[2, 4, 7–18] Ninety per cent of patients who are ambulatory at presentation will be ambulatory after treatment. Only 13% of paraplegic patients will regain function, particularly if paraplegia is present for more than 24 hours before the initiation of therapy. Over 30% of patients who develop spinal cord compression are alive 1 year later and 50% of these patients will remain ambulatory with appropriate therapy. Among 102 consecutive patients with metastatic spinal cord compression, 51% were fully ambulatory at the time of radiotherapy, and 41% were ambulant but with paraparesis. Median survival was 3.5 months, with normal gait returning in 58% 2 weeks after completing radiation and in 71% 2 months after radiation. No paraplegic patient regained function.[4]

Survival after surgery for metastatic spinal cord compression can be accurately predicted by the Tokuhasi and Tomita scores.[41] A Tokuhashi score of 4 or more, or a Tomita score of 6 or less predicted a 76% 3-month survival. Secondary factors include primary site, extent of metastatic disease, performance status, and time between primary diagnosis and diagnosis of spine metastases did not correlate with postoperative survival.

Therapeutic recommendations for spinal cord compression in far advanced cancer

The primary goals of palliative treatment are to efficiently relieve disease-related symptoms and maintain function, while minimizing treatment-related symptoms, and time under therapy. Spine metastases cause significant pain and can result in irreversible paralysis.[42] Patients with known vertebral metastases require frequent clinical evaluation to identify any change in symptoms and/or radiographic findings suggesting risk for spinal cord compromise. Early detection of vertebral compromise is paramount to preventing an oncologic emergency with severe pain and neurologic compromise from spinal cord compression. Emergent oncologic care involves either surgical decompression and/or radiation therapy. Efforts to prevent spinal cord compression due to progression of bone metastases through systemic therapies continue.

Radiation remains an important modality in palliative care.[26] A number of clinical, prognostic and therapeutic factors must be considered to determine the most optimal treatment regimen in palliative radiotherapy. Symptoms that persist after palliative radiation should be evaluated to exclude progression of disease in the treated area, and possible extension of disease outside the radiation portal, especially if there is an associated paraspinal mass. Pain may also persist due to reduced cortical strength after treatment of spinal metastases that can result in vertebral compression or stress microfractures.

Radiation therapy is an important means of treating localized symptoms related to tumour involvement by providing a wide range of therapeutic options. Radiobiological principles, the radiation tolerance of adjacent normal tissues, and the clinical condition influence the selection of radiation technique, dose and fraction size. As a late-reacting tissue, the radiobiological tolerance of the spinal cord to radiation is finite. Technological advances, however, have increased our ability to treat spinal metastases with greater precision, and have allowed consideration of retreatment with radiation to selected patients.

The treatment of bone metastases represents a paradigm for evaluating palliative care in terms of symptom relief, toxicities of therapy, and the financial burden to the patient, caregivers and society. Despite enormous expenditures to treat metastases, patients continue to suffer symptoms and they will die of their disease within 24 months; the prognosis associated with the development of spinal cord compression is even more ominous. As healthcare resources continue to become more limited, our criteria for care must be better defined to provide care that provides effective treatment that fulfils the goals of relieving suffering while avoiding administration of therapy with limited added benefit.

The goals of palliative therapy are very specific for patients with spinal cord compression. The treatment of spinal cord compression is a moral imperative to relieve suffering and attempt to maintain functional integrity and patient dignity. Furthermore, loss of function is among the most significant financial burdens assumed by caregivers and society. More sophisticated and costly radiotherapeutic approaches, like intensity modulated radiation threapy (IMRT) and proton therapy, should be based on prognostic factors and performance status, and reserved for more complicated clinical presentations including retreatment. Similar criteria exist for surgical intervention.

The point and types of intervention for spinal cord compression are clearer than the prevention and early detection of spinal cord compression. Radiation and surgery, both localized therapies, are used in spinal cord compression. Systemic therapies and/or radiation can be used to prevent spinal cord compression. Radiation can be used to treat early vertebral and/or epidural involvement to prevent disease progression resulting in spinal cord compression. Radiopharmaceuticals, administered by a single injection, are an important option with multifocal bone metastases when there is no epidural involvement in the vertebral disease.[43] Spinal cord compression can be prevented in patients at high risk for disease progression with limited treatment-related toxicity and time under therapy.

The role of systemic therapies, such as bisphosphonates, in preventing spinal cord compression is less clear. While systemic therapy with bisphosphonates has reduced the development of skeletal-related events among patients with lytic bone metastases,[44] no analysis has specifically evaluated whether the incidence of spinal cord compression is decreased among patients with lytic bone metastases in the vertebrae at the start of bisphosphonate therapy. The 6 months required before the full benefit of bisphosphonates is realized limits the use of bisphosphonates, because of the poor overall prognosis after the development of spinal cord compression. Furthermore, no clear criteria exist as to when to start or stop bisphosphonate therapy among patients with bone metastases. The current overall financial burden and the opportunity costs, related to the frequent infusions required in bisphosphonate therapy, is high. Cost–utility analyses, which accounts for a broader domain of cost-effectiveness, need to be performed as part of clinical trials in every specialty, especially for palliative care end points. Clinical trials that include these criteria are critical to future practice guidelines development.

Much is accommodated during the course of cancer and its treatment. Prevention or early treatment of symptoms is often the most important care administered. The treatment of vertebral metastases and spinal cord compression to prevent or relieve symptoms of pain and paralysis is among the most important services rendered to cancer patients.

References

1. Earle CC, Neville BA, Landrum MB. *et al*. Evaluating claims-based indicators of the intensity of end-of-life cancer care. *Int J Qual Health Care* 2005; 17(6):505–9.

2. Helweg-Larsen S, Sorensen PS, Kreiner S. Prognostic factors in metastatic spinal cord compression: a prospective study using multivariate analysis of variables influencing survival and gait function in 153 patients. *Int J Radiat Oncol Biol Phys* 2000; 46(5):1163–9.

3. Rades D, Stalpers LJ, Veninga T, Hoskin PJ. Spinal reirradiation after short-course RT for metastatic spinal cord compression. *Int J Radiat Oncol Biol Phys* 2005; 63(3):872–5.

4. Hoskin PJ, Grover A, Bhana R. Metastatic spinal cord compression: radiotherapy outcome and dose fractionation. *Radiother Oncol* 2003; 68(2):175–80.

5. Bates T, Yarnold JR, Blitzer P, Nelson OS, Rubin P, Maher J. Bone metastasis consensus statement. *Int J Radiat Oncol Biol Phys* 1992; 23(1):215–16.

6. Bates T. A review of local radiotherapy in the treatment of bone metastases and cord compression. *Int J Radiat Oncol Biol Phys* 1992; 23(1):217–21.

7. Turner S, Marosszeky B, Timms I, Boyages J. Malignant spinal cord compression: a prospective evaluation. *Int J Radiat Oncol Biol Phys* 1993; 26(1):141–6.

8. Boogerd W, van der Sande JJ, Kroger R. Early diagnosis and treatment of spinal epidural metastasis in breast cancer: a prospective study. *J Neurol Neurosurg Psychiatry* 1992; 55(12):1188–93.

9. Wada E, Yamamoto T, Furuno M, Nakamura M, Yonenobu K. Spinal cord compression secondary to osteoblastic metastasis. *Spine* 1993; 18(10):1380–1.

10. Kim RY, Smith JW, Spencer SA, Meredith RF, Salter MM. Malignant epidural spinal cord compression associated with a paravertebral mass: its radiotherapeutic outcome on radiosensivity. *Int J Radiat Oncol Biol Phys* 1993; 27(5):1079–83.

11. Bach F, Agerlin N, Sorensen JB. *et al*. Metastatic spinal cord compression secondary to lung cancer. *J Clin Oncol* 1992; 10(11):1781–7.

12. Russi EG, Pergolizzi S, Gaeta M, Mesiti M, D'Aquino A, Delia P. Palliative-radiotherapy in lumbosacral carcinomatous neuropathy. *Radiother Oncol* 1993; 26(2):172–3.

13. Saarto T, Janes R, Tenhunen M, Kouri M. Palliative radiotherapy in the treatment of skeletal metastases. *Eur J Pain* 2002; 6(5):323–30.

14. Loblaw DA, Laperriere NJ, Mackillop WJ. A population-based study of malignant spinal cord compression in Ontario. *Clin Oncol (R Coll Radiol)* 2003; 15(4):211–17.

15. Rades D, Blach M, Bremer M, Wildfang I, Karstens JH, Heidenreich F. Prognostic significance of the time of developing motor deficits before radiation therapy in metastatic spinal cord compression: one-year results of a prospective trial. *Int J Radiat Oncol Biol Phys* 2000; 48(5):1403–8.

16. Rades D, Heidenreich F, Karstens JH. Final results of a prospective study of the prognostic value of the time to develop motor deficits before irradiation in metastatic spinal cord compression. *Int J Radiat Oncol Biol Phys* 2002; 53(4):975–9.

17. Altehoefer C, Ghanem N, Hogerle S, Moser E, Langer M. Comparative detectability of bone metastases and impact on therapy of magnetic resonance imaging and bone scintigraphy in patients with breast cancer. *Eur J Radiol* 2001; 40(1):16–23.

18. Algra PR, Bloem JL, Tissing H, Falke TH, Arndt JW, Verboom LJ. Detection of vertebral metastases: comparison between MR imaging and bone scintigraphy. *Radiographics* 1991; 11(2):219–32.

19. Francken AB, Hong AM, Fulham MJ, Millward MJ, McCarthy WH, Thompson JF. Detection of unsuspected spinal cord compression in melanoma patients by 18F-fluorodeoxyglucose-positron emission tomography. *Eur J Surg Oncol* 2005; 31(2):197–204.

20. Conway R, Graham J, Kidd J, Levack P, and other members of the Scottish Cord Compression Group. What happens to people after malignant cord compression? Survival, function, quality of life, emotional well-being and place of care 1 month after diagnosis. *Clinical Oncology* 2007; 19:56–62.

21. Finkelstein JA, Ford MH. Diagnosis and management of pathological fractures of the spine. *Current Orthopedics* 2004; 18:396–405.

22. Tschirhart CE, Nagpurkar A, Whyne CM. Effects of tumor location, shape and surface serration on burst fracture risk in the metastatic spine. *J Biomechanics* 2004; 37:653–60.

23. Tow B, Seang BT, Chong TT, Chen J. Predictors for survival in metastases to the spine. *The Spine Journal* 2005; 5:73S.

24. Nielsen OS, Munro AJ, Tannock IF. Bone metastases: pathophysiology and management policy. *J Clin Oncol* 1991; 9(3):509–24.

25. Moineuse C, Kany M, Fourcade D. *et al.* Magnetic resonance imaging findings in multiple myeloma: Description and predictive value. *Joint, Bone, Spine: Revue du Rhumatisme* 2001; 68(4):334–44.

26. Janjan NA. Radiotherapeutic management of spinal metastases. *J Pain Symptom Manage* 1996; 11(1):47–56.

27. Loblaw DA, Laperriere NJ. Emergency treatment of malignant extradural spinal cord compression: an evidence-based guideline. *J Clin Oncol* 1998; 16(4):1613–24.

28. Morris DE. Clinical experience with retreatment for palliation. *Semin Radiat Oncol* 2000; 10(3):210–21.

29. Minsky BD, Conti JA, Huang Y, Knopf K. Relationship of acute gastrointestinal toxicity and the volume of irradiated small bowel in patients receiving combined modality therapy for rectal cancer. *J Clin Oncol* 1995; 13(6):1409–16.

30. Maranzano E, Bellavita R, Floridi P. *et al.* Radiation-induced myelopathy in long-term surviving metastatic spinal cord compression patients after hypofractionated radiotherapy: a clinical and magnetic resonance imaging analysis. *Radiother Oncol* 2001; 60(3):281–8.

31. Yankelevitz DF, Henschke CI, Knapp PH, Nisce L, Yi Y, Cahill P. Effect of radiation therapy on thoracic and lumbar bone marrow: evaluation with MR imaging. *AJR Am J Roentgenol* 1991; 157(1):87–92.

32. Hortobagyi GN, Libshitz HI, Seabold JE. Osseous metastases of breast cancer. Clinical, biochemical, radiographic, and scintigraphic evaluation of response to therapy. *Cancer* 1984; 53(3):577–82.

33. Cunningham D, Hawthorn J, Pople A, Gazet JC, Ford HT, Challoner T. Prevention of emesis in patients receiving cytotoxic drugs by GR38032F, a selective 5-HT, receptor antagonist. *Lancet* 1987:1461–3.

34. Blitzer PH. Reanalysis of the RTOG study of the palliation of symptomatic osseous metastasis. *Cancer* 1985; 55(7):1468–72.

35. Hatrick NC, Lucas JD, Timothy AR, Smith MA. The surgical treatment of metastatic disease of the spine. *Radiother Oncol* 2000; 56(3):335–9.

36. Landmann C, Hunig R, Gratzl O. The role of laminectomy in the combined treatment of metastatic spinal cord compression. *Int J Radiat Oncol Biol Phys* 1992; 24(4):627–31.

37. Gerszten PC, Germanwala A, Burton SA, Welch WC, Ozhasoglu C, Vogel WJ. Combination kyphoplasty and spinal radiosurgery: a new treatment paradigm for pathological fractures. *J Neurosurg Spine* 2005; 3(4):296–301.

38. Grosu AL, Andratschke N, Nieder C, Molls M. Retreatment of the spinal cord with palliative radiotherapy. *Int J Radiat Oncol Biol Phys* 2002; 52(5):1288–92.

39. Shiu AS, Chang EL, Ye JS. *et al.* Near simultaneous computed tomography image-guided stereotactic spinal radiotherapy: an emerging paradigm for achieving true stereotaxy. *Int J Radiat Oncol Biol Phys* 2003; 57(3):605–13.

40. Tschirhart CE, Roth SE, Whyne CM. Biomechanical assessment of stability in the metastatic spine following percutaneous vertebroplasty: effects of cement distribution patterns and volume. *J Biomech* 2005; 38(8):1582–90.

41. Tokuhashi Y, Matsuzaki H, Oda H, Oshima M, Ryu J. A revised scoring system for preoperative evaluation of metastatic spine tumor prognosis. *Spine* 2005; 30(19):2186–91.

42. Janjan NA, Payne R, Gillis T. *et al.* Presenting symptoms in patients referred to a multidisciplinary clinic for bone metastases. *J Pain Symptom Manage* 1998; 16(3):171–8.

43. Janjan NA. Radiation for bone metastases: conventional techniques and the role of systemic radiopharmaceuticals. *Cancer* 1997; 80(8 Suppl):1628–45.

44. Hortobagyi GN, Theriault RL, Porter L. *et al.* Efficacy of pamidronate in reducing skeletal complications in patients with breast cancer and lytic bone metastases. Protocol 19 Aredia Breast Cancer Study Group. *N Engl J Med* 1996; 335(24):1785–91.

31

Pain relief

Maria Montoya and Eduardo Bruera

Introduction

Pain is one of the major symptoms in patients with advanced cancer, and comprises a hetero-geneous group of more than 100 syndromes with varying underlying pathophysiologies. Although in 80 to 90 per cent of patients, pain can be controlled by methods approved by the World Health Organization, at least 25 per cent of cancer patients die in pain,[1-5] mainly because of inadequate assessment, not enough knowledge about pain and its treatment, and physicians, and patients, misconceptions of opioid use.

Pain relief can be achieved in the hands of a pain specialist in more than 80 per cent of patients during the first week of treatment.[2] Determination of the cause, type, and intensity of pain is essential for appropriate management of cancer pain, because the pain experience is a complex interplay of organic, cognitive, and emotional influences. Figure 31.1 shows the different contributions to pain expression. For patients whose pain persists despite appropriate therapy, multidimensional assessment is mandatory. Table 31.1 summarizes the multidimensional assessment of cancer pain.

Difficult-to-control pain has been described in the literature as paradoxical pain, opioid insensitivity, opioid unresponsiveness, and opioid resistance.[3] Responsiveness to opioids is extremely variable among patients and in individual patients over time.[6] No maximum dose can be specified in defining opioid unresponsiveness and the dose–response for analgesia shows no ceiling effect. Unless important side-effects occur, dose escalation may provide analgesia.[3]

The prognostic factors that indicate to physicians that they may encounter difficulties in con-trolling the patient's pain fall into two major categories: good and poor. Poor prognostic factors include history of somatization, history of alcoholism or drug abuse, development of tolerance to opioids, neuropathic and incidental pain.[1] Other factors that may predict a poor outcome are extent of disease, performance status, prior analgesic therapy, age, and number and severity of other symptoms. They were proposed by several authors, but no association with outcome has been found consistently.[1-3, 7] Table 31.2 summarized the principal prognostic factors.

It is well established that cancer pain is progressive, that is it is more prevalent as the disease progresses and death approaches, with moderately severe pain being reported by approximately one-third of ambulatory patients, three-quarters of patients with advanced cancer and close to 90 per cent of patients in hospices. This pattern suggests that, at a population level, pain is predictive of survival. However, at an individual level, this is less clearly the case. Many years ago, Ventafridda observed that uncontrolled pain (and breathlessness) commonly occurred immediately before death.[8] Maltoni et al.[9] observed that pain and increasing amount of analgesia may be poor predictors of survival, yet others did not confirm this.[10, 11] In fact, a review of the literature of prognostic factors and survival in 2000 found that while there was a positive associa-tion between pain and survival in 5 out of 9 studies looking at this question, in only 1 of 9 studies did pain retain significance after multivariate analysis.[12] The one positive study was a study of

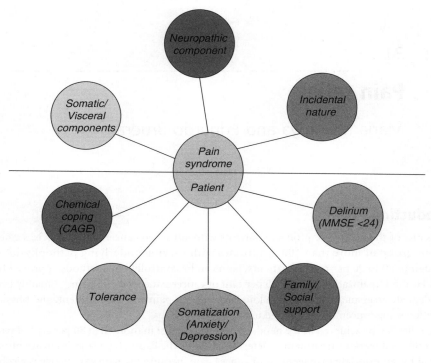

Figure 31.1 Contributions to pain expression, Mini-Mental State Examination (MMSE).

Table 31.1 Multidimensional assessment of cancer pain

Cause (cancer, cancer treatment, not related to cancer)
Intensity (visual analogue, numerical and verbal scales)
Alcoholism/drugs, etc.
Psychosocial distress (somatization)
Cognitive function
Mechanism (neuropathic, non-neuropathic)
Nature (continuous, incidental)
Other related symptoms (ESAS)

ESAS, Edmonton Symptom Assessment System.

Table 31.2 Prognostic factors

Good prognosis	Poor prognosis
Visceral pain	Neuropathic pain
Somatic pain	Mixed pain aetiology
Non-incidental pain	Incidental pain
Absence of somatization	Somatization
Absence of tolerance	Tolerance
Absence of substance abuse	Substance abuse

prognostic factors in US patients with terminal lung cancer referred to hospice more than 10 years ago, and pain was only just significant as a predictor of shortened survival ($p < 0.05$).[13] In 2005, the EAPC working group on prognosis in far advanced cancer determined that pain was one of the prognostic factors 'for which a correlation has been indicated but not confirmed or for which a statistical significance has been identified in patient populations with less advanced disease or for which contradictory data have emerged'.[14] Of note, a survey of Italian doctors found that pain is not one of the criteria they use when formulating a prognosis.[15]

One possible explanation for the lack of association between pain and survival in these studies is the effect of referral bias. Survival studies in the hospice/palliative care literature rarely involve inception cohorts and because of the emphasis on cancer pain management it may be that patients in pain are referred earlier to hospice and live longer on the programme. However, two studies involving true inception cohorts have been published but both failed to find pain as a prognostic factor.[16, 17] It has been suggested that the method of pain management may impact on survival: 202 patients with unrelieved pain rated >/ = 5 on a 0 to 10 scale were enrolled on a random controlled trail (RCT) of spinal opioids versus systemic opioids. Spinal opioid patients had better pain control, less side-effects and improved survival (53.9 per cent alive at 6 months compared with 37.2 per cent) although this difference just failed to reach statistical significance ($p = 0.06$).[18] Similarly, 100 patients with unresectable pancreatic cancer were randomly assigned to receive either neurolytic celiac plexus block (NCPB) or systemic analgesic therapy alone with a sham injection. All patients could receive additional opioids managed by a clinician blinded to the treatment assignment. Although NCPB improved pain relief in patients with pancreatic cancer vs optimized systemic analgesic therapy alone, it did not affect quality of life (QoL) or survival. After 1 year, 16 per cent of NCPB patients and 6 per cent of opioid-only patients were alive, but this survival difference was not significant ($p = 0.26$), probably due to the small sample size.[19]

Recognition of poor prognostic features led to the development of staging systems for different primary tumours. Although these systems require frequent changes as knowledge about the biology of cancer develops, the staging systems allowed researchers to speak a common language and practitioners to apply treatments in a logical and predictable fashion. Precise definition of patient characteristics in clinical trials promotes accurate interpretation of data, successful application of therapies, and subsequent formulation of more advanced clinical studies. An appropriate staging system not only contributes to the execution of clinical trials, it acts as quality control for established and soon to be established therapies.

Two main assessment tools, the Edmonton Staging System for cancer pain (ESS) and the Cancer Pain Prognosis Scale (CPPS), are used to evaluate cancer-related pain prognosis.[1, 2, 20]

The Edmonton Staging System for cancer pain

This is a tool for pain assessment designed by Bruera and associates in 1989.[20] The initial Edmonton Staging System (ESS) included seven parameters: mechanism of pain, pain characteristics, previous opioid dose/exposure, cognitive function, psychological distress, tolerance, past history of addictive personality. The initial analysis of 56 consecutive patients with cancer-related pain was a prospective study in which patients were treated for 21 days and classified in three groups:

1. stage 1 (patients with good prognosis)
2. stage 2 (patients with less predictable outcome)
3. stage 3 (patients with poor prognosis).

Eighteen of twenty-two patients (82 per cent) in the stage 1 group achieved good pain control, compared with two of 22 patients (10 per cent; $p < 0.01$) in the stage 3 group. The staging system's sensitivity (ability to predict good pain control) was 75 per cent, and its specificity (ability to predict poor pain control) was 86 per cent.

In further analysis with a multicentre study that included 276 patients Bruera and associates[21] found that two of the variables – opioid dose and cognitive function – were not independently associated with outcome. The two items were dropped from the system, as was stage II. Now patients are currently classified by the ESS as having good or poor prognosis. A patient is classified as having a poor prognosis when one or more negative prognostic factors are present. In this multicentre study, 93 per cent of patients with good prognosis achieved pain control by day 21, whereas only 55 per cent of the patients considered to have poor prognosis achieved good pain control. Good pain control was defined as no pain most of the time and a need for two or fewer rescue doses per day. The specificity of this tool is low (46 per cent), but its sensitivity is relatively high (93 per cent). According to the specificity of this tool one can expect about 90 per cent of patients with good prognostic factors and nearly 50 per cent of patients with poor prognostic factors to achieve good pain relief.

The ESS may be used after a standard consultation and requires no more than 5–10 minutes to complete. Table 31.3 lists the revised version of the ESS.

The revised Edmonton Staging System for cancer (rESS)

To further test the reliability and predictive value of the ESS, a multicentre study of 619 cancer patients was conducted in Edmonton, Canada.[22] The results showed that patients with

Table 31.3 The Edmonton staging system for cancer pain

Stage	
I: Good prognosis	A1, A2, B1, C1, D1, E1
II: Poor prognosis	A3, A4, A5 (Any B-C-D-E)
	B2 (Any A-C-D-E)
	C2 (Any A-B-D-E)
	D2 (Any A-B-C-E)
	E2 (Any A-B-C-D)

Mechanism of pain
A1. Visceral pain
A2. Bone and soft-tissue pain
A3. Neuropathic pain
A4. Mixed (neuropathic + non-neuropathic pain)
A5. Unknown

Pain characteristics
B1. Non-incidental
B2. Incidental

Psychological distress
C1. Patients without any major psychological distress
C2. Major psychological distress (depression, anxiety, somatization)

Tolerance
D1. Increase of < 5% of initial dose/day
D2. Increase of > 5% of initial dose/day

Past history
E1. Negative history of alcoholism or drug addiction
E2. Positive history of alcoholism or drug addiction

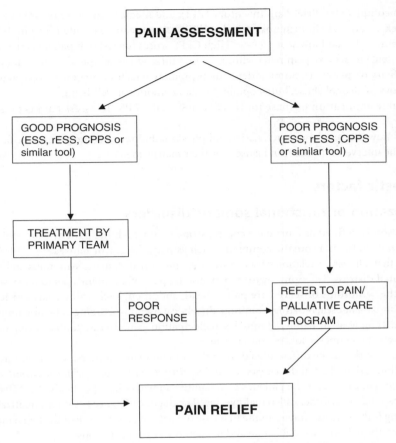

Figure 31.2 Possible applications of the Edmonton Staging System for Cancer Pain (ESS), the revised Edmonton Staging System for Cancer (rESS) and the Cancer Pain Prognostic scale (CPPS).

neuropathic pain, incidental pain, in psychological distress or trouble by addictive behaviour required longer to achieve pain control ($p < 0.05$) and a higher final mean equivalent daily dose (MEDD) of morphine ($p < 0.001$). Impaired cognitive function shortened the time required to achieve stable pain control ($p < 0.05$), and patients with neuropathic or incidental pain used more methods do this ($p < 0.01$). As currently proposed, the system has four prognostic factors: neuropathic pain, incidental pain, psychological distress and addictive behaviour. Drug tolerance is not included. A final, definitive version may prove elusive because knowledge of prognostic factors, diagnosis, and treatment has grown.

The Cancer Pain Prognostic Scale

This four dimensional scale developed by Chang et al.[2] includes pain characteristics, patient's social situation, overall symptom distress, and general overall quality of life with each dimension scored. The system was originally studied in a prospective trial with 74 consecutive patients who experienced cancer-related pain. The patients were treated according to guidelines of the United States Agency for Health Care Policy and Research (AHCPR). Patients were asked weekly to complete the Brief Pain Inventory (BPI), and medications were recorded weekly for three weeks. Cancer Pain Prognostic Scale (CPPS) scores can be divided into high (13–17), intermittent (7–12) and low scores (1–6). High CPPS scores suggest that patients are more likely (> 80 per cent) to achieve pain relief within the first three weeks of opioid treatment (sensitivity 86, specificity 63 per cent). Some independent predictive factors suggested were neuropathic pain, history of alcohol abuse, initial opioid dose, and emotional well-being.

A possible application of these tools (ESS, rESS and CPPS) to assess pain is presented in Figure 31.2.

We will now discuss the characteristics and physiopathology of some prognostic factors and some of the interventions that can be used for their management.

Prognostic factors

Somatization or functional somatic disorders

Somatization is defined as a primary coping strategy in which the patient expresses anxiety, depression or both, as a somatic complaint such as pain, fatigue or nausea.[1, 23–25] It has been suggested that a linear correlation exists between the number of somatic symptoms and measures of emotional distress.[26, 27] Somatization may also be part of a patient's personality structure. Some of the symptoms observed are pain – head, abdomen, back, joints, extremities, chest; gastrointestinal – nausea, bloating, vomiting, diarrhoea; pseudo-neurological – impaired balance or coordination, weak or paralyzed muscles, hallucinations, numbness, double vision, blindness, deafness, seizures, amnesia, loss of consciousness.

Somatization should be differentiated from the somatoform disorders, which are rare psychiatric conditions described in the *Diagnostic and Statistical Manual of Psychiatric Disorders – IV* as having no organic bases for the patient's complaint.[28] Somatization should also be differentiated from the psychiatric disorder called malingering. The major difference between somatization and malingering is the patient's intent: in the first case the patient is not aware of the behaviour, while in the other, the behaviour is deliberate and has a known external purpose.

Somatization is usually the over-expression of an organic problem. All medical subspecialties know at least one unexplained functional symptom: for the rheumatologist prominent muscle pain and tenderness is fibromyalgia; for the gastroenterologist abdominal pain and altered bowel habit is irritable bowel syndrome. Rather than being a specific symptom, somatization is an entity of multiple syndromes, so commonly related that patients with one functional syndrome may meet criteria for other syndrome.[26, 27] The most common functional syndromes are summarized in Table 31.4.

Table 31.4 Functional somatic syndromes by specialty[26]

Gastroenterology	Irritable bowel syndrome, non-ulcer dyspepsia
Gynaecology	Pre-menstrual syndrome, chronic pelvic pain
Rheumatology	Fibromyalgia
Cardiology	Atypical or non-cardiac chest pain
Pulmonary	Hyperventilation syndrome
Infectious diseases	Chronic (post-viral) fatigue syndrome
Neurology	Tension headache
Allergy	Multiple chemical sensitivity

For most cancer patients, somatization is strongly associated with mood disorders. One tool used for screening symptoms of anxiety and depression is the Hospital Anxiety and Depression Scale (HADS); on which a score of 8–21 is considered positive.[7, 29]

Sharpe and colleagues[30] reported that patients with functional somatic syndromes are 'difficult to help patients'; the doctor–patient relationship is frequently unsatisfactory for both. A combination of counselling, distraction, and pharmacological management of affective disorders may be required to decrease the intensity of the patient's pain expression. Regularly scheduled appointments should be maintained to review the patient's symptoms and coping mechanisms.

Opioid tolerance and dose escalation

Cancer pain is often undertreated because of mistaken attitudes about tolerance and dependence. Patients may fear addiction to opioids and for the same reason physicians may be reluctant to prescribe them. To provide rational pain management physicians should know the difference between opioid tolerance, physical dependence and psychological dependence – addiction.

Opioid tolerance is defined as an increase of 5 per cent or more of the initial opioid dose per day.[1, 20] The progression of disease in advanced cancer typically leads to more severe pain that requires higher opioid dosing, but the increasing doses of an opioid needed to yield the same analgesic effect as previous lower doses may signal the development of tolerance.

The physiopathology of this normal physiological phenomenon may include alterations at the opioid receptor level, neural adaptation or changes in opioid metabolism.[3, 25, 31, 32] Development of tolerance varies greatly among patients and opioids; it may occur quickly after acute dosing or more gradually with repeated dosing.[33, 34] Different opioids may produce various opioid responses in the presence of distinct pain mechanisms.

Tolerance to some opioid side-effects including nausea, sedation and respiratory depression, has been well documented in humans.[32] Development of tolerance to adverse effects is usually favourable, because it enlarges the therapeutic window, whereas analgesic tolerance reduces responsiveness to opioids.[3]

Opioid rotation may help to decrease the level of dose escalation because cross-tolerance among opioids is incomplete.[24, 25, 31] Methadone seems to be particularly effective in decreasing tolerance as a result of its N-methyl D-aspartate (NMDA) receptor antagonist properties. Animal studies have suggested that the use of other NMDA receptor antagonist like ketamine and dextrometarphan may help to reverse opioid tolerance.[31, 35] Results in humans have been controversial.[36] The use of steroids may also prevent the development of tolerance by mechanisms related to NMDA action.[31]

Chemical coping

In the patient with cancer-related pain chemical dependence on drugs or alcohol may be a past or present problem. Patients used to coping with different life stressors by using alcohol or illegal drugs will use opioids not only for pain control but also to cope with stress.

Table 31.5 The CAGE screening tool

Have you ever felt that you should **Cut** down on your drinking?
Have you ever been **Annoyed** by people criticizing your drinking?
Have you ever felt bad or **Guilty** about your drinking?
Have you ever had a drink first thing in the morning or a drink to get rid of a hangover (**Eye opener**)?

* The **CAGE** score is positive if two or more of the questions are answered affirmatively.

Drug dependence is defined as the psychological or physical need, or both, to continue taking a substance.[37] It is a common and normal pharmacophysiological effect of opioid use. It has also been found to accompany the use of medications like steroids and beta-blockers.[25] The body simply becomes accustomed to a medication.

Physical dependence is the need to take a substance to prevent occurrence of a withdrawal or abstinence syndrome.[37] For example, upon abrupt reduction or discontinuation of an opioid, the patient will experience agitation, tremulousness, fever, diaphoresis, mydriasis, tachycardia, muscle and abdominal cramping, and diarrhoea. Use of an opioid antagonist may lead to the same syndrome. If reduction of opioid is necessary to avoid this uncomfortable experience, a daily taper of 50 to 75 per cent can be done. Once the tapered dosage is equivalent to 15 mg of morphine per day, the opioid can be stopped.[25, 32]

Psychological dependence – drug-seeking behaviour or addiction – is defined as the psychopathological impulse to use a substance with resulting physical, psychological, or social consequences to the user.[23, 32, 35] Fear of addiction is one of the most common reasons for opioid under-prescription. Addiction to opioids is rare in medical patients[23, 38, 39] and substantial evidence suggests that cancer patients with no history of alcohol or drug dependence who take opioids appropriately are at minimal or no risk for developing psychological dependence.[14, 23]

Alcohol abuse/alcoholism

Alcohol is the most widely available and culturally accepted abusable substance. Ninety per cent of people in most western societies consume alcohol at some time in their lives, but only 30 per cent of drinkers will develop alcohol-related problems.[37] Alcoholism occurs in 5–15 per cent of the general population and in approximately 20 per cent of hospitalized patients; it remains undiagnosed in more than two-thirds of patients.[24, 40, 41] A tool called CAGE may be used to screen for the problem;[42] Table 31.5 shows the CAGE mnemonic.

A CAGE positive score (a yes answer to two or more questions) indicates the possibility of chemical coping. Some studies suggest that a cut-off point score of one affirmative answer should be used, mainly in female patients.[43] Identifying patients who cope chemically is important because opioid analgesics and alcohol have similar reward brain pathways (both are partially mediated by endorphins).[21, 24] Patients with a history of chemical coping are at higher risk, therefore, of using opioid analgesics as a way of coping with stress.

Drug abuse

More than 15 per cent of adults in the US reported a positive lifetime history of drug use. The most commonly abused substances are marijuana, cocaine, hallucinogens such as phencyclidine (PCP), lysergic acid diethylamide (LSD), and heroin.[44, 45]

Substance-abusing patients are often difficult to identify and evaluate because they often fear the consequences of acknowledging the problem. Obtaining information from other sources,

Table 31.6 Strategies of managing coping with chemical use

- First, recognize the problem (assess the patient using the CAGE questionnaire or a similar tool)
- Counsel patient about the difference between nociception and suffering in pain expression (pain versus anxiety, depression)
- Counsel patient about the difference between analgesia and coping chemically
- Restrict treatment to long-acting opioids with limited "prn" doses
- Designate one physician to prescribe opioids for patient.

such as family members, may sometimes be useful. When dealing with these patients, clinicians must present clear, firm and consistent limits, which the patients will frequently test.

Sixty-six to seventy-five per cent of patients with substance abuse disorders have a comorbid psychiatric diagnosis (depression, antisocial personality, anxiety or psychosis),[44–46] which reflects why it is so important for patients to have counselling or formal psychiatric therapy as part of the management of pain and history of substance abuse.[25] Other psychological repercussions are that alcohol and drug use and misuse are frequently associated with family dysfunction, including domestic violence. Patients in such situations are not only dealing with the news of having cancer and being in pain, they also have problems with family support.[45]

Added to the psychological implications of addictive behaviour are the physical implications. Addicted patients have a permanent cognitive deficit related to the chronic use of drugs. Although abstinence leads to recovery of some cognitive functions, with verbal skills returning usually within a month, difficulties with abstraction and problem-solving appear to last longer.[46]

Other physical consequences are the development of multiple comorbidities like human immunodeficiency virus (HIV) and hepatitis C. These may be associated with liver or renal failure that may preclude use of certain opioids because of higher risk of toxicity.[47]

Their greater complexity makes it likely that a significant proportion of patients with a history of alcoholism or drug addiction must be referred to specialized cancer pain or palliative care groups. Strategies for pain control in this population are summarized in Table 31.6.

Neuropathic pain

This type of pain generally originates in compression, invasion, destruction, or dysfunction of the central or peripheral nervous systems.[1, 48, 49] Not only is neuropathic pain commonly seen in cancer patients, but it also occurs in a heterogeneous group, including patients with diabetic neuropathy, trigeminal neuralgia, post-herpetic neuralgia, and spinal cord injury.[49]

The true prevalence of neuropathic pain is largely unknown because of the lack of proper epidemiologic studies. Current estimations suggest that about 1.5 per cent of the general population may be affected.[50]

Neuropathic pain is a constant pain that waxes and wanes in intensity, with some spontaneous paroxysmal exacerbations. It is usually described as a burning, lancinating, electric shock-like, pricking, tingling, or shooting pain.[1, 48, 49] The location follows a dermatomal distribution, to one (trigeminal neuropathy) or several nerves (sacral plexopathy), or to a large region such as the bilateral extremities (peripheral neuropathy or myelopathy of higher origin).

Generally, to achieve analgesia, patients with this kind of pain require higher opioid doses, which are often accompanied by greater toxicity.[3, 5] One-third of patients will require adjuvant drugs such as tricyclic antidepressants, antiepileptics or corticosteroids to achieve pain control.[6, 49, 51, 52]

Neuropathic pain may share common physiopathologic mechanisms with the development of tolerance; both involve NMDA receptors and some intracellular events including nitric oxide production.[31] Medications with NMDA properties like methadone and ketamine could be used as first choice when treating pain of neuropathic origin.[53, 54]

Breakthrough pain

Breakthrough pain is defined as a transitory increase in pain intensity over pain baseline in patients regularly receiving analgesic drugs. It occurs in 64–90 per cent of cancer patients.[3, 55] Some pains may be precipitated by certain events, such as motion (incidental pain); other types of pain may occur without identifiable precipitating events making them less predictable. Different pain mechanisms are at work.

We will mainly discuss incidental pain, because it is even more difficult to control than other kinds of breakthrough pain and because it has been found to have a poor prognosis.

Incidental pain

Incidental pain is characterized by a severe increase in pain intensity with sitting, walking, coughing, defaecating or urinating, and swallowing. Patients with this kind of pain are usually pain free if they avoid pain-causing manoeuvres.[1, 24] The major problem of controlling this kind of pain is its nature. It is short lasting but severely intense, so that by the time the opioid begins to act the pain is resolving. The patient is now sedated or in cognitive failure or has accumulated an opioid, with the higher risk of opioid toxicity. Systemic opioid treatment should be titrated until dose-limiting toxicity is observed; then adjuvant analgesics may be added.

Most patients who have incidental pain have bone metastases, and they may benefit from non-opioid therapies such as: radiation therapy, orthopaedic intervention or bisphosphonates infusion.[3] Neurosurgical procedures, such as percutaneous cordotomy and spinal opioids, can be alternative treatments for these patients.

Radiation therapy may be done with external beam radiation or radioisotopes. Because of these patients' poor performance status and limited life expectancy, external beam radiation is usually given as a single fraction. Most commonly used radioisotopes are strontium-89 and 186-rhenium. Disadvantages of strontium therapy include the potential for haematological toxicity, delay in pain relief, and high cost. Generally, radioisotopes should be considered for patients with refractory multifocal pain caused by metastatic disease, usually of an osteoblastic nature.[53, 56] Orthopaedic interventions may be ised to restore or stabilize a patient's impending fractures; these help to improve the quality of life of bed-bound patients. Results of radiotherapy or surgery for spinal cord compression appear to be similar.[53, 56]

Biphosphonates have been used mainly in patients with breast cancer and myeloma, but their use has also been studied in patients with other solid tumours such as lung, gastrointestinal, and prostate cancer. Besides their clinical analgesic effects, these drugs work for the prevention of fractures and they may also have anti-angiogenic effects.[56–58]

Consensus regarding pain control

Although staging has been widely used in oncology, for example, in lung cancer, stages range from I–IV; each stage implying prognosis for survival and suggesting different types or degrees of treatment, there is no well-structured staging system for pain prognostic factors. Multiple definitions of good pain control have been proposed in recent years. Bruera et al.[20] suggested that patients are considered to be in good pain control when they have no pain most of the time, and need two or fewer rescue doses of opioid per day. The researchers group defined poor pain control as mild to moderate to severe pain most of the time with a need for three or more rescue doses of opioid per day.

Farrar et al.,[59, 60] reviewing pain relief in 130 patients, defined adequate relief in light of the patient's decision not to use another opioid rescue dose in addition to the study medication (which was transmucosal fentanyl citrate), to treat each painful episode. Scales evaluated were absolute pain intensity difference (PID; 0–10 scale); percentage pain intensity difference (PID per cent; 0–100 per cent scale); pain relief (PR; 0 = none, 1 = slight, 2 = moderate, 3 = lots, 4 = complete); sum of pain intensity difference (SIPD over 60 min); percentage of maximum total pain relief (per cent Max; TOTPAR over 60 min); and global medication performance (0 = poor, 1 = fair, 2 = good, 3 = very good, 4 = excellent). The scales converted to a percentage change were most accurate in predicting adequate relief, with 73 per cent of sensitivity and

69 per cent of specificity. Best cut-off point for both the per cent Max TOTPAR and PID per cent was 33 per cent.[59, 60]

Moore et al.[61] chose a 50 per cent cut-off point for the per cent Max TOTPAR. The difference between 33 and 50 per cent does not affect the conclusion of the published studies, because a positive result when using a 50 per cent cut-off for maximum pain relief remain positive with using the 33 per cent cut-off. However, setting the bar too high may result in underestimation of the efficacy of other treatments and has implications for the design of future studies.

An ideal staging system to assess pain relief should allow the patients to integrate into their responses different confounding factors, like mood and expectations, rather than use the investigator's mathematical model. One way of accomplishing this is to count the number of additional rescue doses as an outcome.[60]

Consensus is needed not only regarding the cut-off point for pain relief but also on timing of the assessment. Bruera et al.[20] and Chang et al.[2] assessed the pain response on day 21, a time that will allow titration of opioid and adjuvant analgesic drugs; Farrar et al.[60] assessed patients after each opioid dose. Obviously, standards are needed to compare the effectiveness of one medication or one dose with that of another.

Currently available staging systems for cancer pain are reasonably sensitive; enough to enable us to find patients who will respond well to pain measures, but their specificity is too low to correctly identify patients who are likely to have a poor response. Two possible ways of improving the specificity of current prognostic models are, first, to develop better screening methods of existing factors; even though more sophisticated tools could be difficult to use at bedside (too time-consuming or too complex for a debilitated patient). A second option is to identify new and currently unknown factors that might enhance our prognostic ability.

Both physicians' and patients' misconceptions about opioid administration (too-low doses, long interval between doses, fear of addiction, treatment of pain with only pro re nata ('prn') or 'as needed' doses) not only bring suffering to patients, but they may cause patients to develop pseudo-addictive behaviour (drug-seeking caused by unrelieved pain) and result in unnecessary, rapid medication escalation and subsequent toxicity problems.[1, 25] Table 31.7 shows some of the most common myths about opioids.

The multidimensional approach

A multidimensional and multidisciplinary approach helps patients whose pain syndrome responds poorly to opioids. This concept includes an assessment of the patient's clinical and psychological characteristics, identification of specific prognostic factors related to symptoms and the patient's self-reported symptom burden.

Physicians must work with many other professionals – psychologists, psychiatrists, chaplains, occupational and physical therapists, nutritionists, nurses, and social workers – to provide

Table 31.7 Common Myths About Opioid use for Cancer Pain

◆ Opioid analgesics frequently cause addiction
◆ Physical dependence equal addiction
◆ Tolerance equals addiction
◆ Opioids decrease survival
◆ Opioids frequently cause respiratory depression
◆ Oral opioids are ineffective

care not only to the patients but also to their families. Non-pharmacologic measures may be attempted for patients whose pain is not controlled with pharmacological therapy or when pharmacological therapy results in toxicity.[62]

Five to twenty per cent of patients with cancer-related pain require interventions to achieve analgesia.[63, 64] These include nerve blocks, epidural or intrathecal opioid administration, local anaesthetics for neuropathic or plexopathy pain, nerve stimulation, and percutaneous cordotomy.

Physical therapy (massage, ultrasound, hydrotherapy, electro-acupunture, trigger point injections) is mainly indicated for patients with musculoskeletal pain but can be used as a psychological strategy, keeping patients as mobile as possible allows them to do their regular activities. Psychological techniques include imagery, relaxation, hypnosis and biofeedback.

Conclusion

Pain relief depends on many factors that interact in complex ways. Difficult-to-bear pain due to poor opioid response demands consideration of a range of measures including rotation of opioids, use of adjuvant drugs, use of alternative therapies like radiation and interventional procedures. A disciplined palliative service practice should offer screening tools to identify high-risk patients in order to avoid unnecessary suffering. Appropriate explanation and counselling should be offered to distressed patients and families. Since pain must be treated in different settings, clinicians and investigators must look carefully at definitions of pain control that will be useful for their patients.

References

1. Kim H, Bruera E, Jenkins R (2004). Symptom control and palliative care. In F Cavalli, H Hansen, S Kaye (eds) *Textbook of medical oncology*, pp. 353–70. Abingdon, UK: Taylor and Francis.

2. Hwang S, Chang V, Fairclough D. *et al*. Development of a cancer pain prognostic scale. *J Pain Symptom Manage* 2002; 24:366–78.

3. Mercadante S, Portenoy R. Opioid poorly-responsive cancer pain. Part 1: clinical considerations. *J Pain Symptom Manage* 2001; 21:144–50.

4. Hanks G, Justins D. Cancer pain: management. *Lancet* 1992; 339:1031–36.

5. Zhukovsky D, Abdullah O, Richardson M. *et al*. Clinical evaluation in advanced cancer. *Semin Oncol* 2000; 27:14–23.

6. Portenoy R, Foley K, Inturrisi CE. The nature of opioid responsiveness and its implications for neurophatic pain: new hypothesis derived from studies of opioid infusions. *Pain* 190; 43:273–86.

7. Stromgren A, Groenvold M, Pertensen M. *et al*. Pain characteristics and treatment outcome for advanced cancer patients during the first week of specialized palliative care. *J Pain Symptom Manage* 2004; 27:104–13.

8. Ventafridda V, Ripamonti C, Tamburini M, Cassileth RB, De Conno F. Unendurable symptoms as prognostic indicators of impending death in terminal cancer patients. *Eur.J.Cancer* 1990; 26(9):1000–1001.

9. Maltoni M, Pirovano M, Scarpi E. *et al*. Prediction of survival of patients terminally ill with cancer. Results of an Italian prospective multicenter study. *Cancer* 1995; 10:2613–22.

10. Morita T, Tsunoda J, Satoshi I. *et al*. Survival prediction of terminally ill patients by clinical symptoms: development of a simple indicator. *Jpn J Clin Oncol* 1999; 3:156–9.

11. Bruera E, Miller M, Kuehn N. *et al*. Estimate of survival of patients admitted to a palliative care unit: A prospective study. *J Pain Sympt Manage* 1992; 7:82–6.

12. Vigano A, Dorgan M, Buckingham J, Bruera E, Suarez-Almazor ME. Survival prediction in terminal cancer patients: a systematic review of the medical literature. *Palliat Med* 2000; 14(5):363–74.

13. Schonwetter RS, Robinson BE, Ramirez G. Prognostic factors for survival in terminal lung cancer patients. *J Gen Intern Med* 1994; 9(7):366–71.

14. Maltoni M, Caraceni A, Brunelli C. *et al.* Prognostic factors in advanced cancer patients: evidence-based clinical recommendations – a study by the Steering Committee of the European Association for Palliative Care. *J Clin Oncol* 2005; 23(25):6240–8.

15. Tannenberger S, Malavasi I, Mariano P, Pannuti F, Strocchi E. Planning palliative or terminal care: the dliemma of doctors' prognoses in terminally ill cancer patients. *Annals of Oncology* 2002; 13:1319–1323.

16. Vigano A, Bruera E, Jhangri GS, Newman SC, Fields AL, Suarez-Almazor ME. Clinical survival predictors in patients with advanced cancer. *Arch Intern Med* 2000; 160(6):861–8.

17. Llobera J, Esteva M, Rifa J. *et al.* Terminal cancer: duration and prediction of survival time. *Eur J Cancer* 2000; 36:2036–43.

18. Smith TJ, Staats PS, Deer T. *et al.* Randomized clinical trial of an implantable drug delivery system compared with comprehensive medical management for refractory cancer pain: impact on pain, drug-related toxicity and survival. *Journal of Clinical Oncology* 2003; 20(19):4040–9.

19. Wong GY, Schroeder DR, Carns PE. *et al.* Effect of neurolytic celiac plexus block on pain relief, quality of life, and survival in patients with unresectable pancreatic cancer: a randomized controlled trial. *JAMA* 2004; 291(9):1092–9.

20. Bruera E, MacMillan K, Hanson J. *et al.* The Edmonton staging system for cancer pain: preliminary report. *Pain* 1989; 37:203–9.

21. Bruera E, Schoeller T, Wenk R. *et al.* A prospective multicenter assessment of the Edmonton Staging system for cancer pain. *J Pain Symptom Manage* 1995; 10:348–55.

22. Fainsinger, R, Nekolaichuck C, Neumann C. *et al.* The Revised Edmonton Staging System for Cancer Pain. *Palliat Med* 2004; 18:307.

23. Mai F. Somatization disorder: a practical review. *Can J Psychiatry* 2004; 10:652–62.

24. Bruera E, Walker P, Lawlor P. Opioids in cancer pain. In C Stein (ed.) *Opioids in pain control: Basic and clinical aspects*, pp. 309–24. Cambridge: Cambridge University Press, (1999).

25. Reddy S. Pain management. In A Elsayem, L Driver, E Bruera (eds) *The MD Anderson Symptom control and palliative care handbook,* pp. 15–38. Houston, TX: The University of Texas Health Science Center, 2002.

26. Wessely S, Nimnuan C, Sharpe M. Functional somatic syndromes: one or many? *Lancet.* 1999; 354:936–39.

27. Novy DM, Collins HS, Nelson DV. *et al.* Waddell signs: distributional properties and correlates. *Arch Phys Med Rehabil* 1998; 79, 820–2.

28. Association AP, editor. Diagnostic and statistical manual of mental disorders: DSM-IV Washington, DC: American Psychiatric Association.; 2000.

29. Zigmond AS, Snaith RP. The hospital anxiety and depression scale. *Acta Psychiatr Scand* 1983; 67:361–70.

30. Sharpe M, Mayou R, Seagroatt V. *et al.* Why do doctors find some patients difficult to help? *Quart J Med* 1994; 87:183–87.

31. Mercadante S, Portenoy R. Opioid poorly responsive cancer pain. Part 2: Basic mechanisms that could shift dose response for analgesia. *J Pain Symptom Manage* 2001; 21:255–64.

32. Sweeney C, Bruera E. Opioids. In R Melzack, P Wall (eds) *Handbook of pain management. A clinical companion to Wall and Melzacks textbook of pain*, pp. 377–96. Churchill, Livingstone, 2003.

33. Portenoy R. Tolerance to opioid analgesics: clinical aspects. *Cancer Surv* 1995; 21:49–65.

34. Collin E. Cesselin F. Neurobiological mechanisms of opioid tolerance and dependence. *Clin Pharmacol* 1991; 14:465–88.

35. Bruera E, Watanabe S, Faisinger R. *et al.* Custom-made capsules and suppositories of methadone for patients on high dose opioids for cancer pain. *Pain* 1995; 62:141–6.

36. S.M, Dudgeon J, E. B. A phase III double-blind equivalence study of two different formulations of slow-release morphine followed by a randomization between dextromethorphan or placebo plus Statex SR for chronic cancer pain relief in terminally ill patients. ASCO; 2002; 2002. p. 381a.

37. Sadock B, Sadock V. Alcohol- related disorders. In B Sadock, V Sadock (eds) *Pocket handbook of clinical psychiatry*, 3rd edn, pp. 67–78. Philadelphia, PA: Lippincott, William and Wilkins, 2001.

38. Kanner RM, Foley KM. Patterns of narcotic drug use in cancer pain clinic. *Annals of the New York Academy of Science* 1981; 362:161–72.

39. Porter J, Jick H. Addiction: rare in patients treated with narcotics. *N Engl J Med* 1980; 302: 123.

40. Moore R, Bone L, Geller G. *et al.* Prevalence, detection, and treatment of alcoholism in hospitalized patients. *JAMA* 1989; 261:403–7.

41. Bruera E, Moyano J, Steifert L. *et al.* The frequency of alcoholism among patients with pain due to terminal cancer. *J Pain Symptom Manage* 1995; 10:599–603.

42. Ewing J. Detecting alcoholism: The CAGE questionnaire. *JAMA* 1984; 252:1905–7.

43. Ewing J. Screening for alcoholism using CAGE. *JAMA* 1998; 80:1904–5.

44. Sadock B, Sadock V (2001). Other substance-related disorders In B Sadock, V Sadock (eds) *Pocket handbook of clinical psychiatry*, 3rd edn, pp. 79–99. Philadelphia, PA: Lippincott, William and Wilkins, 2001.

45. Grant B, Dawson D. Epidemiology, etiology and course of substance use disorders. In B McCrady, E Epstein (eds) *Addictions. A comprehensive guidebook*, pp. 9–29. New York: Oxford University Press, 1999.

46. Finney J, Moos R, Timko C. Specific drugs of abuse: pharmacological and clinical aspects. In B McCrady, E Epstein (eds) *Addictions. A comprehensive guidebook*, pp. 30–49. New York: Oxford University Press, 1999.

47. Mercadante S, Arcuri E. Opioids and renal function. *Journal of Pain* 2004; 5:2–19.

48. Namaka M, Gramlich C, Ruhlen D. *et al.* A treatment algorithm for neuropathic pain. *Clinical Ther* 2004 26:951–79.

49. Chong M, Bajwa Z. Diagnosis and treatment of neuropathic pain. *J Pain Symptom Manage* 2003; 25:S4–11.

50. Carter GT, Galer BS. Advances in the management of neuropathic pain. *Eur J Pharmacol* 2004; 12:447–59.

51. Bruera E, Ripamonti C. Adjuvants to opioid analgesics. In R Patt (ed.) *Cancer pain*, pp. 14–149. Philadelphia, PA: JB Lippincott, 1993.

52. Portenoy R. Adjuvant analgesics for pain management. In D Doyle, G Hanks and N MacDonald (eds) *Oxford textbook of palliative medicine*, pp. 187–203. Oxford: Oxford University Press, 1993.

53. Mercadante S, Portenoy R. Opioid poorly-responsive cancer pain. Part 3: Clinical strategies to improve opioid responsiveness. *J Pain Symptom Manage* 2001; 21:338–50.

54. Thomas J, Von Gunten C. Pain in terminally ill patients, guidelines for pharmacological management. *CNS Drugs* 2003; 9:621–31.

55. Portenoy R, Hagen N. Breakthrough pain: definition, prevalence and characteristics. *Pain* 1990; 41:273–81.

56. Oneschuk D, Bruera E. Palliative care of the terminally ill. In Heiner, Kinsella, Zdeblick (eds) *Management of metastatic disease to the musculoskeletal system*, pp. 177–92. St Louis, MO: Quality Medical Publishing, 2002.

57. Conte P, Coleman R. Biphosphonates in the treatment of skeletal metastases. *Semin Oncolo* 2004; 31(5S):59–63.

58. Pereira J, Mancini I, Walker P. The role of biphosphonates in malignant bone pain: a review. *J Palliat Care* 1998; 14:25–36.

59. Farrar J, Berlin J, Strom B. Clinically important changes in acute pain outcome measures: a validation study. *J Pain Symptom Manage* 2003; 25:406–11.

60. Farrar J, Portenoy R, Berlin J. *et al.* Defining the clinically important difference in pain outcome measures. *Pain* 2003; 88:287–94.

61. Moore A, McQuay H, Gavaghan D. Deriving dichotomous outcome measures from continuous data in randomized controlled trails of analgesics. *Pain* 1996; 66:229–37.

62. Crammond T. Invasive techniques for neurophatic pain in cancer. In E Bruera, R Portenoy (eds) *Topics in palliative care*, pp. 63–90. New York: Oxford University Press, 1998.

63. Malone BT, Beye R, Walker J. Management of pain in the terminally ill by administration of epidural narcotics. *Cancer* 1985; 55:438–40.

64. Walker SM, Cousins MJ. Anesthesiological procedures. In: Bruera E, Portenoy R, editors. Cancer Pain: Assessment and Management. Cambridge, UK: Cambridge University Press; 2003. p. 201–27.

32

Malignant bowel obstruction

Sebastiano Mercadante

Introduction

Bowel obstruction is a well-recognized complication in advanced cancer patients with abdominal or pelvic malignancy. Although it may develop at any time of the disease, it occurs more frequently at the advanced stage, with the highest incidence ranging from 5.5 to 42 per cent in ovarian carcinoma. Bowel obstruction ranges from 4.4 to 24 per cent in colorectal cancer.[1, 2]

Natural history

Primary cancer, relapse after surgery, chemotherapy or radiotherapy, and diffuse carcinomatosis are the most common causes of bowel obstruction. The enlargement of the primary tumour or recurrence of abdominal masses, fibrosis or adhesions may produce extrinsic occlusion of the lumen, while polypoid lesions or anular narrowing due to dissemination may cause an intraluminal occlusion of the lumen. Intestinal linitis, due to infiltration of the intestinal muscles, may produce intramural occlusion of the lumen. Furthermore, signs and symptoms of bowel obstruction may present without an evident mechanical obstruction due to intestinal motility disorders frequently associated with advanced cancer patients. This condition, termed pseudo-obstruction, is attributed to the neurologic disorders often observed in diabetics and seen in lung cancer patients with paraneoplastic syndromes as well as patients with previous gastric surgery, affecting extrinsic neural control of the viscera. Contributing factors are constipation, due to the illness or drugs, such as anticholinergics and opioids, and surrounding oedema. Frequently these factors coexist.[1]

Different levels of obstruction due to some specific kinds of cancer can determine a different pattern of symptoms at presentation, slowing or accelerating the progression from partial to complete occlusion. Pelvic tumours not producing diffuse carcinomatosis may have a more slow progression of insidious symptoms, with alternate periods of subacute obstruction. On the contrary, when jejunum is involved, particularly frequent in pancreatic cancer, or fixed tumours extensively infiltrating the small bowel, distension may be minimal, and gastrointestinal symptoms will be precocious.

The time course of pathophysiological events in bowel obstruction is variable, occurring over several days or weeks. In the presence of an obstruction, the bowel continues to contract with an increased peristaltic activity leading to a vicious circle represented by distension–secretion–motor activity and worsening of the clinical picture. The hypertensive state in the lumen is maintained by an inflammatory response and a release of prostaglandins and vasoactive intestinal polypeptide (VIP), producing hyperaemia and oedema of the intestinal wall and an accumulation of fluid in the lumen. A disturbance of the autoregulatory local and neurohumoral control mechanisms of the splanchnic flow may explain the appearance of the multiple organ failure syndrome caused or worsened by systemic hypotension seen in bowel occlusions: circulatory changes such as tachycardia, low central venous pressure and a reduced cardiac output may lead to severe hypotension. The hypovolaemic state may induce a functional renal failure due to a decrease in the renal flow and, as a consequence, of the glomerular filtration. Oliguria, azotaemia and haemoconcentration may accompany dehydration. The increased abdominal distension reduces the venous return and may impair pulmonary ventilation, elevating the diaphragm. Fluids and electrolytes are sequestered in the gut wall and in its lumen in the presence of vasodilatation contributing to hypotension. Sepsis is the consequence of multiple microperforations and leads to multi-organ system failure, which is the cause of death in patients with bowel obstruction.[1, 3]

Factors affecting prognosis

The course described above will depend in time on the rapidity of the progression of disease (locally or at distant sites) and the impact of treatments (Table 32.1). Possible recovery should be considered, and may depend on the type of intervention chosen, both medical or surgical, and its timing.

Bowel obstruction in the patient with a history of cancer remains a vexing problem. Obstruction due to recurrent cancer is commonly associated with poor long-term survival. Surgical attempts to relieve malignant obstruction have a significant morbidity and mortality and variable success in resolving symptoms. The presence of carcinomatosis strongly influences surgical prognosis. Surgical intervention in patients with peritoneal carcinomatosis produces rather short-term success with significant mortality and morbidity rates related to the procedure,[4] ranging between 14–29 per cent, and 37–45 per cent, respectively. Apart from obstruction, peritoneal carcinomatosis may cause motility problems because of intestinal paralysis secondary to extensive tumour involvement of the intestinal mesentery and plexuses, which is not cured by surgical procedures. Survival rates of medically versus surgically treated patients were not significantly different.[5, 6]

The palliative intent, that is the ability to tolerate solid food for remaining lifetime, has been described for as many as 50 per cent of individuals. This was recently confirmed in a study investigating short- and long-term prognosis in 63 patients diagnosed with carcinomatosis as a first presentation of cancer or after a disease-free interval of mean of 15 months, from non-gynaecological primary tumour, who underwent laparotomy. The intent was palliative, to relieve the bowel obstruction, prevent vomiting, and recreate the opportunity of enteral nutrition. Operative procedures included resection, bypass, gastrostomy, and colostomy. Mortality rate at one month was 21 per cent, and the postoperative complication rate was high (44 per cent). The median length of hospital stay was 12 days. The median survival time was 90 days. The ability to tolerate food, defined as successful palliation, led to a significantly longer survival. Small-bowel obstruction, non-colon cancer, and ascites were associated with poor palliation, while type of operation, level of obstruction, disease, and interval from diagnosis had no independent

Table 32.1 Factors affecting surgical prognosis

Carcinomatosis
Ascites
Low performance status, weight loss
Re-obstruction
Other than colorectal cancer

prognostic effect on survival. Of this series, only one-third of patients have prolonged post-operative palliation, at the cost of a significant treatment-related morbidity.[7]

Prognostic factors have been evaluated in patients with carcinomatosis at time of diagnosis of colorectal cancer. The presence of disease at the completation of surgery, presence of ascites, advanced stage, and multiple sites of carcinomatosis were found to have a negative impact on survival, although only the presence of residual disease was found to be an independent predictor of survival.[8] Obstructions caused by colorectal carcinomatosis appeared to have a slightly better prognosis than bowel obstructions caused by carcinomatosis from other tumour types.[9]

Therapies affecting prognosis

Chemotherapy

Chemotherapy has never been considered useful in patients with widespread tumour-inducing bowel obstruction. In heavily pre-treated patients with recurrent disease, chemotherapy associated with parenteral nutrition was ineffective in restoring bowel obstruction, whereas patients with newly diagnosed ovarian cancer may occasionally have temporary response with resolution of obstruction.[10] However, in some circumstances chemotherapy can be a causal treatment, for example when bowel obstruction is maintained by an enlargement of intra-abdominal lymph nodes associated with Hodgkin's disease, which has a good chance of being reversed after a short-term treatment, also providing recovery from bowel obstruction.

Surgery

Surgical assessment is mandatory in any patient presenting symptoms and signs of bowel obstruction.

Until some years ago the treatment was either palliative surgery or continuous intravenous fluids administration with nasogastric drainage. Although surgery should be considered in every cancer patient who develops bowel occlusion, in such an advanced stage of the disease few patients are deemed suitable for surgical procedures. The patient's poor general condition or the extent of the disease, such as large abdominal tumour masses or multiple sites of obstruction, and patient's refusal may preclude surgery. Median survival in patients treated surgically is variable, ranging from 2 to 11 months.[2]

Available retrospective series, mainly not controlled, often suggest inordinately optimistic surgical outcomes because a selection process eliminates patients judged (but not proved) to be inoperable.

The value of operative intervention for bowel obstruction in patients with cancer is derived more from the possibility of a benign cause than alleviation of the consequences of carcinomatosis.[11, 12] Benign adhesions or a single site of obstruction may justify a relatively simple surgery such as forming a loop colostomy or dividing adhesions. Benign adhesions can occur in up to 20 per cent of the patients and are more likely if the abdomen has been previously irradiated and the ileum is obstructed. Indeed, gastrointestinal intubation successfully relieved 81 per cent of small bowel obstructions caused by postoperative adhesions. However, tube suction alone was rarely successful when the obstruction was caused by malignant neoplasms, and no patient with known metastatic disease had a benign obstruction. However, the optimal duration of a trial of medical management remains unclear.

Although operative treatment had a better outcome than nonoperative management in terms of symptom-free interval and reobstruction rates, it is marked by high postoperative morbidity. In one series, 80 per cent of patients were treated by operation, but 47 per cent of these patients had an initial trial of nonoperative treatment. Re-obstruction occurred in 57 per cent of patients who were operated on compared with 72 per cent of patients who were not. The median time to re-obstruction was 17 months for patients who underwent operation compared with 2.5 months for patients who did not. Moreover, 71 per cent of patients were alive and symptom-free 30 days after discharge from operative treatment compared with 52 per cent after nonoperative treatment. Postoperative morbidity and mortality rates were 67 and 13 per cent, respectively.[13] Operative management was associated with 22 per cent hospital mortality, and resolved the obstruction in 76 per cent of patients who survived. Almost half of these survivors continued to have some obstructive symptoms. Nonoperative patients had a hospital mortality of 38 per cent and resolution of obstruction in 90 per cent of survivors, although most of them had gastrointestinal symptoms. Hospital stay was shorter in this latter group of patients.

Long-term survival rates were poor both in operative patients and nonoperative patients (median survival 1 month).[9] Similarly, operative relief was achieved in 70 per cent of patients, mortality rate was 12 per cent, and the median postoperative survival was 5 months, but only 50 per cent of them had at least two months of obstruction-free survival and complication rate was considerable.[14] The 30-day and in-hospital mortality rates for operated patients with small bowel obstruction were 4 and 28 per cent, respectively, and in 36 per cent of patients obstruction failed to resolve. Obstruction secondary to cancer was the only factor predictive of in-hospital mortality.[15]

In another series, higher morbidity and mortality rates, 80 and 40 per cent respectively, were reported among patients with intestinal obstruction who were managed surgically. The poor results of surgery support the conservative management of the intestinal obstruction due to widespread malignancy.[16]

Prognostic indicators, such as age over 65 years associated with severe nutritional depletion, rapidly recurring ascites, palpable abdominal masses, and extensive distant metastases have been subject to statistical scrutiny in the general population with bowel obstruction, and were not selectively associated with a primary cancer diagnosis, unless in association with a poor performance status, which was correlated with the outcome.[14, 17]

In a review assessing the prognostic factors which relate to the results, in terms of survival and quality of life, of palliative surgery in cancer patients presenting with an occlusion, the median survival was 64 days and the peroperative mortality was 21 per cent. The quality of life of patients, assessed by the resumption of transit and the return home,has been improved in 65 per cent of cases. The only factors clearly correlating with survival and the success of the operation were the aetiological diagnosis of the occlusion (local recurrence better than carcinomatosis) and the type of procedure it was possible to carry out (resection better than bypass). Although palliative surgery can, in a certain number of cases, improve the quality of life of patients, it has not been possible to demonstrate prognostic factors which would allow the selection of patients who could benefit from surgery.[18]

Type of surgery

The best type of surgery to be performed for obstructing colorectal cancer is controversial. So far, two principal types of surgical approach have been used for this condition: primary resection (primary anastomosis or Hartmann's procedure) with simultaneous treatment of carcinoma and obstruction, or staged resection (treatment of the obstruction prior to resection). However, neither strategy has been found to have any advantages over the other, when reviewing relevant trials in full. The limited number of identified trials together with their methodological weaknesses do not allow a reliable assessment of the role of either therapeutic strategy in the treatment of patients with bowel obstruction from colorectal carcinoma. Ideally, high-quality large-scale randomized controlled trials (RCT) are needed to establish which treatment is more effective. However, it is doubtful whether they could be carried out in a timely and satisfactory way in this particular surgical context.

Subsequent studies did not clear this issue, presenting contrasting data. Mortality rate in patients with colorectal cancer presenting acute bowel obstruction was about 27 per cent, 47 per cent for the so-called exigency procedures, including colostomy, internal diversion or Hartman colectomy, but only 9 per cent for staged surgery (cecostomy or ileotransversostomy followed by resection and anastomosis after 3 weeks on average). Thus, staged surgery seems to be the safest therapeutical option for colorectal cancers with acute bowel obstruction.[19] However, in another study, mortality and complication rate were higher in staged surgery than one-stage resection and primary anastomoses.[20]

Self-expanding metal stents (SEMS) are now an established treatment for malignant colonic obstruction and have been used increasingly in some selected cases of limited obstructions, such as in the gastric outlet, proximal small bowel and colon-rectum, either as a definitive or as a temporaneous solution for next surgery. While SEMS for preoperative 'bridge to surgery' treatment of obstructive colorectal cancer has been broadly, clinically used with good short-term results, long-term prognosis may be of concern, because of the increased risk of metastasis, invasion, and advancement of the cancer. In an historical comparison with emergency operations, postoperative complications were significantly less frequent in the SEMS group, and survival rate did not differ.[21] About 93 per cent of procedures were successful and good clinical outcome was achieved in about 80 per cent, with a minimal re-obstruction rate by tumour ingrowth occurring after a mean of 183 days. The median survival time for patients with pancreatic cancer who underwent enteral stent placement compared with those who underwent surgical gastrojejunostomy was 94 and 92 days, respectively.[22]

Decompressive gastrostomy is an alternative for long-term nasogastric tube placement in patients who fail medical treatment of gastrointestinal symptoms. Although it is known that the placement of these devices is feasible, there are no prospective trials comparing stent placement for colonic obstruction to routine surgical care.

General view on surgical intervention

Expected survival time is not necessarily an absolute factor for decision-making, as deterioration of patients' condition in the postoperative period, suffering from complications and hospitalization, in other terms quality of life, should be taken also into account. Postoperative complications include wound infections and/or dehiscence, sepsis, enterocutaneous fistula, further obstruction, peritoneal abscess, anastomosis dehiscence, gastrointestinal bleeding, pulmonary embolism, deep venous thrombosis. Successful palliation in terms of duration of maintainance of intestinal transit and gastrointestinal symptom control is the most important outcome. These factors are difficult to explore in comparison with standard key-points of prognosis, like mortality and morbidity rates, while quality of life measurements remain difficult to apply in this context.

Nutrition

The use of parenteral nutrition (PN) in patients with metastatic disease that produces an inoperable intestinal obstruction raises important ethical, moral, and cost issues. In a series of patients with inoperable malignant bowel obstruction, only albumin level and Karnofsky score before starting PN emerged as predictors of survival, although only at a limited extent.[22] Quality of life and length of survival were assessed in advanced cancer patients on PN presenting mostly chronic gastrointestinal obstruction-related symptoms. Patients had a median survival of four months, and approximately one-third of patients had a survival of 7 months. After an initial benefit on quality of life indices in the first months, a progressive decline became evident 1–2 months before death.[23] However, no controlled data, demonstrating that patients not receiving PN would have different survival or quality of life, exist. Moreover, patients with a Karnofskty status > 50 are unlikely to be found in such an advanced status, who are not amenable with therapies and not operable, as described by authors. Others have found that the median survival of patients discharged on home PN to be 63 days with approximately 26 per cent of this time spent in the hospital for treatment of complications.[24] It remains difficult to identify patients that may benefit from PN.

Short- and long-term prognosis

Colorectal cancer

In 8 to 29 per cent of patients with colorectal carcinoma, obstruction is the main symptom at diagnosis, and 85 per cent of patients undergoing emergency colorectal surgery have obstruction from colorectal carcinoma.[25]

Short-term prognosis

Short term-prognosis seems to be influenced by the presence of bowel obstruction. Population studies have shown that 25 per cent of all postoperative deaths after surgery for bowel cancer occur in obstructed patients.[26] Short-term prognosis and risk factors were assessed in multi-centre study during a 1-year period. The average postoperative mortality in patients operated with different techniques for malignant colon obstruction was 16.5 per cent. However, age, anesthesiological risk, operations performed on an emergency basis, and Dukes' classification of colorectal cancer staging were predictors of poor outcome, independently from the operator or hospital, and kind and duration of surgery performed.[27] These data were contradicted by another patients' series in which the perioperative outcomes in patients undergoing definitive surgery for early (Dukes' stages A, B and C) and advanced colorectal cancer were examined. There were no differences in perioperative morbidity or mortality in the groups studied. In the advanced group, more operations were performed as emergencies than in the early group (32.4 vs 17.5 per cent) and more patients presented with bowel obstruction in the advanced group (23.9 vs 10.2 per cent). According to these data, in terms of perioperative outcome, the presence of advanced cancer, per se, should not, therefore, be a justification to decline surgery.[28] While surgery, when indicated, may modify the course of disease, the presence of bowel obstruction at diagnosis, 'per sè' may be able to change both long-term and short-term outcome (Table 32.2).

Long-term prognosis

The occlusive phenomenon by itself represents an independent unfavourable factor negatively affecting long-term prognosis after radical resections. Patients submitted to radical resections had a far poorer prognosis as compared with non-obstructed radically resected ones, the 5-year survival being 41.2 and 78.9 per cent respectively. Radically resected obstructed patients showed an higher and earlier rate of local and distant recurrence with a disease-related death rate of

Table 32.2 Reasons why obstruction per se worsens the prognosis in colorectal cancer

The presence of obstruction negatively affects long term prognosis after radical resection
The occurrence of obstruction reduces long-term survival
Obstruction increases short-term mortality (perioperative)

47.6 vs 16.3 per cent as compared with non-obstructed ones.[29] After one-stage emergency curative treatment, patients presenting with obstructing tumours of the colon had a smaller survival probability than that of patients with nonobstructing lesions. Conversely, obstruction, along with pathologic stage and positive nodes, carries a significantly higher risk of metastatic tumour recurrence and death.[30] Even the development of serious complications may have a poor outcome. In patients developing perforation, survival was worse for patients with obstruction.[26]

A reduction in long-term survival has been demonstrated in patients with obstructing colorectal cancer.[27] Most authors speculated this observation could be explained by the inherent high potential of obstructing tumours to increase permeability and metastasize through the lymphatics, or to spread to visceral peritoneum. In a specific population of patients with right colon cancer, lower survival rates, as well as higher incidence of metastases and decreased curative resection rate, have been described for patients with obstruction when compared with nonobstructed patients at time of diagnosis and operation (about half of the 5-year survival rate).[28] In an observational study performed to identify determinants of survival and to compare recurrence patterns between obstructing and nonobstructing tumours after primary resection and anastomosis as curative treatment, no statistically significant determinant arose out for local recurrence, whereas at multivariate analysis for metastatic and overall relapse, Dukes stage, positive nodes, and obstruction remained independent prognostic factors.[30]

Gynaecological cancer

Almost 50 per cent of patients who die of ovarian cancer are expected to develop bowel obstruction, prevalently of small bowel, during the illness. Bowel obstruction associated with gynaecologic disease has unique features deserving wider recognition, also in terms of the prevalent mechanism or causes of obstruction. The prognosis of these patients is quite unpredictable by comprehensive assessment of risk factors. The prognosis is poor for patients with rapidly accumulating ascites, advanced age, severe mutritional deprivation, liver metastases, or distant metastases, or those who have responded poorly to combination chemotherapy or total abdominal radiation therapy.[11]

Short-term prognosis

About 60 per cent of patients with advanced ovarian cancer who developed bowel obstruction could be discharged with a restored intestinal passage after operation, although no criteria were defined for selecting patients who could benefit from surgical treatment.[31] In a more recent series, surgical correction was performed in 84 per cent of cases. Successful palliation (the ability to tolerate a regular or low-residue diet at least 60 days postoperatively) was achieved in 71 per cent of cases where surgical correction was possible. Perioperative mortality rate was 6 per cent, and the rate of major surgical morbidity was 22 per cent. Postoperative chemotherapy was administered in 79 per cent of cases where surgical correction was possible. The median survival of the entire cohort was 8 months. If surgery resulted in successful palliation, median survival was 11.6 months, versus 3.9 months for all other patients. Thus, the majority of patients undergoing surgery had successful palliation, and were able to receive further chemotherapy.[32]

A larger series has provided important information from the prognostic point of view.[11] Of interest, in this survey patients with terminal illness receiving supportive care and cases of incomplete obstruction were excluded. Gastrointestinal intubation resolved bowel obstruction in 25 per cent of patients who had prevalently postoperative adhesions, possibly occurring less than 30 days after surgery. None of the patients successfully treated by nasogastric suction or having postoperative or postradiation adhesions died. In 9 per cent of patients who underwent exploration, corrective surgical treatment could not be carried out because of carcinomatosis, and 25 per cent of these died. Operative mortality rates were 10 and 19 per cent, for small bowel and large bowel obstruction, respectively.

Although the operative group survived significantly longer than those in the non-operative group, operative mortality was 15 per cent and major postoperative morbidity was 42 per cent.[33] Some factors combined have been identified of prognostic value in patients with malignant bowel obstruction from ovarian cancer. Survival time after operation for bowel obstruction from ovarian cancer was found to be significantly related to the prognostic index, incorporating a multifactorial assessement, including age, nutritional status, tumour spread, ascites, and prior chemotherapy and radiotherapy,[6] confirming previous observations.[4, 11] In gynaecological cancer palpable masses, large volume ascites, multiple sites of obstruction, and pre-operative weight loss were associated with inferior palliation outcome after surgery.[9]

Long-term prognosis

Successful palliation was significantly associated with the following factors: absence of palpable abdominal masses, volumes of ascites less than 3 litres, unifocal obstruction and pre-operative weight loss than 9 kg.[34] Ascites and carcinomatosis may not be absolute contraindications. Paracentesis followed by gastrostomy or gastrojejunostomy were safe and effective in ovarian cancer patients with ascites presenting with small-bowel obstruction. Technical success rate was 98 per cent. Morbidity and mortality rates were 15 and 2 per cent, respectively.[35]

On the other hand, time since the last treatment occurred was also considered. From a retro-spective analysis of patients with bowel obstruction due to advanced ovarian cancer, patients were classified into a favourable group (no previous treatment or interval since last treat-ment exceeding 6 months, without ascites) and a poor prognosis group (interval since last treatment shorter than 6 months, and ascites). Patients with ovarian cancer, who did not receive treatments in the last 6 months or were disease-free had a survival time superior to patients who had received a more recent treatment and having ascites. Surgery did not affect the prognosis, being marginally effective in providing obstruction-free survival in patients with a favourable prognosis, and absolutely ineffective in the poor prognosis patients.[36]

Conclusion

Unfortunately, data reported in literature are confused by several factors, including the retro-spective nature of results and patients' selection bias. In any case, prognostic criteria are difficult to apply in a condition that is highly variable individually, whose assessment is not uniformly recognized, approaches as well as diagnostic and therapeutic choices are dependent on the setting, definition of the outcome is rarely afforded, and available data on survival prognosis of the illness cannot be drawn for practical scoring. The multidisciplinary approach, including the opinion of the oncologist and the surgeon, as well as an expert in palliative medicine, is rarely performed, and despite the possible poor prognosis, surgery is often performed, because it is considered inevitably as an imperative act (otherwise the patient will die). Surgery should be justified on the basis of more benefit than burden to patients, based on the prognostic factors available, and consent to surgery should include discussion of risks, complications, as well as medical alternatives, effective in relieving symptoms.

References

1. Mercadante S. Assessment and management of mechanical bowel obstruction. In R Portenoy, E Bruera (eds) *Topics in palliative care, vol 1*, pp. 113–30. New York, NY: Oxford University Press; 1997.

2. Ripamonti C, Mercadante S. Pathophysiology and management of malignant bowel obstruction. In D Doyle, GW Hanks, N McDonald, N Cherny. *Oxford textbook of palliative medicine*, 3rd edn, pp. 496–506. New York: Oxford University Press, 2005.

3. Mercadante S. Pain in inoperable bowel obstruction. *Pain Digest* 1995; 5:9–13.

4. Krebs HB, Helmkamp F. Management of intestinal obstruction in ovarian cancer. *Oncology (Huntingt)* 1989; 3:25–31.

5. Fernandes JR, Seymour RJ, Suissa S. Bowel obstruction in patients with ovarian cancer: a search for prognostic factors. *Am J Obstet Gynecol* 1988; 158:244–9.

6. Larson JE, Podczaski ES, Manetta A, Whytney CW, Mortel R. Bowel obstruction in patients with ovarian carcinoma: analysis of prognostic factors. *Gynecol Oncol* 1989; 35:61–5.

7. Blair S, Chu D, Schearz R. Outcome of palliative operations for malignant bowel obstruction in patients with peritoneal carcinomatosis from nongynecological cancer. *Ann Surg Oncol* 2001; 8:632–7.

8. Marcus EA, Weber TK, Rodriguez-Bigas MA, Driscoll D, Merepol NJ, Petrelli NJ. Prognostic factors affecting survival in patients with colorectal carcinomatosis. *Cancer Invest* 1999; 17:249–52.

9. Woolfson R, Jennings K, Whalen G. Management of bowel obstruction in patients with abdominal cancer. *Arch Surg* 1997; 132:1093–7.

10. Abu-Rustum N, Barakat R, Venkatraman E, Spriggs D. Chemotherapy and total parenteral nutrition for advanced ovarian cancer with bowel obstruction. *Gynecol Oncol* 1997; 64:493–5.

11. Krebs HB, Goplerud DR. Mechanical intestinal obstruction in patients with gynaecologic disease: a review of 368 patients. *Am J Obstet Gynecol* 1987; 157:577–83.

12. Tang E, Davis J, Silberman H. Bowel obstruction in cancer patients. *Arch Surg* 1995; 130:832–6.

13. Miller G, Boman J, Shrier I, Gordon PH. Small-bowel obstruction secondary to malignant disease: an 11-year audit. *Can J Surg* 2000; 43:353–8.

14. Butler JA, Cameron BL, Morrow M, Kahng K, Tom J. Small bowel obstruction in patients with a prior history of cancer. *Am J Surg* 1991; 162: 624–8.

15. Chan A, Woodruff RK. Intestinal obstruction in patients with widespread intraabdominal malignancy. *J Pain Symptom Manage* 1992; 7:339–42.

16. Weiss SM, Skibber JM, Rosato FE. Bowel obstruction in cancer patients: performance status as a predictor of survival. *J Surg Oncol* 1984; 25:15–17.

17. Legendre H, Vanhuyse F, Caroli-Bosc FX, Pector JC. Survival and quality of life after palliative surgery for neoplastic gastrointestinal obstruction. *Eur J Surg Oncol* 2001; 27:364–7.

18. Nemes R, Vasile I, Curca T, Paraliov T, Pasalega M, Mesina C, Dinca N, Valcea D. Acute bowel obstruction – the main complication of colorectal cancer. Therapeutical options. *Rom J Gastroenterol* 2004; 13:109–12.

19. de Aguilar-Nascimento JE, Caporossi C, Nascimento M. Comparison between resection and primary anastomosis and staged resection in obstructing adenocarcinoma of the left colon. *Arq Gastroenterol* 2002; 39:240–5.

20. Saida Y, Sumiyama Y, Nagao J, Uramatsu M. Long-term prognosis of preoperative 'bridge to surgery' expandable metallic stent insertion for obstructive colorectal cancer: comparison with emergency operation. *Dis Colon Rectum* 2003; 46(10 Suppl):S44–9.

21. Yim HB, Jacobson BC, Saltzman JR. *et al.* Clinical outcome of the use of enteral stents for palliation of patients with malignant upper GI obstruction. *Gastrointest Endosc* 2001; 53:329–32.

22. Pasanisi F, Orban A, Scalfi L, Alfonsi L, Santarpia L, Zurlo E, Celona A, Potenza A, Contaldo F. Predictors of survival in terminal-cancer patients with irreversible bowel obstruction receiving home parenteral nutrition. *Nutrition* 2001; 17:581–4.

23. Bozzetti F, Cozzaglio L, Biganzoli E. *et al.* Quality of life and length of survival in advanced cancer patients on home parenteral nutrition. *Clin Nutrition* 2002; 21:281–8.

24. King L, Carson L, Kostantinides N, et al. Outcome assessement of home patenmteral nutrition in patients with gynecologic malignancies: what have we learned in a decade of experience? Gynecol Oncol 1993;51:377-382.

25. De Salvo GL, Gava C, Pucciarelli S, Lise M. Curative surgery for obstruction from primary left colorectal carcinoma: primary or staged resection? Cochrane Database Syst Rev. 2002;1:CD002101.

26. Mella J, Biffin A, Radcliffe AG, et al. Population-based audit of colorectal cancer management in two heath regions. Br J Surg 1997;84:1731-1736.

27. Tekkis P, Kinsman R, Thompson M. *et al.* The association of coloproctology of Great Britain and Ireland study of large bowel obstruction caused by colorectal cancer. *Ann Surg* 2004; 240:76–81.

28. Isbister WH. Audit of definitive colorectal surgery in patients with early and advanced colorectal cancer. *ANZ J Surg* 2002; 72:271–4

29. Zucchetti F, Negro F, Matera D, Bolognini S, Mafucci S. Colorectal cancer: obstruction is an independent negative prognostic factor after radical resection. *Ann Ital Chir* 2002; 73:421–5.

30. Carraro PG, Segala M, Cesana BM, Tiberio G. Obstructing colonic cancer: failure and survival patterns over a ten-year follow-up after one-stage curative surgery. *Dis Colon Rectum* 2001; 44:243–50.

31. Rubin S, Hoskins W, Benjamin I, Lewis J. Palliative surgery for intestinal obstruction in advanced ovarian cancer. *Gynecol Oncol* 1989; 34:16–19.

32. Pothuri B, Vaidya A, Aghajanian C, Venkatraman E, Barakat RR, Chi DS. Palliative surgery for bowel obstruction in recurrent ovarian cancer:an updated series. *Gynecol Oncol* 2003; 89:306–13.

33. Redman C, Shafi M, Ambrose S. *et al.* Survival following intestinal obstruction in ovarian cancer. *Eur J Surg Oncol* 1988; 14:383–6.

34. Jong P, Sturgeon J, Jamieson CG. Benefit of palliative surgery for bowel obstruction in advanced ovarian cancer. *Can J Surg* 1995; 38:454–7.

35. Ryan JM, Hahn PF, Mueller PR. Performing radiologic gastrostomy or gastrojejunostomy in patients with malignant ascites. *Am J Roentgenol* 1998; 17:1003–6.

36. Zoemulder F, helmerhorst T, Coevorden F, Wolfs P, Leyer J, Hart A. Management of bowel obstruction in patients with advanced cancer. *Eur J Cancer* 1994; 30:1625–8.

33

Breathlessness

Lara Alloway, Vaughan Keeley, and Irene Higginson

Introduction

Breathlessness is a common and often multicausal symptom in patients with advanced cancer. The genesis and pathophysiology is poorly understood and it remains difficult to treat effectively. Studies[1, 2, 3, 4] show that breathlessness occurs in between 21–71 per cent of patients with cancer, with increasing prevalence and severity towards death. Hence breathlessness is often seen as a sign of impending death. The inability to breathe frightens many patients, and their families. It can lead to significant disability, social isolation and financial burden. It may result in hospital admission, either from an acute exacerbation or gradually increasing symptoms.

Definition

Breathlessness is the term often used to describe an unpleasant sensation of being unable to breathe easily. The sensation of dyspnoea is subjective and includes both the perception of laboured breathing by the patient and their reaction to that sensation. Much controversy exists over the precise definitions of 'breathlessness' and 'dyspnoea'. As with definitions of pain, many have their favoured definition. Dyspnoea originates from the Greek '*dys*' which means abnormal or disordered and '*pnoia*' meaning breath; hence literally disordered breathing. Breathlessness may indicate a different sensation felt during exercise or excitement, which may not be unpleasant. The terms breathlessness, dyspnoea and shortness of breath are often used interchangeably. For the purposes of this chapter we have chosen to concentrate on the term breathlessness (as in the title), which is defined as the subjective feeling of laboured breathing.

Prevalence

The prevalence of breathlessness in patients with advanced cancer, particularly lung cancer, can be found in four studies in different countries.

In the American National Hospice Study,[1] which followed patients during their last 6 weeks of life, Reuben and Mor found that 70.2 per cent of the 1754 cancer patients studied, suffered from breathlessness during this time. The severity of this symptom was at least moderate in 28 per cent of patients able to grade their breathlessness. Only pain and eating problems exceeded the prevalence of breathlessness: 75 per cent of patients with lung involvement from their cancer reported breathlessness at some point during their disease trajectory.

In a UK study of patients dying in the community[2] the authors reported breathlessness to be the main symptom in the terminal phase for 21 per cent of 86 cancer patients. A further UK study[3] showed that 60 per cent of 289 patients with non-small cell lung cancer were breathless at presentation, rising to 90 per cent just prior to death.

A study of 923 cancer patients in Canada[4] found that 46 per cent patients had some degree of breathlessness. However this population is uncharacteristic; only 4 per cent had lung cancer and 5.4 per cent lung metastases. Risk factors found to be significantly related to the presence of breathlessness were a history of smoking, asthma or chronic obstructive pulmonary disease (COPD), lung irradiation or a history of exposure to asbestos or other industrial dusts.

The differences in the figures from the above studies probably represent a variety of definitions and methods of detecting the symptom[5] as opposed to true differences in the populations, other than perhaps the slight variation in disease demographics. Roberts *et al.* in a qualitative study[6] showed that there is a tendency of under reporting of breathlessness as a symptom. There were also discrepancies between the rates reported by patients and those observed by nursing staff. Patients with cancer outside the lungs were less likely to have their breathlessness identified, perhaps because this symptom is associated with carcinoma of the lung and not, as the above data would suggest; a common symptom in advanced cancer.

Aetiology

Mechanism of breathlessness

No one universal theory has been found to explain the generation of the sensation of breathlessness. In advanced cancer it is likely to be multifactorial.[7] However, four principal mechanisms exist:

1. An increase in the respiratory effort to overcome an imposed load e.g. COPD, restrictive lung disease or pleural effusion.

2. An increase in the proportion of respiratory muscle required to maintain a normal workload, due to muscle fatigue.

3. An increase in ventilatory requirements (e.g. hypoxaemia, anaemia, metabolic acidosis).

4. Higher cortical experience to the sensation, influenced by pathways from different areas in the central nervous system.

Pathophysiology

The pathophysiology of breathlessness in advanced cancer is manifold (Table 33.1).[8] The mechanisms can be broadly divided into the following categories: direct effects of cancer in the chest,

Table 33.1 Main causes of breathlessness in advanced cancer.[8]

Effect of the cancer	Systemic non-metastatic disease	Secondary to treatment	Coexistent disease
Large/small airways obstruction	Weakness/cachexia	Radiation pneumonitis/fibrosis	COPD/asthma
Lymphangitis carcinomatosa	Anaemia	Chemotherapy Fibrosis	Heart failure/dysarythymia
Lung/segmental collapse	Pain	Infection	Ischaemic heart disease
Pleural effusion	Paraneoplastic syndromes		Motor neurone disease
Pericardial/cardiac infiltration	Pulmonary embolism		Etc.
Hepatomegaly			
Infection			
Rib/spinal metastases			

This table has been reproduced, with permission from the Royal Society of Medicine, from Booth S and Wade R. Oxygen or air for palliation of breathlessness in advanced cancer. *J R Soc Med* 2003; 96: 215–218.

systemic non-metastatic effects of cancer, sequelae of anti-cancer treatment and coexistent non-malignant disease.[8]

Commonly a patient will have several of these aetiological factors, and these will be influenced by higher cortical effects; previous experience of breathlessness as well as fear and anxiety which modify the sensation. Although the relative importance of each coexisting factor in a patient's breathlessness may not always be identifiable, it is essential to recognize potentially reversible causes.

Assessment

Breathlessness is notoriously difficult to assess, due to the multidimensionality and subjective nature of the symptom. Although accurate diagnosis of the cause remains the best guide to effective treatment of the symptom, the appropriateness of investigations will depend on the clinical condition of the patient at the time. There is no gold standard for the measurement of breathlessness; however the same rules for assessment of any clinical situation still apply.

In assessing the cause, severity and effect of breathlessness, a detailed clinical history should be taken. Patients describe breathlessness, as with many of their symptoms, in unique ways. These can range from: tightness in the chest, or the need to gasp or pant to extreme fear of drowning or suffocating. The descriptors used may have therapeutic significance and should be explored with the patient.[15] However it remains doubtful that these descriptors help differentiate between different aetiologies of breathlessness. It is also important to explore the functional effect of the breathlessness. This may include exercise tolerance, remembering to one person that may mean distance walked, but to another may be measured in ability to hold a conversation.

As with all symptoms physical examination will give a significant amount of information. This together with the clinical history will enable the clinician to diagnose most reversible causes of breathlessness (see Table 33.2). If the cause is still uncertain, further information may be derived from simple blood tests (full blood count), chest X-ray and pulse oximetry; however the need and appropriateness of each of these should be assessed on an individual basis.

It is widely accepted that oxygen saturation or pulmonary function tests correspond poorly to the individual's perception of breathlessness in many conditions, particularly advanced cancer. Such investigations do have a place in assessment of coexistent disease such as COPD, whereby within patient correlation can give information on treatment efficacy. Measurement of the intensity of breathlessness provides useful data on the effectiveness of therapeutic interventions. Commonly used scales for the subjective measurement of breathlessness include: the visual analogue, modified Borg and verbal rating scales.[9]

The visual analogue scale (VAS) is a horizontal or vertical line anchored with terms that categorize two extremes of a possible subjective status, such as 'no breathlessness' and 'worst possible breathlessness'. The patient is asked to place a mark on the line (creating an interval scale) that best reflects the intensity of the breathlessness at the time. This has been validated; it is reproducible and sensitive and is now widely used in clinical practice and research. The modified Borg scale is a vertical scale labelled 0 to 10, with corresponding verbal expressions of progressively increasing sensation intensity, such as 'nothing at all' to 'maximal'. Because of the established categories it is more convenient for comparison of individuals than the VAS. Verbal rating scores such as 'absent', 'mild', 'moderate', 'severe' or 'excruciating' are often easier to understand and useful when the patient is very unwell or too distressed by their symptoms to be able to concentrate on a written scale.

Breathlessness can also be measured using quality of life and outcome questionnaires e.g. The Edmonton Symptom assessment Schedule (ESAS), McGill Quality of Life Questionnaire (MQOL), Palliative Care Assessment (PACA) and European Organisation on Research and

Therapy of Cancer (EORTC QLQ-C30) which has a specific lung cancer (QLQ-LC13) module that includes a multi-stem breathlessness scale. The Palliative Care Outcome Scale (POS)[10] measures the subjective effect on the patient of their symptoms, including breathlessness, by means of a Likert scale (a set of statements where each is given a numerical value from one to five. Thus a total numerical value can be calculated from all the responses). This scale also allows objective assessment by staff, for comparison or as a substitute when the patients are too unwell to complete the questionnaire themselves. A symptom module has been developed, to be used in addition to the core POS: this will specifically assess the affect on patients of their symptoms, including breathlessness. This is currently being validated (personal communication). However one study[6] found significant differences in objective reporting of breathlessness, with nursing staff reporting more severe breathlessness than that found by the patient's self-reporting. This is particularly interesting as frequently in other symptoms, e.g. pain, the reverse is observed, whereby the staff report symptoms to be more significant to the patients than they report themselves.

Ultimately the most appropriate tool for the assessment of breathlessness depends on the information required and what the patient is capable of at the time. It is important to remember that it is likely that a combination of history, clinical examination and self-report of the symptom provides sufficient information in most clinical settings.

Natural history of breathlessness in cancer

Studies have shown a trend towards increasing prevalence of breathlessness towards the end of life. Figures range from 21–70.2 per cent[1, 2] in the last 6 weeks of life. In a multi-centre Spanish study[11] where symptoms were assessed in the last 48 hours of life in patients in an oncology centre, community and hospice, 46.6 per cent of patients reported significant breathlessness. A study of an English specialist palliative care unit 55.5 per cent of patients complained of breathlessness on admission and this rose to 78.6 per cent in patients who died within one day.[12] The reason for the increase in prevalence towards death is likely to be due to either progression of the cancer itself in the lungs and/or general debility caused by the disease. Psychosocial factors affecting breathlessness may well have greater influence as the patient realizes death is imminent.

Progression of primary or secondary cancer in the lungs

As the disease progresses the likelihood of ventilation/perfusion mismatches increases, with the replacement of normal lung tissue by tumour causing a restrictive defect. Corresponding with tumour growth is an increased likelihood of an occluded primary or segmental bronchus causing atelectasis or collapse of a lobe or lung. Lymphatic spread of disease or interstitial oedema also reduces the compliance of the lungs. Paralysis of the diaphragm can occur due to phrenic nerve damage by tumour-replaced mediastinal nodes. Although outside the lungs, splinting of the diaphragm by hepatomegaly, ascites or direct tumour invasion is likely to cause breathlessness. Pleural effusions are more prevalent as cancer progresses due to pleural spread and it becomes less likely that the patient will be strong enough to tolerate aspiration of the effusion.

General debility

Universal muscle weakness is a common feature of advanced cancer and this will affect not only the skeletal muscles, causing immobility, but also those required for respiration; the diaphragm, intercostal and sternomastoid muscles. The cause of this is probably multifactorial: patients with advanced cancer are frequently malnourished. Low serum albumin and loss of 10 per cent of normal body weight can be used as indicators of poor nutritional status and this has been shown to affect ventilation[13] by up to 40 per cent.

Immobility often means the patient is lying flat in bed and therefore gravity is not aiding respiration. The bases of the lungs are not aerated and patients are at increased risk of atelectasis and pneumonia. Anaemia is common in advanced cancer due to treatment effects on bone marrow, bone marrow infiltration by tumour or by blood loss. Anaemia increases the patient's ventilatory requirements, by causing respiratory muscle dysfunction and fatigue. In patients with advanced disease the prevalence of clinically detectable pulmonary emboli is 15 per cent, with undetected pulmonary emboli found in up to 50 per cent of post-mortems. Pulmonary emboli cause ventilation perfusion mismatches and are a common cause of acute breathlessness or acute deterioration in an already dyspnoeic patient.

Psychosocial factors

The impairment of a person's breathing has life-threatening connotations; it has an impact on their very existence, the essence of their being, and on life itself. It can be a difficult and distressing symptom for those with cancer, as well as for carers and health professionals alike.[14]

It is widely accepted that the sensation of breathlessness, like pain, can be modified by the patient's own perception of the origin and seriousness of the underlying cause. Anxiety has been found to be a predictor for intensity of breathlessness.[4] However, the relationship is complex in that anxiety is also a contributory factor for breathlessness. A feature of panic attacks is frequently breathlessness and breathlessness can commonly incite panic attacks. The combination of the physical, psychological, social and spiritual dimensions can be referred to as 'total breathlessness'.[15] The longer the duration of the symptom, the more likely it is that the non-physical elements assume significance in its perception and expression.

Patients with breathlessness may frequently be admitted to hospital or a palliative care unit, either due to an acute exacerbation or gradual increase in their symptoms. The patient and family's anxiety is likely to be a significant factor in precipitating this admission. Hence breathlessness has significant impact, not only on the patient but also their family.

Breathlessness has also been associated with diminishing will to live.[16] A study in a palliative care centre in Canada found that as death approached dyspnoea became the variable most predictive of fluctuation of will to live.

Factors affecting prognosis

As we have discussed, breathlessness is an individualized sensation determined by much more than just the pathophysiological cause. Unlike some other symptoms or clinical states, it is difficult to break it down to determine in which patients it indicates very poor prognosis and for which the prognosis may not be so poor. Escalate and Martin[17] looked at risk factors for imminent death (within 2 weeks) in cancer patients presenting with breathlessness. A random sample of 122 patients presenting to the emergency centre in the USA with acute breathlessness was analysed retrospectively. Variables were collected and analysed in univariate and logistic regression models. Statistically significant indicators of death within 2 weeks were: triage respiration rate of greater than 28 per minute, triage pulse greater than or equal to 110 beats per minute, uncontrolled progressive disease and history of metastases.

Short-term survival indicators – up to three months in this study – were found using the same models. These were response to treatment and cancer diagnosis.

Therapies affecting the course of breathlessness and prognosis

Some causes of breathlessness in a patient with advanced cancer will be potentially reversible, others will not. Table 33.2 shows those that may be reversible.

However, in the cases of breathlessness caused directly by primary or secondary cancer, although the breathlessness may be improved, there is very little evidence for the majority of the interventions that the overall prognosis is altered. This includes the use of systemic therapies, such as chemotherapy or corticosteroids. In the majority of cases the aim of the treatment, although specific to the cause, is to improve the patient's comfort.

In some situations, particularly in the treatment of causes of breathlessness not directly caused by the cancer; such as anticoagulation for pulmonary emboli, antibiotics for a chest infection or treatment of acute cardiac failure, the prognosis of the patient may be improved by the aforementioned intervention. Hence it is more likely that therapies altering acute, reversible problems will influence survival.

A judgement on the appropriateness of such interventions needs to be made for each individual at the time of presentation, with as much information on their likely prognosis and wishes

Table 33.2 Treatment options for reversible causes of breathlessness

Cause of breathlessness	Treatment options
Bronchial obstruction/lung collapse	Corticosteroids Endoscopic radiotherapy (brachytherapy) External beam radiotherapy LASER therapy Stenting Systemic anticancer therapy (in sensitive tumours)
Pleural effusions	Drainage Pleurodesis Systemic anticancer therapy
Pericardial effusions	Drainage Corticosteroids Fenestration
Lymphangitis carcinomatosa	Corticosteroids
Pneumonitis	Corticosteroids
Ascites	Diuretics Drainage
Anaemia	Blood transfusion
Cardiac failure	Diuretics ACE inhibitors
Chest infection	Antibiotic Physiotherapy
COPD/asthma	Bronchodilators Corticosteroids
Haemorrhage	Treatment of systemic bleeding diathesis
Pulmonary emboli	Anticoagulation

as possible. Even when a patient is very close to death, in some cases it may be appropriate to treat a potentially reversible condition, for example if the patient was desperately hoping to be alive for a significant family event in the near future.

When it is not possible or appropriate to reverse the cause of the patient's breathlessness, or while waiting for the intervention to improve the symptom, there are a number of methods for palliating the symptom. Palliation of breathlessness, like any other symptom, aims to maintain and improve the quality of life of the patient and their families. The central tenets of palliative care are physical, social, spiritual and psychological and therefore all must be considered when treating breathlessness. The main stays of treatment can be divided into non-pharmacological and pharmacological interventions.

Non-pharmacological methods include: cool draught across the face, breathing exercises, oxygen, relaxation therapy and complementary therapies such as massage, visualization, acupuncture and hypnosis. Improvements in breathlessness were also reported in a multi-centre randomized controlled trial of nursing interventions.[18] The intervention consisted of a range of strategies combining breathing control, activity pacing, relaxation techniques and psychological support. There is no evidence to suggest that these techniques alter prognosis, but much to suggest they improve the sensation of breathlessness.

The main aim of drug treatment for the palliation of breathlessness is to suppress respiratory awareness. This should not be confused with respiratory suppression.[13] When used in appropriate doses, drugs such as opioids, benzodiazepines and phenothiazines can improve the sensation of breathlessness and may reduce the metabolic requirements of the body (e.g. by overall sedation) so that a lower level of ventilation is actually appropriate. There is no evidence that in patients with advanced cancer when used in doses appropriately titrated, these drugs alter the survival of the patient.

Breathlessness as a prognostic factor

Breathlessness has been associated with a short prognosis, compared with other prognostic factors, in a number of studies. Hardy et al.[12] in a study of patients admitted to a palliative care unit in a cancer hospital showed the factors with the highest relative risk of death in multivariate analysis were breathlessness and immobility. They concluded that particularly when the breathless patient had a diagnosis of carcinoma of the lung they were very likely to die in the unit. Another study[19] found that patients who are breathless at rest are very ill. Of 38 patients breathless at rest, the median survival was 19 days.

In a qualitative systematic review of literature on survival prediction in terminal cancer patients, Vigano et al.[20] found 22 studies fulfilling their inclusion criteria: this included a total of 7089 patients, with median survival ranges of 1.8–11 weeks. Breathlessness was identified as being definitely associated with a decreased survival in 6 out of 7 studies, with only one study showing no association with worse survival. Patients with lung cancer were consistently associated with worse prognoses in all studies.

In recent years several prognostic tools have been developed to try to improve the accuracy of prognostication. These have been developed using a two-stage design: first, identifying likely predictive factors from a population using multiple regression analysis. The factors are then incorporated into a score with relative weightings. The second stage is to test the score in a comparable population, to determine accuracy.

Both the Palliative Prognostic Score (PaP) [21] and Palliative Prognostic Index (PPI)[22] include breathlessness as a prognostic factor. The PaP score[21] classifies patients with advanced cancer into homogenous risk groups for survival based on various clinical and laboratory parameters: presence or absence of breathlessness and anorexia, Karnofsky Performance Status, clinician's prediction of survival and white cell blood count and lymphocyte differential. The presence of breathlessness is the lowest weighted factor in the score. It is not specified whether the breathlessness is at rest or on exertion.

The PPI score[22] uses performance status and the clinical symptoms: presence of breathlessness at rest, presence of oedema, delirium and a measure of oral intake with weighted scores for each. The authors concluded that whether patients live longer than weeks can be acceptably predicted by the PPI score.

Conclusion

Breathlessness is a common symptom in patients with advanced cancer.[1, 2, 3] It has also been noted that it is frequently under reported, so the figures given are likely to be an underestimate. The genesis and pathophysiology is poorly understood and it remains difficult to treat effectively, in part because of the complex interaction between the physical cause and the patient's psychological response to it.

There is much evidence to suggest patients who are breathless, particularly at rest, have short prognoses, frequently measured in days or a short number of weeks. For this reason the presence or absence of the breathlessness occurs in existing prognostic scales: PaP and PPI. Breathlessness is likely to feature in the development of further scales to aid prognostication. It would therefore be useful to further analyse the symptom, e.g., is it the severity of breathlessness that has the impact on prognosis? Studies[19] have shown that cancer patients who are breathless at rest may only live for a matter of days, however patients who are breathless at rest from long-standing chest disease, for example COPD, are more likely to live longer, so perhaps the duration of breathlessness at rest, the cause or speed of onset may be significant.

There is also a need to address the under reporting of the symptom. Is this because of a lack of awareness amongst some health care professionals of the prevalence of breathlessness in any advanced cancer, so that patients are not asked about the symptom? Or are current symptom assessment tools or history taking techniques not sensitive enough to elucidate the symptom? Is this due to the varied descriptors that patients use to describe their symptomatology? If the presence or absence of breathlessness as a symptom is going to be used for aiding prognostication, it must be ensured that there is a simple and effective method to elucidate this symptom.

References

1. Reuben DB, Mor V. Dyspnoea in terminally ill cancer patients. *Chest* 1986; 89:234–6.
2. Higginson I, McCarthy M. Measuring symptoms in terminal cancer: are pain and dyspnoea controlled? *J R Soc Med* 1989; 82:264–7.
3. Muers MF, Round CE. Palliation of symptoms in non-small cell lung cancer: a study by the Yorkshire Regional Cancer Organisation Thoracic Group. *Thorax* 1989; 4:339–43.
4. Dudgeon DJ, Kristjanson L, Sloan JA, Lertzman M, Clement K. Dyspnea in cancer patients: Prevalence and associated factors. *J Pain Symptom Manage* 2001; 2:195–102.
5. Potter J, Higginson IJ. Pain experienced by lung cancer patients: a review of prevalence, causes and pathophysiology. *Lung Cancer* 2004; 43(3):247–57.
6. Roberts DK, Thorne SE, Pearson C. The experience of dyspnoea in late stage cancer: patients' and nurses' perspectives. *Cancer Nurs* 1993; 16(4):310–20.
7. Carreri VK, Janson-Bjerklie S, Jacobs S. The sensation of dyspnoea: a review. *Clin Rev Critic Care* 1984; 13:437–46.

8. Booth S, Wade R. Oxygen or air for the palliation of breathlessness sin advanced cancer. *J R Soc Med* 2003; 96:215–18.

9. Ripamonti C, Bruera E. Dyspnoea: pathophysiology and assessment. *J Pain Symptom Manage* 1997; 13:220–31.

10. Hearn J, Higginson IJ. Development and validation of a core outcome measure for palliative care: the palliative care outcome scale. *Quality in Health Care* 1998; 8:219–27.

11. Conill C, Verger E, Henriquez I. *et al*. Symptom prevalence in the last week of life. *J Pain Symptom Manage* 1997; 14:328–331.

12. Hardy JR, Turner R, Saunders M, A'Hern R. Prediction of survival in a hospital-based continuing care unit. *Eur J Cancer* 1994; 30A:284–8.

13. Arora NS, Rochester DF. Effect of body weight and muscularity on human diaphragm muscle mass, thickness and area. *J Appl Physiol* 1982; 52, 64–70.

14. O'Driscoll M, Corner J, Bailey C. The experience of breathlessness in lung cancer. *Eur J Cancer Care* 1999; 8:37–43.

15. Ahmedzai S. Palliation of respiratory symptoms. In D Doyle, GWC Hanks, N MacDonald (eds) *Oxford textbook of palliative medicine*, pp. 583–617. Oxford: Oxford University Press, 1999.

16. Chochinov HM. *et al*. (1999) Will to live in the terminally ill. *The Lancet* 354:816–19.

17. Escalante CP, Martin CG, Elting LS *et al*. Identifying risk factors for imminent death in cancer patients with acute dyspnea. *J Pain Symptom Manage* 2000; 20:318–25.

18. Bredin M, Corner J, Krishnasamy M, Plant H, Bailey C, A'Hern R. Multicentre randomised controlled trial of nursing intervention for breathlessness in patients with lung cancer. *BMJ* 1999; 318:901.

19. Booth S, Kelly MJ, Cox MP, Adams L, Guz A. Does oxygen help dyspnoea in patients with cancer? *Am Resp Cit Care Med* 1996; 153:1515–18.

20. Vigano A, Dorgan M, Buckingham J, Bruera E, Suarez-Almazor ME. Survival prediction in terminal cancer patients: a systematic review of the medical literature. *Pall Med* 2000; 14:363–74.

21. Pirovano M, Maltoni M, Nanni O. *et al*. A new palliative prognostic score: a first step for the staging of terminally ill cancer patients. Italian Multicenter and Study Group on Palliative Care. *J Pain Symptom Manage* 1999; 17:231–9.

22. Morita T, Tsunoda J, Inoue S, Chihara S. The Palliative Prognostic Index: a scoring system for survival prediction of terminally ill cancer patients. *Supp Care Cancer* 1999; 7:128–33.

34

Delirium

Miriam Friedlander and David Kissane

Introduction

While sometimes associated with wild excitement or ecstasy, the term 'delirium' is derived from the Latin *delirare*, meaning 'to become deranged, incoherent or raving mad'.[1] In the setting of the medically ill, the diagnosis 'delirium' represents an acutely disordered state of mind involving disturbances of consciousness and either perception or cognition, including confusion, disorientation, and changes in attention, memory, psychomotor behaviour, emotion and the sleep–wake cycle. Its abrupt onset and fluctuating course are important features in helping distinguish it from dementia, while its presentation can be agitated or hypoactive in nature. Delirium is an extremely common neuropsychiatric manifestation of the dying process and, as such, can be a useful predictor of the imminence of death.

Epidemiology and diagnostic challenges

Rates of delirium among hospitalized, medically ill patients have varied between 25–50 per cent,[2–4] while in terminally ill patients, rates rise to between 30–88 per cent.[5–8] Diagnostic criteria as defined by DSM-IV are shown in Table 34.1.[9] The absence of a minimum duration of symptoms means that very transient episodes, such as transient sedation from a newly administered opioid analgesic regimen, constitute delirium. In this context, it is important to understand the mechanism of development of delirium.

Multiple pathways can induce a reversible deterioration in the state of consciousness, in which the brain must focus attention on selected stimuli and discriminate what is relevant from 'noise'. Selective attention is dependent on neuronal interconnections that are susceptible to direct neuronal trauma and indirectly through actions on the glia and vasculature.[10] Neurotransmission within networks occurs through a variety of chemicals, including acetylcholine, dopamine, serotonin, norepinephrine, gamma-aminobutyric acid and histamine, and processes that interfere with the availability and balance of these substrates, including related oxygenation and blood flow, might induce delirium.[11, 12] Alternatively, inflammatory cytokines and glucocorticoids, which are released during sepsis and advanced cancer, might act on cerebral vasculature, stimulate glial cells, alter regulation of neurotransmission and impact on the hypothalamic–pituitary–adrenal axis at several levels.[13]

These several pathways to the development of delirium explain the multiple aetiologies involved in its precipitation and necessitate consideration of multifactorial processes in the clinical investigation of the delirious patient.[8] Studies of delirium in palliative care reveal that only one-third have a single cause, with common overlapping contributors including opioids (64 per cent), metabolic disorders (53 per cent), infection (46 per cent), recent anaesthetic/surgery (32 per cent) and structural lesions (15 per cent).[14] Other causes include dehydration, pre-existing dementia, organ failure (hepatic, pulmonary, renal, cardiac), substance withdrawal, corticosteroid

Table 34.1 DSM-IV* diagnostic criteria for delirium

Delirium due to general medical condition, multiple aetiologies, substance intoxication (multiple codes are used and the causes are listed after the word delirium)
A. Disturbance of consciousness with reduced ability to focus, sustain or shift attention
B. Change in cognition (disorientation, memory, language) or development of perceptual disturbance that are not better accounted for by pre-existing dementia
C. Onset over a short period of time and tends to fluctuate during the day

*DSM-IV, Diagnostic and Statistical Manual of Mental Disorders, 4th edition (Association 1994)

therapy and a variety of other medications – anti-emetics, anti-convulsants, anti-cholinergics, anti-histamines, chemotherapeutics and psychotropics (Table 34.2).

Vigilance about the recognition of delirium is vital in cancer and palliative care, particularly given the under recognition of the hypoactive subtype[15] and the distress that delirium causes.[16] A key clinical task is the recognition and treatment of reversible causes of delirium, for such management provides vital information about the ultimate prognosis.

Table 34.2 Causes of delirium in palliative medicine

Medications	Opioids, corticosteroids, anti-cholinergics, anti-parkinsonians, anti-emetics, anticonvulsants, NSAID and COX-2 inhibitors, proton pump inhibitors, antihistamines, antidepressants, antipsychotics, bronchodilators, antiarrhythmics, chemotherapeutic agents
Substance withdrawal	Alcohol, benzodiazepines, corticosteroids, opioids
Organ failure	Hepatic encephalopathy Uraemia Hypoxic encephalopathy Cardiac failure
Metabolic	Dehydration Hypercalcaemia Hypoglycaemia Hyponatraemia Hypernatraemia
Septic	Urinary tract infection Septicaemia CNS infections Chest and other infections
Intracerebral	Primary or metastatic cancer Pre-existing dementia syndromes
Immunologic	Paraneoplastic syndromes Cytokines in anorexia cachexia syndrome
Haematologic	Anaemia Disseminated intravascular coagulopathies
Nutritional	Scurvy Pellagra Thiamine deficiency Vitamin B12 deficiency

The natural history of delirium

Brief episodes of delirium, especially associated with medications in patients with normal renal and hepatic function, can resolve within hours, the patient noting their bewilderment, confusion and recalling any hallucinations experienced during the event. Such spontaneous resolution carries a good prognosis, and beyond explanation about the sequence of events, may not be of great clinical concern.

In contrast, agitated delirium typically precipitates a crisis, in which confusion induces alarm in relatives, removal of intravenous or other catheters alerts nursing staff, paranoid or frightened behaviour leads the patient to request help from the police – in short, attention is rapidly drawn to the predicament.

More problematic clinically is the patient with hypoactive delirium, where quiet confusion and self-neglect could be recognized by caregivers/nurses, yet readily passes without further attention as the patient has been that way from admission or transfer.[15] As dehydration, further medications and delayed diagnosis occur, there is risk of deterioration and grave illness.

In circumstances of advanced illness with progressive organ failure, delirium can certainly be part of the normal dying process. A common example is liver failure due to widespread metastatic disease, where jaundice and hepatic encephalopathy occurs. As the altered conscious state deteriorates, progressive obtundation, stupor, coma and a peaceful death can evolve. With less advanced disease, and typically post anesthetic (where shunting processes within the lungs lead to hypoxic episodes), confusion might become symptomatic, but be clearly reversible within a few days. A portion of such patients will be seen as having early cognitive deficits, with an emerging early dementia. For others, overt cognitive problems will not appear for several more years, but the vulnerability to delirium represents a warning sign for the development of dementia in the future.

Studies of psychotropic medication as an adjunct to the treatment of delirium have shown an ability to ameliorate the course and lessen any related distress.[17–19] Of particular note is the beneficial contribution of neuroleptics over benzodiazepines and other sedative medications in improving cognitive function.[20, 21] Nevertheless, the age-old adage of treating the cause of the delirium prevails if ultimate recovery is to be achieved.

Let us explore the predisposing and precipitating factors affecting the prognosis of a patient with delirium, so that we can better discuss this prognosis with relatives and the care team.

Factors affecting prognosis

A number of studies provide support that delirium impacts unfavourably on the short-term survival of patients with advanced cancer. Bruera and colleagues demonstrated a significant association between cognitive failure and the probability of dying within 4 weeks.[22] In Japan, Morita's group found that delirium predicted poor short-term prognosis in patients admitted to hospice.[23] Morita included delirium in the Palliative Prognostic Index (PPI) score, also incorporating performance status, oral intake, oedema, and dyspnoea at rest to classify patients into three distinct survival profiles and establish threshold points to predict whether any individual patient was likely to survive longer than 3 or 6 weeks. Similarly, Caraceni et al. evaluated the impact of delirium on patients for whom chemotherapy was no longer considered effective and had been referred to palliative care programmes: the survival curve of patients with delirium differed significantly from those without.[24] Compared with an overall median of 39 days in their study, the survival of delirious patients reduced to 21 days. Moreover, delirium retained an independent association with decreased survival. If the Palliative Prognostic (PaP) score was used to assign patients to three different prognostic groups to predict the likelihood of 30 days survival, the presence of delirium influenced the survival curves adversely for each group. The impact of delirium on median survival was particularly relevant for patients with a relatively favourable prognosis.[24]

Reversibility

An important challenge is the clinical differentiation of delirium as either a reversible complication of cancer or an integral element of the dying process. Lawlor and colleagues explored the aetiologic precipitants and potential reversibility of delirium in advanced cancer patients admitted to a palliative care unit for symptom control and found an overall reversibility rate of 49 per cent.[7] No difference was found in reversibility rates for delirium present on admission and that which developed subsequently. However, a significant difference existed in the reversibility of initial (56 per cent) compared to repeated episodes (6 per cent). The median duration of reversible delirium (3.5 days) contrasted with irreversible delirium (6 days). The median number of precipitating factors for both reversible and irreversible delirium was 3 (range 1–6). The application of standardized criteria resulted in a classification of aetiologic factors in 78 per cent of episodes of reversible delirium and 59 per cent of irreversible cases. Reversibility of delirium was significantly associated with opioids, other psychoactive medications and dehydration. In contrast, irreversibility of delirium was significantly associated with hypoxic encephalopathy and metabolic factors related to major organ failure, including hepatic and renal insufficiency, and refractory hypercalcaemia. [7]

Morita examined factors associated with reversibility of delirium in another population of advanced cancer patients admitted to hospice for terminal care.[25] This study's overall delirium reversibility rate was 20 per cent, lower than that reported in prior studies. Patients with delirium had a 30-day mortality rate of 83 per cent and a 50-day mortality rate of 91 per cent. While reversibility of delirium was significantly associated with medication (37 per cent) or hypercalcaemia (38 per cent), irreversibility was associated with infection (12 per cent), hepatic failure, hypoxia, disseminated intravascular coagulation, and dehydration (< 10 per cent).

These studies highlight that the prognosis of patients who develop delirium is defined by the interaction of the patient's baseline physiologic susceptibility to delirium, the precipitating etiologies, and any response to treatment. If a patient's susceptibility or resilience is modifiable, then targeted interventions may reduce the risk of experiencing delirium upon exposure to a precipitant and enhance the capacity to respond to treatment. Conversely, if a patient's vulnerability is high and resistant to modification, then exposure to precipitants enhances the likelihood of developing delirium and may diminish the probability of a complete restoration of cognitive function.

Predisposing or vulnerability factors

In medically ill populations, advanced age, pre-existing cognitive impairment, disease severity, and burden of other comorbid illnesses constitute increased susceptibility to developing delirium.[26, 27] These basic vulnerabilities also apply to patients with advanced cancer. Cognitive impairment related to neurotoxic chemotherapy regimens or brain irradiation elevates risk. Primary central nervous system tumors, cerebral metastases, or leptomeningeal disease further increase vulnerability.

Cerebrovascular injury sustained secondary to hemorrhage, coagulopathy, or hyperviscosity increases physiologic susceptibility to the development of delirium. Furthermore, extensive disease, represented not only by metastases involving multiple sites, but also its progression contributing to multiorgan insufficiency increase a patient's vulnerability to developing delirium.

Previous treatments with chemotherapeutics may add to hepatic, renal, pulmonary or cardiac insufficiency, resulting in reduced physiologic reserve. Patients exposed to immunosuppressants may have enduring and enhanced risk of infections. Finally, vulnerability may result from toxicities incurred by chronic cytokine and endocrine activation. The concurrent presence of other poor prognostic indicators including anorexia and cachexia, dyspnoea, oedema, impaired immunoreactive status, and poor performance status creates a relatively high baseline vulnerability. In the palliative care setting, these factors are generally related to progressive disease and likely to be irreversible.

Precipitating factors

Identification of acute precipitants is more likely to yield potentially reversible factors. The capacity to identify an aetiology may influence prognosis, although this has been elusive in several studies. If an aetiology is identifiable, the physician can target treatment, but if not, the physician may have to explore multiple interventions to achieve benefit. If early enough in the course of illness, accurate identification of offensive precipitants is more likely; in contrast, when the disease has advanced extensively, any investigations may be excessively burdensome. An isolated, single aetiology may be more amenable to identification and treatment than multiple aetiologies. If an insult is isolated or infrequent, the patient resists becoming overwhelmed and equilibrium may be re-established quickly. In the terminal phase, however, reserves will be inevitably depleted and unable to weather even slight insults. Although hospice studies have not demonstrated any difference in mean number of precipitants for reversible or irreversible delirium, these cohorts have been close to death.[7, 28] This finding may not extend to patients seen earlier in the course of illness.

The pattern of exposure to precipitants also influences the prognosis. If re-exposure to a precipitant is a rare or singular occurrence, the patient is likely to have a more favourable prognosis than those with repeated exposures or sustained contact with an aggravating factor. The source of the precipitant is relevant. Extrinsic factors triggering delirium tend to be modifiable, whereas intrinsic factors, consequent upon progression of advancing disease, prove more resistant.

Course of illness

Ultimately, the inherent reversibility of any aetiology determines the significance of delirium as a contributor to prognosis. Prompt reduction, discontinuation, and selection of less injurious alternative medications may be accomplished readily. In contrast, reversing the progression of metastases precipitating hepatic or pulmonary insufficiency is unlikely, even impossible to accomplish. Therefore, the best prognosis is afforded by low baseline vulnerability, reversible aetiology and complete remission following treatment of the cause. Increasing baseline vulnerability with only temporarily or partially reversible aetiologies and a limited response to treatment confers an intermediate prognosis. High baseline susceptibility, the presence of multiple irreversible aetiologies, and lack of response to treatment generate the poorest prognosis.

Repeated episodes of delirium induce resistance to remission. The duration, severity, and subtype of delirium experienced clearly influence prognosis. Thus, patients experiencing briefer episodes with mild symptoms will fare better than patients suffering extended episodes with severe symptomatology. The subtype of delirium experienced may also influence a physician's ability to diagnose the disorder, implement an effective clinical evaluation and treatment strategy, and select appropriate pharmacologic management of symptoms.

The availability of appropriate, tolerable treatments and adequacy of response influences the ultimate prognosis. If an available treatment exists, presents minimal burden to the patient, and corrects the precipitating factor, the prognosis improves. Lack of available treatment, therapies that represent a prohibitive burden to the patient, an inability to reverse the precipitating element temporarily or permanently, or incapacity to provide symptomatic relief indicates a poorer prognosis (Table 34.3).

Clinical evaluation, management, and estimation of prognosis

The intensity of the clinical search for reversible aetiologic factors and the extent of treatment employed to pursue reversal must be individualized. The purpose of the clinical assessment is to identify and eliminate reversible aetiologies or recognize the presence of irreversible aetiologies signifying progression of disease. A clinically informed model of evaluation that recognizes the goals of care pursues investigations and provides treatments that are acceptable, tolerable, improve quality of life, and minimize the burden or distress experienced by the patient.

Obtaining an accurate history from the patient and caregivers provides crucial information regarding baseline cognitive function and context of presentation. A review of the medication record is necessary to identify a number of potential precipitants. The patient assessment includes a comprehensive physical examination, which most patients will be able to tolerate with minimal distress. Observation of specific findings may indicate usefulness for complementary investigations or identify signs of imminent death, refocusing interventions on providing comfort.

Table 34.3 Influence of vulnerability, etiology, course and treatment response factors on prognostic outcomes

Good prognosis	1. Low baseline vulnerability	Younger age, free of CNS comorbidity, few other medical comorbidities
	2. Reversible etiology	Medications like opioids, readily identifiable infection, hypercalcaemia, mild dehydration
	3. Course – brief	Single, brief episode: readily corrects and does not recur
	4. Remission with treatment	Treatment of cause straightforward and relative ease of symptomatic amelioration
Intermediate prognosis	1. Greater baseline vulnerability	CNS comorbidity, immunosuppressed, toxic anti-cancer therapies, anorexia cachexia syndrome, limited performance status
	2. Partially reversible etiologies	More serious infection, early organ insufficiency, severe dehydration
	3. Course – lingering	May have repeated episodes, with slow recovery from each
	4. Limited treatment response	Partial improvement, higher dosage of neuroleptic medication needed
Poor prognosis	1. High baseline susceptibility	High tumour load in multiple sites, advanced cachexia, bed bound with very poor performance status
	2. Multiple irreversible etiologies	Organ failures dominate, fulminant sepsis, refractory hypercalcaemia
	3. Course – chronic	Persisting delirium, no hint of improvement
	4. Absence of treatment response	Persists or warrants deep sedation to ameliorate until death

Investigations

The ordering of complementary investigations depends on the patient's prior wishes, current clinical status, likelihood of reversibility of presumed aetiology, and availability of resources. Information obtained from the clinical history and physical examination will also assist this decision. Earlier in the course of disease, patients benefit from and tolerate more extensive, invasive investigations if necessary to identify aetiologies. Later in the course of disease, such investigations induce distress and are less likely to yield identifiable, reversible aetiologies.

Most patients will accept and tolerate venipuncture to assist in identifying or excluding reversible aetiologies. Consider a simple laboratory appraisal that includes a complete blood count and analyses of electrolytes, hepatic enzymes, blood urea nitrogen, creatinine, glucose, calcium, phosphate, and magnesium. Oxygen saturation may be readily and non-invasively obtained from a pulse oximeter. If infection is suspected based on clinical exam or laboratory evidence of leukocytosis, inspect wounds, examine indwelling catheters, and obtain cultures of urine, sputum, and blood. Chest X-ray may assist in the identification of pneumonia. A 12-lead electrocardiogram may be analysed to monitor for arrhythmias or ischemia.

Patients with lateralizing neurologic signs on examination or clinical suspicion of intracranial hemorrhage may require neuroimaging, either computed tomography (CT) or magnetic resonance imaging (MRI) of the brain. Lumbar puncture and cerebrospinal fluid examination may identify meningitis or leptomeningeal disease. Electroencephalography is indicated if seizures are suspected. These latter examinations and procedures require more cooperation from the patient. All have the potential to place additional duress on the patient. Remember that the burden of diagnostic investigations and treatments should be balanced with the expected benefit for quality of life.

Management

Treatment of delirium is directed at identification and elimination of the underlying aetiologies. If a medication is identified as a precipitant, consider dose reduction, withdrawal, or substitution. For opiates, consider rotation at an equianalgesic dose with a 20–30 per cent reduction.[29–31] Active metabolites of morphine are hydrosoluble and accumulate with renal insufficiency or volume depletion.[32] Adequate hydration may reduce the severity and duration of delirium, however parenteral hydration is not always appropriate as intravenous lines may impose additional distress on the patient. Although hypodermoclysis may be less burdensome, hydration may not be appropriate if there is a risk of fluid overload or not consistent with goals of care.[8] Electrolyte abnormalities may be corrected and infections treated with antibiotics.

Physicians should assess potential problems associated with correction of aetiologies and the impact on quality of life. Consider with the patient and caregivers the advantages and disadvantages of intervention versus no intervention. Discuss treatment options, allow informed decision-making, and develop consensus on an appropriate level of intervention. During the interval during which an identifiable aetiology is sought and corrected, the patient will benefit from both non-pharmacologic and pharmacologic treatment. For patients in whom the delirium is irreversible, symptomatic relief will be the main intervention.

Non-pharmacologic treatments, though not systematically evaluated, are recommended based on modest evidence, clinical experience, and lack of adverse effects. Supportive measures contribute to good care: these are unlikely to alter prognosis but likely to improve quality of life. Providing reassurance and reorientation to the patient is comforting; continue to treat the patient with courtesy and respect. Encourage engagement in simple tasks, while avoiding excessive demands. Attempt to mollify or allay the patient's fears and provide a safe, comfortable, and relaxing environment. Surround the patient with familiar people and objects. Provide structure and routine, while avoiding physical restraints if at all possible.

Pharmacologic therapy can provide patients with symptomatic relief of distressing symptoms, while an underlying aetiology is identified and reversed or provide comfort if the aetiology is irreversible. Most physicians will select an antipsychotic to provide symptomatic relief. Haloperidol is a frequent initial choice as it is easy to administer by a variety of routes and provides high-potency dopamine blockade with minimal active metabolites, anticholinergic effects, and sedation.[20] Potential extrapyramidal adverse effects may be managed with dose reduction or the addition of benztropine. If haloperidol provides inadequate relief of symptoms, consider alternatives with more sedation such as chlorpromazine to provide relief of more severe agitation. Newer atypical antipsychotics are available especially for patients vulnerable to extrapyramidal adverse effects. Case reports and small case series suggest efficacy in reducing distressing delirium symptomatology. Risperidone or olanzapine may provide relief from distressing symptoms.[21]

Alternative medications will provide enhanced sedation, but not directly modify the symptoms of delirium. Benzodiazepines have an advantage of a more predictable dose–effect relationship. Midazolam provides a rapid induction and its short half-life permits reversal of sedation, allowing easy titration and frequent reassessment of delirium reversibility as potential etiologies are addressed and corrected. Routes of administration include intravenous and subcutaneous.

Complicated delirium may not respond to antipsychotics or benzodiazepines. The need for sedation emerges in the presence of refractory symptoms (e.g. agitation) and in the final days may be the only means for relieving distress and providing comfort. Delirium is the most frequent cause of palliative sedation.[31] Deep palliative sedation is 'the deliberate intent to induce sleep but not cause death deliberately'.[26] A reported 10–52 per cent of patients require some level of sedation at the end of life.[33–36] The fundamentals of using palliative sedation include: verification of the diagnosis of delirium; assurance of appropriate efforts to evaluate reversibility within the context of goals of care; clarification of the intent of sedation; and appropriate communication with family and staff. Phenobarbital is useful for inducing deep palliative sedation for resistant agitation in terminal delirium, as is propofol, a short-acting anaesthetic.[31] The mean time to death after initiating sedation for control of refractory symptoms is 2.0–3.9 days.[34–36] Morita examined the effects of sedatives on survival in terminally ill patients. Such sedative pharmacologic agents included opioids, benzodiazepines, haloperidol, chlorpromazine, barbiturates, and propofol. Interestingly, Morita and colleagues did not find any significant difference in patient survival between the group receiving sedation versus the group that did not receive sedation[25] (Figure 34.1).

Communication of prognosis and support of caregivers

Three clinical scenarios have emerged for the delirious patient which will lead to subsequent clinical discussions as part of the overall care:

1. Reversible delirium from which the patient recovers and for whom the task of making sense of what has happened is integral to their psychosocial adaptation and healing – often here the prognosis can be optimistic, but risks for the future are part of the clinical remit;

2. Reversible or only partially controlled delirium where the prognosis is poor, and potentially only weeks to months of life remain;

3. Irreversible delirium where the patient is dying and the prognosis is merely days to weeks. This subtype has in the past been called 'terminal restlessness', but hypoactive delirium also lies within this group.

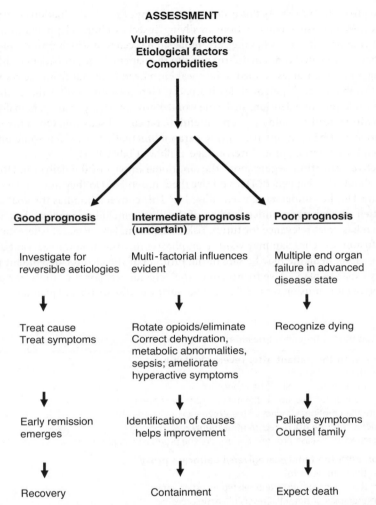

Figure 34.1 Flow chart depicting the influence of disease trajectory and delirium management on outcome.

Discussing delirium and its prognosis with the patient

In the first clinical scenario, a series of steps can be laid out to guide what is discussed with the patient. First, the word 'delirium' is generally worthwhile teaching to patients and relatives who are seeking to integrate what has happened – many understand the association between confusion and a delirious mental state as they recall old movies in which the prognostic question was 'Will the fever break?'

Second, the phenomenology should be addressed, reviewing what the patient recalls. 'How much do you remember about what you experienced? It's usually helpful to discuss this.' Perceptual disturbances including hallucinations and any resultant paranoid delusions need to be explained as a component of the delirium, real at the time to the patient yet disordered, irrational and resulting from the illness. As this is done, the content of any hallucinations merits sensitive consideration. While visual hallucinations involving 'insects' or 'pink elephants running up the wall' are easily appreciated for what they are, more subtle scenes in which misinterpretation and confusion have dominated can remain troubling to the patient. Thus, in patients with advanced cancer, images like 'the nurses seemed to be sneaking a dead body out from the room opposite mine' point to the patient's personal death anxiety. Here a comment like 'the content of your experiences while you were delirious make me wonder how anxious you are personally about any prospect of future death?' could open up a useful therapeutic discussion. Often the tone of fear or the experience of being frightened during paranoid mental states reflects some inner level of anxiety about the operation, procedure, or stage of illness (Table 34.4).

Herein active evaluation begins about the emotional impact of the delirium. How does the patient feel about what happened? Does it leave them unsettled? Do they now understand that it was delirium? Do they understand what caused it? This conversation has the goal of ensuring that the patient integrates an understanding of the illness, including medical data about likely causes, which has great relevance for future risk of delirium. For instance, where an opioid has caused confusion, the clinician may want to emphasize that the dose was relevant and smaller doses of the same medicine may be safe in the future. For the alcohol-dependent patient, an opportunity exists to plan active treatment of the dependence. For the family, the question of future caregiving if confusion returned might be worthy of discussion and planning.

Table 34.4 Communicating about delirium and its prognosis

A. Discussion with the patient after reversible delirium:
1. Explain the term delirium
2. Review the patient's recall of the experience
3. Promote understanding about the meaning of the content
4. Evaluate the emotional impact of the experience
5. Consider any future risk of recurrent delirium
6. With respect to disease progression, explore the prognostic implications

B. Discussion with the family/caregivers/healthcare proxy
1. Explain the term delirium
2. Review the potential causes and related investigations
3. Explain therapies of potential reversible aetiologies
4. Explain supportive treatment to maintain safety and comfort
5. Review the goals of care with reversible and irreversible delirium
6. Review how caregivers relate to the delirious patient
7. Evaluate the emotional impact of the experience
8. Discuss the decision-making process

C. Guidelines in discussing prognosis
1. Identify preference for level of information
2. Review understanding of disease progression and seriousness
3. Discuss results of investigations and resultant prognosis
4. Use mixed framing (with best and worst scenarios)
5. Use a variety of media: words, graphs, figures
6. Ask about emotional response to the information
7. Empathize with these feelings
8. Reconsider goals of care and restate commitment to care
9. Ask the patient/relatives to summarize their understanding of the discussion
10. Consider balance between hope and grief

Finally, if the episode is in some way related to overall disease progression and the patient's ultimate prognosis, consideration should be given to discussion of this.[36] Guidelines about this strategy include:

- before offering prognostic information, identify the patient's preference for the level of information they want;[37, 38]

- include in the prognostic statement the extent of disease and it's recent response to treatment, the current goals of care and anticipated course of future illness;

- explain the limitations of statistics when applied to any one person;[39]

- use mixed framing in estimating prognosis, including a better and then a worse case scenario, and a variety of media – words, graphs and figures;[40, 41]

- ask how the patient feels about the information provided[42, 43]

- empathize with the patient's feelings, acknowledging their reasonableness and return to the goals of care, emphasizing commitment to care and continuing treatment;

- ask the patient to summarize what they have understood, using their feedback as a stepping stone to a final clinical summary that seeks to keep an appropriate balance between realistic hope and support for grief.[44]

The model presented here can help transition patients to an acceptance of hospice care through the gradual development of their understanding of the clinical reality, a process dependent on continuity of care.

Discussing delirium and its prognosis with the family

Onlookers find the experience of delirium when it affects their loved one to be alarming. They need considerable explanation and support regarding the nature of this mental state and associated disinhibition or aggression; its cause and potential for reversal; the risk of harm to the patient from impaired judgments; and the decision-making capacity of the patient.[31] How caregivers should respond to the patient, when to seek to reorient, when not to contradict and how to reduce sensorial stimuli and calm the person – all of these practical concerns merit discussion.[45]

The clinical judgement for the physician is not only whether this episode of delirium might be reversible, but also whether weeks to months of future life can still be anticipated, or whether this is a terminal development. In some ways, recognition that the patient is dying creates a more manageable scenario, given the relative predictability of the clinical course. When the clinical prognostic factors point to a prognosis of just hours to days, the focus of family discussion is about comfort measures and keeping watch, alongside supporting relatives empathically in their distress. Goals of care focus on treating patient's symptoms, including avoiding episodes of agitation through sustained sedation if this is indicated clinically. When dying patients can be kept peaceful, their loved ones have time to come to terms with their dying, eventually helping their overall adaptation. Cultural variations in the importance of sentience and clear cognition are pronounced and impact on the value attached to sedative medications at the end of life.[46]

A series of conversations with family over days to weeks are needed where the delirium persists, even if ameliorated by psychotropic medication. Early in this sequence, relatives are advised of the planned investigations in search for reversible aetiologic factors, while supportive therapies like oxygenation, rehydration, and medications such as antibiotics and psychotropics are introduced. If the delirium persists, its very chronicity becomes an additional prognostic factor. The healthcare proxy is of course consulted about treatment recommendations, and frequently clinical teams need to reach consensus about decisions like opioid rotation and any revision in the goals of care. The course of the delirium helps ultimately to guide this process, and frequent communication is vital to sustain understanding and support for the caregivers involved.

Conclusion

Delirium is not only a medical crisis in which protection and safety of the patient are crucial, but also a clear predictor of prognosis and therefore of ultimate outcome. The clinician is invited to evaluate predisposing and precipitating factors, searching for reversible aetiologies, while monitoring the course of illness as treatment is offered to ameliorate the phenomenology. Delirium can certainly occur in good prognostic situations, but when accompanied by very advanced disease, multiple comorbidities, poor physical performance and imminently failing organs, it can be a clear pointer to the closeness of death. Clinical skill is needed to deliver comprehensive and sensitive care, which typically involves all members of the multidisciplinary team. Relatives are readily distressed by the agitated form of delirium and warrant care and support in their own right. Accurate prognostication increases the possibility of minimizing the distress experienced by the patient and family and enhances the opportunity to provide the patient with a 'good' death.

References

1. Marchant J, Charles JF (1917) *Cassell's Latin dictionary*. London: Cassell.

2. Massie M, Holland J. *et al*. Delirium in terminally ill cancer patients. *American Journal of Psychiatry* 1983; 140:1048–50.

3. Stiefel F, Fainsinger R. *et al*. Acute confusional states in patients with advanced cancer. *Journal of Pain and Symptom Management* 1992; 7:94–8.

4. Fann, J. The epidemiology of delirium. *Seminars in Clinical Neuropsychiatry* 2000; 5:64–74.

5. Minagawa H, Uchitomi Y. *et al*. Psychiatric morbidity in terminally ill cancer patients. *Cancer* 1996; 78:1131–7.

6. Gagnon P, Allard P. *et al*. Delirium in terminally ill cancer patients. *Journal of Pain and Symptom Management* 2000; 19:412–26.

7. Lawlor P, Gagnon B. *et al*. Occurences, causes, and outcome of delirium in patients with advanced cancer. *Archives of Internal Medicine* 2000; 160:786–94.

8. Casarett D, Inouye S. Diagnosis and management of delirium near the end of life. *Annals of Internal Medicine* 2001; 135:32–40.

9. American Psychiatric Association. *DSM-IV. Diagnostic and statistical manual of mental disorders*, 4th edn. Washington, DC: American Psychiatric Association, 1994.

10. Landis, D. (1996). Brain as tissue: the interacting cell populations of the nervous system. In R Rabsohoff and E Benveniste *Cytokines and the CNS*, pp. 63–83. Boca Raton, FL: CRC Press Inc., 1996.

11. Trzepacz P. Is there a final common neural pathway in delirium? Focus on acetylcholine and dopamine. *Seminars in Clinical Neuropsychiatry* 2000; 5:132–48.

12. Van der Mast R, Fekkes D. Serotonin and amino acids: partners in delirium pathophysiology? *Seminars in Clinical Neuropsychiatry* 2000; 5:125–31.

13. Olsson T. Activity of the hypothalamic–pituitary–adrenal axis and delirium. *Dementia Geriatric Cognitive Disorders* 1999; 10:345–9.

14. Tuma R, DeAngelis L. Altered mental status in patients with cancer. *Archives of Neurology* 2000; 57:1727–31.

15. Olofsson S, Weitzner M. *et al*. A retrospective study of the psychiatric management and outcome of delirium in the cancer patient. *Supportive Care in Cancer* 1996; 4:351–7.

16. Breitbart W, Gibson C. *et al.* The delirium experience: delirium recall and delirium-related distress in hospitalized patients with cancer, their spouses/caregivers, and their nurses. *Psychosomatics* 2002; 43:183–94.

17. Rosen J. Double-blind comparison of haloperidol and thioridazine in geriatric outpatients. *Journal of Clinical Psychiatry* 1979; 40:17–20.

18. Fainsinger R. Bruera E. Treatment of delirium in a terminally ill patient. *Journal of Pain and Symptom Management* 1992; 7:54–56.

19. Akecki, T., Y. Uchitomi, *et al.* Usage of haloperidol for delirium in cancer patients. *Supportive Care in Cancer* 1996; 4:390–2.

20. Breitbart W, Marotta R. *et al.* A double-blinded trial of haloperidol, chlorpromazine, and lorazepam in the treatment of delirium in hospitalized AIDS patients. *American Journal of Psychiatry* 1996; 153:231–7.

21. Breitbart W, Tremblay A. *et al.* An open trial of olanzapine for the treatment of delirium in hospitalized cancer patients. *Psychosomatics* 2002; 43:175–82.

22. Bruera E, Miller M. *et al.* Estimate of survival of patients admitted to a palliative care unit: a prospective study. *Journal of Pain and Symptom Management* 1992; 7:82–6.

23. Morita T, Tsunoda J. *et al.* The Palliative Prognostic Index: a scoring system for survival prediction of terminally ill cancer patients. *Support Care Cancer* 1999; 7:128–33.

24. Caraceni A, Nanni O. *et al.* Impact of delirium on the short term prognois of advanced cancer patients. *Cancer* 2000; 89:1145–9.

25. Morita T, Tsunoda J. *et al.* Effects of high dose opioids and sedatives on survival in terminally ill cancer patients. *Journal of Pain and Symptom Management* 2001; 21:282–9.

26. Lawlor P, Bruera E. Delirium in patients with advanced cancer. *Hematology Oncology Clinics of North America* 2002; 16:701–14.

27. Michaud L, Burnand B. *et al.* Taking care of the terminally ill cancer patient: delirium as a symptom of terminal disease. *Annals of Oncology* 2004; 15:199–203.

28. Morita T, Tsunoda J. *et al.* Underlying pathologies and their associations with clinical features in terminal delirium of cancer patients. *Journal of Pain and Symptom Management* 2001; 22(6):997–1006.

29. Bruera E, Franco J. *et al.* (1995). Changing pattern of agitated impaired mental status in patients with advanced cancer: Association with cognitive monitoring, hydration, and opioid rotation. *Journal of Pain and Symptom Management* 1995; 10:287–91.

30. de Stoutz N, Bruera E. *et al.* Opioid rotation for toxicity reduction in terminal cancer patients. *Journal of Pain and Symptom Management* 1995; 10:378–84.

31. Centeno C, Sanz A. *et al.* Delirium in advanced cancer patients. *Palliative Medicine* 2004; 18:184–94.

32. Morita T, Tei Y. *et al.* Increased plasma morphine metabolites in terminally ill cancer patients with delirium: an intra-individual comparison. *Journal of Pain and Symptom Management* 2002; 23:107–13.

33. Fainsinger R, Miller M. *et al.* Symptom control during the last week of life on a palliative care unit. *Journal of Palliative Care* 1991; 7:5–11.

34. Fainsinger R, Landman W. *et al.* Sedation for uncontrolled symptoms in a South African hospice. *Journal of Pain and Symptom Management* 1998; 16:145–52.

35. Ventafridda V, Ripamonti C. *et al.* Symptom prevalence and control during cancer patients last days of life. *Journal of Palliative Care* 1990; 6:7–11.

36. Butow P, Dowsett S. *et al.* Communicating prognosis to patients with metastatic disease: What do they really want to know? *Supportive Care in Cancer* 2002; 10:161–8.

36. Morita T, Inoue S. *et al.* Sedation for symptom control in Japan: the importance of intermittent use and communication with family members. *Journal of Pain and Symptom Management* 1996; 12:32–8.

37. Parker P, Baile W. *et al.* Breaking bad news about cancer: patients' preferences for communication. *Journal of Clinical Oncology* 2001; 19:2049–56.

38. Gattellar M, Voight K. *et al*. When the treatment goal is not cure: are cancer patients equipped to make profound decisions? *Supportive Care in Cancer* 2002; 10:314–21.

39. Sutherland H, Lockwood G. *et al*. Communicating probabilistic information to cancer patients: is there noise on the line? *Social Science in Medicine* 1991; 32:725–31.

40. Nakao M, Axelrod S. Numbers are better than words. Verbal specifications of frequency have no place in medicine. *American Journal of Medicine* 1983; 74:1061–5.

41. Marteau T. Framing of information: its influence upon decisions of doctors and patients. *British Journal of Social Psychology* 1989; 28:89–94.

42. Mazur D, and Merz J. How the manner of presentation of data influences older patients in determining their treatment preferences. *Journal of the American Geriatric Society* 1993; 41:223–38.

43. Fogarty L, Curbow B. *et al*. Can 40 seconds of compassion reduce patient anxiety? *Journal of Clinical Oncology* 1999; 17:371–9.

44. Australia, NBCCo and NCC Initiative. *Clinical practice guidelines for the psychosocial care of adults with cancer*. Camperdown, NSW: National Breast Cancer Centre of Australia, 2003.

45. Ingham J, Caraceni A. Delirium. In A Berger, R Portenoy, R Weissman (eds) *Principles and practice of supportive oncology*, pp. 477–95. Philadelphia, PA: Lippincott-Raven, 1998.

46. Fainsinger R, Nunez-Olarte J. *et al*. The cultural differences in perceived value of disclosure and cognition: Spain and Canada. *Journal of Palliative Care* 2003; 19:43–8.

35

Weight loss

Aminah Jatoi and Phuong L. Nguyen

Prediction is very difficult, especially about the future.[1]

Introduction

Studies clearly show that cancer patients and their families seek professional assessment of life expectancy and look for clues that might help in estimating it. Kirk and others recently observed that among a group of 72 cancer patients from Australia and Canada, nearly all sought information on prognosis.[2] Indeed, lack of provision of such information was often met with consternation, as one patient recalled:

> I asked how much time and he said he couldn't tell me because he wasn't God. I didn't care for that answer very much. I thought maybe he could be a little more specific. Sometimes it seems that the information is strictly for the medical staff and not for the people.

In this context, weight loss can by viewed as an important and unique prognosticator. As discussed below, as little as > 5% of premorbid weight loss carries prognostic significance. Unlike perhaps all other cancer prognosticators, weight loss does not require cutting edge instrumentation – outside of an ordinary household scale – or special questionnaires to document its presence. In fact, when patients are markedly emaciated, weight loss is readily apparent. Patients and family members recognize this finding and see it for what it is: an ominous sign of early demise. Poole and Froggatt recently reviewed the literature on cancer patients' and their family members' perceptions of weight loss.[3] Although these investigators acknowledge that research on patients' and family members' perceptions of weight loss is limited, they nonetheless point out that most available studies suggest that weight loss is a cause of emotional distress, based on its perceived, negative prognostic impact.

A sizeable number of studies provide firm data to substantiate these perceptions from patients and family members. DeWys and others provide one of the most seminal studies on the prognostic effect of weight loss[4] in which 3047 cancer patients, all of whom were participating in Eastern Cooperative Oncology Group trials, were assessed for survival in the context of weight loss. In a multivariate analysis, these investigators found that patient-reported weight loss of >5% over the preceding 6 months was associated with a shortened survival. These investigators observed that this prognostic effect occurred independently of performance status, tumour type, and tumour stage. In short, weight loss was a very powerful prognostic tool and predicted an early demise. In addition, there also appeared to be some evidence that weight loss was associated with a lower likelihood of tumour response, but, to our knowledge, previous studies have not yet explained this phenomenon. Since this seminal study, several others have provided confirmatory findings.

Natural history of weight loss in cancer patients and factors affecting prognosis

This prognostic effect carries even greater impact when one realizes that weight loss is common among patients with cancer. This sign occurs in the majority of patients with incurable malignancies. Sarhill and others evaluated 352 cancer patients, who had been referred to the Cleveland Clinic Palliative Care Program.[5] Three hundred and seven of these patients experienced weight loss. Among patients with weight loss, the extent of weight loss was dramatic: 71% had lost >/ = 10% of their pre-illness weight. Other studies have confirmed such high rates of weight loss, and, taken together, such data suggest that weight loss is a prevalent sign of end of life in cancer patients, a finding that further underscores the importance of its prognostic significance.

Does the relationship between weight loss and survival represent a cause and effect connection? To our knowledge, there are no previous studies that demonstrate irrefutably that weight loss directly causes an early death. However, several indirect lines of evidence have established a strong link between weight loss and early demise. First, it is important to point out that weight loss in cancer patients is a separate, unique process from simple starvation and that, in contrast to starvation, where lean tissue is relatively preserved, cancer-associated weight loss leads to an excess wasting of lean tissue. Case–control studies between cancer patients and non-cancer individuals clearly demonstrate that the former erode their lean tissue compartment excessively[6] (Figure 35.1). Second, the importance of this first observation rests in the fact that lean tissue comprises a vital body compartment. Moore and others summarized the function of lean tissue based on energy exchange mechanisms.[7] They concluded that lean tissue, or more specifically lean body mass, is a highly functional compartment that holds the infrastructure for cellular metabolism, blood circulation, integumentary protection, as well as a variety of other activities critical to the sustenance of life. Thus, if a small wasting of lean tissue translates into diminished function, it follows that a dramatic loss of lean tissue – estimated at 40% by some – might translate into death. Third, in patients with other, non-malignant/non-oncologic diseases, a direct relationship between lean tissue and survival has been observed. Kotler and others analysed data from 32 AIDS patients who were, in retrospect, within 100 days of death.[8] These investigators measured whole body ^{40}K, a naturally occurring isotope that is particularly relevant here because over 97% of potassium is found in non-adipose tissue, thereby allowing for a reasonable estimate of body cell mass with the detection of ^{40}K. This study reported a direct association between total body potassium, which approximates body cell mass, and survival (r = 0.48; p = 0.0013). This study once again suggests a potential cause and effect relationship between loss of lean tissue and diminished survival. When all three of these lines of investigation are taken together, it appears

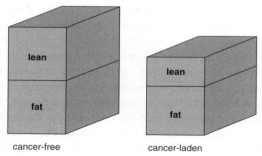

cancer-free   cancer-laden

Figure 35.1 The importance of lean tissue.

plausible that weight loss, perhaps by means of a true cause and effect relationship, leads to an early demise in patients with advanced cancer.

Therapies affecting prognosis

If weight loss leads to an early demise, it might follow that regaining weight summons an improved prognosis. At first glance, this argument seems logical. Indeed, some clinical trials that have employed effective antineoplastic agents have documented weight gain and in turn have demonstrated a solid survival advantage with the use of these agents. However, in the absence of such an impressive antineoplastic effect, the majority of previous studies that have evaluated commonly used agents for treating cancer-induced weight loss, that do not otherwise alter cancer growth, have not demonstrated that reversal of weight loss leads to improvements in survival.

One example to make this point centres around the use of megestrol acetate, a frequently used appetite stimulant that is associated with weight gain in end-stage cancer patients, sometimes as high as > 10% of baseline weight. Early studies in breast cancer patients identified weight gain as a noxious side effect of megestrol acetate, only to find later that this side effect might be used to the advantage of some cancer patients who were suffering as a result of weight loss. In one of the largest and in the first published placebo-controlled trial on megestrol acetate as an agent to promote weight gain in patients with weight loss and/or anorexia, Loprinzi and others demonstrated the efficacy of this agent. These investigators observed that in a cohort of 133 advanced cancer patients with hormone-insensitive tumours, a statistically significant percentage of patients were gaining weight when compared to placebo-exposed patients. Despite this statistically significant difference in weight gain between treatment groups, no survival advantage was observed with the use of this hormonal agent.

The disappointing survival outcome may seem counterintuitive. How might we explain it? Subsequent studies have clearly shown that megestrol acetate does relatively little to promote an augmentation of lean tissue. Detailed body composition assessment in megestrol acetate-treated cancer patients point out that much of the weight gain derived from this progestational agent must be attributed to an increase in fat mass. Loprinzi and others studied seven of twelve cancer patients who had gained weight on this hormone. It is important to point out that these patients were receiving megestrol acetate as a means of cancer treatment, not as a means to treat weight loss. Utilizing dual X-ray absorptiometry and tritiated body water, these investigators observed that the bulk of weight gain in this small cohort represented fat. When one considers the importance of lean tissue and the fact that megestrol acetate does not appear to augment it, the observation that megestrol acetate does little to improve survival appears both plausible and reasonable.

Short- and long-term prognosis

The study by DeWys and others, as discussed above, provides firm data on outcome in the setting of weight loss (Table 35.1). The outcomes of patients with metastatic disease appear sobering, but they are even more so in the presence of weight loss. For example, weight-losing metastatic breast cancer patients lived for 45 weeks, as opposed to 70 weeks among metastatic breast cancer patients without weight loss (p < 0.01). Similarly, weight-losing metastatic colon cancer patients lived for 21 weeks, as opposed to 43 weeks (p < 0.01). Weight-losing metastatic prostate cancer patients lived for 24 weeks, as opposed to 46 weeks (p < 0.05). Similar differences in survival were observed among patients with a variety of cancer types with the exception of pancreatic cancer, where the prognosis appears to be poor overall regardless of whether or not weight loss is present.

Table 35.1 Effect of Weight Loss on Survival

Tumor Type	Median Survival (weeks)		P-Value
	No Weight Loss	Weight Loss	
Lung, small cell	*34*	*27*	*<0.05*
Lung, non-small cell	*20*	*14*	*<0.01*
Breast	70	45	<0.01
Colon	43	21	<0.01
Prostate	46	24	<0.05

Although a few studies have been divergent in their findings, the majority appears to be in agreement with the findings reported by DeWys and others.

In cancer patients with potentially curable malignancies, these survival differences appear magnified in their importance. Jeremic and Shibamoto showed that chances of cure are improved in patients who have not suffered weight loss prior to the initiation of treatment.[9] These investigators studied 169 patients with locally advanced non-small cell lung cancer. Patients who had lost > 5% of their weight prior to treatment had survival rates of 33, 12, 4, 3, and 3% at years 1, 2, 3, 4, and 5, respectively. In contrast, patients who had maintained their weight manifested survival rates of 87, 56, 33, 31, and 31% prior to the initiation of cancer treatment (p = 0.00000 and p = 0.00013, by univariate and multivariate analyses, respectively). In short, these findings show that the prognostic effect of weight loss pertains not only to patients with metastatic cancer but also to patients with locally advanced cancer. Moreover, they suggest that weight loss impacts the likelihood for cure.

In addition to this prognostic effect, there are clearly other findings that accompany weight loss and contribute to the poor outcome associated with this sign of weight loss (Table 35.2). In the study mentioned earlier, DeWys and others also reported on performance status.[4] These investigators observed that the percentage of cancer patients with weight loss was significantly lower among patients with an Eastern Cooperative Oncology Group performance status of 0–1 versus 2–4 (p < 0.01 among all nine tumour types). In short, weight loss and a decline in performance score, or functional status, were intimately interconnected. Demonstrating the same point, Finkelstein and others also studied the relationship between functional status and weight loss.[10] With the use of questionnaires that assessed patients' activity level, these investigators observed

Table 35.2 Ramifications of weight loss

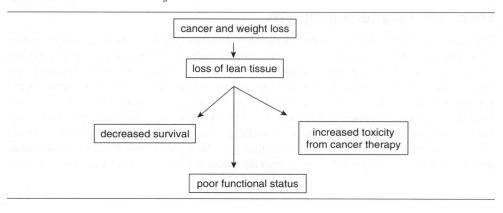

that weight loss of > 5% was associated with a poor functional status (p = 0.004). These observations are an important because they emphasize once again the importance of lean tissue in maintaining function. Thus, the prognostic effect of weight loss not only translates into a shortened survival but also into a decline in functional status.

Socinski and others recently observed that weight loss of > 5% also predicted increased toxicity from cancer treatment, as specifically observed with higher rates of mucositis.[11] These invetigators pooled multiple clinical trials that focused on the treatment of locally advanced non-small cell lung cancer and that included trials from the Cancer and Leukemia Group B. Including 694 such patients, these investigators observed that > 5% weight loss predicted grade 3 or worse mucositis (OR 2.9; 95% CI: 1.3, 6.6; p = 0.008). Thus, it appears that weight loss not only predicts a diminished survival and a decline in functional status but also a more severe toxicity from cancer therapy.

In summary, weight loss carries widespread ramifications in cancer patients. Both short- and long-term survival differences have been observed based on weight loss. Additionally, the impact of weight loss in terms of worsening side effects of cancer treatment and in terms if negatively impacting functional status have also been reported. The disappointing results of such interventions as megestrol acetate should provide a strong impetus to move forward with novel clinical trials in this area.

References

1. Niehls Bohr, quote.
2. Kirk P, Kirk I, Kristjanson LJ. What do patients receiving palliative care for cancer and their families want to be told? A Canadian and Australian qualitative study. *BMJ* 32004; 10:1136.
3. Poole K, Froggett K. Loss of weight and loss of appetite in advanced cancer: a problem for the patient, the carer, or the health professional? *Palliative Medicine* 2002; 16:499–506.
4. Dewys WD, Begg C, Lavin PT. *et al.* Prognostic effect of weight loss prior to chemotherapy in cancer patients. Eastern Cooperative Oncology Group. *American Journal of Medicine* 1980; 69:491–7.
5. Sarhill N, Mahmoud F, Walsh D. *et al.* Evaluation of nutritional status in advanced metastatic cancer. *Supportive Care in Cancer* 2003; 11:652–9.
6. Cohn SH, Gartenhaus W, Sawitsky A. *et al.* Compartmental body composition of cancer patients by measurement of total body nitrogen, potassium, and water. *Metabolism* 1981; 30:222–9.
7. Moore FD. Energy and the maintenance of the body cell mass. *JPEN* 1980; 4:228–60.
8. Kotler DP, Tierney AR, Wang J, Pierson RN. Magnitude of body cell mass depletion and the timing of death from wasting in AIDS. *Am J Clin Nutrition* 1989; 50:444–7.
9. Jeremic B, Shibamoto Y. Pre-treatment prognostic factors in patients with stage III non-small cell lung cancer treated with hyperfractionated radiation therapy with or without concurrent chemotherapy. *Lung Cancer* 1995; 13:21–30.
10. Finkelstein DM, Cassileth BR, Bonomi PD. *et al.* A pilot study of the Functional Living Index-Cancer (FLIC) Scale for the assessment of quality of life for metastatic lung cancer patients. An Eastern Cooperative Oncology Group study. *American Journal of Clinical Oncology* 1988; 11:630–3.
11. Socinski MA, Zhang C, Herndon JE. *et al.* Combined modality trials of the Cancer and Leukemia Group B in stage III non-small cell lung cancer: analysis of factors influencing survival and toxicity. *Annals of Oncology* 2004; 15:1033–41.

36

Cancer-related fatigue

Tugba Yavuzsen and Mellar P. Davis

Introduction

Fatigue is a non-specific subjective symptom that is often associated with many chronic illnesses and psychiatric disorders. It is one of the most prevalent cancer related symptoms and has a significant adverse impact on daily function, quality of life (QoL), and survival. There are a limited number of studies addressing the prevalence of fatigue in cancer which varies between 4 to 91 per cent, depending on the diagnostic criteria.[1]

Fatigue adversely influences tolerance to chemotherapy and impairs self-care, therefore an assessment of fatigue should be part of routine cancer care.[2] Fatigue is poorly managed by physicians and there are few truly evidence based treatments.

An expert panel of the National Comprehensive Cancer Network (NCCN) recently proposed the following definition of cancer-related fatigue (CRF): 'a common persistent and subjective sense of tiredness related to cancer or cancer treatment that interferes with usual functioning'.[3] CRF differs from normal fatigue, which is usually transient, related to exertion and relieved by rest. CRF is severe, disabling, unrelated to activity, and not relieved by rest. Cancer fatigue as a subjective, multidimensional symptom differs from normal fatigue in severity and chronicity. There is no consensus about the optimal approach to assessing fatigue in cancer, but there are several validated multidimensional scales for detecting fatigue and measuring its severity.[4]

A large national study involving 379 patients found fatigue a major negative factor to quality of life. Eight per cent of patients actually never discuss fatigue with their physicians. The detrimental influence of fatigue on QoL is more marked and longer lasting than nausea, depression, and pain, yet rarely addressed adequately in the patient–physician encounter.[2]

Fatigue is often the initial symptom cancer patients' experience, the prevalence and severity increases with cancer treatment and disease course. Donnelly et al. found that 48 per cent rate fatigue as 'clinically important'.[5] Moreover, cancer fatigue persists for months or years in cancer survivors. In a study of Cella and colleagues fatigue was reported in 17 per cent of cancer survivors more than one year after treatment.[6] Okuyama and colleagues studied women with stage I–III breast cancer. After more than 2 years from adjuvant treatment (789 days on average) fatigue was still present in 28 per cent who had received chemotherapy and 9 per cent after radiation.[7] A recently published study found that fatigue was still prevalent 8 years after successful treatment for Hodgkin's disease.[8]

Fatigue and prognosis

Fatigue has prognostic significance.[2, 3, 6, 9, 10] Prognosis in cancer is based upon a constellation of disease and patient characteristics. Prognostication of life expectancy is important to oncology and palliative care, since both tumor and end of life decisions depend upon projected survival.

Several studies have examined prognostic factors in advanced cancer. The Palliative Prognostic Index (PPI) was recently developed to improve the ability to predict short-term (30 days) survival.[11] The PPI score subdivides patients into three specific survival risk classes based on six predictive factors. Anorexia and performance are the most important factors; fatigue is not included in the PPI. Most studies predicting survival in palliative care involve groups of patients who have an average survival of 30 days and fail to find fatigue a major prognostic factor. This is probably due to the very high prevalence of fatigue at the end of life, which would negate the ability to predict 'short-term' survival. In a prospective study in which the average patient survived nearly 100 days; asthaenia (fatigue) was a negative predictor of survival and after multivariate analysis, fatigue, quality life index, and predicted survival by treating oncologists remained independent predictive factors.[12]

In a study by Vigano and colleagues factors prognosis in cancer were related to high tumor burden, visceral metastases, moderate to severe fatigue, anorexia, and an impaired sense of well-being. The primary diagnosis, liver metastasis, moderate to severe comorbidities, estimated survival by the treating physicians of less than 30 days, weight loss, serum albumin and lactate dehydrogenase levels were also independently associated with shorter survival.[13]

Prognosis was gauged by combining quality of life (Therapy Impact Questionnaire) and clinical variables in multiple Italian palliative units. Fatigue from the quality of life scale showed a strong prognostic relevance. However, it was outweighed by clinical variables. Fatigue in this study was a weak prognostic factor, which did not contribute to overall predictability when other factors are added to the model.[14] This is further evidenced by the working group of the Research Network of the European Association for Palliative Care recommendations regarding prognostication.[15] The working group did a systematic review of prognostication in cancer. Studies reviewed involved patients with survivals < 90 days on average. Performance score, indices of activity, functional autonomy, anorexia, cachexia, delirium, and dyspnoea were consistently predictive of a shortened survival whereas fatigue, malaise, and weakness were not mentioned (and we assume not prognostic).

Symptoms associated with fatigue

Cancer and its treatments produces multiple symptoms, which are summated as 'symptom burden'. The most common burdensome symptoms are anxiety, cognitive impairment, depression, fatigue, pain, and wasting. Most of these symptoms appear in clusters and are proposed to share a similar biologic mechanism.[16]

In a study by Cleeland[16] and colleagues fatigue-related symptoms clustered more closely to affective disturbances (depression, anxiety), and cognitive impairment (poor problem-solving, memory, attention) than gastrointestinal and respiratory symptoms.

Anorexia and cachexia

The specific etiology to fatigue is often attributed to multiple factors, which coexist (depression, weight loss, anaemia, hormone abnormalities). Cancer-related anorexia and cachexia are a known to contribute to fatigue in cancer.[17]

There is a relationship between pro-inflammatory cytokine activity, anorexia, cachexia, and fatigue. Anaemia, anorexia, cachexia, infection, metabolic abnormalities, and paraneoplastic syndromes association with fatigue are related to pro-inflammatory cytokine upregulation.[18]

Cytokines play an important role in the function of the immune system. Tumors promote expression of cytokines such as interleukin-1, 6, and tumor necrosis factor alpha, which are released to a greater extent in cancer than in healthy individuals. The characteristics of cytokine-induced sickness behaviour in animal models have much in common with those of fatigue in cancer.[16] Fatigue is commonly observed during cytokine therapy (interferon, interleukin-2).[19, 20] These cytokines contribute to the development of fatigue by altering neuroendocrine modulators and by amplifying pro-inflammatory cytokine production in the central nervous system as a feed-forward process.[21] The result is altered neurotransmitter release with a pro-inflammatory central nervous system (CNS) response. The activation of the CNS immune system is one of the plausible mechanisms by which tumor or treatment of disease may induce fatigue.

Few prospective studies have investigated the effects of improvement in nutritional state on fatigue.[22, 23] Progestins (megestrol acetate and medroxyprogesterone acetate) are the most common drugs used to treat anorexia. These drugs alleviate anorexia, improve weight and in some studies progestins significantly improved fatigue.[24, 25]

Cognitive impairment

Fatigue has a cognitive component. Cognitive impairment and difficulty in concentration are common components to fatigue, which resemble delirium in terminally ill cancer patients.[26] The relationship between delirium and short survival in cancer is well-documented.[27] Cognitive decline and inability to concentrate, fatigue, pain, and dyspnoea are associated with high symptom burden. Patients whose cognitive status is failing will likely have fatigue, nausea and/or vomiting, anxiety, depression, confusion, and a shortened survival.[28]

Depression

Symptoms of depression such as sadness, crying, and lack of interest in family and friends are common in cancer. Patients with cancer have an increased risk for depression.[29] The prevalence of depression in cancer patients ranges from as low as 1 per cent to 50 per cent depending on diagnostic criteria and increases with stage and with certain symptoms such as fatigue and pain.[30]

Fatigue is strongly linked to depression in cancer.[29, 31] It is often difficult to distinguish fatigue and depression using validated screening tools because of overlapping characteristics. Assessment tools for fatigue do not clearly separate fatigue symptoms from depression. Psychosocial factors components of depression such as anxiety, difficulty sleeping, and social withdrawal influence the severity of fatigue. Psychosocial support reduces anxiety, depression, and pain may also increase survival with cancer (though this is controversial).[32] It is not known if improved social support also improves fatigue.

Several studies evaluated the effect psychostimulants and psychological interventions in fatigue.[18, 33] Methylphenidate is a mild psychostimulant, which successfully reduces opioid induced sedation, cognitive failure, hiccups, and depression.[34]

Randomized clinical trials of methylphenidate for fatigue in cancer have not been performed, though cohort trials are positive.[19, 35, 36] These cohort studies found a significant rapid improvement in fatigue within 7 days.[35, 36] A pilot project investigated fatigue as measured by exercise programme and methylphenidate treatment in patients with melanoma receiving interferon therapy. Less fatigue was seen in all treated subjects, which appeared better than historic control groups.[19]

Depression in cancer may not different from depression associated with other conditions, but treatment needs to be adapted to the particular needs of cancer patients. There are a number randomized clinical trials using antidepressants in cancer that show a benefit, which is subject to dose, timing, and duration of treatment in cancer patients.[37, 38] In a study by Marrow et al. paroxetine did not improve fatigue but did improve depression in patients receiving chemotherapy.[37]

A different pathophysiology for fatigue and depression may exist during chemotherapy such that fatigue and depression though closely associated do not share a common pathophysiology. Selective serotonin receptor inhibitors may be simply ineffective in the management of fatigue but reduce depression as opposed to psychostimulants, which improve fatigue and depression. Other pharmacologic treatments and perhaps non-pharmacologic interventions have been reported to be effective.[19, 33–36]

Metabolic and hormone abnormalities

Disorders such as diabetes mellitus, hypothyroidism, and electrolyte disorders (low sodium, potassium, or magnesium, or hypercalcemia) are often accompanied by fatigue. These metabolic complications are potential reversible causes of fatigue in cancer. Chemotherapy may adversely influence thyroid function in breast cancer and progressively worsen fatigue and performance status.[39] Patients with fatigue and hypothyroidism should be treated with thyroid replacement therapy, even if the hypothyroidism is mild or compensated. Metabolic disorders (hypokalaemia or hypomagnesemia etc.) require correction before treating fatigue.

Anaemia

Anaemia is an important contributor to cancer related fatigue.[40, 41] Cancer patients often have low hemoglobin levels owing to the inflammatory nature of cancer or cancer treatments. Anaemia often progresses during chemotherapy and is probably the most reversible factor contributing to fatigue.

The pathogenesis of cancer-associated anaemia is complex. Haemolysis, haemorrhage, nutritional deficiencies, and production of cytokines are major factors.[42]

Anaemia is often caused by reduced erythropoietin and impaired iron use in cancer. The relationship between haemoglobin levels and severity of fatigue is complex and not linear. Improvements in fatigue is greatest when the haemoglobin rises from 11 to 12 gram/dl.[41] Treatment of anaemia with recombinant erythropoetin improves anaemia, fatigue and reduces the necessity for blood transfusions. The treatment of anaemia and improvement of fatigue with erythropoietin does not correlate well with survival or tumor response in all cancers.[41] The outlook for head and neck cancer and cervical cancer under treatment may improve with improvement in haemoglobin.[41] However, two studies suggest worsened survival and increased risk for tumor progression in erythropoietin-treated patients.[43, 44] An improved well-being after transfusion may not correlate with the degree of anaemia and performance status.[45] Blood transfusion for prompt symptom relief must be weighed against cost and logistical issues in the terminally ill, which are factors that govern the choice of treatments. To date there is no evidence to prove that transfusions improve survival even if fatigue is improved.

Pain

The prevalence of pain increases throughout the course of cancer. Pain is related to the underlying disease, therapy or comorbities and may persist in cancer survivors. Fatigue will worsen with uncontrolled pain. Effective treatment of pain may result in relief of fatigue.[46] However, at the present time the evidence that demonstrates a clear relationship between fatigue and pain is tenuous.

Analgesics (opioids, steroids, nonsteroidal anti-inflammatory drugs etc.) or adjuvants to analgesics (anti-depressants, anti-convulsants, psychostimulants etc.) are frequently administered for relief pain. Fatigue symptoms have been associated with decreased function of the hypothalamic–pituitary–adrenal axis as has been opioid therapy. Hypotension occurs more frequently with chronic fatigue than in controls.[47]

Corticosteroids reverse fatigue, usually for a short period of time and as a side benefit also increases appetite and increase a sense of well-being for a brief period of time.[48, 49] There is an interplay between cytokine signaling pathways in the hypothalamic–pituitary–adrenal axis and fatigue that may be altered by exogenous corticosteroids. However, there is no evidence that the improvement in fatigue with corticosteroids will improve survival in cancer.[50]

Performance status

Recently two systematic reviews have been published regarding predictions of survival.[51, 52] Performance status is the most important prognostic factor in terminally ill patients. Karnofsky Performance Status (KPS) has proven to be a reliable prognostic parameter in all cancers. Several studies have shown that the strength of correlation between performance status and survival vary with length of follow-up.[12, 13] KPS has increased prognostic significance when integrated with specific symptoms. Symptom burden contributes to KPS and fatigue. Reduced performance status correlates with symptom severity. Loss of energy and motivation due to reduce perform-ance status may be interpreted as fatigue.[29] In a study by Dimeo et al.[29] fatigue in relapse-free patients with hematological malignancy was associated with reduced performance status, and depressed mood. Fatigue may contribute to other prominent symptoms and reduced performance status, which are predictive of survival.

The management of fatigue in cancer patients

The management of fatigue requires identifying reversible factors. The first essential step is to educate patients and relatives on the difference between normal and cancer-related fatigue so that they may recognize and anticipate it patterns in connection with specific treatment regimens. Screening for specific treatable causes of fatigue should occur with initial assessment and if identified (anaemia, depression, metabolic disorders, and insomnia etc.), treated. Exercise to prevent de-conditioning and erythropoietin for anaemia have the greatest evidence for improving fatigue in cancer.[19, 33, 41]

The NCCN proposed an algorithm in their Fatigue Practice Guidelines,[3] which identified seven reversible factors:

1. anaemia
2. certain comorbidities
3. emotional stress
4. nutrition
5. pain
6. sedentary lifestyle
7. sleep disturbance.

The management of these factors may improve fatigue but it is unknown whether improve-ment in fatigue actually improves survival.

Non-pharmacological (psychosocial) interventions

Non-pharmacological interventions include exercise programmes, improved sleep hygiene, and restorative therapies. Most non-pharmacologic studies have examined the effect of exercise in patients on fatigue.[19, 33] Physical exercise as an intervention in cancer patients has attracted increasing interest and support through persuasive clinical evidence.[19, 29, 33] Paradoxically energy conservation is a frequently recommended by physicians as a non-pharmacologic therapy, but evidence for such a recommendation is lacking.

Sleep disturbances may worsen fatigue, however the association has been inadequately investigated.[53, 54] Sleep quality may be more significantly related to fatigue than sleep quantity. Sleep disturbances are influenced by factors such as depression, anxiety, pain, and the type and timing of food and beverage.

Stress reduction is an important factor in managing cancer fatigue. A strong correlation exists between emotional stress and fatigue, but the precise relationship between stress reduction and improved fatigue is not nearly as well understood.[7, 55, 56, 57]

Nutrition should be assessed in cancer-related fatigue. Patients with poor dietary intake may need assessment by a dietician. However, neither weight loss nor laboratory markers of impaired nutritional status (prealbumin) correlate significantly with fatigue and should not be used as a justification for nutritional intervention in fatigue.[23]

Restorative therapies include gardening, quiet time (meditation etc.), volunteer activities, and walking in a natural environment are said to reduce fatigue but evidence is lacking.

Summary

Cancer-related fatigue has been described as 'the commonest and most debilitating symptoms in patients with cancer'.[1, 5–7] There are many causes of cancer related fatigue including physical and psychological symptoms and the sequelae of cancer treatment. Fatigue severity does not correlate with stage or type of cancer.

Fatigue worsens during cancer treatment and may continue after treatment in cancer survivors. Persistent fatigue during the treatment is associated with psychological and physical factors. Interventions to improve these factors may improve fatigue but may not influence prognosis. Studies regarding prognosis in cancer related fatigue are very limited. The evidence for the influence of fatigue on the short- and long-term prognosis in cancer is mixed. An individualized treatment plan should include different therapy modalities, but at the moment there is lack of well-designed randomized clinical trials to evaluate pharmacologic treatment in fatigue and its influence on survival.

A number of pharmacologic or non-pharmacologic interventions in the management of fatigue have been investigated. The treatment of reversible factors associated with fatigue such as anaemia, pain, depression, and anorexia/cachexia, and non-pharmacological interventions that improve sleep hygiene may improve fatigue in cancer but it is not known if the treatment of fatigue influences survival. We need a more systematic approach to the study and management of fatigue in cancer.

Many gaps in our understanding of fatigue occur across the cancer experience. We still do not understand why fatigue is a presenting symptom in early stage cancer in some individuals or why it persists after cancer treatment. The neuromuscular changes associated with fatigue in cancer are poorly understood. Fatigue should be a priority symptom for future research due to its prevalence and influence on quality of life, even if prognostically unimportant.

References

1. Lawrence DP, Kupelnick B, Miller K, Devine D, Lau J. Evidence report on the occurrence, assessment, and treatment of fatigue in cancer patients. *J Natl Cancer Inst Monogr* 2004; 32:40–50.
2. Curt GA, Breibart W, Cella D. et al. Impact of cancer-related fatigue on the lives of patients: new findings from the fatigue coalition. *Oncologist* 2000; 5:353–60.

3. Mock V, Atkinson A, Barsevick A. et al. National Comprehensive Cancer Network. NCCN practice guidelines for cancer-related fatigue. Version 1.2004

4. Jacobsen PB. Assessment of fatigue in cancer patients. *J Natl Cancer Ins Monogr* 2004; 32:93–7.

5. Donnelly S, Walsh D, Rybicki L. The symptoms of advanced cancer: identification of clinical and research priorities by assessment of prevalence and severity. *J Palliat Care* 1995; 11:27–32.

6. Cella D, Davis K, Breitbart W, Curt G. Cancer-related fatigue: prevalence of proposed diagnostic criteria in United States sample of cancer survivors. *J Clin Oncol* 2001; 19:3385–91.

7. Okuyama T, Akechi T, Kugaya A. et al. Factors correlated with fatigue in disease-free breast cancer patients: Application of the Cancer Fatigue Scale. *Support Care Cancer* 2000; 8:215–22.

8. Hjermstad MJ, Fossa SD, Oldervoll L. et al. Fatigue in long-term Hodgkin's disease survivors: a follow-up study. *J Clin Oncol* 2005; 23:6587–95.

9. Vogelzang NJ, Breitbart W, Cella D. et al. The Fatigue Coalition. Patient, caregiver, and oncologist perceptions cancer-related fatigue: results of a tripart assessment survey. *Seminars in Oncology* 1997; 34:4–12.

10. Cella D, Paul D, Yount S. et al. What are the most important symptoms targets when treating advanced cancer? Survey of providers in the National Comprehensive Cancer Network (NCCN). *Cancer Investigation* 2003; 21:526–35.

11. Maltoni M, Nanni O, Scarpi E. et al. Successful validation of the palliative prognostic score in terminally ill cancer patients *J Pain Symptom Manage* 1999; 17:240–7.

12. Llobera J, Esteva M, Rifa J. et al. Terminal cancer: duration and prediction of survival time. *European J of Cancer* 2000; 36:2036–43.

13. Vigano A, Bruera E, Jhangri GS, Newman SC, Fields AL, Suarez-Almazor ME. Clinical survival predictors in patients with advanced cancer. *Arch Intern Med* 2000; 160:861–8.

14. Toscani F, Brunelli C, Miccinesi G. Predicting survival in terminal cancer patients: clinical observation or quality-of-life evaluation? *Palliative Medicine* 2005; 19:220–7.

15. Maltoni M, Caraceni A, Brunelli C. et al. Prognostic factors in advanced cancer patients: evidence-based clinical recommendations – a study by the Steering Committee of the European Association for Palliative Care. *J Clin Oncol* 2005; 23:6240–8.

16. Cleeland CS, Bennett GJ, Dantzer R. et al. Are the symptoms of cancer and cancer treatment due to a shared biologic mechanism? A cytokine-immunologic model of cancer symptoms. *Cancer* 2003; 97:2919–25.

17. Laviano A, Meguid MM, Rossi-Fanelli F. Cancer anorexia: clinical implications, pathogenesis, and therapeutic strategies. *The Lancet Oncology* 2003; 4:686–94.

18. Gutstein HB. The biologic basis of fatigue. *Cancer* 2001; 92:1678–83.

19. Schwartz AL, Thompson JA, Masood N. Interferon induced fatigue in patienst with melanoma: a pilot study of exercise and methylphenidate. *Oncol Nursing Forum* 2002; 29:E85–E90.

20. Naglieri E, Lopez M, Lellli G. et al. Interleukin-2, interferon-alpha and medroxyprogesterone acetate in metastatic renal cell carcinoma. *Anticancer Res* 2002; 22:3045–51.

21. Demitrac MA. Neuroendocrine aspects of chronic fatigue syndrome: a commentary. *The American J of Medicine* 1998; 105:11S–14S.

22. Stone P, Hardy J, Broadley K. et al. Fatigue in advanced cancer: a prospective controlled cross-sectional study. *Br J Cancer* 1999; 79:1479–86.

23. Beach P, Siebeneck B, Buderer NF, Ferner T. The relationship between fatigue and nutritional status in patients receiving radiation therapy to treat lung cancer. *Oncol Nurs Forum* 2001; 28:1027–31.

24. Bruera E, Ernst S, Hagen N. et al. Effectiveness of megestrol acetate in patients with advanced cancer: a randomized, double-blind, crossover study. *Prevention and Controle en Cancerologie* 1998; 2:74–8.

25. Westman G, Bergman B, Albertsson M. et al. Megestrol acetate in advanced, progressive, hormone insensitive cancer. Effects on the quality of life: a placebo-controlled, randomized, multicentre trial. *Eur J Cancer* 1999; 35:586–95.

26. Tamburini M, Brunelli C, Rosso S, Ventafridda V. Prognostic value of quality of life scores in terminal cancer patients. *J Pain Symptom Manage* 1996; 11:32–41.

27. Lawlor PG, Gagnon B, Mancini IL. et al. Delirium a predictor of survival in older patients with advanced cancer. *Arch Intern Med* 2000; 160:2866–8.

28. Klinkenberg M, Willems DL, van der Wal G, Deeg DJH. Symptom burden in the last week of life. *J Pain Symptom Manage* 2004; 27:5–13.

29. Dimeo F, Schmittel A, Fietz T. et al. Physical performance, depression, immune status and fatigue in patients with hematological malignancies after treatment. *Annals of Oncology* 2004; 15:1237–42.

30. Winell J, Roth AJ. Depression in cancer patients. *Oncology* 2004; 18:1554–60.

31. Jacobsen PB, Weitzner MA. Evaluating the relationship of fatigue to depression and anxiety in cancer patients. In R Portenoy, E Bruera (eds) *Issues in palliative care research*, pp. 127–50. New York (NY): Oxford University Press, 2003.

32. Spiegel D, Giese-Davis J. Depression and cancer: mechanism and disease progression. *Biol Psychiatry* 2003; 54:269–82.

33. Schwartz AL. Daily fatigue patterns and effect of exercise in women with breast cancer. *Cancer Pract* 2000; 160:526–34.

34. Homsi J, Nelson KA, Sarhill N. et al. A phase II study of methylphenidate for depression in advanced cancer. *Am J Hospice & Palliative Care* 2001; 18:403–7.

35. Sarhill N, Walsh D, Nelson KA, Homsi J, LeGrand S, Davis MP. Methylphenidate for fatigue in advanced cancer: A prospective open-label pilot study. *Am J Hospice & Palliative Care* 2001; 18:187–92.

36. Bruera E, Driver L, Barnes EA. et al. Patient-controlled methylphenidate for the management of fatigue in patients with advanced cancer: A preliminary report. *J Clin Oncol* 2003; 21:4439–43.

37. Marrow GR, Hickok JT, Roscoe JA. et al. Differential effects of paroxetine on fatigue and depression: a randomized, double-blind trial from The University of Rochester Cancer Center Community Clinical Oncology Program. *J Clin Oncol* 2003; 21:4635–41.

38. Fisch MJ, Loehrer PJ, Kristeller J. et al. Fluoxetine versus placebo in advanced cancer outpatients: A double-blinded trial of the Hoosier Oncology Group. *J Clin Oncol* 2003; 21:1937–43.

39. Kumar N, Allen KA, Riccardi D. et al. Fatigue, weight gain, lethargy and amenorrhea in breast cancer patients on chemotherapy: is subclinical hypothyroidsm the culprit? *Breast Cancer Research and Treatment* 2004; 83:149–59.

40. Turner R, Anglin P, Burkes R. et al. Epoetin alfa in cancer patients: evidence-based guidelines. *J Pain Symptom Manage* 2001; 22:954–65.

41. Harper P, Littlewood T. Anemia of cancer: impact on patient fatigue and long-term outcome. *Oncology* 2005; 69(Suppl 2):2–7.

42. Stasi R, Abriani L, Beccaglia P, Terzoli E, Amadori S. Cancer-related fatigue. *Cancer* 2003; 98:1786–801.

43. Leyland-Jones B, Semiglazov V, Pawlicki M. et al. Maintaining normal hemoglobin levels with epoetin alfa in mainly nonanemic patients with metastatic breast cancer receiving first-line chemotherapy: a survival study. *J Clin Oncol* 2005; 23:5960–72.

44. Henke M, Laszig R, Rube C. et al. Erythropoietin to treat head and neck cancer patients with anemia undergoing radiotherapy: randomized, double-blind, placebo-controlled trial. *Lancet* 2005; 362:1255–60.

45. Monti M, Castellani L, Berlusconi A. et al. Use of red blood cell transfusions in terminally ill cancer patients admitted to a palliative care unit. *J Pain Symptom Manage* 1997; 13:18–22.

46. Fleishman SB. Treatment of symptom clusters: Pain, depression, and fatigue. *J Natl Cancer Inst Monogr* 2004; 32:119–23.

47. Rowe PC, Calkins H. Neurally mediated hypotension and chronic fatigue syndrome. *Am J Med* 1998; 105:15S–21S.

48. Bruera E, Roca E, Cedaro L, Carraro S, Chacon R. Action of oral methylprednisone in terminal cancer patients: a prospective randomized double blind study. *Cancer Treat Reports* 1985; 69:751–4.

49. Willox JC, Corr J, Shaw J, Richardson M, Calman CK, Drennan M. Prednisolone as an appetite stimulant in patients with cancer. *BMJ* 1984; 288:27.

50. Rich T, Innominato PF, Boerner J. et al. Elevated serum cytokines correlated with altered behavior, serum cortisol rhythm, and dampened 24-hour rest-activity patterns in patients with metastatic colorectal cancer. *Clin Cancer Res* 2005; 11:1757–64.

51. Glare P, Virik K, Jones M. et al. A systematic review of physicians' survival predictions in terminally ill cancer patients. *BMJ* 2003; 327:195–8.

52. Vigano A, Dorgan M, Buckingham J, Bruera E, Suarez-Almazor ME. Survival prediction in terminal cancer patients: a systematic review of medical literature. *Palliat Med* 2000; 14:363–74.

53. Dodd MJ, Miaskowski C, Paul SM. Symptom clusters and their effect on the functional status of patients with cancer. *Oncol Nurs Forum* 2001; 28:465–70.

54. Mercandate S, Girelli D, Casuccio A. Sleep disorders in advanced cancer patients: prevalence and factors associated. *Support Care Cancer* 2004; 12:355–9.

55. Bruera E, Brenneis C, Michaud M. et al. Association between asthenia and nutritional status, lean body mass, anemia, psychological status, and tumor mass in patients with advanced cancer. *J Pain Symptom Manage* 1989; 4:59–63.

56. Derogatis LR, Abeloff MD, Melisaratos N. Psychological coping mechanism and survival time in metastatic breast cancer. *JAMA* 1979; 242:1504–8.

57. Bower JE, Ganz PA, Desmond KA. et al. Fatigue in breast cancer survivors: Occurrence, correlates, and impact on quality of life. *J Clin Oncol* 2000; 18:743–53.

Prognostication in the imminently dying patient

James Stevenson and John Ellershaw

Introduction

In many of the preceding chapters of this book there have been discussions related to prognosis in a variety of cancer-related states, from early through to metastatic disease, as well as a number of clinical conditions which occur as complications of advancing cancer. Statistics are available which, in conjunction with clinical assessment, assist clinicians with calculating prognosis and communicating this to patients, their families and other healthcare professionals. In the broad sense, it is now possible to discuss prognosis from the time of diagnosis for many of these conditions in terms of mean and median survivals for all those who have been diagnosed with the same condition. Ranges can also be quoted, covering the spectrum from worst-case to best-case scenarios. The same process applies to non-cancer diagnoses too.

This final chapter is concerned with prognostication in the imminently dying patient, and the key step is to be able diagnose dying. Specifically the focus is where reversible causes of deterioration have been excluded and death is expected within hours to days.

Diagnosing dying

It has previously been stated that the three key clinical skills in medicine are diagnosis, treatment and prognosis. Modern acute medicine generally focuses on making a diagnosis so that treatment can be provided to cure; with cure, there is little need to focus greatly on prognosis. Despite all the advances in medicine, people ultimately die, often due to chronic diseases where cure is not possible. Treatment can control symptoms and sometimes delay death without curing. For these diseases, prognostication is recognized as an important skill, as outlined at the beginning of this text.[1]

The therapeutic goals of palliative medicine emphasize care rather than cure, and generally the clinical priority is treatment rather than diagnosis. Symptoms and complications of advanced disease are considered for treatment with the aim of improving patients' well-being. As can be seen from section two of this text, much of the work of 'diagnosing the disease' is done before patients are referred to palliative care services. Patients already have a diagnosis of incurable cancer which may include the presence of metastases. Information may have been provided about prognosis for these conditions with an understanding that there is uncertainty for an individual's exact length of survival.

However, a key skill in the palliative phase of any disease is diagnosing dying. It can be difficult to differentiate a decline in health due to an acute reversible problem, from the natural progression of a life-limiting illness towards death. What follows is a review of the traditional model of clinical assessment, focusing on those features that may help make the diagnosis of dying.

More than using intuition, or experience, one needs to be able to actively use the skills of history taking and examination, with the possible addition of investigations, and formulate the findings into a diagnosis.

Studies assessing clinicians' predictions of survival do suggest that despite being generally inaccurate, these predictions are more accurate the closer patients are to death, a finding which has been termed the 'horizon effect'.[2, 3, 4] In addition to reviewing important aspects of history taking and examination in relation to prognostication in the imminently dying patient, there will be a brief review of existing performance scales and measurements in terms of how they may add helpful information to the diagnostic and prognostic process.

History

A key decision to be made is whether the presenting problem is an acute reversible one or part of the progressive nature of an individual's life-limiting illness. The classical model of history taking usually commences with asking about the presenting complaint or complaints, followed by obtaining a more detailed description of these complaints before moving onto areas such as medication and allergy history, past medical history, systems review and other issues. This classical model may not always be the most appropriate in the setting of advanced cancer and it is worth considering some variations.

Within the specialties of oncology and palliative care it can be helpful to begin by obtaining important background details, especially with respect to the primary diagnosis as well as information on treatments, complications, spread and extent of disease before moving on to the presenting issue. From the history alone, it is often possible to determine a list of probable diagnoses, and sometimes a definitive diagnosis. In particular, it is now recognized that there are several possible trajectories for diseases and that determining which one applies to an individual will enhance the process of prognostication. These different disease trajectories will be explored below. Collateral history from family and other carers provides further valuable information.

Background history

The most common cancers have been discussed in Part II of this book and the earlier chapters of this section have discussed many of the complications of advanced disease. Outlining these aspects of history first enables the assessing clinician to understand what this individual has experienced to this point as well as consider the likely ongoing problems which could be caused by their disease. This allows the assessing clinician to create a framework for that individual based on their disease history. Although cancer can cause death for many different reasons, some complications are more likely with certain types and locations of malignancy. Having a thorough understanding of an individual's background should enable one to actively consider these possibilities when a significant deterioration occurs.

The following examples are not intended to be comprehensive but rather to illustrate some of these potential complications:

- Haematological disease – acute sepsis, haemorrhagic events, anaemia
- Cerebral disease – seizures, strokes, falling Glasgow Coma Score
- Pulmonary – obstructive pneumonia, respiratory failure
- Intra-abdominal disease – bowel obstruction, pulmonary embolism
- Bony metastases – hypercalcaemia, spinal cord compression.

In addition it is important to remember that for many people cachexia plays a significant role in their overall deterioration. Far more than a problem of weight loss, it is an irreversible process of total body involution with a wide range of effects on several organs and metabolic processes. The effects of cachexia play an important role in death for many people.[5, 6]

Other features of background history will provide further help to detect those situations where a severe decline may be due to a potentially treatable problem. Beyond the problems surrounding advanced malignancy, it is always important to gather information on comorbidities, particularly those that continue to be active. This should also help differentiate whether an acute decline is due to progressive malignancy or a non-malignant and potentially reversible problem. Cardiovascular disease remains the leading cause of adult death in developed countries and some patients with both malignancy and cardiac disease die due to an acute cardiac event which may be unrelated to their malignancy. Linked to medical comorbidities is the issue of polypharmacy, which becomes more likely in advanced disease where drugs for symptom control are added to other long-standing medications used for conditions such as hypertension and diabetes.[7] There will be situations where a patient's decline is caused by adverse drug reactions and interactions and it is important to obtain information about all the medications a person is taking to exclude and address this cause.

Different disease trajectories

The natural history of disease is not a straightforward matter of constant and steady decline from diagnosis to death. Rather, there are several possible disease trajectories which are influenced by the diagnosis itself as well as individual patient factors such as age, comorbidities, complications of the disease or its treatment, and health prior to the diagnosis of a life-limiting illness. In general, there are now a number of recognized disease trajectories into which most diseases can be classified. Although conditions other than cancer are not the principle focus of this text, it is worth considering 'disease' as a generic term briefly. The different trajectories result in different consequences not only in terms of diagnosis, prognosis and treatment, but also in terms of providing patients and their families the opportunity to prepare for death. Patients with cancer can still die from other causes which complicates the issue of prognostication.

The following different trajectories to death are worth reviewing:

- Sudden death
- Death from acute illness
- Death from chronic illness which includes:

  (i) Slow and steady decline

  (ii) Chronic limitations with intermittent acute episodes of decline

  (iii) Period of reasonable health followed by a relatively acute decline.[8]

Sudden death

Sudden death usually refers to death which is unexpected or unforseen. The event is so overwhelming that death usually occurs within a few seconds to a couple of minutes. Some examples are listed in Box 37.1. In most situations, sudden death implies that relatives and friends do not have time to prepare for the person's death.

Death from acute illness

Acute illnesses develop over a period of hours to days and can put a massive strain on one or many body systems, potentially leading to death. In western countries the most common types of illness which cause death acutely include infections and organ failure where death is slower than

Box 37.1 Examples of causes of sudden death

Brain

Massive stroke

- haemorrhagic
- ischaemic – (embolic, thrombotic)

Head injury:

- with or without bleeding (motor accidents, gunshot injuries)

Toxic brain injury:

- hypoxia - lack of oxygen (circulatory or respiratory failure)
- hypoglycaemia
- drugs (alcohol, heroin, stimulant drugs e.g. ecstasy, speed)

Heart

Cardiac arrest

- myocardial infarction
- arrhythmia (congenital, biochemical disturbance)
- brain death

Cardiac rupture:

- usually caused by another underlying problem

Lungs and airways

Physical obstruction:

- food bolus aspiration, laryngeal oedema from anaphylaxis,
- laryngeal spasm (e.g. drowning)

Small airway spasm:

- severe asthma

Failure of muscles:

- failure of neurological output, fatigue of respiration

Lung collapse:

- pneumothorax, haemothorax

Circulation

Massive pulmonary embolism:

- usually in association with deep vein thrombosis

Shock

hypovolaemic:

- haemorrhage

Box 37.1 Examples of causes of sudden death *(continued)*

cardiogenic:

- post myocardial infarction
- neurological failure

septic:

- infection

anaphylactic:

- e.g. drug reaction

---

sudden death indicated above. Most of the causes for sudden death can also follow a slower, that is, acute course too. The process can be seen to evolve anywhere from several minutes to a few days, and will often be accompanied by a range of symptoms and signs which allow a diagnosis to be made, and for treatment to be initiated. Even if treatment is appropriate, the illness may still be overwhelming and lead to death. Severe failure of one organ can lead to multi-organ failure which is difficult to survive, even with the most intensive care available. As the person deteriorates it is often possible to see the changes clearly enough to allow the diagnosis of dying to be made. Eventually, some sudden event happens as described above and the person dies. Unlike sudden death however, relatives and friends usually have some time to prepare for the person's death, although this may not be more than a few minutes or hours.

In some circumstance, a person may recover from an acute illness, with or without treatment, even when death seemed the most likely outcome. This point is particularly important to consider in the context of this chapter, as there are occasions when it is clearly believed and communicated that someone is imminently dying only for their condition to stabilize or even improve. The uncertainty of diagnosing dying and communicating information on prognosis will be discussed later in this chapter.

Death from chronic illness

People live years and even decades with some chronic illnesses. With medical advances, some previously fatal chronic diseases can now be survived but many still lead to death. A person with a chronic illness may well die from a sudden or acute event, totally unrelated to their chronic illness, as outlined above. When chronic illnesses cause death, they tend to follow one of three main pathways:

- Slow and steady decline
- Chronic limitations with intermittent acute episodes of decline
- Period of reasonable health followed by a relatively acute decline.

Slow and steady decline

Some conditions progress slowly over time and lead to death due to a gradual failure of multiple bodily functions. There may never be a specific event which heralds the start or even the final stages of the illness, but rather gradual changes which progress and eventually make it more obvious that the person is dying. Treatments may slow the underlying disease or at the very least help maintain as many of the person's functions for as long as possible. A common example of such conditions is dementia. There comes a time where the combinations of problems make it clear the person with the condition is dying and often there is a long period of time where the patient and their family can prepare for this.

Chronic limitations with intermittent acute episodes of decline

With other illnesses, there can be acute exacerbations of the chronic illness which require more intense treatment, and sometimes these episodes can prove fatal. Common examples of this include chronic lung diseases, cardiac failure and HIV/AIDS where episodes may require hospital admission. Even when someone becomes critically ill, treatment may resolve the crisis and even allow the patient to return to the previous level of function. Over time, it is often recognized that an episode may result in a decline in health and recovery may not be complete. This progressive weakness reduces their ability to then survive an acute exacerbation. At any one of the acute episodes, a more severe decline can occur and the person may die. Again, some sudden event occurs resulting in death. Compared to the examples above, the person as well as their relatives and friends may have months or even years to prepare for death. Despite this, the exact moment can not be predicted and the moment of death may still come unexpectedly.

Period of reasonable health followed by a relatively acute decline

The most common disease which follows this pattern is cancer. As more people survive chronic illness such as ischaemic heart disease and diabetes there has been an increase in the number of people who now develop cancer and in western countries, approximately one in three people will develop cancer in their lifetime. As a result, more people now die of cancer than in past decades and a little over one in four deaths in developed countries are due to cancer.

Even though treatment and survival figures are improving, statistics show more people are dying from cancer due to the absolute increase in cancer diagnoses. In the past, a diagnosis of cancer often meant that death would occur within a few weeks or at most months. In this sense, it was seen as a severe acute illness with few or no treatment options. The modern reality is that many cancers now behave more like a chronic illness.

Even when cancer cannot be cured, good palliative care allows people to maintain a good level of health and independence for a period of time until the disease progresses. Some treatments clearly prolong survival, even without cure. This period varies between individuals and can be anywhere from a few weeks up to many years. In this time there may be no obvious signs of disease activity.

When cancer progresses and can no longer be treated, a person's health usually deteriorates over a period of weeks, sometimes months, in a steady and predictable way. At this time, it becomes clearer that death is approaching although the exact time may not be predicted in terms any more accurate than some 'weeks' or 'months'. For people living with incurable cancer, there is often time for them, their relatives and friends to prepare for death. In this sense, it is a chronic illness more than an acute illness. Prognostication is this setting has been described in detail throughout the preceding chapters of this book.

When death is imminent

The remainder of this chapter will focus on the imminently dying patient. Although there are many different ways to define dying, the following discussions will refer to the last hours to days of life.

Presenting complaint

The nature of advanced disease may make it impossible to obtain much detail directly from the patient, as they may be semicomatose or comatose and this feature in itself may be an important factor in determining whether or not someone may be dying. The observations of other health professionals such as nursing staff, trained carers and family members may be the only history available. Even if the patient can communicate well, they may not be aware of the signs witnessed by others, and the combination of reported symptoms and observed signs will provide valuable additional information. Communication may still be possible, however, and there are a number of symptoms a patient may report which provide important information for the assessment. Most of these symptoms can occur at earlier stages of cancer or even in acute illnesses, but it is the formulation of these features of history with knowledge of the patient's background history that will make the diagnosis of dying more likely.

There have been many studies and reviews which have highlighted several symptoms, as well as examination findings and laboratory investigations which are correlated with poor survival. A good history alone will help identify many of these features.

The following are symptoms which may be encountered in the dying phase. Many of these have been suggested as valuable factors when determining if death is approaching.[9] This list is not meant to be exhaustive and it is not exclusive to the dying phase. Some evolve over a long time whilst others occur in the setting of acute problems.

◆ Weakness: the dying person is usually profoundly weak, usually bed bound and unable to manage any of their self cares. Many of the other symptoms are exacerbated by this. Weakness is a good example of a symptom which can evolve over months of living with cancer but becomes extreme at the end of life.

◆ Fatigue: even if a dying person is not unconscious, they tire easily and rarely stay awake for long periods.

◆ Delirium: although often an acute medical problem, some studies suggest delirium is present in over 80 per cent of dying patients, a situation in which it is difficult to reverse.[10]

◆ Breathing issues: collateral history from carers and family may reveal there have been changes in a patient's breathing pattern, such as continuous deep breaths from worsening metabolic acidosis (Kussmaul's respiration) or the varying pattern caused by brainstem dysfunction (Cheyne-Stokes). Others develop progressively shallower breathing towards the end of life, whilst others develop periods of apnoea as the respiratory drive fails. With shallow breathing, there is insufficient tidal volume to allow adequate gas exchange with the alveoli, leading to both hypoxia and hypercapnia. The effects of these changes affect all other organs including the brain and contribute to decreased consciousness.

◆ Chest secretions: secretions may accumulate within the airways leading to the characteristic 'death rattle' and this is often reported by observers, worried that it may be causing respiratory distress for the patient. Although one of the only terms that includes the word 'death', it may begin up to a few days before death.

◆ Anxiety/fear/premonition: some patients become aware they may be dying, but not all are fearful. Although there are many studies assessing clinicians' ability to predict dying, there is not thorough research assessing patients' own abilities in this area. There are times where patients clearly articulate these feelings and it may be an important piece of information for clinicians to factor into their assessments. Further research in this area would be valuable.

◆ Anorexia: although most people with malignancy experience anorexia for a variety of reasons, it becomes more pronounced towards death such that it is rare for a dying person to desire any food.

◆ Dysphagia/aspiration: with progressive weakness, it becomes more difficult to control swallowing and people become unable to swallow anything safely. They become unable to take oral drugs or have great difficulty swallowing them. In addition, they may be unable to take any more than sips of water. These are common finding in the dying phase.[11]

♦ Decreased fluid intake/dehydration: as death approaches, weakness and loss of hunger result in many people not drinking fluid. Although often worrying for relatives and even healthcare workers, it is not always associated with patient distress even if dehydration develops. Dehydration may make the appearances of cachexia even more obvious, such as the eyes looking more sunken. As dying patients become dehydrated there may be a history of decreased urine output, with increased urinary concentration.

♦ Dry or sore mouth: there are many reasons these symptoms might occur even in persons who are not dying but they are common in the last days of life.

♦ Myoclonus and/or asterixis: further symptoms which can occur in people who are not dying, these may be noticed in the last few hours to days of life for a range of reasons including drug accumulation in the setting of organ failure and dehydration or hypoxia.

♦ Skin changes: as the circulatory system fails, carers may report that the patient's skin develops irregular patterns of colours and changes in temperature, the commonest of which is cold hands and feet. Oedema may also be noted especially if it develops in the upper limbs (often in association with severe weakness in the last hours to days of life) such as when relatives notice rings becoming stuck on the patient's fingers.

♦ Withdrawing: as the patient becomes severely weakened and fatigued, there is usually a loss of normal social interactions, which may be reported by family or carers concerned the person is 'giving up' or becoming suddenly depressed.

♦ Somnolence: as death approaches, patients spend more time sleeping as the body aims to conserve energy for the vital internal organs. This partial loss of consciousness is very common in dying patients.

Of the many features outlined above, four are commonly seen in the dying phase, and should at least raise the possibility that someone is dying. These are patients who are:

♦ Bed bound

♦ Semicomatose

♦ Unable to take oral drugs or having great difficulty swallowing them

♦ Unable to take any more than sips of water.[11]

Patient preferences

Open communication is an important aspect of good palliative care and, where possible, patients are generally encouraged to participate in discussions regarding treatment wishes and plans. In addition, it is also important to know how much information patients want to know at any time. It is desirable for such discussions to occur before patients becoming acutely unwell, especially with regard to how far to investigate or treat such declines in their health. Clearly, if someone is dying, treatments aimed at reversing the process will be futile, regardless of the patient's wishes, and the active focus of treatment should be on avoiding distress and maximizing comfort. When there is a possibility that decline is due to a reversible problem, ongoing assessment and treatment should provide patients with the option of attempting to reverse the problem should they desire it.

As the burden of disease increases, patients may decide they do not want to have new problems actively pursued and treated. Discussions about treatment wishes need to be an ongoing process involving the patient and those closely involved with their care as individuals' wishes can change over time. When someone is possibly dying they may be unable to communicate their wishes. At this time it is important to have access to either a record of their most recent wishes and/or another person who they have asked to represent them at such times. This will help guide not only the assessment and management processes but also communication required.[12]

If a patient has clearly expressed a wish not to undergo further investigations then assessment and management can focus on history and examination alone. With a good understanding of the patient's background history, it may be possible to make the definitive diagnosis of dying without investigations. The more important aspect of patient wishes at this time relate to preferences of type and location of care whilst they are dying.[13]

Examination

The aims of a physical examination are to exclude reversible pathology or to confirm the diagnosis of dying. It is also important to look for signs of distress which need specific treatments to maximize patient comfort. In most cases, the findings of examination should complement the information obtained from the history. Like history taking, most findings can be found when patients are not dying and it is the formulation of multiple findings which guides diagnosis.

The steps of physical examination

Following the classical steps of clinical examination is useful when diagnosing dying.

◆ **Inspection**. Inspection is an essential part of any examination and in dying patients may be the only step required to make the diagnosis. Assessments can be made on the patient's conscious state, respiratory pattern and rate, respiratory secretions, skin colour and perfusion. Certain observations will make it clear an acute catastrophic event is happening such as massive haemorrhage or status epilepticus.

◆ **Palpation**. The simple things that can be assessed with palpation include pulse rate and characteristics, skin perfusion and oedema, and signs of an intra-abdominal problem such as a perforated viscous.

◆ **Percussion**. Percussion would rarely be needed to diagnose dying but will detect problems such as significant pleural effusions and chest consolidation.

◆ **Auscultation**. Auscultation may provide extra information to confirm the diagnosis. The stethoscope can confirm hypotension, weakening heart sounds and decreased air entry.

The following discussion will focus on easily measurable findings which do not usually require one to be invasive or even greatly intrusive on the patient and their family. In general, the examination can focus on those aspects required to confirm the diagnosis of dying, and it would rarely be necessary or appropriate to do a complete physical examination as is required in a more acute setting.

Physical findings in the dying phase

Dying is the process of transition from life to death. The range of life-sustaining physiological body processes go through a transition at this time from normal, or near normal functioning, to no function. Many of the findings on examination which may indicate that death is approaching can be thought of as part of this transition. It may be necessary to repeat the examination over a period of time to detect this process of change.

Although detailed research on predicting death is rare, a range of easily recordable and objective signs should provide information to assist in this process. A prospective multicentre cohort designed study in eight palliative care units suggest in the 4 days before death that there is an increased incidence of cold and/or white nose, cold extremities, livid spots, cyanotic lips, death rattle, apnoea (> 15 sec/minute), oliguria (< 300 mls/day) and somnolence (> 15 hrs/day). Apnoea and death rattle generally occurred closer to death, whilst oliguria and livid spots occurred earlier in the dying process.[14]

In the following section, a range of physical findings which may be found on examining a dying patient will be discussed in terms of different bodily systems. As with those features discussed in the history section earlier, this is not intended to be a fully inclusive or exclusive list.

Cardiovascular

As the cardiovascular system shuts down in the dying phase, a range of clinical findings may be apparent depending on the proportionality of forward and/or backward cardiac failure. These findings can be summarized as follows:

1. Forward failure:
   - hypotension, cool skin, soft heart sounds,
   - decreased or no urine output, drowsiness.
2. Backward failure:
   - peripheral oedema, pulmonary oedema.

Peripheral signs

Pulse and blood pressure

In the dying phase, signs of shock are likely. The peripheral pulse can become weaker to palpate and tachycardia may develop over time. Systolic blood pressure tends to fall at the same time. These findings are well recognized as risk factors for an acute deterioration in health. The types of shock may be varied but can include:

- Hypovolaemic: due to decreased fluid intake or increased loss (e.g. vomiting, diaphoresis)
- Cardiogenic: as part of multi-organ failure, acute myocardial infarction
- Septic: acute infection such as pneumonia.

When death is close central pulses such as those of the femoral or carotid arteries can also become difficult to palpate.

Peripheral circulation

With failing cardiac output there are a number of possible changes seen in the circulation. Falling arterial pressure results in the peripheries such as fingers and toes becoming cool and even cyanotic, and over time these changes can involve the entirety of the limbs. In a similar way the ears and nose can also show the same changes. Capillary refill time can become prolonged, and the skin can develop irregular blotchy patterns. Slowing of venous return can result in the acute development of oedema, which can also be exacerbated by the decrease in limb movement caused by profound weakness. Symmetrical oedema of the upper limbs should raise a strong suspicion of failing circulation in the last hours to days of life.

Cardiac signs

Even in the presence of cachexia the apex beat can become more difficult to palpate. On auscultation, the presence of tachycardia may again be noted, and extra systole may be heard. As death approaches, not only is tachycardia likely to increase but the heart sounds become softer as cardiac effort fails. Irregular beats are more likely and in the minutes before death the heart sounds may become very difficult to distinguish.

Respiratory system

Peripheral signs

Respiratory patterns

Several different changes may be observed. Most of these were discussed in the history section above, as they may be seen by family and carers and reported to medical staff. These include Kussmaul's breathing, Cheyne–Stokes breathing, periods of apnoea without Cheyne–Stokes breathing and progressively more rapid and shallow breaths. During the last hours to days of life the build-up of secretions in the upper airways can be heard as loud moist breath sounds of the 'death rattle'. In the last minutes of life, breathing can become very irregular and it may be noted the little or no air is heard to be moving despite the muscular effort.

Oxygenation

With failing respiratory effort, due to factors such as falling tidal volumes, irregular frequency of breaths, poor intrapulmonary gas exchange and concomitant cardiovascular failure, it is possible for both peripheral and central cyanosis to develop. Sometimes, the development of type 2 respiratory failure with hypercapnia may mask cyanosis even when hypoxia is present. Dyspnoea may not be present even with severe hypoxia.

Breath sounds

As the respiratory drive fails, auscultation will reveal decreasing intensity of breath sounds throughout the lung fields. Initially this will be most noticeable at the lung bases, but can eventually result in difficulty hearing breath sounds throughout the entire lung fields in the minutes before death. When there are secretions present then transmitted sounds will be heard throughout the lung fields.

Cor pulmonale

With the progression of respiratory failure there may be signs of right heart failure including raised Jugular Venous Pressure, parasternal heave and loud pulmonary component of the second heart sound.

Neurological system

Consciousness

In the hours to days before death, it is common for a patient's conscious state to fall and this can be formally yet easily assessed with tools such as the Glasgow Coma Score (GCS). This feature can be inconsistent and variable and there may be times when a dying patient can be very alert and interactive between prolonged periods of somnolence. Delirium is common in dying patients and may be noted in > 80 per cent of cases.[10]

Sensory changes

When the conscious level falls, there may be a loss of response to noisy and painful stimuli. At these times previously distressing symptoms, such as pain, may decrease.

Autonomic changes

In addition to the above cardiovascular changes, other irregularities in autonomic function may be noted such as temperature dysregulation and diaphoresis. In the acute setting, hypothermia is noted to be a more significant risk factor for deterioration than hyperthermia. More commonly noted are disorders of the genitourinary system such as incontinence or retention.

Musculoskeletal output

As death approaches patients are less likely to move spontaneously, even if feeling discomfort from pressure, due to the extreme levels of weakness and fatigue. Involuntary jerking movements can occur for a number of reasons. These can be either myoclonus (transient contractions, e.g. drug accumulation) or asterixis (transient relaxations in tone, e.g. hepatic or renal failure, hypercapnia). Muscle tone can become more flaccid and reflexes reduced or absent. Loss of power results in an inability to swallow safely. It may be inappropriate or impossible to thoroughly examine all the cranial nerves when someone is dying.

The eyes

As autonomic function deteriorates in the last minutes to hours of life, normal pupillary reflexes become slower to both light and accommodation and the pupils may begin to dilate. This is the precursor to the fixed and dilated pupils found when diagnosing death.

Gastrointestinal

A thorough examination is rarely necessary to make the diagnosis of dying, but acute pathology such as bowel perforation or massive gastrointestinal haemorrhage may be the cause of death in some patients. Bowel obstruction is another cause of acute deterioration. If these complications are not present then the main findings will pertain to decreasing intestinal activity, such as decreased bowel sounds.

Genitourinary

This is another body system where a thorough examination is rarely required to diagnose dying. There may be decreased urine output due to renal and/or cardiac insufficiency and loss of normal urinary control. An important aspect of caring of the dying is to assess whether a urinary catheter is required for comfort reasons, particularly if there is evidence of urinary retention.

Diagnosing death

In most countries a medical professional is required to examine someone when they die to confirm that death has occurred. Most doctors have performed this task at sometime during their careers. There is usually a minimum set of examinable features which need to be confirmed to diagnose death. In the setting of an expected death, this process is usually straightforward and, fortunately, mistakes are rare.

However, the process is not always clear-cut, especially in terms of unexpected death where there may be the prospect of successful resuscitation. In addition, the exact moment of death is not always clear and it is recognized that there are few reliable criteria in this regard. It is recognized that life may no longer be possible even if certain physiological functions continue and there are several different guidelines surrounding issues such as diagnosing brain death. There is not the scope in this text to elaborate on this topic.

For the purposes of this chapter, concerning expected deaths from a known cause such as advanced cancer, there are some simply measured findings which confirm death. At a simplistic level death can be described as the moment when the body stops living as a whole being. When life cannot continue, the brain stops sending the impulses necessary to sustain the function of all organs necessary for life. Without this control, the heart stops beating and circulation stops. Without the circulation of oxygen, most organs cease meaningful function within seconds to a few minutes. This includes the lungs, the sensory nervous system, the musculoskeletal system and the brain itself.[15] Without either voluntary or involuntary (autonomic) bodily functions, there are several easily detected findings:

- No heart sounds
- No peripheral pulses
- Lack of skin perfusion and capillary refill
- No respiratory effort
- No response to noise or pain
- No voluntary movement
- No pupillary reaction to light; pupils dilated and fixed,

Over time as molecular processes end, other findings include:

- Purpuric death spots from hypostasis
- Muscle stiffness and rigor mortis (after 3 hours)
- Decreasing body temperature.[16]

Performance scales and prognostic models

In the earlier sections of this text, there have been discussions on different tools available which help in the formulation of prognosis at different times of a life-limiting illness. Performance scales such as the Karnofsky Performance Score (KPS), the Palliative Prognostic Index (PPI) and Palliative Performance Scale (PSS) have been developed and studied over recent decades. They focus on a range of physical and functional parameters making them easy to apply without invasive tests. In general, these are not specifically targeted at predicting the last hours to days of life but longer timeframes.

Although it is noted that good scores do not necessarily correlate with prolonged survival, it is generally accepted that poor performance scores are associated with shorter survival. It is also recognized that a fall in an individual's performance scale over time is associated with a worse prognosis. It may not be necessary to use these scales when diagnosing dying, but they can be helpful to reinforce the formulation, particularly if the score is very low or if it has dropped significantly for that patient. Various studies have demonstrated the association of worse scores with shortened survival. KPS scores under 20 are associated with median survivals ranging from 7–16 days.[17, 18] PPI scores greater than 4 confer a median survival of 12 days.[19] A previous study of PPS showed that patients admitted to a hospice with a score of 10 survived an average of less than 2 days, whilst over half of those with a score of 40 at admission never left the unit and their average survival was 10 days.[20, 21] The PPS appears to be a useful tool in the clinical assessment of patients dying from non-cancer causes too.[22]

So whilst they do not focus purely on the last days of life, very poor performance scales can strengthen the above findings from history and examination to reinforce the likelihood that a patient is dying. If there is some discrepancy between these, then further investigations may be necessary. For example, if there is little in history or examination to explain a sudden fall in PPS to 10 per cent, an acute problem should be excluded. If, however, a patient has a clearly known metastatic process with cachexia and has steadily been deteriorating, then a determination that their PPS is 10 per cent will provide additional support to the probability that they are dying, with survival measured in days at most.

The more detailed prognostic models, which incorporate combinations of physical, functional and biological parameters, are also not specifically able to help make the diagnosis of dying as the results are usually divided into survival groups with magnitudes of weeks or even months. These scales are better than clinical prediction alone at improving the accuracy of prognostication and they do highlight those whose survival is likely to be short.[23] One study found that patients with a combination of poor ECOG performance, need for admission at first referral, elevated serum bilirubin and low systolic blood pressure were unlikely to survive longer than one week.[24] However, if the findings of clinical assessment raise the strong likelihood that someone is dying, it would be unlikely for these scales to predict a long survival. As with performance scales above, a prognostic model would help reinforce the diagnosis if that patient scores very badly. For example patients with a Palliative Prognostic (PaP) Score > 11.0 have a median survival of 7–14 days.[25]

Investigations

In most cases, a diagnosis of dying can be made by history and physical examination alone, and in this setting further investigations are unnecessary and usually an inappropriate burden. Investigations are important if the diagnosis is uncertain and there is the possibility of a reversible pathological process. This is most likely in the situation of a sudden, unanticipated decline.

Bedside investigations are usually seen as an extension of physical examination and include determination of blood pressure, temperature, pulse oximetry, blood glucose reading and a ward test of urine.

Some examples of treatable conditions to be excluded and possible investigations

- Infection: cultures (blood, urine and sputum), leucocyte count
- Biochemical: renal and hepatic function, electrolytes (Na, K) and minerals (Ca)
- Drug causes: anticonvulsants, digoxin levels
- Blood loss: haemoglobin.

Box 37.2 Summarises the key points of assessment used to determine if someone is dying, as has been outlined in the first half of this chapter.

Box 37.2 Key points of assessment

Aims

- Exclude a reversible cause for the deterioration
- Confirm the diagnosis of dying
- Determine patient needs

Box 37.2 Key points of assessment *(continued)*

History

- Background:
  - Malignancy: primary site, past treatments and complications, extent of disease
  - Comorbidities: active vs inactive problems
  - Medications: polypharmacy
- Disease trajectory for this malignancy for this patient: is this decline expected?
- Presenting complaint: from patient, family and carers
- Patient preferences: extent of investigations and treatment, preferred place of care and dying

Examination

- Complement the findings from history
- Thoroughness depends on need and appropriateness
- Inspection is the key element
- Palpation, percussion and auscultation as required

Investigations

- Rarely required if diagnosis already certain
- Aimed at finding a reversible cause if the diagnosis is in doubt

Communication and care in the dying phase

Once a diagnosis of dying is suspected, important decisions need to follow regarding the communication of this diagnosis and the ongoing active care required. The diagnosis of dying implies a short period of survival, normally somewhere between a few hours to a few days. Important discussions may be needed between various individuals including the patient, their family and friends, the clinician making the diagnosis and all health workers involved in their care. This need is not restricted to patient's immediate location but may involve others less directly involved at that instant, such as family who live far away, the patient's general practitioner or other specialists. Ongoing care of the dying patient may well mean a change in care, but it does not mean a decrease in care. Rather, the best care of the dying involves active ongoing care which is planned and delivered at the same level of excellence expected for all other phases in life.

Communicating the diagnosis and prognosis

As was discussed earlier in this text, there are many reasons for needing to communicate prognosis, and many of these are equally valid for patients who are dying. There are many aspects of good communication, including listening and understanding, which should be considered as important as any words spoken and the manner in which they are delivered. Before providing information to a patient or their relatives, it is essential to determine their level of understanding and need for information. Not every person wants or needs to know every detail of their illness, and this applies in the dying phase too. Discussions need to be tailored to the individual person and their circumstances. The right information, provided well, should allow patients to gain understanding about their condition and reset their priorities for the time they have left to live in a way that is the best possible for them.

The needs of patients may be different from their families. Whilst it is rarely possible to predict the exact moment of death, evidence suggests over one-third of patients and closer to half of their relatives want to know the timing of death.[12] This information would allow people to make plans, such as contacting relatives who need to travel long distances, notifying employers to arrange time off work and to prepare emotionally for the approaching death. Even if the exact timing is not sought, being made aware that death is approaching allows people the opportunity to ask further questions and refocus their goals. If death was not expected, people may still plan longer-term strategies such as active treatments for their cancer or other activities which may not be the most important of their goals.

A patient's needs, when they are dying, will not be restricted to purely physical ones and in fact many physical problems decrease in importance at this time. The total care of a patient involves addressing their total needs, including emotional and spiritual support. In addition, families too need increased support at this same time, including being given the opportunity to ask questions and express concerns. Much of the process of bereavement can be recognized as having begun before a patient dies, particularly where families can no longer talk with the dying person. Physical symptoms, especially fatigue, weakness and delirium, will interfere with communication in the dying phase, such that it is no longer possible to hold normal conversations. It also becomes more difficult to determine a patient's wishes. By optimizing open communication throughout the entire duration of a patient's illness, it would be hoped that at least some of these needs would be known before they became too weak to communicate.

For health professionals, knowing that a patient is dying also allows care to be focused appropriately. Unnecessary and futile treatments can decrease the quality of care provided by diverting time and resources away from those strategies which are most important. This is not to say that all treatments should be stopped when someone is dying. Rather, certain treatments could be stopped but others started or enhanced which would improve the patient's comfort at physical, emotional, spiritual and psychological levels. Without good communication between the various members of the multidisciplinary team, there is a risk that inappropriate or even harmful treatments could be pursued. Decision-making can be better coordinated if there is agreement that a patient is dying. It is also important for healthcare professionals who know them to be prepared for their death, not only at a practical or work level but also emotionally.

In the hospital setting, it is unfortunately common for treating teams to not keep the patient's primary care clinicians informed regarding the patient's progress. It must not be forgotten that general practitioners and community-based nurses and carers are involved not only in the patient's care but also their families. When a patient is dying, or has died, the relatives may well go to their primary care service assuming this information has been shared. Without being actively informed, these professionals will be unaware and therefore less than ideally prepared to help these people.

Communicating diagnostic uncertainty

As with any situation where a diagnosis is made and a prognosis formulated, there is always a degree of uncertainty and there are many reasons for this. Estimations are purely that, and whether formulated through objective scales, clinical assessment, intuition, or a combination of all, they are created on past evidence not future events. The instant a clinical assessment is finished, it becomes a past event. Estimates based on past averages are made up of figures above and below the end result, meaning that the average result will be inaccurate for most individuals. Even when we strongly believe someone is dying and survival is only expected to be hours to days, errors can occur in that some patients get better again or they may even die faster than predicted.

Reflecting again on the different disease trajectories, people can die suddenly and therefore unexpectedly. Even if it has been communicated that someone may die in the next few days a sudden event could occur, as listed in Box 37.1, before relatives can be informed or arrive. In clinical settings, the more likely problem is one of dying not being anticipated or readily accepted, meaning it is not diagnosed and therefore not discussed.

People can also live longer than expected and may even recover when it was expected they would die. Whilst this recovery may be only short-lived, as in a few more days, it is possible for someone to improve dramatically. Again, there are many reasons why this may occur. The person may have suffered an acute problem, and then recovered even though it appeared they would die. If polypharmacy is inadvertently contributing to someone's decline and they stop receiving those medications because they cannot swallow, then they might also recover. In many instances, no explanation is found. The fear of making a wrong diagnosis may be one reason the diagnosis is missed or at least not communicated.

The fear of a wrong diagnosis should be not accepted as a good enough reason for failing to make the diagnosis. As with any diagnosis, it is far easier to accept that uncertainty exists and make that issue clear in any discussion. There are times when families are advised to expect the relative's death only to have that person recover. This will be easier to accept if that possibility was raised clearly, whereas problems with trust may develop if the outcome was completely unexpected either way. Individual patient variation will mean that even the best science can be wrong at times, and the issue of diagnosing dying will remain one area where medicine is a mixture of science and art for the foreseeable future.

Box 37.3 outlines a range of possible barriers to diagnosing dying, the effects that may result and some strategies for overcoming these barriers.

Care of the dying

In addition to issues of communication, the other essential reason to be able to diagnose dying is to provide the best possible care for the dying patient. As has been stated, one of the key aims of assessment is to determine the patient's needs and optimize their care at a time when it is clearly needed. Even is someone is not dying, it would be hoped that distressing symptoms and concerns can be identified and managed.

There are usually several objectives and goals for optimizing the care of the dying patient and overall care needs to be active at this time, not withdrawn as is unfortunately too often the case in acute settings. Consciously thinking about the fact that care goes beyond the physical aspects is an important step in being able to care well for dying patients.

Before care of the dying can be successful two important and interrelated steps need to occur. First, the diagnosis which has been the principle focus of this chapter has to be made. The diagnosis, as has already been stated, needs to ensure there is not a reversible cause to the patient's decline. The second crucial factor required is that the members of the multidisciplinary team caring for the patient agree that the patient is likely to die. Without agreement, the goals of care will not be consistent across the team and communication will be confused between healthcare professionals, the patient and their relatives. It is hard to imagine that good outcomes will be easy to achieve in this environment.

Box 37.3 Overcoming barriers to caring for dying patients[11]

Barriers to 'diagnosing dying'

- Hope that the patient may get better
- No definitive diagnosis
- Pursuance of unrealistic or futile interventions
- Disagreement about the patients condition
- Failure to recognize key symptoms and signs
- Lack of knowledge about how to prescribe
- Poor ability to communicate with the family and patient
- Concerns about withdrawing or withholding treatment
- Fear of foreshortening life
- Concerns about resuscitation
- Cultural and spiritual barriers
- Medico–legal issues

Effects of patients and families if the diagnosis of dying is not made

- Patient and family are unaware that death is imminent
- Patient loses trust in doctor as their condition deteriorates without acknowledgement that this is happening
- Patient and relatives get conflicting messages from the multiprofessional team
- Patient dies with uncontrolled symptoms, leading to a distressing and undignified death
- Patient and family feel dissatisfied
- At death, cardiopulmonary resuscitation may be inappropriately initiated
- Cultural and spiritual needs are not met.

All the above can lead to contribute to complex bereavement problems and formal complaints about care.

Educational objectives for overcoming barriers to diagnosing dying

- Communicate sensitively on issues related to death and dying
- Work as a member of a multidisciplinary team
- Prescribe appropriately for dying patients to:
  - Discontinue inappropriate drugs
  - Convert oral to subcutaneous drugs
  - Prescribe as required drugs as appropriate e.g. pain, agitation
  - Prescribe subcutaneous drugs for delivery by a syringe driver

Box 37.3 Overcoming barriers to caring for dying patients *(continued)*

- Use a syringe driver competently
- Recognize key symptoms and signs of the dying patient
- Describe an ethical framework that deals with issues related to dying such as resuscitation, withholding/withdrawing treatment, foreshortening life, and futility
- Appreciate cultural and religious traditions related to the dying phase
- Be aware of medico–legal issues
- Refer appropriately to a specialist palliative care team.

Once the diagnosis is agreed, then consistent plans and communication can occur, and care can be appropriately focused for the patient. In many modern institutions formalized care plans and strategies have been developed for many aspects of patient care, including care of the dying. For a plan to be comprehensive, it needs to address the combination of unique physical, psychological, social, spiritual and religious needs of the patient and their relatives. It should acknowledge and integrate the various roles and input from the multidisciplinary team in an ongoing way. It should be a plan that is accessible and approachable for all those who provide input to and benefit from it, and should not be difficult to follow.

Care of the dying needs to be an ongoing process. After an initial assessment to confirm the diagnosis and to ascertain the individual's needs, there should be provision for ongoing assessment of the patient and their response to treatment and care provided. As well as providing what is needed, it is also important to discontinue actions that are unnecessary and ensure futile measures are not initiated, such as attempting cardiopulmonary resuscitation. When the patient does die, there are ongoing care issues which need to be performed well, and it is advisable for care plans for the dying to consider these aspects as routine. The lives of the bereaved continue and their ongoing needs should be incorporated into the care of their dying relative. Formalized care plans and pathways set such plans out in a clearly written and formatted way, which provides a consistent pattern of strategies to prompt care workers of varying experience and skill to ensure a minimum standard is achieved and documented. Whilst not directly making any health worker better at their job, it should provide helpful guidance and reminders as to what is required to deliver an excellent level of care.

One such example of an integrated care pathway for the dying is the Liverpool Care Pathway for the Dying Patient (LCP) developed by the Royal Liverpool University Hospitals Trust and the Marie Curie Centre Liverpool in the UK. This pathway is an innovative model that translates best practice for care of the dying from the hospice setting to other venues such as acute hospitals, care homes and community settings. It provides a template outlining best practice and can be used by the entire multidisciplinary team. It is regularly reviewed and modified to meet the needs of dying patients being cared for in a continually evolving health system (www.lcp-mariecurie.org.uk). It contains three sections: initial assessment, ongoing care and care after death. The document acts as a guide for best care of the dying and is the central document for care completed by all members of the team. It has been demonstrated that the LCP can be used in the majority of patients dying of cancer and is also transferable to patients dying from non-cancer diagnoses. The LCP is supported by guidelines for symptom control and supporting information for relatives and healthcare professionals. By completing the document, the goals of care can also be audited to demonstrate outcomes of care and also highlight areas for further educational initiatives and resource issues.

Box 37.4 Goals of care for patients in the dying phase

Comfort measures

Goal 1 Current medications assessed and non-essentials discontinued

Goal 2 As required subcutaneous drugs written up according to protocol (pain, agitation, respiratory tract secretions, dyspnoea, nausea, vomiting)

Goal 3 Discontinue inappropriate interventions (blood tests, antibiotics, intravenous fluids or drugs, turning regimens, vital signs)

- – Document not for cardiopulmonary resuscitation
- – Deactivate implantable cardiac defibrillators (ICDs)
- – A syringe driver, if required, available within four hours of a doctor's prescription

Psychological and insight measures

Goal 4 Ability to communicate in English assessed as adequate

Goal 5 Insight into condition assessed

Religious and spiritual support

Goal 6 Religious and spiritual needs assessed with patient and family

Communications with family or others

Goal 7 Identify how family or other people involved are to be informed of patient's impending death

Goal 8 Family or other people involved given relevant hospital information

Communications with primary healthcare team

Goal 9 General practitioner is aware of patient's condition

Summary

Goal 10 Plan of care explained and discussed with patient and family

Goal 11 Family or other people involved express understanding of plan of care

Box 37.4 outlines the key goals of patient care in the dying phase and is an adaptation of the initial assessment of the LCP. Figure 37.1 illustrates the relationship between advancing life-limiting illness, the diagnosis of dying and how care is continually provided through to and beyond death. This care is continuous, even if the patient does not die as expected. It is important to remember that the LCP documentation can be discontinued if it becomes clear the diagnosis of dying was wrong. The goals of care, however, should be applicable to most patients with the complex needs that occur throughout the course of advanced cancer and other life-limiting illnesses.

Conclusion

Although the majority of patients with advanced cancer will die as a result of their disease, being able to diagnose dying and formulating a prognosis in the imminently dying patient remains a great challenge. In the future there may be tools to improve the accuracy of this diagnosis, but for

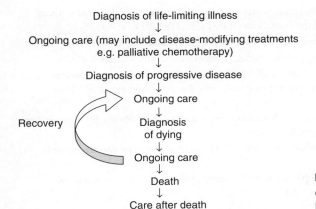

Diagnosis of life-limiting illness
↓
Ongoing care (may include disease-modifying treatments
e.g. palliative chemotherapy)
↓
Diagnosis of progressive disease
↓
Ongoing care
↓
Recovery
Diagnosis
of dying
↓
Ongoing care
↓
Death
↓
Care after death

Figure 37.1 Clinical trajectory of the care patients with life-limiting illness.

now clinical assessment remains a key skill. Through the combination of good history taking, physical examination and investigations as appropriate it should be possible to make the diagnosis in many circumstances. It is recognized that there remains a degree of uncertainty with the diagnosis of dying in many situations, particularly where the decline is quicker than had been expected.

When the diagnosis of dying is made it is important to be able to communicate this, and any unrelated uncertainty, to the patient, their relatives and other healthcare professionals. It is important for the skills of diagnosis and communication to be developed and used effectively in order to avoid unnecessary treatment, unrealistic expectations of patients, their families and other carers and the risk of low self-esteem in healthcare workers, who may feel opportunities for optimum care were missed.

The ability to diagnose dying should be seen as a potentially rewarding challenge rather than an unpleasant or daunting task. When combined with good communication and agreement between all healthcare workers, patients and their families, it will result in better outcomes, the most important of which is providing the best possible care for the dying patient.

References

1. Glare P and Christakis N. Predicting survival in patients with advanced cancer. In D Doyle, G Hanks, N Cherny, K Calman (eds). *The oxford textbook of palliative medicine*, 3rd edn, pp. 29–42. Oxford: Oxford University Press, 2004.

2. Oxenham D, Cornbleet MA. Accuracy of prediction of survival by different professional groups in a hospice. *Palliat Med* 1998; 12:117–18.

3. Higginson IJ, Costantini M. Accuracy of prognosis estimates by four palliative care teams: a prospective cohort study. *J Clin Oncol* 2002; 20(17):3647–82.

4. Glare P, Virik K, Jones M *et al*. A systematic review of physicians' survival predictions in terminally ill cancer patients. *BMJ* 2003; 327:195–8.

5. Kotler DP. Cachexia. *Ann Intern Med* 2000; 133(8):622–34.

6. Stevenson JP, Abernethy AP, Millar C, Currow DC. Confidently managing comorbidities at the end of life. *BMJ* 2004; 329:909–12.

7. Currow DC, Stevenson JP, Abernethy A, Plummer J and Shelby-James T. Prescribing in Palliative Care as death approaches. *J Am Geriatr* 2007; 55(4): 590–5.

8. Lynn J, Adamson DM. *Living well at the end of life. Adapting health care to serious chronic illness in old age*. RAND Health Santa Monica, California, 2003.

9. Vigano A, Dorgan M, Buckingham J, Bruera E, Suarez-Almazor ME. Survival prediction in terminal cancer patients: a systematic review of the medical literature *Palliat Med* 2000; 14:363–74.

10. Centeno C, Sanz A, Bruera E. Delirium in advanced cancer patients. *Palliat Med* 2004; 18:184–94.

11. Ellershaw JE, Ward C. Care of the dying patient: the last hours or days of life. *BMJ* 2003; 326:30–4.

12. Steinhauser KE, Christakis NA, Clipp EC, McNeilly M, McIntyre L, Tulsky JA. Factors considered important at the end of life by patients, family, physicians, and other care providers. *JAMA* 2000; 284:2476–82.

13. Higginson IJ, Sen-Gupta GJ. Place of care in advanced cancer: a qualitative systematic literature review of patient preferences. *J Palliat Med* 2000; 3:287–300.

14. Menten J and Hufkens K. Objectively observable signs of imminently dying in palliative patients. *Palliat Med* 2004; 18:351.

15. Stevenson JP, Ellershaw JE. How do people die? In D Beckerman (ed.) *How to have a good death*, Chapter 1. London: Dorling Kindersley, 2006.

16. Charlton R. Diagnosing death. *BMJ* 1996; 313:956–7.

17. Llobera J, Esteva M, Rifa J. *et al.* Terminal cancer: duration and prediction of survival time. *Eur J Cancer* 2000; 36:2036–43.

18. Lamont EB, Christakis NA Prognostication in advanced disease. In AM Berger, RK Portenoy, DE Weissman. *Principle and practice of palliative care and supportive oncology*, 2nd edn, Chapter 42. Philadelphia, PA: Lippincott, Williams & Wilkins, 2002.

19. Morita T, Tsunoda J, Inoue S, Chihara S. The Palliative Prognostic Index: a scoring system for survival prediction of terminally ill cancer patients. *Support Care Cancer* 1999; 7(3):128–33.

20. Anderson F, Downing GM, Hill J, Casoro L, Lerch N. Palliative Performance Scale (PPS): a new tool. *J Palliat Care* 1996; 12(1):5–11.

21. Virik K, Glare P. Validation of the Palliative Performance Scale for inpatients admitted to a palliative care unit in Sydney, Australia. *J Pain Symptom Manage* 2002; 23(6):455–7.

22. Glare P. The use of the palliative prognostic score in patients with diagnoses other than cancer. *J Pain Symptom Manage* 2003; 26(4):883–5.

23. Chow E, Harth T, Hruby G, Finkelstein J, Wu J, Danjoux C. How accurate are physicians' clinical predictions of survival and the available prognostic tools in estimating survival times in terminally ill cancer patients? A systematic review. *Clin Oncol R Coll Radiol* 2001; 13:209–18.

24. Rosenthal MA, Gebski VJ, Kefford RF, Stuart-Harris RC. Prediction of life-expectancy in hospice patients: identification of novel prognostic factors. *Palliat Med* 1993; 7:199–204.

25. Pirovano M, Maltoni M, Nanni O *et al.* A new palliative prognostic score: a first step for the staging of terminally ill cancer patients. *J Pain Symptom Manage* 1999; 17(4):231–9.

Index

The index entries appear in word-by-word alphabetical order.
Page references in italics indicate information in figures and tables.